Physiolo
and Nur

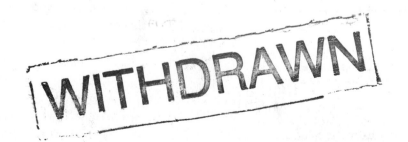

For Churchill Livingstone:

Senior Commissioning Editor: Sarena Wolfaard
Project Development Manager: Claire Wilson
Project Manager: Samantha Ross
Design: Judith Wright
Illustration Manager: Bruce Hogarth

Physiology for Health Care and Nursing

Edited by

Sheenan Kindlen BSc MSc MRSC SRD

Former Lecturer in Physiology and Coordinator Biological Sciences, Department of Health and Nursing, Queen Margaret University College, Edinburgh, UK

Foreword by

Professor Patricia Peattie BSc RSCN RGN RNT MHSM FRSA

Napier University, Edinburgh, UK

SECOND EDITION

Developed from Rutishauser's *Physiology and Anatomy – A Basis for Nursing and Health Care*

With special thanks to MARKS for the reuse of illustrations borrowed from the first edition

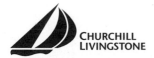
CHURCHILL
LIVINGSTONE

EDINBURGH LONDON NEW YORK OXFORD PHILADELPHIA ST LOUIS SYDNEY TORONTO 2003

CHURCHILL LIVINGSTONE
An imprint of Elsevier Science Limited

First published 1994
Reprinted 1997
Reprinted 1999
Second edition 2003

ISBN 0 443 07116 0

British Library Cataloguing in Publication Data
A catalogue record for this book is available from the British Library

Library of Congress Cataloging in Publication Data
A catalog record for this book is available from the Library of Congress

Note
Medical knowledge is constantly changing. Standard safety precautions must be
followed, but as new research and clinical experience broaden our knowledge,
changes in treatment and drug therapy may become necessary or appropriate.
Readers are advised to check the most current product information provided by the
manufacturer of each drug to be administered to verify the recommended dose, the
method and duration of administration, and contraindications. It is the
responsibility of the practitioner, relying on experience and knowledge of the
patient, to determine dosages and the best treatment for each individual patient.
Neither the Publisher nor the editor assumes any liability for any injury and/or
damage to persons or property arising from this publication.

The Publisher

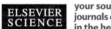

your source for books,
journals and multimedia
in the health sciences

www.elsevierhealth.com

The
publisher's
policy is to use
**paper manufactured
from sustainable forests**

Printed in UK

Contents

SECTION 1
THE BODY AND ITS INTERNAL ENVIRONMENT   *3*

SECTION 2
INTERACTION WITH THE
EXTERNAL ENVIRONMENT *351*

SECTION 3
THE LIFE SPAN *479*

Contributors

Philip Docherty BN RGN OND RCNT DipN
Lecturer in Nursing, Dept of Health and Nursing,
Queen Margaret University College, Edinburgh, UK

Sheena Douglas BA(Hons) MSc SRD
Senior Dietician, Metabolic Unit, Western General
Hospital, Edinburgh, UK

Jan S. Gill BSc(Hons) PhD
Lecturer (Physiology), Faculty of Health and
Social Sciences, Queen Margaret University College,
Edinburgh, UK

Christine M. Harris RGN
Clinical Nurse Specialist (Urology), Nurse Urology
Unit, Western General Hospital, Edinburgh, UK

Simon J.H. Hettle BSc(Hons) PhD AIBMS MILT HE
Lecturer in Biological Sciences, Department of
Biological Sciences, University of Paisley, UK

Catriona M. Kennedy PhD BA(Hons) RN DN RNT DNT PWT
Senior Lecturer, School of Acute and Continuing Care
Nursing, Napier University, Edinburgh, UK

Sheenan Kindlen BSc MSc MRSC SRD
Former Lecturer in Physiology, and Coordinator
Biological Sciences, Department of Health and Nursing,
Queen Margaret University College, Edinburgh, UK

Dawn Lowe BSc RGN
Senior Nurse and Manager in the NHS

Douglas E. McBean BSc(Hons) PhD
Lecturer in Physiology and Neuroscience, School of
Health Sciences, Queen Margaret University College,
Edinburgh, UK

Allan MacDonald BSc(Hons) PhD
Reader in Pharmacology, School of Biological and
Biomedical Sciences, Glasgow Caledonian University,
Glasgow, UK

Professor Patricia Peattie BSc RSCN RGN RNT MHSM FRSA
Napier University, Edinburgh, UK

Margaret H. Parker BA RGN RNT OHNC Cert Ed.
Lecturer in Nursing, Queen Margaret University
College, Edinburgh, UK

Frank Prior BPharm MSc MBA PhD MRPharmS MIBiol
The Osmosis Unit, Longniddry, East Lothian, UK

Jane Renton MRPharmS, MSc(Clin Pharm) PGDip(Wound
Healing & Tissue Repair)
Principal Pharmacist, Medicines Information, Lothian
Primary Care NHS Trust, Royal Edinburgh Hospital,
Edinburgh, UK

Heather Shaw MSc BA RGN RM RMT ADM
Senior Lecturer, University of Paisley Ayr Campus,
Ayr, UK

Graeme D. Smith PhD BA RGN
Lecturer in Nursing Studies, Department of Nursing
Studies, University of Edinburgh, Edinburgh, UK

Mary Warnock PhD
Lecturer in Microbiology and Immunology,
Department of Dietetics, Nutrition and Biological
Sciences, Queen Margaret University College,
Edinburgh, UK

Roger Watson BSc PhD RGN CBiol FIBiol ILTM FRSA
Professor of Nursing, School of Nursing, Social Work
and Applied Health Studies, The University of Hull,
UK

Foreword

It is a privilege to be invited to contribute the foreword to this revised text, which should prove immensely useful to all healthcare professionals.

There has been an increasingly rapid expansion of knowledge over the past 50 years, and no more so than in those areas of scientific endeavour which impinge on health care. Some of the research has been driven by the health needs of populations, as direct consequences of changes in health status create new challenges for investigation, care and cure. Some research has been in quite distinct fields, but has provided solutions to some of the diagnostic and therapeutic difficulties faced in the latter part of the 20th century. Much of the novel drug development and DNA research falls into this category. And yet other research, resulting in major environmental change, has facilitated international travel, transformed communication and opened up individual choices which can threaten health on an individual or collective basis.

In the early days of the National Health Service in Britain, it was initially thought by some that the illnesses which threatened society at the time could be cured within a few years, and subsequent attention need only to be paid to health education and promotion. But of course, it hasn't been like that. As fast as clinical care brings about improvements, for example, in the management of pregnancy and childbirth resulting in fewer maternal and neonatal deaths, the challenge now, both clinical and ethical, is the care of very small babies; and technological advances give rise to the dilemmas of assisted fertilisation. Many of the diseases from which young adults and the middle aged died in the 1960s, have indeed become part of history, but today the challenges arise from chronic, degenerative disease, often in older people, or acute, complex critical care interventions, when seconds to make a clinical decision can make a difference to outcomes.

To be a safe practitioner in any healthcare profession today, requires an intellectual rigour, applied to a body of knowledge which is ever expanding. It is no longer enough to know something – understanding derived from a sound appreciation of fundamental principles, skills and application in different circumstances and the recognition of the responsibility to become engaged in lifelong learning are key to the development of autonomous practitioners within a multi-disciplinary team.

This book, in its second edition, recognises the complex nature of the knowledge base for such a team member. It is not fully comprehensive – much of the original text in anatomy is properly removed and the reader referred elsewhere. Nor does it seek to address in detail the psychological or ethical issues that face practitioners. It does seek to underpin the choices that have to be made as a result of the increasing potential derived from an enhanced understanding of how the human body works, how it responds to internal and external stresses, how such knowledge can be used to bring about change and the implications of such applications for individuals and society.

These may be choices for the individual patient, or the clinical practitioners, for the researcher or for representatives of society. Fundamental to informing such choices is an understanding of the issues, and an ability to communicate in an appropriate manner. As changes in care delivery occur, and professional boundaries become less rigid, new roles develop in all fields. Responsibility for decision making, for discriminating between different information sources within the plethora freely available, is no longer solely the province of the medical consultant.

In revising a valued text, the authors have provided an up-to-date book, in a format which provides the foundation knowledge to underpin evidence-based practice. The questions challenge the reader's understanding and promote application reflecting realistic issues faced on a daily basis, with further reading recommended for those who need more detail. As such, it provides an excellent source book which I am pleased to commend to students and newly qualified practitioners in all fields of healthcare.

Edinburgh 2003   Professor Patricia Peattie

Preface

The first edition, edited by Dr Sigrid Rutishauser, was published in 1994. It proved to be a popular choice, respected by its readers. This second edition has a new editor, new contributors and new material, but hopefully retains some of the character of the first edition. The contributors come mainly from biological science backgrounds with specialist areas identified by their chapters. All work in health care or teach health-care practitioners and students.

Apart from the continual requirement to update scientific and technical material, many of the changes in this edition have been guided by changes in healthcare professions themselves. Over recent years, increasing autonomy has meant increasing individual professional responsibility on the part of those who work in health care. Nurses, physiotherapists, dieticians and others, must know more than just *how to*, they must be able to work out the rationale for their actions – and the effects. Patients and clients make much more use of the word *why* (as they should) and often have bundles of downloaded material to check the answers. We have therefore included in the explanations of mechanisms some of the intermediate steps often omitted from applied texts. These intermediate steps are frequently targets of therapeutic agents such as drugs and so we have also included a short chapter on the mechanisms of drug action.

The extended section concerned with the internal environment concentrates on those aspects of homeostasis, such as blood pressure and body temperature, which are routinely assessed in clinical practice. The concepts developed in the maintenance of the normal state are then applied to the events brought about by its disturbance.

In order to accommodate the new material yet maintain the size of the book, some of the sections in the first edition have been omitted. Anatomy, for example, is a highly specialized discipline and, to give it the space it deserves, a different kind of book and different contributors would have been required. The anatomy which has been included allows the reader to navigate the systems easily. The more psychological aspects of the central nervous system and the work on bones and joints were similarly felt to be deserving of fuller treatment elsewhere.

Physiology is a fascinating subject. Its principles are logical and dependable. Once learned, they can be relied on. Like any other subject, however, to most of us, physiology only becomes real when applied. Applications of the theory have been included in many of the chapters, along with explanations of dysfunction and the rationale for treatment systems.

The questions which introduce the chapters in Section 1, *The body and its internal environment*, include examples of incidents and queries from practice where the application of physiology can provide an answer. Just as in the real world, there may be several different answers of varying levels of complexity.

I would like to thank all the contributors, the authors who gave their time and expertise, the many others who gave advice and well considered opinions, and information on technical and current clinical practice. Many thanks to all who responded constructively when we tried out our early drafts on them. We would all like to thank our copy-editor Laila Grieg-Gran who took in good part all (my) queries and numerous edits upon edits.

Finally, we would like to thank Dr Rutishauser and her colleagues without whose hard work in the first edition, there would have been no second edition. We would like to acknowledge the original contributors, some of whose chapters have simply been revised and updated. We were certainly grateful for their efforts and hope that they will approve of our amendments.

Edinburgh 2003   Sheenan Kindlen

Introduction

PHYSIOLOGICAL NORMALITY OR GOOD HEALTH?

The two phrases may seem to be interchangeable but, in fact, they are very different. Physiological normality is a state made up of numerous individual but related components, such as blood pressure, body temperature, fluid balance, the plasma electrolytes and so on. Taken as a whole, they make up the internal climate in which the cells live. These components can be measured and are therefore sometimes referred to as parameters. The parameters in the internal climate are not constant values: they are, instead, constantly adjusted to remain within limits so that a steady state is achieved. If one considers the challenges of activity, feeding, and changes in the external climate, it is surprising how steady the state of the internal environment remains. The maintenance of this steady state of normality is referred to as homeostasis, a term coined to describe the physiological actions which restore the normal state once it has been disturbed. The topic of homeostasis is expanded in Section 1, Part B.

Each parameter is controlled by many mechanisms. These may work on different time scales and have different signalling systems, but many have the common characteristic of working on a feedback system. Each parameter has a range of normal values. The range may be relatively wide or so narrow that it might be regarded as a set point. As a parameter value begins to move to one or the other end of its range, this acts as a signal triggering the appropriate mechanism which will correct the deviation. When the value is again within range, the signal is removed and the correcting mechanism ceases its activity. The mechanism has responded to a stimulus (the deviation) and has been inhibited by negative feedback (correction of the deviation). The mechanisms may be neural or hormonal or, in many instances, both. The neural mechanisms give a rapid response while a slower, but longer lasting response can be provided by the endocrine systems. This general rule of stimulus and negative feedback applies to a very large part of homeostatic regulation.

Where the stimulus comes from the external rather than the internal environment, this is sometimes referred to as an open-loop system. An example might be a drop in external temperature which has to be compensated by the retention or production of extra body heat. The principle, however, is the same: a sensory signal leading to action to preserve an internal parameter. When the signal is removed, the action ceases.

The limits of the ranges for the parameters are common to any humans in a group matched for age, sex and stage of development. In any group, the values within a given range change predictably with activity, feeding etc. Where an error develops in the system, for example if it fails to respond to negative feedback, or the deviation is too large to be corrected by the adjustment systems, the evidence can be found in an abnormal result when the parameter is measured. This may be, for example, a high or low body temperature or an abnormal reading for a plasma electrolyte. When the error remains beyond the capacity of the mechanisms to correct it, it may cause clinical symptoms associated with disorder.

The useful thing about physiological responses is that they are highly predictable: a specific stimulus will give rise to a specific effect. It follows that a good knowledge of how the mechanisms work enables you to interpret the signs and symptoms as they happen. It also indicates which pieces of information, for example which electrolyte level or which physical response, to look for as evidence. Even more valuable, knowledge and understanding make it possible to predict the next steps – *if this has happened, that will happen next*. In clinical practice, an ability to predict can save lives.

Unlike the parameters associated with a normal homeostatic environment, which can be objectively measured and which respond predictably to deviation from their normal values, health is a much less definable state. It is difficult to find an acceptable definition of health: even the dictionary definitions are many and varied. Words such as soundness and integrity are offered and longer versions tend to use negatives such as absence of disease. Absence of symptoms does not necessarily preclude the presence of disease. The usual guidelines of defining, measuring and studying the subjects in a group are difficult to apply. The equivalent of the measurements possible with the homeostatic parameters does not seem to be possible either. There are complex indices but these reflect the problem of clearly identifying health since most are attempts to make some assessment of the quality of life.

An individual asked about their health is likely to give a subjective response. Most people can only say how they feel at that time. The answer to *how do you feel?* is affected by factors such as state of mind, the external environment, physical surroundings, the quality of food and company, even the weather. A view of health is highly individual. A patient who has been unwell will often respond to a small improvement by saying how well they feel. The healthy, very fit athlete views giving a less than standard performance as a sign of being unfit, even when that performance is far in excess of anything that most people could manage.

People are unlikely to have any clue as to their physiological parameters although we can all detect even small changes in our feelings of well-being. Deciding where and what the *unwellness* is, however, might be another matter. The concepts of physiological norms and health come together when *well* becomes *unwell*. When clinical practice is faced with questions about health, it begins to assess the physiological norms.

General principles

Cells need a controlled environment which can meet all their requirements. Cells have become specialized as functional units of the organs and systems, so, in fact, they contribute specific components of their own total environment.

The systems have become specialized to exchange gases, digest food, process nutrients and so on, therefore neural and endocrine control systems are required to organize these nominally separate systems into a cohesive and efficient whole.

Homeostasis is the term given to the maintenance of the internal environment by this organized assembly of systems. Any disturbance in the environment will be met by compensatory responses from the systems, each contributing part of the total response.

In normal circumstances, we have little sense of any of this continuous activity, however a larger disturbance can produce conscious or measurable effects of the mechanisms at work. Some of the effects are so predictable that they are viewed, not as evidence of compensatory responses, but as clinical signs or symptoms. When they are produced in response to an effect caused by a drug, they are sometimes even described as *side effects*.

The overall management of the internal environment is under the control of the central nervous system. As well as initiating new actions, thoughts and ideas, the central nervous system must be able to interpret signals from the external environment, make the appropriate responses and, if necessary, adjust the internal environment to suit. In other words, brain and body must be able to live in the outside world.

A fundamental requirement for the continuation of a species is the ability to reproduce. Individuals are born, live their lives and die, but because of the processes of reproduction, the new individuals born will ensure the continued existence of the group.

How the book is arranged

Section 1 consists of three parts:
Part 1A deals with cells, the systems they make up and the mechanisms by which the systems are regulated.
Part 1B puts the systems together, showing how they cooperate to produce and maintain a stable internal environment by constantly responding to and correcting disturbance.
Part 1C is about the causes and effects of disturbance of this normally stable state.

Section 2 consists of two parts:
Part 2A covers the role of the central nervous system in managing and controlling the internal environment, and responding and interacting with the external environment.
Part 2B considers learning and memory, and aspects of experience such as pain.

Section 3 considers the generation of new individuals, their development and maturation and the processes and events surrounding the end of life.

Chapter questions

The chapters in Section 1 are introduced by a series of questions. Some of these are derived from happenings and queries which might be encountered in practice. The solutions might be derived from the immediate chapter or might need to be developed from several chapters. Many of the questions are open-ended, so that your own knowledge and experience can take a solution even further.

Blue-edged text and boxes

- Where dysfunction or disorder has been used to illustrate and expand on normal function or control, this text is shown with a blue edge. Similarly, pharmacology related to the topic is highlighted with blue at the edge of the text.
- Healthcare applications and items of additional information are shown as blue text boxes.
- More general additional information related to the topic is shown as a yellow text box.

SECTION 1
The body and its internal environment

Section 1 is made up of three parts:

Part 1A – Cells and systems

Part 1A begins with cells and their many structures and functions. Cell division and the role of DNA and RNA are considered in some detail. The chapters on blood, neurones and muscle, in addition to considering these as tissues, illustrate the principles of specialization in blood cells and excitable cells.

The cellular systems are applied in the chapter on drug action. This shows how receptor sites, membrane channels and the cell's chemical systems can be manipulated for therapeutic purposes.

Other chapters are concerned with the major organ systems and their control by the autonomic and endocrine systems.

Part 1B – Maintaining the internal environment – systems working together

Chapters in this part put together the separate systems and show how they cooperate to maintain particular aspects of the internal environment. The homeostatic parameters selected are those routinely assessed as part of clinical practice, e.g. blood pressure, body temperature, fluid and electrolyte balance. Chapters on other important topics, such as nutrition and the body's defence systems, are included here. Disorder and dysfunction of the cells, systems and overall homeostasis are used to illustrate normal function throughout Section 1.

Part 1C – Disturbance of the internal environment

This chapter examines the cellular and system responses at a wound site and the whole body response to the event of a wound or some other form of physiological stress. Illness is considered as a state of increasing deviation from the norm with the early disturbance adequately compensated, then with the emergence of the uncompensated effects and eventual progression to a state of frank disorder.

1 Cells

In practice you may be asked to consider the following:

1. Explain how changes in the genetic information of the cell can bring about the development of disease.

2. In type 2 (non-insulin dependent) diabetes mellitus, glucose is unable to enter cells despite adequate levels of the hormone (insulin) that drives this process. What might be the cellular defect that causes this problem?

3. What happens in the liver following an injury involving loss of tissue? What if a similar injury were to occur in the heart muscle?

4. Some drugs act as channel blockers. What would be the effects of a calcium channel blocker on the cells of the myocardium?

5. When intravenous rehydration is required, water as such is not used. Why not? What can be used?

6. Cells are specialized to allow them to fulfil their function. What would be the role of cells with microvilli? Where can they be found ?

7. The ciliated cells in the respiratory tract are also highly specialized. What function does their specialized structure serve?

8. A student describes a laboratory practical where water was added to blood in a sample tube. The liquid in the tube became a transparent pink colour, with no sign of the red cells. What happened?

9. Drugs of the mustine group prevent separation of the DNA strands in the cell. What is the clinical application of this property?

10. A child with phenylketonuria (PKU) must adhere to dietary restrictions imposed by the condition. What is the cellular fault which leads to PKU?

Each human being begins life as a single cell (the zygote) which is created by the fusion of two sex cells (or gametes): an ovum (from the mother) and a sperm (from the father). Contained within the zygote (in the form of coded instructions in its genetic material) is all the information necessary to determine the form and function of all the many different types of cells from which the body is ultimately composed. The process of development from zygote to fully mature adult is characterized by two processes: a huge increase in the number of cells (achieved by many, many rounds of cell division), and specialization of different cells for particular functions in the body (e.g. liver cell, muscle cell). Thus, the mature body is composed of a huge number of individual cells of many different types.

Every cell, whatever its exact type, is made up of a huge number of individual component parts: atoms, molecules and ions (Fig. 1.1). There is a huge number of individual molecules of many different types (e.g. lipids, proteins, nucleic acids) in each cell, and the characteristics of and interactions between these molecules determine the structures and thus the function(s) of both the different parts of the cell (e.g. membranes) and the cell as a whole. The importance of this relationship between structure and function within the cell can hardly be overstated and, indeed, such relationships are seen at all levels in biological systems (e.g. within organs such as the heart) and are always important, as will be illustrated later.

Cells are dynamic structures and their activities (e.g. turnover of individual parts, movements of components into and out of membranes, division) are influenced both by the genetic information they contain and also by their environment (e.g. specific regulatory factors released by other cells). It is important to note that, despite their dynamic nature, both the basic organization (structure) and activities (function) of the cell remain intact (though function can be modified in response to changing conditions, e.g. secretion of a hormone in response to the appropriate stimulus). This maintenance of structure and function in a changing environment (usually referred to by the term 'homeostasis') is also a very important feature of living systems and is evident at all levels of biological organization, from the individual cell to the whole, intact organism.

Clearly, the cells of the body do not exist in isolation, but rather exist together, being supported and maintained by the extracellular matrix in which they are embedded and being physically linked together to form tissues (which are joined together to form organs, which, in turn, are associated together to form organ systems). Moreover, cells interact with one other, in ways that are often intricate and complex, to ensure the appropriate operation of each tissue, organ and organ system, and thus the well-being of the individual person as a whole organism.

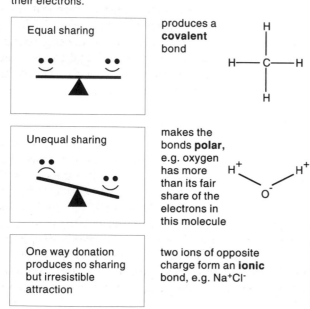

Atoms
Atoms consist of:
   protons (positively charged)
   neutrons
   electrons (negatively charged).
Number of protons = number of electrons therefore an atom is uncharged overall.

Ions
An **atom** that gains or loses an electron is an **ion**. Ions may have a positive charge (+) **cations** or a negative charge (-) **anions.**

Atom	Symbol		Ion
Sodium	Na	Na minus an electron	Na$^+$
Chorine	Cl	Cl plus an electron	Cl$^-$
Hydrogen	H	H minus an electron	H$^+$
Carbon	C	C does not form an ion	

Molecules
A molecule consists of atoms linked together by chemical bonds caused by the interchange of electrons.
The type of bond formed depends on how the atoms share their electrons.

Equal sharing	produces a **covalent** bond
Unequal sharing	makes the bonds **polar,** e.g. oxygen has more than its fair share of the electrons in this molecule
One way donation produces no sharing but irresistible attraction	two ions of opposite charge form an **ionic** bond, e.g. Na$^+$Cl$^-$

Figure 1.1 Structure of an atom and meaning of the terms ion and molecule. The bonds formed between atoms and molecules are of several different types: covalent, polar and ionic.

CELLULAR COMPONENTS

MOLECULES AND MOLECULAR INTERACTIONS

Atoms combine together chemically to form molecules by forming bonds with each other, and these bonds involve interactions between the electrons of atoms

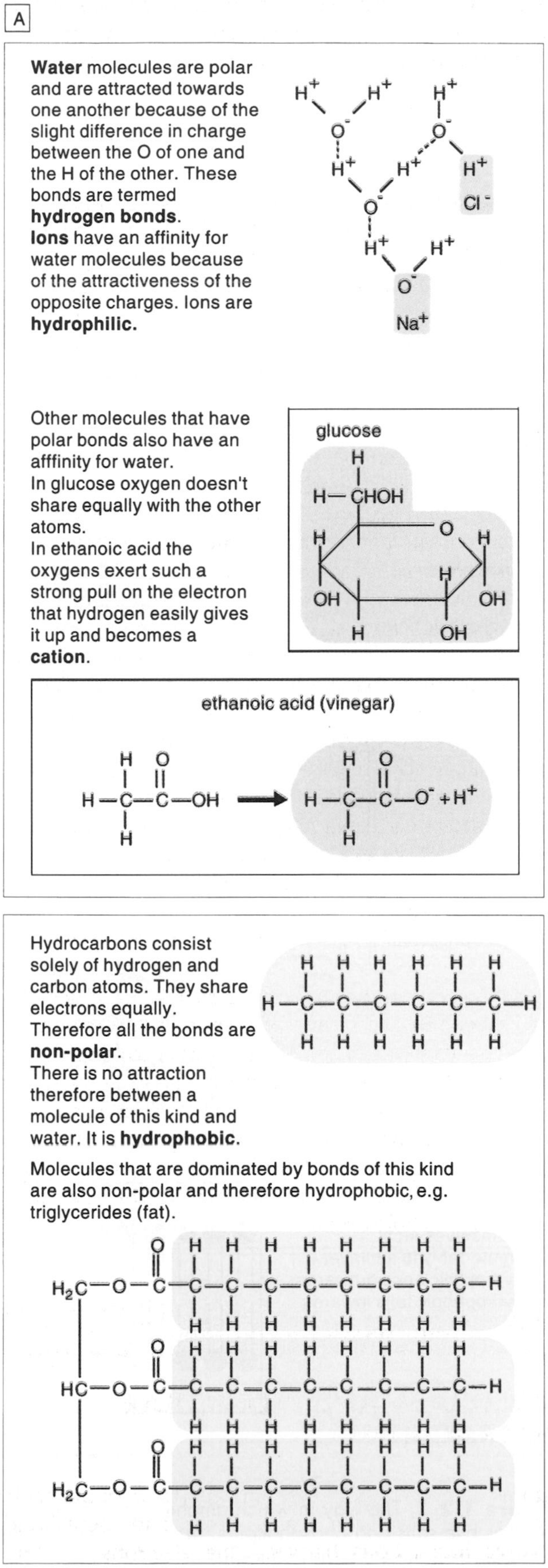

(Fig. 1.1). The interactions between molecules depend upon the properties of those molecules and these, in turn, are determined by the properties of the molecule's constituent atoms.

Hydrophilic and hydrophobic molecules

Molecules in biological systems can be divided into two broad groups (Fig. 1.2A):

- *hydrophilic* (water-loving) – have an affinity for an aqueous (watery) environment
- *hydrophobic* (water-hating) – prefer to associate with fatty substances and thus may also be called *lipophilic* (fat-loving).

If the interactions between the component atoms of a molecule involve unequal sharing of electrons, the molecule will have differing electrical charges at different points on its surfaces, i.e. it will be polar; such molecules are hydrophilic. The water molecule itself is polar (Fig. 1.1) and (obviously) is thus hydrophilic. Any other molecules that are polar (e.g. glucose; ethanoic (acetic) acid – vinegar) will have an affinity for water (or other hydrophilic molecules) because of the electrostatic attraction between positive and negative electrical charged regions of the molecules (Fig. 1.2A).

If the interactions between atoms in a molecule involve equal sharing of electrons, however, then there will be no variation in electrical charge over the surface of the molecule, i.e. it will be non-polar. Such molecules (e.g. hydrocarbons) are hydrophobic since there is no electrical attraction possible between them and polar water molecules. Thus, a triglyceride, which possesses three very long hydrocarbon chains (Fig. 1.2A), is almost completely insoluble in water, the triglyceride molecules preferring to associate with one another and to form a layer distinct from the water molecules, as can be seen when oil separates from water.

Amphipathic molecules

Wholly hydrophilic and hydrophobic molecules represent two extremes. Other molecules (e.g. phospholipids, sodium glycocholate – Fig. 1.2B) possess both hydrophobic and hydrophilic characteristics in different parts of the same molecule – these are said to be amphipathic. They can thus act as a 'bridge' or 'link' between wholly hydrophilic and wholly hydrophobic molecules. Such molecules are extremely important in living systems, as they permit the dispersion of hydrophobic molecules (e.g. lipids) in an aqueous

A

Water molecules are polar and are attracted towards one another because of the slight difference in charge between the O of one and the H of the other. These bonds are termed **hydrogen bonds**.
Ions have an affinity for water molecules because of the attractiveness of the opposite charges. Ions are **hydrophilic**.

Other molecules that have polar bonds also have an afffinity for water.
In glucose oxygen doesn't share equally with the other atoms.
In ethanoic acid the oxygens exert such a strong pull on the electron that hydrogen easily gives it up and becomes a **cation**.

glucose

ethanoic acid (vinegar)

Hydrocarbons consist solely of hydrogen and carbon atoms. They share electrons equally.
Therefore all the bonds are **non-polar**.
There is no attraction therefore between a molecule of this kind and water. It is **hydrophobic**.

Molecules that are dominated by bonds of this kind are also non-polar and therefore hydrophobic, e.g. triglycerides (fat).

Figure 1.2 Water-loving (hydrophilic) and water-hating (hydrophobic) molecules, and those with sympathies both ways (amphipathic). A, Characteristics and examples of each type. (B overleaf)

Phospholipids are **amphipathic**. Part of the molecule is hydrophilic; part is hydrophobic.

Hydrophilic

Hydrophobic

B

Sodium glycocholate (a bile salt)

lipophilic side

In its three-dimensional structure all the polar groups are on the same side of the molecule. These molecules are most comfortably arranged with their lipophilic side facing a fatty environment and their hydrophilic side facing a water environment.

hydrophilic side

Phospholipid-bile salt **micelle**

Longitudinal section

Cross-section

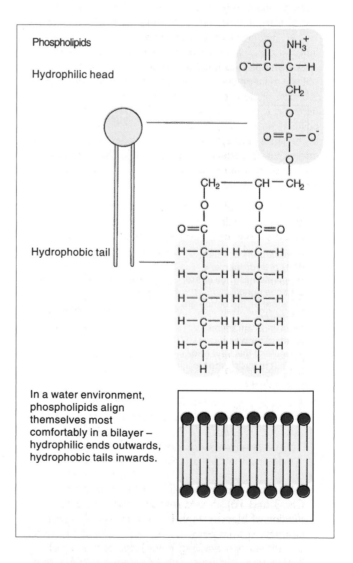

Phospholipids

Hydrophilic head

Hydrophobic tail

In a water environment, phospholipids align themselves most comfortably in a bilayer – hydrophilic ends outwards, hydrophobic tails inwards.

Figure 1.2 B, The way in which amphipathic molecules, such as bile salts and phospholipids, arrange themselves in a water environment to form micelles and bilayers.

(hydrophilic) environment: e.g. phospholipids are very important in the formation of cell membranes (see below), forming sheet-like structures ('phospholipid bilayers') with a hydrophobic interior and hydrophilic surfaces (Fig. 1.2B); sodium glycocholate (one of the bile salts, used in the digestion and absorption of fats – see Ch. 9) promotes the dispersion of lipid material in the digestive tract in the form of tiny droplets (micelles), thus enabling this material to be efficiently absorbed into the body.

Cells and healthcare practice

A cell has been defined as the basic living, structural and functional unit of all organisms. The human body consists of approximately 100 million million (1×10^{14}) cells of approximately 200 different types, the activities of which are largely outwith our control. It is remarkable that, for most of the time, individual cells function normally despite encountering situations that might damage them: e.g. natural wear and tear; various toxic/allergenic agents; pathogenic organisms (such as viruses, bacteria) which gain entry to the body; self-inflicted problems such as overeating. Should cells become unable to function normally, however, then altered cellular and whole body function is noticeable in the form of signs and symptoms of disease – indeed, in all disease processes there is ultimately an underlying cellular abnormality. People often ask for explanations of the signs and symptoms of their disease and a sound and accurate understanding of cellular function makes such explanation easier. The following simplified examples illustrate this:

- The symptom of pain may be experienced as a result of altered cellular activity in response to restricted blood supply: cells are deprived of their source of oxygen and normal metabolism is impaired. Cell damage results in the release of chemicals which stimulate pain receptors. To demonstrate this, put on a blood pressure cuff, inflate it to restrict arterial blood flow, then exercise your forearm – pain will be experienced very rapidly. (This is worth remembering when difficulty is experienced in recording blood pressures. Do not maintain inflation of the cuff for too long, otherwise you will increase the patient's discomfort.)

- An increasing number of people are sensitive to substances entering the bloodstream. Certain foods (e.g. shellfish, strawberries) and drugs (e.g. penicillin, aspirin) may cause skin rashes and more serious symptoms. The allergen to which the person is allergic (sensitive) causes histamine and other substances to be released from tissue mast cells (see Chs 3 and 16). A mild response may cause local dilation of blood vessels in the skin, with leakage of fluid into spaces between the cells causing signs such as redness and swelling (hives) and symptoms of itching and mild pain. This knowledge enables us to explain why antihistamine tablets are more effective than antihistamine ointment which will temporarily relieve local itching but not prevent the more generalized release of histamine.

When people ask for information and explanation it may not be useful to offer detailed accounts of cellular function. However, that knowledge must be there to provide reliable information if the questioner is to learn from the information. The following examples indicate applications of scientific theory to practical situations. One must be guided by the questioner as to how much theoretical background is appropriate.

- There is a move towards the use of unleaded petrol in cars as a result of reports that high concentrations of atmospheric lead may retard mental development in young children. Think about the proximity of babies and toddlers in push chairs to exhaust fumes from cars when out shopping with adults! The organic lead alkyls which escape into the atmosphere in exhaust fumes are more toxic than the inorganic compounds (e.g. lead bromide) because their lipophilic property allows them to cross the blood–brain barrier (see Ch. 20) and enter cells within the brain. Organic lead is capable of interfering with the proper function of some cells, including those of the brain. Fortunately, the majority of the body's unwanted lead usually accumulates in bone, where damage is less likely to be serious.

- It is well known that chronic alcoholism causes damage to the liver (cirrhosis). Many families support and care for heavy drinkers and consult healthcare workers such as the community dietician or community nurse for advice. Liver cells require adequate protein in the diet to function properly, particularly to metabolize fat. The body is not able to synthesize all amino acids (Table 1.1) and the amino acid methionine is essential to liver cells for fat metabolism. Its absence from the diet causes fat to accumulate with eventual damage to the structure of the liver. One of the factors affecting food intake in chronic alcoholism is the large alcohol intake which reduces interest in food. The high energy value of alcohol, or perhaps the presence of large amounts of alcohol metabolites, suppresses appetite, often with a large enough effect to cause malnutrition. This information may help to explain the dietary advice offered or, at least, make the frequent refusal of food more understandable.

PROTEINS

Composition

Proteins are macromolecules (large molecules) and are polymers, consisting of chains of many individual units known as amino acids linked together by peptide bonds (Fig. 1.3A). Twenty different amino acids are found commonly in biological systems (Table 1.1). They differ from one another in various ways in that they may be:

- acidic, basic or neutral
- predominantly hydrophilic or hydrophobic.

An almost infinite number of different proteins can be formed from these 20 different units since they can be combined together in any number and in any combination.

Following injuries such as burns where tissue has to be renewed, a high protein diet may be prescribed. This will supplement the body's production of amino acids.

Conformation

The very long chains of amino acids can fold up in a variety of ways into distinctive three-dimensional shapes ('conformations' – Fig. 1.3B) because of the affinity of different chemical groups on the amino acids for each other. The conformation adopted by any particular protein is both unique to that protein and crucial to its function (again illustrating the importance of the relationship between structure and function). However, the conformation of a protein can change

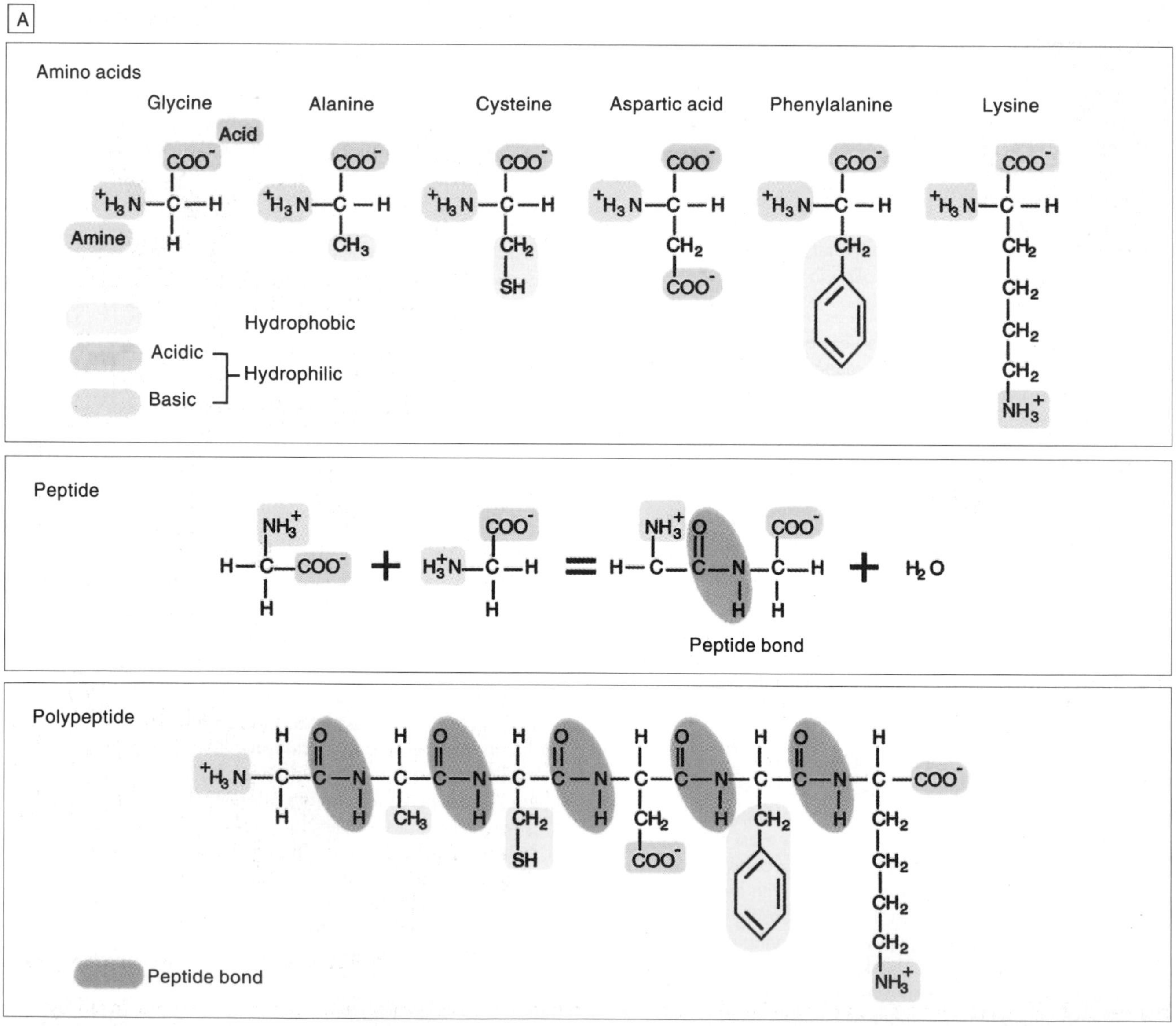

Figure 1.3 A

Table 1.1 Amino acids

Acidic	Basic	Neutral		
Aspartic acid	Arginine	Alanine	Valine	Phenylalanine
Glutamic acid	Histidine	Glycine	Leucine	Tryptophan
	Lysine	Serine	Isoleucine	
		Threonine	Cysteine	
		Asparagine	Methionine	
		Glutamine	Tyrosine	
		Proline		
STRONGLY HYDROPHILIC		MIXED PROPERTIES		STRONGLY HYDROPHOBIC

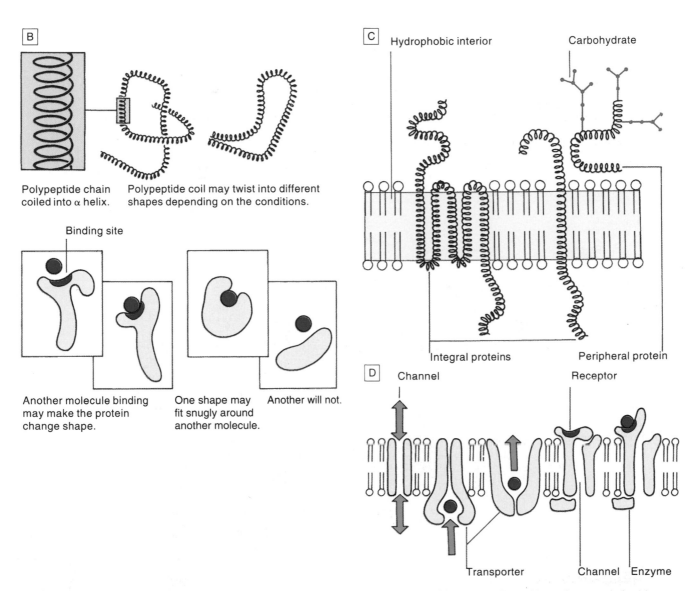

B Polypeptide chain coiled into α helix. Polypeptide coil may twist into different shapes depending on the conditions.

Binding site

Another molecule binding may make the protein change shape. One shape may fit snugly around another molecule. Another will not.

C Hydrophobic interior Carbohydrate

Integral proteins Peripheral protein

D Channel Receptor

Transporter Channel Enzyme

Figure 1.3 Structure and function of proteins. A, Examples of different types of amino acids and how they are linked by peptide bonds to form polypeptides. B, Shapes adopted by proteins; how they change and why it matters. C, Position and arrangement of proteins in cell membranes. D, Some of the functions performed by proteins in cell membranes.

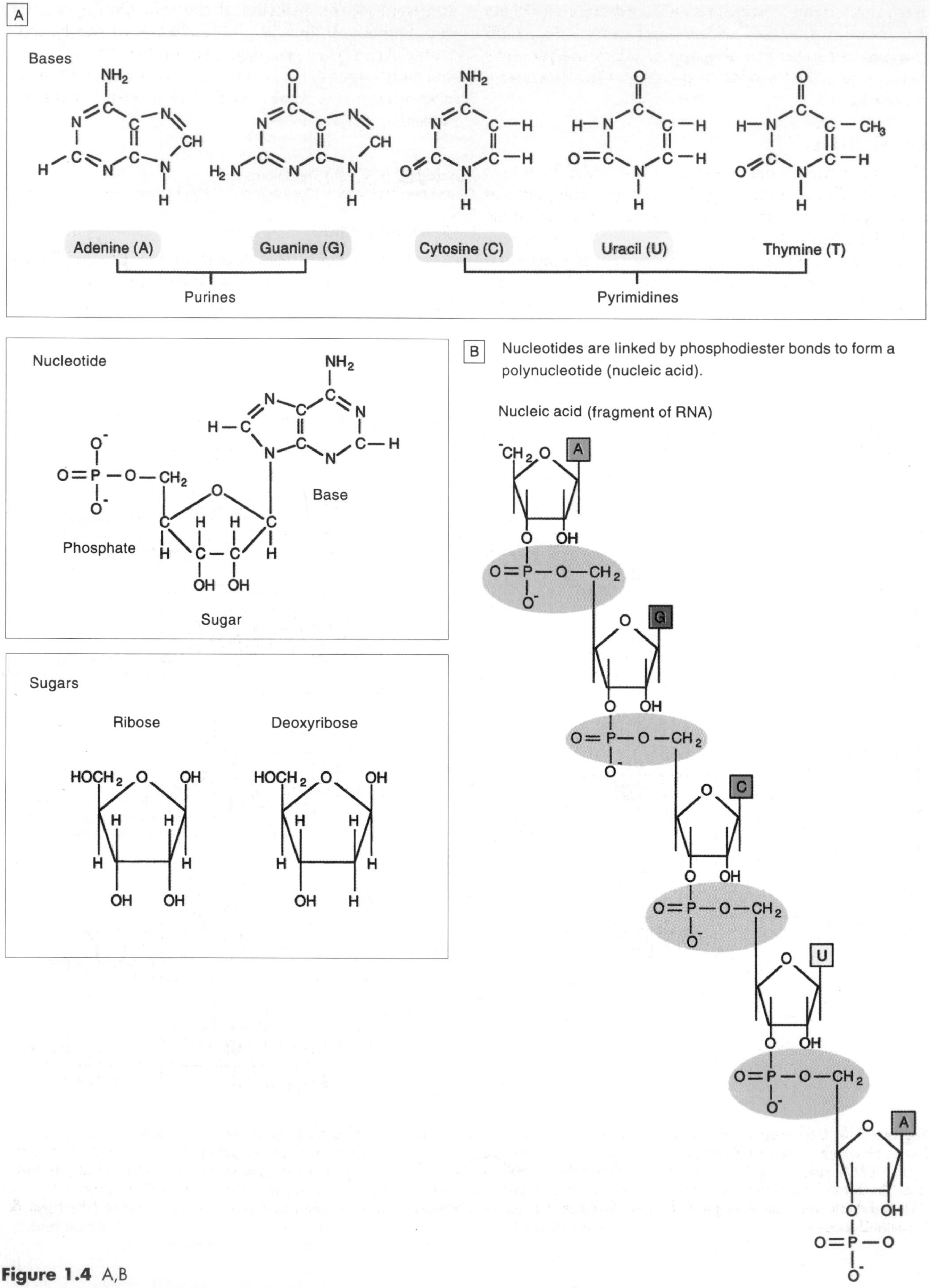

A — Bases: Adenine (A), Guanine (G) [Purines]; Cytosine (C), Uracil (U), Thymine (T) [Pyrimidines]. Nucleotide (Phosphate, Base, Sugar). Sugars: Ribose, Deoxyribose.

B — Nucleotides are linked by phosphodiester bonds to form a polynucleotide (nucleic acid). Nucleic acid (fragment of RNA).

Figure 1.4 A,B

according to the environmental conditions in which it is found (e.g. altered acidity or alkalinity – Fig. 1.3B) and such changes can also be crucial to the protein's function (e.g. the transport of oxygen by haemoglobin – see Ch. 7).

Production

The 'instructions' that determine the order in which amino acids are linked together to form polypeptides and proteins are contained in the genetic material of the cell. The details of the processes by which this genetic information is utilized are given below, but notice that there is a very important link between the genetic material of the cell and the structure (and hence function) of the proteins of the cell. One important consequence of this is that a change to the genetic material can produce a change in protein structure and function, sometimes with very serious pathological consequences, e.g. sickle-cell anaemia or Duchenne muscular dystrophy.

NUCLEIC ACIDS

Composition

The two nucleic acids found in the cell are DNA (deoxyribonucleic acid) and RNA (ribonucleic acid). DNA is confined to the chromosomes in the nucleus of

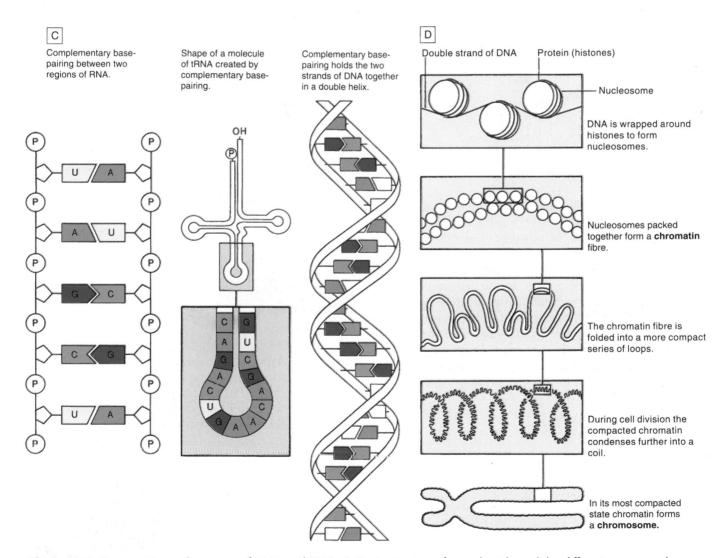

Figure 1.4 Composition and structure of DNA and RNA. A, Basic structure of a nucleotide and the different sugars and bases of which it may be composed. B, Structure of a nucleic acid. C, Complementary base-pairing in RNA and DNA. (Note that in DNA, adenine (A) pairs with thymine (coded white) in place of uracil (coded yellow) present in RNA.) D, Composition and structure of chromatin and how it is twisted and folded into a very compact form as a chromosome. (After copyright 1983. From Molecular Biology of the cell IE, Alberts et al. Reproduced with permission of Routledge, Inc., part of the Taylor & Francis Group.)

the cell and acts as an information storage molecule, holding all the information required to specify the structure, function and development of the cell (and organism). RNA molecules are found in both the nucleus and cytoplasm and are crucial in expressing the information stored in DNA.

Both DNA and RNA are macromolecular polymers and both consist of chains of individual units known as nucleotides.

A nucleotide consists of three component parts (Fig. 1.4A):

$$sugar + base + phosphate\ group(s)$$

The sugar present in DNA is deoxyribose; in RNA it is ribose.

There are five different bases found in total in DNA and RNA (Fig. 1.4A):

- two purines
  - guanine (G)
  - adenine (A)
- three pyrimidines
  - cytosine (C)
  - uracil (U)
  - thymine (T).

Adenine, guanine and cytosine are found in both DNA and RNA; thymine is found only in DNA, uracil only in RNA.

Nucleotides are linked together in different combinations by phosphodiester bonds between the sugar and phosphate parts of adjacent nucleotides to form long strands – nucleic acid molecules (Fig. 1.4B). The linked, alternating sugar and phosphate groups form what is usually referred to as the 'sugar–phosphate backbone' of the strand, whilst the bases of the nucleotides protrude out to the side of this backbone.

Molecules of DNA are typically double-stranded (see below) and very long, whereas those of RNA are typically single-stranded and much shorter. There are three different forms of RNA found in the cell:

- messenger RNA (mRNA)
- ribosomal RNA (rRNA)
- transfer RNA (tRNA).

Each of these forms has a crucial role to play in the expression of the genetic information that is stored in the DNA (see below).

Conformation

A key feature of nucleic acids is the specific associations that exist between the different purine and pyrimidine bases. Each pyrimidine associates most readily with only one of the purines through hydrogen bonds (Fig. 1.4C) and thus very specific base-pairing relationships are found:

Pyrimidine		Purine
cytosine	pairs with	guanine
thymine (in DNA)	pairs with	adenine
uracil (in RNA)	pairs with	adenine

These specific associations between the bases of nucleic acids are referred to as complementary base-pairing and they have important consequences. For example, they determine the conformation of a nucleic acid molecule; they enable the information stored in DNA to be expressed (usually in the form of a particular protein) and they enable a nucleic acid molecule to act as a template for its own replication and thus enable it to transmit genetic information from one individual cell or organism to another.

DNA and the various forms of RNA differ in terms of conformation and, again, a clear relationship between structure and function can be seen in these molecules. DNA is typically double-stranded, the two strands being held together principally by complementary base-pairing: this double-stranded molecule is rather like a ladder, with the two 'uprights' of the ladder being the sugar–phosphate backbones of the two strands and the 'rungs' being the complementary base pairs. The molecule is not flat, however – rather, the two strands wind round each other to form a double-helical structure (Fig. 1.4C). tRNA molecules, which are a crucial link between nucleic acid and protein structure, have a unique 'clover-leaf' shape that is essential to their function (Fig. 1.4C). rRNA molecules also have very particular conformations that are crucial in determining the structure of the ribosome, one of the subcellular organelles (see below).

Chromatin and chromosomes

DNA molecules are too long to fit inside the nucleus of the cell without extensive folding and packaging; e.g. if all the DNA molecules in one human cell were allowed to uncoil to their full relaxed length, the total length of these molecules would be almost two metres! Each very long macromolecule of DNA is therefore condensed through extensive intricate folding into a form which is much more compact (Fig. 1.4D).

Initially in the folding of DNA, each double-stranded DNA molecule is wrapped around multiple units of basic proteins (histones) to form nucleosomes. These nucleosomes are then twisted and folded in further ways to form even more compact structures to ensure that the DNA can be contained within the cell nucleus.

A chromosome is a single molecule of DNA with protein molecules of many different kinds associated with it – many of these proteins are involved in the folding of DNA. Thus, chromosomes are composed of both DNA and protein; this combination is sometimes referred to as chromatin.

Each human cell contains 46 chromosomes and these are arranged in 23 pairs. One pair of these are the sex chromosomes (the X and Y chromosomes in the human); the remainder are the non-sex chromosomes (or autosomes).

THE CELL IN ACTION

As previously stated, the cell is a dynamic structure, made up of many different components, and it functions as an integrated whole. Its life-cycle and activities are influenced both by the genetic information it contains and also by its environment (e.g. specific regulatory factors released by other cells).

EXPRESSION OF GENETIC INFORMATION

Storage of information

Information is stored in DNA in the form of the sequence of nucleotides on the strands of the molecule: it is the precise nucleotide sequence of (part of) a DNA molecule that specifies the precise sequence of amino acids in a particular protein. Different DNA molecules differ only in the sequence of the nucleotides of which they are composed, and these differences have profound consequences for the cell and organism which possess particular DNA molecules. Thus, the DNA molecules of a plant (e.g. lily) and of an animal (e.g. horse) are constructed in basically the same way, as described above – the only difference between these DNA molecules is in the order of nucleotides on their constituent strands.

A gene is the sequence of nucleotides coding for a specific protein. The nucleotide sequence is organized in groups of three nucleotides (known as codons), each set of three nucleotides specifying a single amino acid in a protein. For example, the codon GGG specifies glycine; the codon GCA specifies alanine. The relationship between particular codons and particular amino acids is known as the genetic code (Fig. 1.5). It can be seen that many amino acids can be specified by more than one codon (e.g. six different codons specify leucine; four different codons specify valine), this is described as 'degenerate' or 'redundant'; however, each codon specifies only one amino acid, i.e. it is not 'ambiguous'. The code is therefore referred to as being degenerate, but not ambiguous.

Expression of information

The expression of the information stored in DNA is a two-stage process: firstly, in transcription, part of the DNA molecule is used as a template for the production of an mRNA molecule; this occurs in the nucleus. Secondly, in translation, this mRNA molecule is used to specify the sequence of amino acids in a protein molecule; this occurs on the ribosome in the cytoplasm.

Thus, again, it can be seen that the order of amino acids in a protein is ultimately determined by the sequence of bases in the DNA molecule.

Transcription

In the formation of mRNA, the two strands of the DNA molecule separate for a small part of their length, and ribonucleotides assemble on the DNA template in the sequence determined by the complementarity of base-pairing (Fig. 1.5). The mRNA formed then dissociates from the DNA and passes to the ribosomes in the cytosol.

Translation

As an mRNA molecule passes through the ribosomes (Fig. 1.5), molecules of tRNA, each bearing a specific amino acid, associate in turn with successive codons on the mRNA molecule. It is important to notice that it is the tRNA molecules which act as a link between nucleic acid (RNA) structure and protein structure: each possesses a different three base-pair region (known as the anti-codon) that attaches to a codon on mRNA according to the complementarity of base-pairing. As each tRNA molecule also carries only one specific amino acid, the accuracy of the translation process is thus assured. Ribosomal enzymes then catalyse the formation of bonds between adjacent amino acids and protein synthesis thus proceeds.

COMPONENT PARTS AND FUNCTIONS

Membranes

The membranes of the cell are very important in biological systems as they form boundaries between

The DNA of some bacteria (e.g. *Escherichia coli*) can be altered in several ways, e.g. by inserting genes from other organisms. This recombinant DNA makes the bacterial cells synthesize proteins which they do not normally produce; e.g. insulin to treat people with diabetes mellitus is now produced biosynthetically using *E. coli* cells that have had the gene for human insulin inserted into them. Thus, a plentiful source of human insulin is now available, without any of the infection risks of using material isolated from human sources. Other semi-synthetic insulin is also produced by altering the amino acid sequence of porcine (pig) insulin.

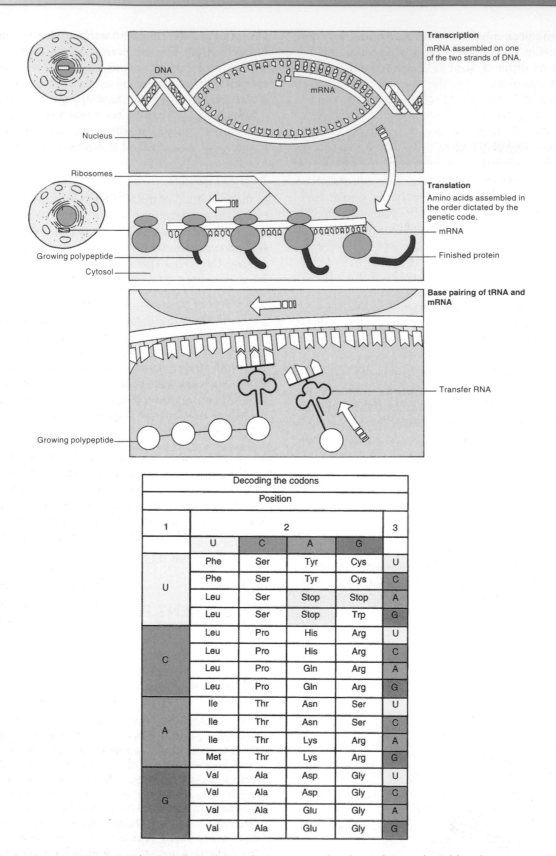

Figure 1.5 Transcribing and translating the genetic code. The codons in the table relate to RNA. Phe, Ser, Tyr etc. are abbreviations for different amino acids (phenylalanine, serine, tyrosine etc.). The codon sequence UUU codes for phenylalanine, UCU for serine etc. UAA signals the end of a polypeptide.

different compartments, both within cells and between cells and their environment which, in turn, allows localization of different functions to different parts of the cell and organism.

As mentioned above, phospholipids are very important in the formation of cell membranes: the hydrocarbon chains of these molecules are hydrophobic, whereas their phosphate groups (localized together at one end of the molecule) are strongly hydrophilic. Thus, when these molecules are placed in an aqueous environment, the phosphate groups associate with water molecules and the hydrocarbon chains face one another, thus forming a phospholipid bilayer with a hydrophobic interior and hydrophilic surfaces (Fig. 1.2B). Bilayers of this kind are found in many places in the cell and are very important in compartmentalizing the cell's interior.

Note that the term 'membrane' is also used to mean a quite different sort of structure in biology – a boundary that consists of cells or tissue, such as the cells lining the mouth (a mucous membrane), or the vibrating membrane of the inner ear (basilar membrane; see Ch. 23).

The outer boundary of the cell itself is the plasma (or cell) membrane. Other membranes are organized into different structures (organelles) within the cell (Figs 1.6 and 1.7). These organelles include:

- nucleus
- endoplasmic reticulum
- Golgi apparatus (complex)
- mitochondria
- lysosomes
- peroxisomes.

The space between the organelles is filled with cytosol, which consists chiefly of proteins of many types (see below), water and ions.

Although diagrams frequently give the impression that cell organelles are completely distinct from one another, this is not always true. The membrane surrounding the nucleus is in fact continuous with that of the endoplasmic reticulum. Also, membrane-bound vesicles are continually being incorporated into the plasma membrane, and being formed from it as a result of the twin processes of exocytosis and endocytosis (Fig. 1.8).

Movement across membranes

It is obviously important that materials are able to pass across cell membranes (e.g. for the secretion of cellular products). Materials can pass across membranes by a variety of means, including the following:

- diffusion (simple or facilitated, occurring from a region of high to low concentration, i.e. down a concentration gradient; does not require energy)
- active transport (movement occurring from a region of low to high concentration, i.e. against a concentration gradient and thus requiring energy)
- two processes that involve gain or loss of part of the membrane: exocytosis (moves material out of the cell) and endocytosis (moves material into the cell) (Fig. 1.8).

In exocytosis, a vesicle from inside the cell fuses with the plasma membrane and its contents are released to the cell exterior. The membrane of the vesicle becomes part of the existing plasma membrane. Clearly, the plasma membrane would grow ever larger if membrane were not being removed simultaneously at other sites by endocytosis.

In endocytosis a small area of plasma membrane is drawn inwards (invaginates) and the membrane at the mouth of the invagination fuses to form a vesicle enclosing a tiny droplet of fluid from outside the cell.

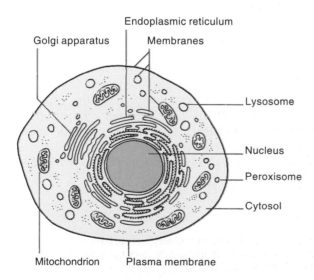

Figure 1.6 The cell and its structures.

Absorption of drugs

The phospholipid bilayer enables some drugs to pass through cell membranes into the cell interior. Highly liposoluble drugs like thiopental, dicoumarol and griseofulvin diffuse rapidly though the bilayer and readily attain a high concentration inside cells. It is important to note, however, that such drugs must also be sufficiently water-soluble to dissolve in body fluids if they are to reach their target cells. Liposoluble drugs taken orally need to dissolve in the fluids of the gastrointestinal tract to be available for absorption. Controlled release drugs are designed to dissolve slowly in the gastrointestinal fluids to provide uniform absorption over a long period.

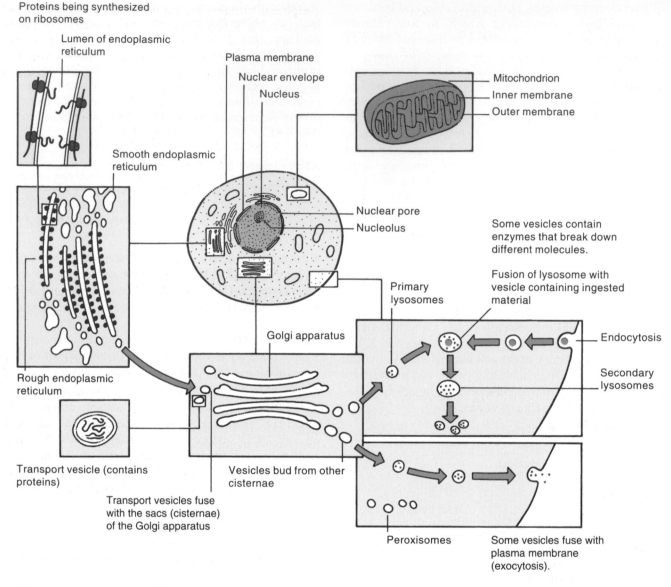

Figure 1.7 Structure and function of cellular organelles.

Secretory cells in the digestive glands (see Ch. 9) secrete digestive enzymes by exocytosis. White blood cells (leucocytes; see Chs 3 and 16) are able to engulf relatively large particles, bacteria and even other cells by a modified form of endocytosis known as phagocytosis.

Membrane proteins

Cell membranes do not consist just of a phospholipid bilayer. If they did, they would act as a very effective barrier to the movement of water-soluble substances, but they would permit very little else to happen. It is found that, inserted into and associated with the various membranes of the cell, are numerous proteins. This is possible because parts of the protein molecules are hydrophobic and can interact with the lipid bilayer. Membrane proteins are thus very important and convert phospholipid bilayers into highly selective, sensitive and active systems.

The proteins which associate with cell membranes (Fig. 1.3C) are divided into two groups:

- integral
- peripheral.

The integral proteins are lodged relatively firmly within the phospholipid bilayer, anchored by hydrophobic groups on parts of their external surfaces; many of these proteins span the membrane from side to side.

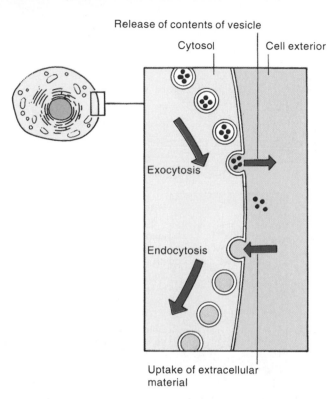

Figure 1.8 Fusion of vesicles with the cell membrane expelling contents from the cell (exocytosis) and formation of new vesicles by invagination of the cell membrane (endocytosis).

How drugs act

Some drugs act by binding to proteins. In so doing they alter the functional ability of the protein and thereby increase or decrease the processes reliant on it. The name of one group of drugs, the monoamine oxidase inhibitors (MAOIs), explains how they act. These drugs, which are used in the treatment of depression, inhibit the oxidation (one form of processing) of monoamines by binding to the enzyme monoamine oxidase (MAO). Some of the amines concerned are the neurohormone adrenaline (epinephrine), and the neurotransmitters noradrenaline (norepinephrine), serotonin and dopamine (see Chs 5 and 20) The result is an increase in the concentrations of these amines and stimulation of their receptors; for some people there is an improvement in mood. However, excess adrenaline also causes a marked rise in blood pressure (hypertension), headache and abnormalities of heart activity. Other amines, which are taken into the body in food and proprietary cold cures, also accumulate because they too cannot be broken down. Patients for whom these drugs are prescribed are therefore given a list of banned foods and medications (e.g. cheese, yeast and meat extracts, broad beans, alcohol, proprietary cold cures) all of which contain high proportions of amines.

Peripheral proteins are more loosely associated; most are bound to integral proteins either outside or inside the cell; some of these are glycoproteins (proteins with carbohydrate molecules attached). Membrane proteins collectively perform a range of very important functions (Fig. 1.3D), including acting as:

- *channels* through which small water-soluble molecules and ions can pass through the hydrophobic core of the membrane – often important in simple diffusion
- *transporters* that bind to molecules dissolved in the water environment on one side of the membrane and carry them through the membrane to the other side – often important in facilitated diffusion and active transport
- *enzymes* which catalyse specific chemical reactions
- *receptors* which detect hormones and neurotransmitters and control cell activity (see later)
- *markers* of cell identity.

Cytosol proteins

There are very many different proteins found in the cytosol: some are enzymes which catalyse specific chemical reactions (e.g. glycogen synthase catalyses the formation of glycogen from glucose); others form structures which act as a 'skeleton' for the cell (cytoskeleton). These include tubulin, which forms microtubules, and actin, which forms microfilaments. These structures are also involved in causing movement, both of the cell as a whole and of structures within the cell, in:

- cell division (see below)
- muscle contraction (see Ch. 4B)
- movement of vesicles from place to place inside the cell
- movement of white cells through the tissues (see Ch. 16).

A pair of structures known as the centriole pair, formed of tubulin, is believed to be involved in organizing the cytoskeleton. It is important also in cell division (Fig. 1.9).

ORGANELLES

See Figures 1.6 and 1.7.

Plasma (cell) membrane

This is the barrier between the cell and its environment. It has many very important functions, including the following: it determines what substance may enter and leave the cell; it acts as the communication link between the inside of the cell and the outside; it is

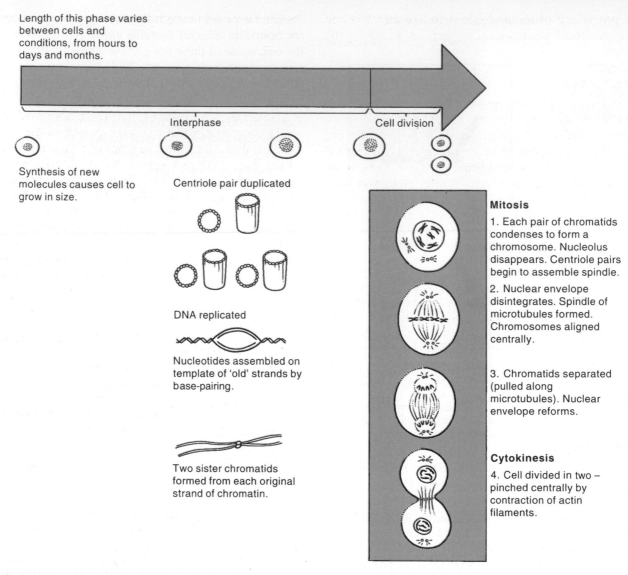

Length of this phase varies between cells and conditions, from hours to days and months.

Interphase   Cell division

Synthesis of new molecules causes cell to grow in size.

Centriole pair duplicated

DNA replicated

Nucleotides assembled on template of 'old' strands by base-pairing.

Two sister chromatids formed from each original strand of chromatin.

Mitosis

1. Each pair of chromatids condenses to form a chromosome. Nucleolus disappears. Centriole pairs begin to assemble spindle.

2. Nuclear envelope disintegrates. Spindle of microtubules formed. Chromosomes aligned centrally.

3. Chromatids separated (pulled along microtubules). Nuclear envelope reforms.

Cytokinesis

4. Cell divided in two – pinched centrally by contraction of actin filaments.

Figure 1.9 The sequence of changes (cell cycle) undergone by a cell as it grows, duplicates its constituents and then divides to form two new daughter cells.

the means by which the cell is recognized by other cells.

Endoplasmic reticulum

This is a network of membranes engaged in the manufacture and processing of many different molecules, such as proteins, lipids, steroids and phospholipids. It is also the place where many waste materials are broken down and converted into products that can be excreted.

There are two forms of endoplasmic reticulum (ER): the ER that is studded with ribosomes is referred to as rough (RER); ER that has no ribosomes is known as smooth (SER). RER is involved in the synthesis of proteins which are to be inserted into the membranes of the cell or exported from it. SER is the site of synthesis

of phospholipids, lipids and steroids, and is also where waste materials are broken down.

Golgi apparatus or Golgi complex

This consists of a stack of membranous sacs and is closely associated with the endoplasmic reticulum. It is a site for the processing and packaging of certain molecules in the cell. It receives products (e.g. proteins synthesized on the endoplasmic reticulum) and adds components (e.g. sugar groups) to this basic product to form a modified derivative (e.g. glycoprotein). It then packages the modified derivative in vesicles which are either taken to the plasma membrane, so that the product can be secreted from the cell, or shunted to another place in the cell as required. In certain diseases, this processing of molecules is defective and this can have profound pathological consequences, e.g. cystic fibrosis.

Lysosomes

These are sacs of varying sizes that contain enzymes (acid hydrolases) that are capable of breaking down a wide variety of molecules, including those of the cell itself. They are involved in the digestion of unwanted material (e.g. bacteria engulfed by phagocytosis; worn out organelles), the products of such digestion then being made available for further use by the cell. Thus, they can be thought of as organelles involved in waste disposal and recycling.

Peroxisomes

These are similar in appearance to lysosomes but contain a different set of enzymes (oxidative enzymes) that break down some molecules in the normal course of metabolism (e.g. certain lipids) and detoxify other foreign substances (e.g. alcohol). In these processes, the toxic material hydrogen peroxide is produced, but this is then immediately destroyed by the enzyme catalase that these organelles also contain. Hence, no damage is sustained by the cell.

Mitochondria

Mitochondria (singular = mitochondrion) have both an outer and an inner membrane; the inner one is highly folded and studded with many enzymes. These are involved in the chemical reactions which convert the energy contained in molecules like glucose and fats into an immediately available form (adenosine triphosphate – ATP) that can be used to provide the energy directly for different cellular activities (see Chs 10, 15, 18), such as the synthesis of new molecules, the secretion of products, or the movement of the cell itself. The number of mitochondria varies greatly from one cell type to another – physiologically active cells (e.g. liver, muscle, kidney) possess a very large number; less active cells (e.g. resting cells of connective tissues, such as fibroblasts) have only a few.

Nucleus

The nucleus is a spherical or ovoid structure and is usually the most prominent organelle in the cell. It is enclosed by a double layer of membrane (nuclear envelope) which is perforated by holes (nuclear pores) that control the movement of materials between the nucleus and the cytoplasm. The principal contents of the nucleus are the chromosomes (see above), which are the cell's genetic material. Often, one or more spherical bodies can be distinguished within the nucleus – these nucleoli are the sites where ribosomes are assembled

before they pass through the nuclear pores to enter the cytoplasm.

CELL SPECIALIZATION

Although each nucleated cell of the body contains the same components and the same genetic material, it is obvious that there is a wide range of different cell types in the body. There are approximately 200 different cell types altogether and they differ from one another in size, form and function (Fig. 1.10). These differences arise because the different cell types each express different parts of the genetic information stored in their chromosomes. Whilst there are certain genes that all cells need to express in order to ensure their survival (e.g. genes for the proteins involved in cellular

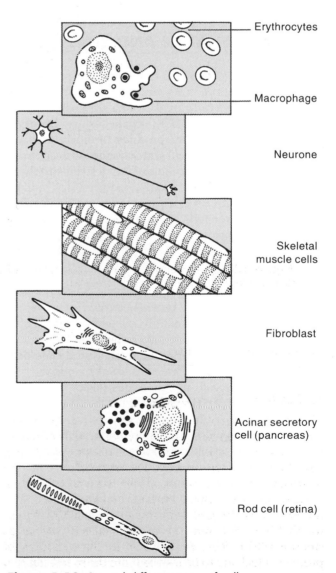

Erythrocytes

Macrophage

Neurone

Skeletal muscle cells

Fibroblast

Acinar secretory cell (pancreas)

Rod cell (retina)

Figure 1.10 Several different types of cell.

respiration, which generates energy for the cell), there are others that are only expressed in certain cell types in a manner that is consistent with their function (e.g. the genes for the visual pigment proteins are only expressed in the cells of the retina of the eye).

Thus, in each different cell type, some structures and activities are more prominent whilst others are less so. In muscle cells, for example (Fig. 1.10), the actin present in all cells is developed into a sophisticated system which can develop a powerful contractile force (see Ch. 4B). In enzyme-secreting cells of the digestive glands (see Ch. 9), the synthesis and packaging of proteins for export dominates cell activity, and so the rough endoplasmic reticulum is particularly prominent and many secretory vesicles (zymogen granules) are present. Mature red cells (see Ch. 3. – 'Erythrocytes'), in contrast, have no cell organelles at all, but instead are packed full of the oxygen-transporting protein haemoglobin (see Ch. 7).

CELL MAINTENANCE AND RENEWAL

Within all living cells there is a continual production and turnover of molecules and cellular components: e.g. new proteins are formed by the ribosomes; lipids are manufactured in the SER; organelles are damaged and degraded. Many of the products of breakdown are recycled and re-used (e.g. amino acids derived from proteins; iron from haemoglobin), but a fresh supply of some materials is continually required to replace substances that are used up or which are irreversibly degraded and excreted. This, of course, is ultimately why we need to eat.

Wound healing

Wound healing is a natural, automatic process. It has been said that the body provides its own intensive care when healing is required, but understanding of the processes allows us to help rather than hinder. Most people have experienced a cut from a knife or other sharp instrument; the cut is usually made in clean conditions with straight edges similar to that made during an operation. Provided that the wound is not too deep, it usually heals very quickly because the gap is negligible, there is no irritant such as a splinter or pathogenic organisms, the supply of nutrients is uninterrupted and the temperature is unchanged. In other words, all the requirements for normal cell division and healing are being met. Where the injury is large or not made under ideal conditions, i.e. as with most accidents, more cell systems are recruited to deal with the injury. For details of the processes involved in wound healing, see Chapter 19 at 'Wounds and wound healing'.

THE CELL CYCLE

The cell cycle (Fig. 1.9) is an orderly sequence of events by which a cell duplicates its contents and divides in two. It has two principal phases:

- interphase – cell preparing for division
- mitotic phase – cell dividing.

Interphase

In interphase, the cell replicates its DNA and also manufactures additional organelles and cytosolic components in preparation for cell division. It is a phase of high metabolic activity and the phase in which the cell does most of its growing.

Maintenance of the genetic material

It is crucial that the genetic information carried by DNA is maintained and passed on from cell to cell without error. If a mistake (mutation) occurs and is not corrected then not only may it have very serious consequences for the cell in which it occurred (and thus possibly for the individual of which the cell is a part, e.g. cancer), but also it will be reproduced in all succeeding generations of cells (and of individuals if the mistake occurs in the DNA of the gametes – sperm and ova).

Many different factors can produce changes in DNA molecules; e.g. cytosine can be converted to uracil, ultraviolet (UV) light can make adjacent thymines bond together. Normally these changes are repaired by enzymes that cut out the abnormal part of the damaged DNA strand and replace it with new nucleotides, using the undamaged strand as a template (DNA repair) and thus there is no persistent damage. However, these repair processes can sometimes fail, and then a mutation is stably established.

The replication of DNA is a complex process involving the activity of several enzymes including DNA polymerase. New strands are assembled using the old strands as templates, and the complementarity of base-pairing ensures that the two new molecules are exact copies of the original molecule. If errors do occur, mechanisms exist to allow these to be corrected. Following replication, the new DNA molecules become complexed with the proteins of chromatin (e.g. the

All newborn babies in the UK are screened for the disease phenylketonuria (PKU). The abnormal (mutated) DNA is unable to direct the synthesis of the enzyme phenylalanine hydroxylase which converts phenylalanine to tyrosine. As a result, phenylalanine accumulates in the blood; it is toxic to the brain cells in early life and causes mental retardation. A special diet limiting phenylalanine intake prevents retardation.

histones) and thus duplicated chromosomes (sometimes referred to as chromatids) are formed (Fig. 1.9).

Mitotic phase

Once all the cell's constituents have been replicated the mitotic ('M') phase begins and the cell divides. This occurs in two stages (Fig. 1.9):

- Mitosis – nuclear division: distribution of the two sets of chromosomes, one set into each of two separate nuclei. Thus, the genetic material is exactly partitioned between the two new cells.
- Cytokinesis – cytoplasmic division: distribution of the cytosol and organelles of the two new cells. This does not always result in an equal distribution of these structures between the two new cells.

A crucial role is played in mitosis by components of the cell's cytoskeleton. These become reorganized to form assemblies of fibres, some of which draw the chromosomes to each pole of the cell (the mitotic spindle), and others of which (the contractile ring) contract around the middle of the cell to split it into two new cells.

The time that it takes for a cell to pass through the cell cycle varies from one cell type to another. Amongst the cells with the shortest cycle times are the surface cells of the digestive tract (see Ch. 9): these cells are continually being eroded from the gut wall and so need to be replaced. They complete the cell cycle in about 8 hours. Other types take approximately 2 months to pass through the cycle, whilst still others, like nerve cells, skeletal muscle cells and red blood cells, no longer divide at all once they are mature.

Use of cytotoxic drugs and radiation

Cancer cells do not always form a well-defined tumour that can be removed by surgery, neither are they always all confined to the tumour mass. Diffuse malignant disease is often treated with cytotoxic drugs. These kill cells by preventing the formation of new DNA or by blocking some other essential function of the cell. Cells which divide rapidly are most susceptible to cytotoxic drugs. However, they also kill healthy dividing cells, e.g. those in the hair follicles, lining the intestines and blood cells in the bone marrow. This causes the side effects which often accompany therapy in some patients, i.e. hair loss, ulceration of the mouth, irritation of the gastrointestinal tract and suppression of blood cell production.

The main classes of cytotoxic drugs are alkylating agents, cytotoxic antibiotics, antimetabolites and vinca alkaloids.

- *Alkylating agents*, e.g. cyclophosphamide, chlorambucil, lomustine. The compounds are chemically similar to mustard gas. They work by preventing normal DNA synthesis and thus halting replication. Alkylating agents particularly cause nausea and vomiting (although anti-emetic drugs such as ondansetron can significantly reduce these effects). They can also cause cystitis and bone marrow depression. Male infertility and premature menopause may occur.
- *Cytotoxic antibiotics*, e.g. bleomycin, doxorubicin, mitomycin. These antibiotics interfere with DNA/RNA synthesis. The effects of some of these drugs are radiomimetic and the simultaneous use of radiotherapy should be avoided as it may markedly enhance toxicity.
- *Antimetabolites*, e.g. methotrexate, cytarabine, fluorouracil, mercaptopurine. These are synthetic analogues of normal metabolites which become incorporated into new nuclear material or combine irreversibly with vital cellular enzymes, thus preventing normal cellular division.
- *Vinca alkaloids*, e.g. vincristine, vinblastine. These are derived from the periwinkle (*Vinca rosea*) and inhibit cell division by preventing the formation of microtubules critical to mitosis.

Ionizing radiation (radiotherapy) is also used to kill malignant cells and can be directed at a specific tumour. Radiation dissociates molecules, causing disruption of chromosomes leading to mutation, and damaging or altering components of the cytoplasm. Ionizing radiation is used in carefully controlled doses and at highly targeted sites. The developments in radiography and radiotherapy have greatly improved diagnosis and treatment. However, radiation can damage all cells, healthy and otherwise. Great skill and care is essential in therapeutic radiography and adequate protection must always be given to patients and any persons involved in the use of radiation.

Controlling factors

Two factors can affect the cycle of cell growth and division:

- cellular environment
- availability of space.

If the conditions around the cells are not optimal then the cycle of growth and division may be slowed or even completely arrested. Factors which slow or arrest the cycle include a shortage of nutrients (e.g. a lack of amino acids will cause protein synthesis to be inhibited) or other essential resources (e.g. if there is insufficient oxygen, energy production will be limited) and lack of growth factors. Further, if the temperature of the environment is lowered, the rate at which chemical reactions occur in the cell is reduced and cells will not grow and divide as rapidly.

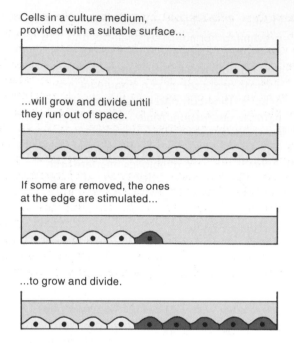

Cells in a culture medium,
provided with a suitable surface...

...will grow and divide until
they run out of space.

If some are removed, the ones
at the edge are stimulated...

...to grow and divide.

Figure 1.11 Factors controlling the growth and reproduction of cells.

Cells also normally stop dividing if they run out of space and come into close contact with one another (contact inhibition) (Fig. 1.11). This is important in healing for, if a tissue is injured, the contact between cells is broken, and the cells at the margins are thus stimulated to grow and divide again until the gap is repaired.

REGULATION OF CELL ACTIVITY

In general terms, the activity of cells is regulated largely by many different chemical regulators. These regulators

---

Patients who are immobile for long periods are at risk of developing pressure sores. Tissues that are compressed lack a good blood supply. Insufficient nutrients are supplied to maintain the cells and replace those that are lost.

One of the ways that cancer cells differ from normal cells is that their growth lacks contact inhibition. When cultured, these cells pile up on top of one another and continue to grow and divide. Should they have acquired a good blood supply they grow exceedingly fast because of the abundance of nutrients. A growing mass of cancerous tissue makes increasing demands on the nutrient supplies available to the body as a whole. In time, other tissues are progressively starved and their growth and renewal is arrested.

---

not only affect metabolic processes in the cytoplasm, but can also affect which parts of the cell's genetic material are expressed.

Chemical regulators and their modes of action

Chemical regulators of cell activity are manufactured and secreted by many cells including:

- endocrine cells
- nerve cells.

Chemical regulators which are secreted into the bloodstream (often by ductless, or endocrine, glands) and are carried to many target tissues through the circulation are termed hormones (see Ch. 11), whereas those which are secreted by nerves in close contact with the target cells are called neurotransmitters (see Chs 4A, 5 and 20).

Another large group of regulatory factors, the cytokines, are produced by many types of cell and can have their effects locally, or can be carried in the bloodstream to affect more distant cells (see Ch. 11). The group includes a number of factors which are growth promoters and growth inhibitors.

Several modes of action of chemical regulators are summarized in Figure 1.12. A fundamental principle of these various modes of action is that each regulator interacts only with its own specific receptor(s) (most commonly a protein) present in the cell – this ensures very specific responses to each different regulator. Many of these receptor molecules are embedded in the plasma membrane; others are found in the cytosol.

Following an interaction between a regulator and its membrane-bound receptor, there can be one of several outcomes. For example, this interaction may:

- open a protein channel in the membrane which allows specific ions, such as calcium, to move into the cell
- stimulate endocytosis (receptor-mediated endocytosis) and the uptake of the regulator, such as nerve growth factor, into the cell
- activate an enzyme located on the inner surface of the cell membrane which catalyses the formation of an intracellular regulator, such as cyclic AMP (cAMP).

This latter result is an example of the use of what is known as a second messenger, i.e. the interaction between receptor and regulator does not directly cause the regulator's ultimate effect, but rather it causes an intracellular change that then, in turn, affects the cellular process being controlled. A variety of substances have been found to act as second messengers, e.g. calcium, cAMP, guanosine monophosphate (GMP), inositol trisphosphate (IP_3) and diacylglycerol (DG). All of them act as links between the first messengers (hormones and neurotransmitters) and the cellular processes which are being controlled. These mechanisms usually produce rapid changes in the cell's behaviour since the various constituent steps can all be quickly completed.

Calcium acts intracellularly by binding to specific proteins, altering their conformation and changing their activities; e.g. in muscle cells, calcium binds to the proteins which affect the association between the contractile proteins actin and myosin and thus alters the degree of contraction of the cells (see Ch. 4B).

cAMP (formed from adenosine triphosphate (ATP) by the action of the enzyme adenylate cyclase) activates a group of enzymes called protein kinases which catalyse the addition of phosphate to specific intracellular proteins. This phosphorylation of these proteins, which are often enzymes themselves, in turn alters their activity and thus changes the rate of the chemical reaction(s) which they catalyse. It is by such a means that cAMP, for example, regulates the breakdown of glycogen to glucose (see Chs 10 and 18).

Some chemical regulators (e.g. lipophilic substances, such as steroid hormones) do not bind to receptors on the plasma membrane, but are able to enter the cell and bind to receptor proteins in the cytosol. Typically, these regulators act by modifying the pattern of gene expression: the hormone/receptor complex enters the nucleus where it binds to chromatin and modifies gene transcription. This changes the type(s) and/or quantities of proteins synthesized by the cell and this, in turn, alters the capacity of the cell to perform specific functions. For example, anabolic steroids stimulate protein synthesis in muscle cells; the cells therefore enlarge and are able to generate a greater contractile force.

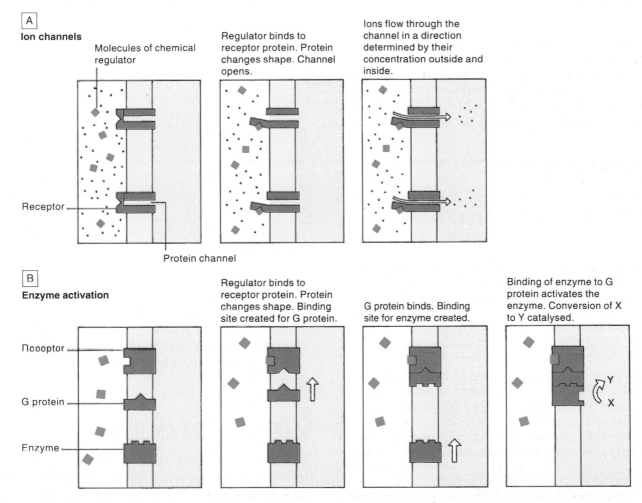

Figure 1.12 Ways in which chemical regulators affect cell activity by controlling: A, ion channels; B, enzyme activation; (C, D overleaf.)

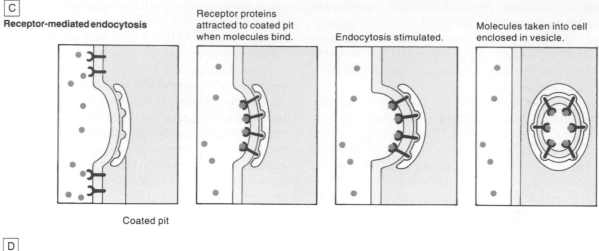

C
Receptor-mediated endocytosis

Receptor proteins attracted to coated pit when molecules bind.

Endocytosis stimulated.

Molecules taken into cell enclosed in vesicle.

Coated pit

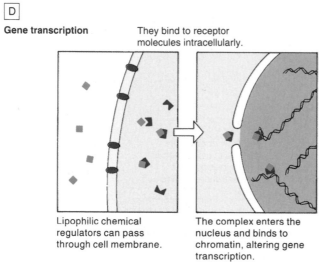

D
Gene transcription

They bind to receptor molecules intracellularly.

Lipophilic chemical regulators can pass through cell membrane.

The complex enters the nucleus and binds to chromatin, altering gene transcription.

Figure 1.12 (Cont'd) C, receptor-mediated endocytosis; D, gene transcription.

As protein synthesis takes some time to complete, these changes in cell behaviour do not occur immediately.

CELLS AND TISSUES

The cells of the body do not exist in isolation, but rather exist together, being supported and maintained by the extracellular matrix in which they are embedded and being physically linked together to form tissues. These are joined together to form organs, which, in turn, are associated together to form organ systems.

There are four basic types of tissue described according to their structure and function, though several subtypes of each are also described:

1. Epithelial tissue – covers body surfaces and lines hollow organs, body cavities and ducts, e.g. skin; lining of blood vessels. Epithelial tissue also forms glands.

2. Connective tissue – protects and supports the body and its organs, e.g. tendons; ligaments; bones; cartilage; blood.

3. Muscle tissue – generates the physical force needed to make body structures move, e.g. muscles attached to the skeleton (voluntary muscle); muscle of the digestive tract (involuntary muscle).

4. Nervous tissue – detects changes in a variety of conditions inside and outside the body and responds by generating nerve impulses, e.g. touch receptors in skin.

EXTRACELLULAR MATRIX

This material provides both the correct biochemical environment and physical support for the appropriate function of cells and is thus a vital component of the body. The precise nature of the extracellular matrix (ECM) varies from one tissue to another (e.g. it can be

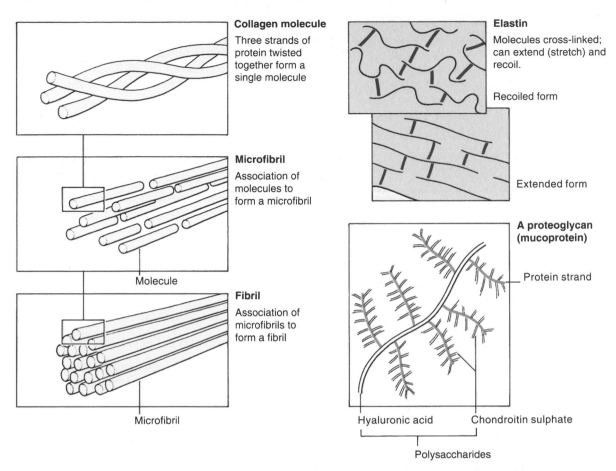

Figure 1.13 Composition and structure of three major constituents of the extracellular matrix: collagen, elastin and a proteoglycan.

fluid, gel-like or solid) but its role is consistently important – it helps to hold cells together, influences their activity and guides the migration of certain cell types.

Formation and constituents

The ECM is formed chiefly by fibroblasts, though other cells (e.g. in bone – osteoblasts; in cartilage – chondroblasts) may contribute too.

Typically, the ECM consists of a ground substance in which are embedded protein fibres of different types (Fig. 1.13). Proteins commonly found in the ECM include:

- collagen – very widespread (e.g. in tendons); an extremely strong, rope-like protein that gives great mechanical strength
- elastin – also widely found (e.g. in the skin); can both stretch and recoil

- fibronectin – promotes adhesion of collagen to cells and ground substance.

Both the absolute and relative amounts of each of these proteins can vary greatly, and other proteins are found in the ECM of some tissues.

A very extensively found form of ECM is the gel form in which the ground substance consists of a variety of complex macromolecules known as glycosaminoglycans (e.g. hyaluronic acid, heparin, chondroitin sulphate) and proteoglycans (glycosaminoglycans linked to proteins). Both glycosaminoglycans and proteoglycans are strongly hydrophilic and thus attract water and form a gel. Dissolved in the water of the gel are salts and other materials (e.g. glucose and amino acids).

Physically different forms of ECM are found in other tissues; e.g. the ECM of blood is fluid; in bone it is solid (calcified). These variations again reflect the link between structure and function in different tissues.

One particular specialization of the ECM is found wherever an epithelial tissue is attached to underlying connective tissue: this is known as a basement membrane. Generally, the basement membrane serves to support the epithelial layer above it and acts to guide cells as they migrate during growth and tissue repair; in certain areas, however, it has other, more specialized, functions – e.g. in the kidney, it acts as a filter (Fig. 1.14).

TISSUE CELLS

Just as the precise nature of the ECM varies from tissue to tissue according to that tissue's function, so the precise cell type(s) found also varies from tissue to tissue. For example, the retina contains light-sensitive cells; the lining of the gastrointestinal tract includes cells that are highly specialized for the absorption of materials from digested food. The exact details of both the structures and functions of the many different cell types that are found in different tissues will be considered in the chapters on each of the systems of the body.

CELL JUNCTIONS

Most epithelial cells and some nerve and muscle cells are tightly joined into functional units; cell junctions are the points of contact between the plasma membranes of tissue cells. There are three main functions of such junctions:

- to anchor cells to each other or to the ECM
- to act as channels to allow the passage of ions and molecules to pass from cell to cell
- to form fluid-tight seals between cells.

The three principal types of cell junction are (Fig. 1.15):

- desmosomes – hold cells firmly together, and thus contribute to the overall stability of tissues; found extensively in the epidermis and also between cardiac muscle cells
- tight junctions – prevent passage of material between cells; join together those cells that line the

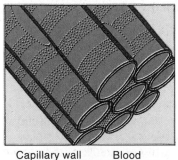

Blood capillaries
Basement membrane

Absorptive cells of the digestive tract (see Ch. 9)

Skeletal muscle (see Ch. 4B)

Basement membrane surrounds each cell. Guides the regeneration of damaged tissue.

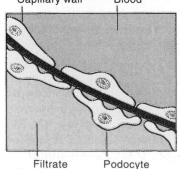

Capillary wall   Blood

Filtration barrier: kidney glomerulus (see Ch. 8)

Substances filtered by the kidney have to pass through the basement membrane

Filtrate   Podocyte

Figure 1.14 The basement membrane in three different tissues.

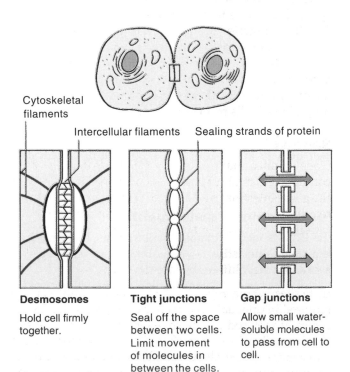

Cytoskeletal filaments

Intercellular filaments   Sealing strands of protein

Desmosomes

Hold cell firmly together.

Tight junctions

Seal off the space between two cells. Limit movement of molecules in between the cells.

Gap junctions

Allow small water-soluble molecules to pass from cell to cell.

Figure 1.15 Structure and function of three different types of linkages between cells: desmosomes, tight junctions and gap junctions.

surfaces of organs and body cavities, e.g. epithelial cells of the intestine, urinary bladder

- gap junctions – allow passage of small molecules and ions between cells and thus allow cells in a tissue to communicate with one another; important in rapid transmission of nerve and muscle impulses between cells.

TISSUE FORMATION AND RENEWAL

Formation

The process of development from zygote (single cell) to fully mature adult (composed of a huge number of individual cells of many different types) is characterized by two processes: a huge increase in the number of cells (achieved by many, many rounds of cell division), and specialization (differentiation) of different cells for particular functions in the body (e.g. liver cell, muscle cell). Commonly, relatively unspecialized cells proliferate at the site in the body in which their derivatives are ultimately to be found and the cells resulting from these divisions then differentiate there into the variety of cells of which the tissue is composed. Although the process of differentiation is controlled genetically, it is important to note that the maintenance of the differentiated state depends also on the ECM.

Not all cells arise in the body at the site at which they will ultimately be found – some cells arise in one place and then migrate to another; e.g. primitive neurones migrate from nervous tissue to colonize organs and tissues some distance away, forming parts of the autonomic nervous system (see Ch. 5). The cytokine factors in the ECM are important in guiding the migration of cells from one site to another.

Renewal

Once tissues have been formed, many undergo continual renewal (e.g. red blood cells, epithelial cells of the gastrointestinal tract). Others can form new tissue if required to do so (e.g. the liver, following injury).

Cells are replaced in two ways, either by:

- division of existing cells
- division and differentiation of stem cells.

In tissues where replacement of cells is only usually required in unusual circumstances (e.g. injury), cells are typically replaced by the division of existing cells; e.g. if some cells of the liver (see Ch. 10) or those of the inner lining of the blood vessels (endothelium) are lost through injury, some of the remaining cells are stimulated to divide and make good the tissue deficit.

In tissues where replacement is a normal physiological process, however (e.g. blood – see Ch. 3),

replacement is usually achieved by the division and differentiation of precursor cells known as stem cells. Stem cells have the particular feature that they both maintain their own numbers and give rise to more differentiated progeny cells; they can thus produce a steady supply of replacement cells indefinitely. There are two types of stem cell:

- *unipotent* (gives rise to only one cell type)
- *pluripotent* (gives rise to several types, e.g. the stem cell that gives rise to the cells of the blood; see Ch. 3).

However, stem cells can also be involved in regeneration of tissue following damage – e.g. in muscle, stem cells exist, but are normally inactive (quiescent); only in the event of damage to the muscle tissue are they stimulated to divide.

Non-renewable cells

Not all cells, however, can be replaced. Some, once formed, no longer divide. The molecules of which they are composed undergo renewal and repair, but the cell itself cannot be replaced by division of adjacent cells, or by differentiation of stem cells. This applies, for example, to nerve cells and the muscle cells of the heart: if they are irreversibly damaged they cannot be replaced. This has obvious, and potentially very serious, consequences if these tissues suffer damage.

> When a person suffers a myocardial infarction (heart attack) the heart muscle (myocardium) is damaged and as heart muscle cells cannot be replaced, there is a thinning of the heart wall, which may rupture.

Tumours

The renewal and replacement of normal cells occurs in a controlled way, the control being exerted by many factors including the genetic material of the cells themselves and various regulatory influences exerted on them (e.g. growth-promoting and growth-inhibiting factors).

The growth of neoplastic cells is not controlled in the same way and, indeed, it is this escape from the normal processes of growth control that is the common diagnostic feature of the group of diseases known as tumours or neoplasms. Neoplastic cells proliferate freely, without any control, and thus an excess of these cells accumulates in the body.

There are two basic types of tumour: the benign tumour typically grows slowly, does not aggressively invade adjacent tissues and remains localized to one place; the malignant tumour typically grows rapidly, does aggressively invade adjacent tissues and also spreads (or has the potential to spread) to other, distant sites in the body (often by the blood or lymph).

Malignant tumours, if untreated, are always fatal; benign tumours are usually less serious, but can be very serious in some circumstances (e.g. if growing in a confined space, such as within the skull).

REFERENCES AND FURTHER READING

Alberts B, Bray D, Johnson A, Lewis J, Raff M, Roberts K, Walter P 1998 Essential cell biology. Garland Publishing, New York & London
An up-to-date and comprehensive introduction to the molecular biology of the cell

Atkins P W 1987 Molecules. Scientific American Library, New York
Interesting facts about molecules that matter in everyday life. A beautifully illustrated compendium for leisure-time reading as well as reference

De Duve C 1985 A guided tour of the living cell. W H Freeman, Oxford
Cell biology with a difference. A beautifully illustrated expedition through the intricacies and marvels of cellular life

Gartner L P, Hiatt J L 1990 Color atlas of histology. Williams & Wilkins, Baltimore
Very clearly presented pictures of cells and tissues

Hinwood B 1992 A textbook of science for the health professions. Chapman & Hall, London
Excellent book for getting to grips with the basic science of atoms and molecules

Klug W S, Cummings M R 2000 Concepts of genetics, 6th edn. Prentice Hall, Upper Saddle River, WJ
A well-presented and comprehensive in-depth textbook of genetics

Tortora G J, Grabowski S R 2000 Principles of anatomy and physiology, 9th edn. John Wiley, New York
An excellent anatomy and physiology text with very good chapters on molecules and cells

2 How drugs work – cellular and molecular systems

Pharmacology is the study of the manner in which drugs affect the function of living biological systems. The word 'pharmacology' comes from the Greek word *pharmakon*, meaning a 'medicine' or 'drug' and *ology* meaning 'study of'. A 'drug' can be defined as a chemical which affects the activity of a living biological system and can include endogenous substances, i.e. chemicals produced by the body. For example, adrenaline (epinephrine) is a hormone produced in the body, secreted into the blood from the adrenal medulla. It can also be used therapeutically to raise blood pressure in patients with circulatory collapse, to localize the effects of local anaesthetics and to ease breathing during asthmatic attacks.

Historically, the earliest drugs were extracts of natural materials that people found around them. The treatment of disease was, for a long time, tied up with magic, spells, potions and the like and the effectiveness of many remedies was doubtful. On the other hand, the usefulness of some of these extracts has been known for centuries. Extracts of willow bark have been used as a treatment of pain, rheumatism and fevers since the time of the Pharaohs. Willow bark contains salicin, a glycoside very similar in structure to aspirin. Extracts of the foxglove plant were used by the physician William Withering in the seventeenth century to treat 'the dropsy', now known as congestive heart failure. The foxglove plant contains the cardiac glycosides, digitoxin, gitoxin and gitalotoxin which slow and strengthen the heart beat. Digoxin, a derivative of digitoxin, is still widely used to control cardiac arrhythmias. A final example of a powerful drug known for some time, in this case millennia, is opium, the extracts of the poppy *Papaver somniferum*. Opium contains 25 alkaloids including morphine, codeine and papaverine. All three of these agents are used therapeutically. Diamorphine (heroin), chemically derived from morphine, is a very good analgesic although its abuse causes many problems to society. In conclusion, although some drugs have been in common use for a long time, the ways in which they worked and the doses which should be given were often not understood and as a result many of the remedies were of doubtful value. The scientific study of drugs did not begin until the mid–late nineteenth century.

Today pharmacology can be thought of as having three main branches: *pharmacodynamics*, the study of the mechanism of action of drugs, encompassing their physiological, biochemical and, increasingly, molecular effects; *pharmacokinetics*, the study of how the body handles drugs, encompassing their absorption, distribution, metabolism and excretion; *therapeutics*, the use of drugs in the prevention, diagnosis and treatment of disease. The remainder of this chapter will deal with how drugs act (pharmacodynamics), with therapeutic examples being given wherever appropriate.

HOW DRUGS ACT (PHARMACODYNAMICS)

Broadly speaking, drugs actions can be classified into

- non-specific physico-chemical interactions
- interactions with specific macromolecular targets.

Relatively few drugs fall into the first category but a few examples are as follows. Bulk laxatives, such as fibre, work by drawing water into the gastrointestinal tract by osmosis. The increased fluid softens the stools and increases their volume, thus promoting peristalsis and hence defecation. A second example of drugs working through non-specific physico-chemical interactions is antacids, taken by the population in great amounts to relieve indigestion. Antacids work by chemically neutralizing the hydrochloric acid produced by the stomach, a simple acid–alkali reaction. The majority of therapeutically important drugs, however, work by binding to specific large molecules, proteins, and influencing their function.

These macromolecular protein targets are:

- enzymes
- carrier molecules
- ion channels
- receptors.

Other macromolecular targets are known. For example, antibiotics, which are used to attack invading microorganisms, or chemotherapeutic agents, which attack cancer cells, bind to DNA and thus affect cell division.

ENZYMES AS DRUG TARGETS

One important drug target is a group of enzymes, the cyclo-oxygenases (COX). These enzymes are responsible for the synthesis of prostacyclins, prostaglandins and thromboxanes (Fig. 2.1) which have important roles in pain sensation, inflammation and blood clotting. The discovery that COX was the macromolecular target for aspirin was made by the pharmacologist John Vane in 1971. Vane later received the Nobel Prize for Medicine and a knighthood for his work in this area. It is now well known that aspirin and other non-steroidal anti-inflammatory drugs (NSAID) (see Chs 11, 29) non-competitively inhibit this enzyme. The prevention of

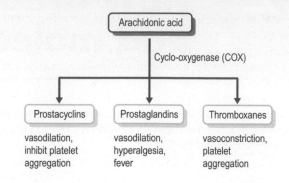

Figure 2.1 Enzymes as drug targets – cyclo-oxygenase.

the synthesis of prostaglandins largely accounts for the anti-inflammatory, anti-pyretic and analgesic effects of aspirin (see Ch. 29). Interference with the blood-clotting mechanism provided a new use for aspirin, beginning in the 1970s: aspirin, in relatively low doses compared with that required for its anti-inflammatory and analgesic effects, reduced the incidence of myocardial infarction (heart attack) in patients at risk by reducing the tendency of the blood to clot (see Ch. 3). The rationale for this treatment is not obvious from Figure 2.1 – aspirin inhibits the formation of both prostacyclins (anti-clotting) and thromboxanes (pro-clotting). However, prostacyclins are secreted by the lining endothelial cells of blood vessels and the cells can resynthesize COX. Thromboxanes, however, are released from platelets which are not complete cells and lack the necessary machinery to make new COX. Thus the balance is shifted in favour of prostacyclins and the tendency for platelets to aggregate is reduced.

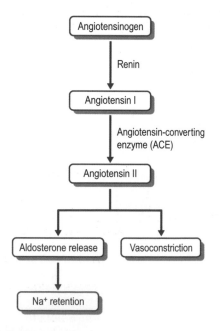

Figure 2.2 Enzymes as drug targets – angiotensin-converting enzyme (ACE).

Another example of drugs having their effect through enzymes is provided by drugs which inhibit angiotensin-converting enzyme (ACE inhibitors). Angiotensin II is a powerful vasoconstrictor and also stimulates the release of aldosterone, which promotes sodium retention (Fig. 2.2). Both effects lead to an increase in blood pressure and therefore drugs which inhibit ACE are used therapeutically in the treatment of hypertension (see Chs 8 and 12).

A third example of a drug which targets an enzyme for its action is sildenafil (Viagra), which inhibits the action of an enzyme called phosphodiesterase 5. It was originally thought that inhibition of this enzyme might be beneficial in patients with heart failure and during a clinical trial with a phosphodiesterase 5 inhibitor to investigate this, male patients reported an unexpected side effect leading to an entirely different therapeutic use – treatment of male erectile dysfunction. Normally, erection is initiated by the release of nitric oxide (NO) from nerves in the penis (Fig. 2.3). Nitric oxide causes relaxation of vascular smooth muscle and this causes engorgement of blood and hence erection. Nitric oxide works by stimulating the formation of a substance called cyclic GMP (cGMP) inside the vascular smooth muscle cells (see Chs 6 and 12). This cGMP is eventually broken down by an enzyme, phosphodiesterase 5, and prevention of this breakdown by sildenafil enhances erection.

CARRIER MOLECULES AS DRUG TARGETS

An example of a carrier molecule as a drug target is the noradrenaline (norepinephrine) transporter (Fig. 2.4).

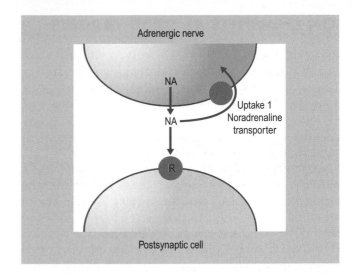

Figure 2.4 Carrier molecules as drug targets – the noradrenaline transporter.

Noradrenaline released from neurones is normally removed from the synapse by re-uptake into the pre-synaptic nerve. Drugs such as cocaine can inhibit the noradrenaline transporter and thus lead to accumulation of noradrenaline in the synapse and excess stimulation of postsynaptic cell membranes. The stimulant effects of cocaine are due to this action at noradrenergic synapses in the brain.

A further example of an action at a carrier molecule is provided by drugs known as proton pump inhibitors. These drugs target the carrier molecule in gastric parietal cells responsible for transporting H^+ into the gastric lumen against a very high concentration gradient (Fig. 2.5). The proton pump exchanges H^+ for K^+ and uses ATP as a source of energy and is thus also known as an H^+/K^+ ATPase. Proton pump inhibitors, e.g. omeprazole (Losec), produce a profound inhibition of gastric acid secretion and are used therapeutically for the treatment of peptic ulcer and reflux oesophagitis (see Ch. 9).

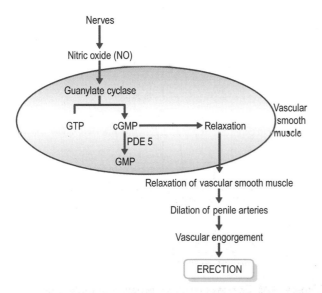

Figure 2.3 Enzymes as drug targets – phosphodiesterase 5.

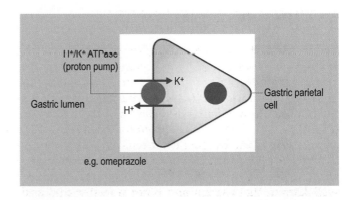

Figure 2.5 Carrier molecules as drug targets – the proton pump.

ION CHANNELS AS DRUG TARGETS

Charged ions are unable to diffuse through cell membranes and thus ions pass in and out of cells via protein channels in their membranes. Drugs can affect the operation of ion channels in different ways (Fig. 2.6). Ion channels can be physically blocked by drugs or their opening can be modulated, either to decrease or to increase it.

Local anaesthetics, e.g. lidocaine (lignocaine), block sodium channels in nerves, thus preventing the conduction of nerve impulses leading to the loss of sensation in the affected part (see Ch. 4A). Calcium channel blockers, e.g. nifedipine, decrease the opening of calcium channels, preventing calcium entry and thus contraction in smooth and cardiac muscle cells. Calcium channel blockers are used in the prophylaxis of angina, where they act by improving perfusion of the heart (by vasodilation of coronary vessels) and by reducing the workload of the heart (by reduction in cardiac contractility) (see Ch. 6). Finally, potassium channel activators, e.g. nicorandil, work by increasing the opening of potassium channels in smooth muscle, leading to entry of potassium and hyperpolarization of the smooth muscle cells. These drugs are vasodilators (see Ch. 6).

RECEPTORS

Receptors are the targets for endogenous hormones and neurotransmitters and they are the site of action of many therapeutic drugs. Drugs may activate a receptor and mimic the effect of the endogenous hormone or neurotransmitter (agonists) or block the receptor and prevent the endogenous hormone or neurotransmitter from having its usual effect (antagonists). Drugs have

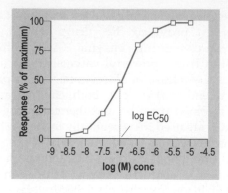

Figure 2.7 Relationship between drug concentration and biological response – the log concentration–response curve.

two properties which govern their interaction with receptors. *Affinity* is the ability of the drug to bind to a specific receptor whereas *efficacy* is the ability of the drug to activate a receptor after binding and thus produce a biological response. Thus an agonist has both affinity and efficacy while an antagonist also possesses affinity but has zero efficacy (see Ch. 5). The biological response to an agonist drug is frequently represented quantitatively by a log concentration–response curve, which has a characteristic sigmoid shape (S-shaped curve) (Fig. 2.7). The log concentration–response curve shows that as the concentration of the agonist at the receptor increases then the biological response increases, until a maximum response is reached. A quantitative measure of the efficacy of an agonist obtained from the log concentration–response curve is the EC_{50} – the concentration of agonist required to produce 50% of the maximum response. An antagonist drug may compete with an agonist for the same receptor. In most cases the binding of the antagonist is reversible and *reversible competitive antagonism* is the commonest and most important form of drug antagonism. The

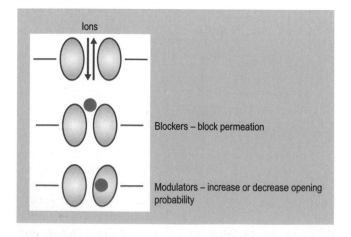

Figure 2.6 Ion channels as drug targets.

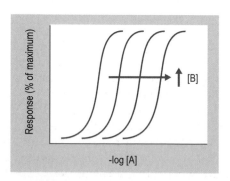

Figure 2.8 Reversible competitive antagonism. Log concentration–response curve to an agonist (A) in the presence of increasing concentrations of antagonist (B).

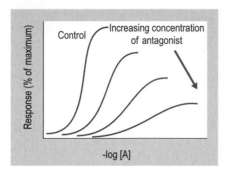

Figure 2.9 Irreversible competitive antagonism.

effect of this type of antagonism on the agonist log concentration–response curve is to shift the curve to the right with no change in the slope or the maximum response (Fig. 2.8). In some cases the antagonist may bind irreversibly. *Irreversible competitive antagonism* is characterized by a reduction in the slope and maximum of the agonist log concentration–response curve (Fig. 2.9). This type of antagonism occurs with drugs that form covalent bonds with the receptor. The effects of these drugs are long-lasting and they are likely to be toxic and not useful therapeutically.

Receptors are usually named according to the hormone or neurotransmitter that normally activates them, e.g. acetylcholine receptors, histamine receptors, adrenoceptors (receptors for noradrenaline and adrenaline). Agonist drugs can sometimes distinguish between subtypes of these receptors; e.g. some of the actions of acetylcholine can be mimicked by the plant alkaloid muscarine, and the receptors which mediate these effects are named muscarinic acetylcholine receptors. Other effects are mimicked by another plant alkaloid, nicotine, and the receptors involved are named nicotinic acetylcholine receptors. Adrenoceptors also divide into two major subtypes, α adrenoceptors and β adrenoceptors, according to the relative potencies of the catecholamines, noradrenaline, adrenaline and isoprenaline (a synthetic catecholamine):

Receptor	Agonist potency
α	Noradrenaline > adrenaline > isoprenaline
β	Isoprenaline > adrenaline > noradrenaline

An important further distinction made with regard to adrenoceptors was that β adrenoceptor agonists could distinguish between different types of β adrenoceptors (confirmed by selective antagonists, see below). Three subtypes of β adrenoceptors have now been identified, β_1, β_2 and β_3 adrenoceptors. β_1 adrenoceptors are found in the heart whereas β_2 adrenoceptors are found in airway smooth muscle. β adrenoceptor agonists which are selective for β_2 adrenoceptors are widely used in the treatment of asthma since they activate β_2 adreno-

ceptors on the airway smooth muscle to cause bronchodilation with minimal undesirable effects on the β_1 adrenoceptors of the heart (e.g. salbutamol). The concept of selectivity is an important one in pharmacology: the greater the selectivity of a drug for one particular receptor subtype, then the less likely it is to produce side effects. However, it should be noted that selectivity is only relative; e.g. at high concentrations β_2 adrenoceptor agonists can also activate β_1 adrenoceptors (a side effect of bronchodilator treatment can be tachycardia) (see Ch. 5).

Receptor subtypes may also be distinguished by antagonist drugs. The division of β adrenoceptors into β_1 and β_2 subtypes (see above) was confirmed by the discovery of drugs which could selectively antagonize each subtype. Thus β_1 adrenoceptor antagonists are clinically useful for their effects on the heart while minimizing the side effects of bronchoconstriction produced by non-selective β adrenoceptor antagonists (thus sometimes referred to as cardioselective β blockers).

Another important example of subtype selectivity of antagonist drugs is that the effect of histamine to stimulate gastric acid secretion is not prevented by drugs which block effects of histamine seen in allergic responses, e.g. increased vascular permeability, contraction of smooth muscle. Thus the conventional antihistamines, developed to relieve the troublesome effects of histamine released during allergic responses, have no effect on histamine-induced gastric acid secretion. This led to the realization that there must be more than one type of histamine receptor (designated H_1 and H_2 histamine receptors) and to the subsequent development of drugs which selectively blocked the effects of histamine on gastric acid secretion. The drugs, histamine H_2 receptor antagonists (e.g. cimetidine (Tagamet)), revolutionized the treatment of peptic ulcer which, up until the time of the introduction of H_2-antagonists in the 1970s, was largely surgical.

There are many hundreds of different receptors for hormones and neurotransmitters in the body. The receptors can be grouped into four large families (superfamilies):

- ionotropic receptors
- G-protein-coupled receptors
- kinase-linked receptors
- intracellular receptors.

The first three superfamilies are located in the cell membrane; hormones and neurotransmitters outside the cell can bind to the receptors on the cell surface, resulting in changes inside the cell. The fourth superfamily of receptors is located intracellularly, either in the nucleus (usually) or in the cytosol, and hormones which activate these receptors have to be lipid soluble in order to pass through the cell membrane.

IONOTROPIC RECEPTORS

These receptors consist of a number of protein subunits which together form an ion channel. Agonists binding to the receptor cause the channel to open, allowing the flow of ions (these receptors are sometimes referred to as agonist-gated or ligand-gated ion channels to differentiate them from voltage-gated channels (Fig. 2.10). Opening and closing of ion channels are very fast events (milliseconds), and these receptors are the receptors for fast-acting neurotransmitters (see Ch. 4A). The best studied example of this type of receptor is the nicotinic acetylcholine receptor, located in skeletal muscle, in autonomic ganglia and in central nervous system neurones. Activation of the receptor by the neurotransmitter acetylcholine allows the channel to open, allowing Na^+ ions to flow into the postsynaptic cell with resultant depolarization and excitation of the postsynaptic cell. An important group of drugs acting at this receptor are the neuromuscular blocking drugs. These drugs are competitive antagonists at the nicotinic acetylcholine receptor and their main action is to cause relaxation of skeletal muscle. They are used clinically during surgical anaesthesia – before the advent of these drugs much higher doses of anaesthetic had to be given to perform surgical operations and anaesthesia was much more risky. The first neuromuscular blocking drug used clinically, tubocurarine, was obtained from 'curare', a mixture of plant alkaloids used as arrow poisons by South American Indians. This is now rarely used clinically but synthetic drugs with similar actions, e.g. pancuronium, have been developed.

Other examples of ionotropic receptors are the $GABA_A$ receptor and the glutamate receptor (see Chs 4A and 20). GABA and glutamate are the main inhibitory and excitatory amino acid neurotransmitters, respectively, in the central nervous system.

G-PROTEIN-COUPLED RECEPTORS

These receptors are single proteins which are coupled to intracellular effectors via a protein known as a G-protein (guanine nucleotide binding protein). Activation of the receptor by an agonist causes activation of a G-protein and this in turn activates a cellular effector, either an enzyme or an ion channel (Fig. 2.11). Activation of enzymes results in the production of molecules inside the cell, referred to as second messengers (the hormone or neurotransmitter is the first messenger). Many G-protein-coupled receptors (GPCRs) couple to the enzyme adenylyl cyclase, activation of which results in the production of the second messenger, cyclic AMP, inside the cell. For example, β_2 adrenoceptors are GPCRs which activate adenylyl cyclase. Bronchodilator drugs of the β_2 adrenoceptor agonist class, e.g. salbutamol (Ventolin), act on β_2 adrenoceptors in airway smooth muscle and cause relaxation by elevating intracellular cAMP levels. Another common target of GPCRs is the enzyme phospholipase C which breaks down membrane phospholipids to produce second messengers inositol trisphosphate (IP_3) and diacylglycerol. IP_3 releases Ca^{2+} from intracellular stores, a signal for contraction in smooth and cardiac muscle cells. Muscarinic acetylcholine receptors are GPCRs and some types of these receptors activate receptors coupled to phospholipase C, e.g. the receptors for acetylcholine in smooth muscle. Tropicamide is a muscarinic antagonist which is used clinically in eye drops to dilate the pupil. It binds to

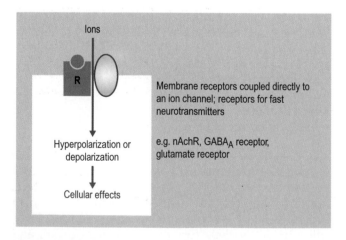

Figure 2.10 Ionotropic receptors.

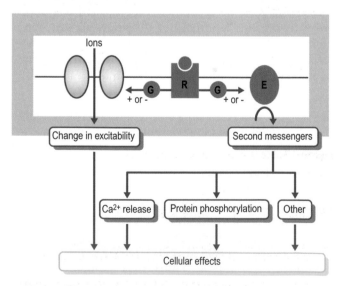

Figure 2.11 G-protein-coupled receptors.

muscarinic receptors and prevents the normal action of acetylcholine on smooth muscle.

KINASE-LINKED RECEPTORS

These are membrane receptors which themselves have enzyme (usually tyrosine kinase) activity (Fig. 2.12). The tyrosine kinase activity phosphorylates intracellular proteins, thus leading to cellular effects, mainly on cell growth and differentiation. These receptors are involved in the action of growth factors and cytokines and certain hormones such as insulin and leptin (see Ch. 11).

INTRACELLULAR RECEPTORS

These receptors differ from the other groups of receptors in that they are located intracellularly, usually in the nucleus (Fig. 2.13). Thus the hormones which activate these receptors, steroid and thyroid hormones, are lipophilic, i.e. they can cross the cell membrane. The receptors are proteins which have hormone and DNA binding sites. Binding of hormone affects DNA transcription and hence mRNA and, ultimately, protein synthesis. These effects are slow in onset and can be highly diverse. An example of a drug acting on this type of receptor is tamoxifen, an oestrogen antagonist which is used in the treatment of oestrogen-dependent breast cancer. Steroid and thyroid hormones are also themselves used clinically in various situations (see Ch. 11).

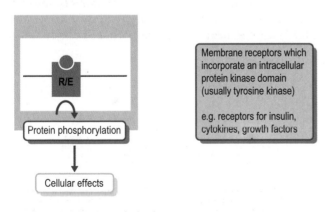

Figure 2.12 Kinase-linked receptors.

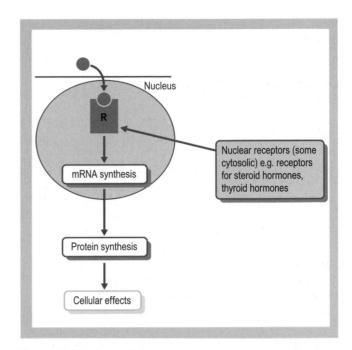

Figure 2.13 Intracellular receptors.

NEW THERAPIES

Many of the recent advances in our understanding of how drugs work have been made due to knowledge gained from the application of molecular biology to pharmacology. This 'molecular pharmacology' has not only contributed greatly to our understanding of drug action but has pointed the way to new therapeutic possibilities. One exciting new potential treatment is gene therapy – the genetic modification of cells to cure or alleviate disease. The basic principle is straightforward – introduction of a cloned gene or altered DNA or RNA into cells in order to change their activity. In practice there are technical difficulties which have not yet been completely overcome but it is hoped that we can look forward to safe and effective gene therapies in the future. These therapies offer great hope not only in the treatment of single gene diseases such as cystic fibrosis but also in the therapeutic management of many other diseases which have a genetic component. There is even the potential for treatment of disease with no genetic component if we have the means of controlling gene expression.

REFERENCES AND FURTHER READING

Galbraith A, Bullock S, Manias E, Richards A, Hunt B 1999 Fundamentals of pharmacology. Addison Wesley Longman, Harlow

Page C P, Curtis M J, Sutter M C, Walker M J A, Hoffman B B 2002 Integrated pharmacology, 2nd edn. Mosby, Edinburgh

Rang H P, Dale M, Ritter J M 2003 Pharmacology, 5th edn. Churchill Livingstone, Edinburgh

3 Blood and related tissues

In practice you may be asked to consider the following:

1. A haematology report indicates that a female patient has a low haematocrit result. What is a normal haematocrit value?

2. What is the difference between plasma and serum?

3. A sample of blood left to stand in an untreated tube will clot. What has initiated the coagulation mechanism?

4. An elderly woman is found to have several bruises and is subsequently found to be thrombocytopenic. Please explain.

5. A patient who has appendicitis has a raised white cell count. His haematology results show neutrophilic leucocytosis. Please explain.

6. A cardiac patient has been given a plasminogen activator. What is this and why was it administered?

7. What are the risks associated with plasminogen activators?

8. In a research study, samples of lymph were taken before and after a meal. One set of samples was found to be 'milky' in appearance. Were these samples from before or after, and what has caused the milky appearance?

9. Heparin and warfarin are both anticoagulants. Why is one of the two rapid acting and rapidly reversed, and the other slow in onset and slow to reverse? And which is which?

10. A 30-year-old woman has had one uneventful pregnancy. Her blood group is A Rh negative. If she becomes pregnant again should she be concerned?

Blood is composed of many constituents, cellular and non-cellular. The cellular components, erythrocytes, leucocytes and platelets, are formed in haemopoietic (i.e. blood producing) and lymphoid tissues (bone marrow, thymus gland and lymph nodes), and are disposed of by phagocytic cells mainly in the spleen and the liver. The non-cellular component (plasma) consists of water and dissolved substances, e.g. salts, nutrients and proteins.

Blood is usually liquid. It is therefore a mobile tissue and it is this distinctive property which enables it to circulate between all other tissues of the body acting as a transport system. It can, however, be converted very quickly into a gel. This helps to seal off damaged blood vessels and limits the leakage of blood from the circulation (see Ch. 19 at 'Wounds and wound healing').

HAEMOPOIETIC AND LYMPHOID TISSUES

Several tissues and organs are involved in the formation and disposal of blood cells (Fig. 3.1). In the adult person, blood cells develop in the bone marrow from stem cells (primitive precursor cells) (see Ch. 1). Some of the cells (leucocytes; see p. 50) undergo further maturation and proliferation in lymphoid tissues such as the thymus gland and lymph nodes.

Aged and injured cells are engulfed and so removed from the circulation by large phagocytic cells (macrophages), many of which are lodged in blood vessels of the spleen and the liver.

BONE MARROW

Marrow is the soft tissue that fills the cavities present in bone (Fig. 3.2). It consists of:

- blood cell precursors (in various stages of development)
- fat cells
- macrophages (large phagocytic cells)
- fibroblasts (which produce collagen fibres).

The blood capillaries (sinusoids) that supply the marrow are relatively leaky. Blood cells formed in the

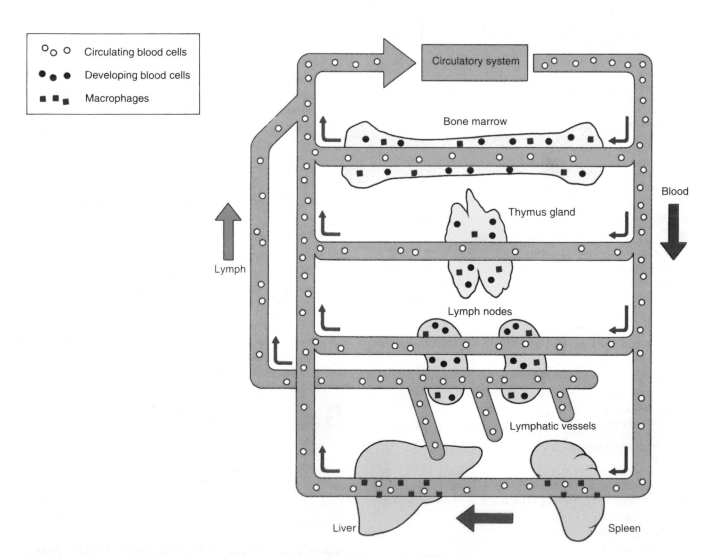

Figure 3.1 Tissues and organs involved in the formation and disposal of blood cells.

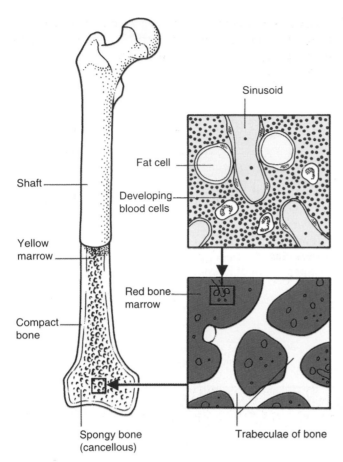

Figure 3.2 Structure of an immature long bone (femur) showing sites of red and yellow marrow.

In certain dyscrasias (blood disorders) specimens of red bone marrow are obtained by needle biopsy from the sternum or iliac crest. The number, size, shape and characteristics of cells in the various developmental and maturational phases are noted. This aids distinction of the different forms of dyscrasias. This procedure can be a valuable diagnostic aid but is an unpleasant experience for the patient because of the pressure needed to penetrate the hard bony cortex, although local anaesthetic is used.

LYMPHOID TISSUE

Lymphocytes formed in the bone marrow are carried in the blood to all other tissues. Tissue that processes or contains exceptionally large congregations of lymphocytes is termed lymphoid. Examples include:

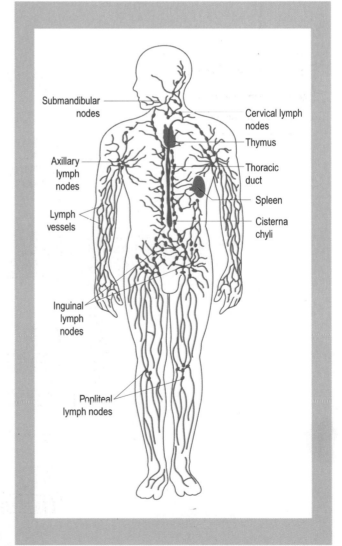

Figure 3.3 Principal organs of the lymphatic system. (After Thibodeau & Patton 2000, with permission of Elsevier.)

marrow can squeeze through spaces in the walls of the sinusoids to enter the circulatory system.

When the marrow is very active it looks red because of the huge number of developing red cells (erythrocytes) present. It can become yellowish when its blood-cell-producing (haemopoietic) activity decreases, and then fat cells predominate.

In a newborn baby all bones contain red bone marrow. As the child grows, more and more marrow in the limb bones becomes yellow, until in the adult only the marrow of the flat bones (sternum, vertebrae, ribs, clavicles, pelvis and skull) is still active in blood cell production (haemopoiesis).

The stem cells (see Ch. 1) present in the bone marrow are precursors for all the cellular constituents of blood:

- red cells (erythrocytes)
- white cells (leucocytes), which are subdivided into:
  – granulocytes
  – lymphocytes
  – monocytes
- platelets (thrombocytes).

- thymus gland
- lymph nodes
- tonsils
- tissue present in the spleen.

Thymus gland

The thymus is a small bi-lobed gland situated at the top of the chest underneath the breast bone (sternum) and on top of the major vessels entering and leaving the heart (Fig. 3.3). It is a very large gland at birth and continues to grow slightly throughout childhood. Around puberty it begins to shrink and by adulthood it has decreased in size significantly.

The thymus contains an enormous population of developing lymphocytes. Immature lymphocytes from the bone marrow migrate into the thymus, where they mature and proliferate. Most of the cells live for only a short time and are disposed of by macrophages within the thymus. Some leave the gland and enter the

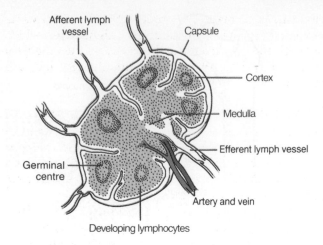

Figure 3.4 Structure of a lymph node. (From Rogers 1992, with permission of Elsevier.)

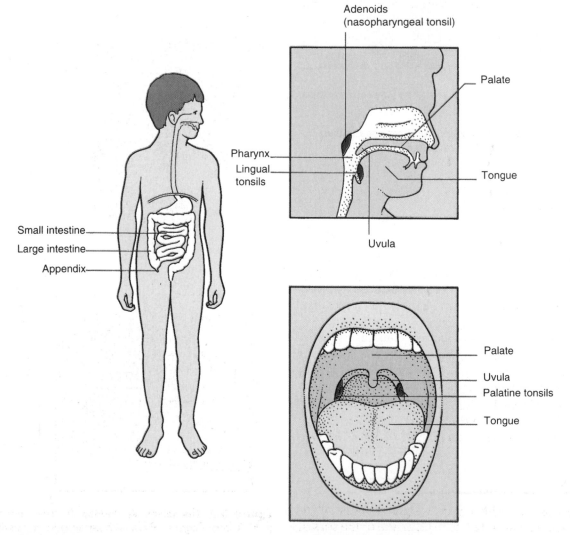

Figure 3.5 Lymphoid tissue of the digestive tract. Small and large clumps of tissue are scattered throughout the tract. There are several large clumps (the 'tonsils') at the back of the mouth.

bloodstream as mature T lymphocytes; also, the thymus secretes hormones (lymphopoietin, thymosins) which regulate the production and activity of lymphocytes in the thymus, other lymphoid tissues and the circulation.

Lymph nodes

Lymph nodes are similar in structure to the thymus but are much smaller. Several hundred are found throughout the body (Figs 3.3, 3.4). They are especially numerous in the thorax and abdomen. Other key sites include the neck, axilla and groin.

They are permeated by lymph, which is tissue fluid carried away from the tissue spaces in lymphatic vessels. Lymphatic vessels are blind-ending tubes originating in the tissue spaces, which act as an overflow for interstitial fluid, and carry it back into the circulatory system (see Ch. 6 and Fig. 6.21). Lymph nodes occur at intervals along these vessels and are well placed to respond to undesirable bacteria etc. present in the fluid, for they contain lymphocytes and macrophages. Thus the nodes effectively cleanse the interstitial fluid before it is returned to the circulation.

Lymph nodes are the 'glands' that swell up when there is infection, for example when you have a sore throat.

> As part of the body's defence system, lymphoid tissue filters out invading organisms but can be overwhelmed by repeated or very acute infections and, in the case of tonsils and the appendix, may have to be removed surgically. This depletes the body's defences and is only done when essential.

Tonsils

Tonsils are clumps of unencapsulated lymphoid tissue lying just below the surface covering (epithelium) of the digestive tract. They too contain lymphocytes. The uppermost of these are the adenoids (nasopharyngeal tonsils), which are prominent in young children (Fig. 3.5). Other tonsils are found at the back of the mouth (palatine tonsils – most frequently infected and removed by tonsillectomy) and around the base of the tongue (lingual tonsils). Similar lymphoid tissue is also found in the appendix, and scattered in small and large clumps (Peyer's patches) throughout the digestive tract.

SPLEEN

The spleen is a sizeable organ, weighing about 200 to 250 g. In the neonate (see Ch. 31) it is one of the sites of red cell production. The spleen is situated to the left in the abdomen, tucked between the stomach and the left

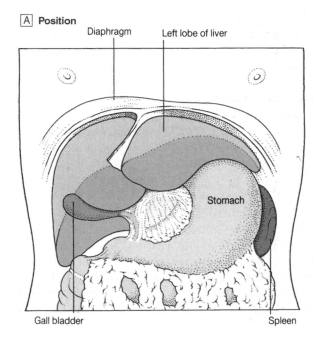

A Position

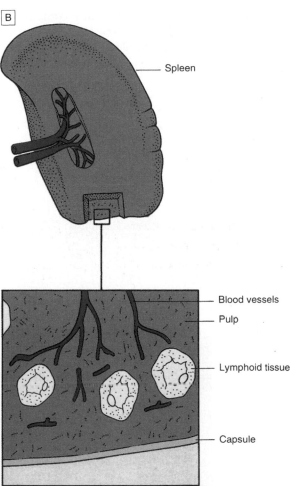

Figure 3.6 The spleen. A, Position. B, Tissue structure. (Part A from Rogers 1992, with permission of Elsevier.)

kidney (Fig. 3.6A & B). It is enclosed by a capsule of connective tissue and is richly supplied with blood, which gives it its dark red appearance. Blood seeps through the tissue (pulp) of the spleen rather like water through a sponge. The leaky splenic capillaries (sinusoids) allow blood cells to pass easily out of the circulation into the tissue spaces of the spleen, and then to move back again via different sinusoids.

It was noted above that the lymph nodes act to cleanse the interstitial fluid of potentially dangerous bacteria etc. Macrophages and lymphocytes resident within the spleen pulp perform a similar role on blood. In addition, damaged and aged erythrocytes (red blood cells) are also removed.

BLOOD

COMPOSITION

The adult circulatory system normally contains about 5 litres of blood (about 7% of the body weight in an adult, up to 8% in a 3-month-old child). About 3 litres of this is plasma, a water-based solution of proteins,

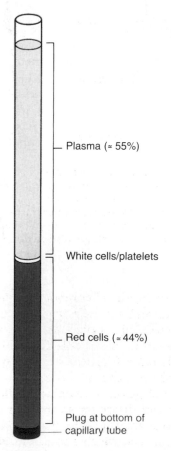

Plasma (≈ 55%)

White cells/platelets

Red cells (≈ 44%)

Plug at bottom of capillary tube

Figure 3.7 Appearance of a sample of blood in a capillary tube that has been centrifuged at high speed for 3 minutes.

electrolytes and other dissolved constituents. The remainder is cellular, and consists of:

- erythrocytes (red cells)
- leucocytes (white cells)
- thrombocytes (platelets).

If a sample of blood is spun in a tube in a centrifuge, the heavier constituents (the cellular components) are driven to the bottom of the tube leaving most of the plasma as a clear area at the top (Fig. 3.7). If the tube is the same diameter all the way up, the lengths of the cellular and plasma components can be measured, and

Blood components and their uses

Donated blood can be separated into its component parts and each can be used to treat a particular blood deficiency. It is worth noting that all donated blood in the UK is tested for the presence of several viruses while preparations of plasma, platelets and red blood cells have white cells removed to reduce the risk of transmitting the infectious agents associated with Creutzfeldt–Jakob disease (CJD). White cells can also be inactivated in blood products by irradiation. To reduce infection risk, autologous blood transfusion (self donated) is becoming more common. This may involve preoperative donation of blood or its salvage at the operation site.

- Red blood cells – whole blood with 0% of the plasma removed; used to:
  - correct red blood cell deficiency and improve oxygen-carrying capacity of the blood
  - transfuse organ transplant patients who have repeated febrile (feverish) reactions to blood transfusions containing active white cells.
- White blood cells (leucocyte concentrate) – whole blood with all red cells and 80% of the plasma removed; used to treat patients with life-threatening granulocytopenia (decreased granulocytes) when infections do not respond to antibiotics.
- Plasma (fresh frozen) – plasma separated from whole blood; used to:
  - treat a clotting factor deficiency when that factor is unknown
  - maintain normal clotting ability following massive intravenous infusions of stored blood
  - prepare blood protein fractions.
- Platelets – platelets sedimented out from platelet-rich plasma and resuspended in 30 to 50 ml of plasma; used to treat the patient with thrombocytopenia (decreased platelets) whose bleeding is caused by decreased platelet production, aplastic anaemia, acute leukaemia, cytotoxic drug therapy or radiotherapy, causing increased platelet destruction, functionally abnormal platelets or massive transfusion of stored blood (dilutional thrombocytopenia).

Note that the terms serum and plasma are not identical. Plasma refers to the fluid component of blood. It contains all the dissolved substances including plasma proteins. Serum is the fluid that can be separated from blood which has been allowed to clot. Thus serum is plasma minus factors important to clot formation such as the protein fibrinogen.

the percentage of the total blood volume occupied by each can be calculated. The cellular fraction (packed cell volume or PCV, also called the haematocrit (hct)) is between 40 and 54% in men and 36 and 48% in women. It consists almost entirely of erythrocytes. Leucocytes and platelets form a very small fraction of the blood in health (no more than 1% of the total blood sample). They may be seen as the small white band at the top of the packed red cells.

The haematocrit (hct) is now routinely measured automatically by a cell counter. This reduces the need for laboratory staff to handle human blood samples. The hct figure is usually reported as a decimal figure: 0.40 to 0.54 for males or 0.36 to 0.48 for females.

ERYTHROCYTES

Erythrocytes are quite different from any other cells in the body in that when they mature they do not possess any cellular organelles, not even a nucleus. Instead, they can be viewed as a membrane bag containing a very large amount of the protein haemoglobin which is involved in the transport of oxygen and carbon dioxide between the lungs and the tissues (see Ch. 7).

Development

In the adult, erythrocytes are formed in the bone marrow from pluripotent stem cells (see Ch. 1). The rate of production of red cells is controlled by the hormone erythropoietin (see Chs 9 and 11). Many developmental changes occur as red cells mature (Fig. 3.8). Each time the cells divide the daughter cells are slightly smaller than the parent cells. The synthesis of DNA for the nucleus requires the presence of vitamin B_{12} and folic acid. If these vitamins are deficient the erythrocytes formed are larger than normal (macrocytic).

During development the cell begins to manufacture one protein, haemoglobin, in very large amounts, so that eventually a large proportion of the cell is occupied by this substance. Each molecule of haemoglobin (see Fig. 7.18) consists of four units, each of which is made up of:

• a polypeptide chain
• a haem unit
• an iron atom.

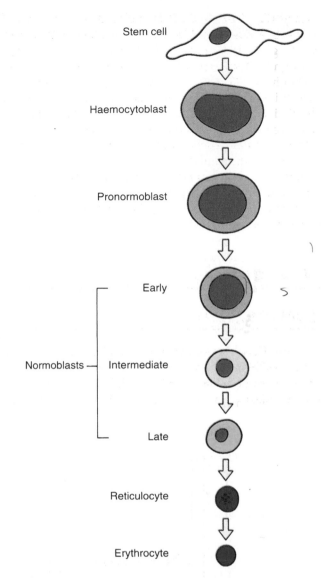

Figure 3.8 Stages in the development of the red cell from stem cells in the bone marrow to mature erythrocytes in the circulation. Cell division (mitosis; see Ch. 1) occurs at each stage as far as the late normoblast so that each pronormoblast gives rise to very many erythrocytes. (After McDonald et al 1988, with permission of Elsevier.)

If iron is deficient, the cells cannot manufacture as much haemoglobin, and the cells tend to be smaller than normal in size (microcytic). As haemoglobin makes erythrocytes red in colour, cells that contain less of this protein look paler (hypochromic) than normal cells, when viewed through a microscope.

In the later stages of development cellular organelles disintegrate and disappear so that the cells emerging from the bone marrow into the blood contain only residual fragments, which also soon disappear. These fragments stain in a distinctive way, giving these first immature erythrocytes the name of reticulocytes

Table 3.1 Red cell characteristics: normal and abnormal

	Normal	Megaloblastic anaemia	Iron deficiency anaemia
Mean cell volume (MCV)	86 ± 10 fl	High	Low
Mean cell haemoglobin (MCH)	29.5 ± 2.5 pg	High	Low
Mean cell haemoglobin concentration (MCHC)	325 ± 25 g/l	Normal	Low

because of the network (reticulum) of residual fragments that is visible. Normally, reticulocytes make up 1% (the reference range is 0.2 to 2%) of the total numbers of red cells in the blood. However, if the need for erythrocytes increases, e.g. after significant loss of blood, the number of reticulocytes in blood will increase.

Normal values

There are about 5×10^{12} red cells and 150 g haemoglobin per litre of blood (average range in women: 4.2 to 5.4×10^{12} and 120 to 160 g/l; average in men: 4.6 to 6.2×10^{12} and 130 to 180 g/l). An increase in cell numbers above normal is polycythaemia, a decrease is

anaemia. Clinically, anaemia is said to exist if the haemoglobin concentration in blood is less than an agreed reference value, although the decision to correct with red blood cell transfusion will be influenced by the age and condition of the patient.

Using the figures for red cell count, haemoglobin concentration and hct 0.45, other factors which characterize red blood cells can be calculated, for example see below. They can be used in distinguishing between different types of anaemia (Table 3.1).

$$\text{Mean cell volume (MCV)} = \frac{\text{hct}}{\text{red cell count}}$$

$$= \frac{45}{100} \times \frac{1}{5 \times 10^{12}}$$

Anaemias

In anaemia there is a reduction in the number of circulating erythrocytes in the blood or a decrease in the concentration of haemoglobin. This results in a reduction in the capacity of the blood to carry oxygen. There are three ways in which anaemias can arise.

Anaemias secondary to decreased erythropoiesis:

- Nutritional deficiency anaemias – essential nutrients for erythrocyte production, such as iron, vitamin B_{12}, folic acid or protein, may be lacking due to dietary insufficiency or defective absorption. Treatment depends on cause and includes making good the deficit by dietary advice or supplement, or by injection.

- Aplastic anaemia – due to depressed bone marrow activity and usually involving decreased production of leucocytes and thrombocytes as well as red cells. The condition is caused by toxins from various drugs, chronic infection, excessive radiation or invasion by malignant cells. Treatment includes removal of the cause, transfusion of packed cells and platelets and possibly bone marrow transplant.

Anaemias secondary to increased destruction of red cells (haemolytic anaemias):

- Haemolytic anaemias resulting from intrinsic congenital defects where the cells do not have the

ability to survive for their normal life span. These include hereditary spherocytosis, sickle cell anaemia and thalassaemia. Treatment may be removal of the spleen to reduce the excessive destruction of abnormal blood cells, and frequent blood transfusions.

- Haemolytic anaemias due to extrinsic factors, such as acquired antibodies, some infections and certain drugs and chemicals.

- Mechanical effects of, for example, artificial heart valves.

Anaemias secondary to blood loss:

- The loss of blood from the circulation through haemorrhage reduces the number of erythrocytes and therefore the oxygen-carrying capacity of the blood. Bone marrow normally responds quickly to the hormone erythropoietin whose production is stimulated by tissue hypoxia (see Chs 8, 9, 11), and blood loss can be replaced in 2 to 4 weeks. However, if over 20% of circulating volume is lost, the potential detrimental effect on the renal and cardiovascular systems must be considered (see Ch. 12). Again the patient's age and clinical history are relevant but there is a move away from the transfusion of blood to replace the lost volume because of the associated risk of transferring infectious agents. In this case volume expanders are used.

$$= 90 \times 10^{-15} \, l$$
$$= 90 \text{ femtolitres (fl)}$$

This is the average volume of a single red blood cell. Where for example there is a lack of vitamin B_{12}, red blood cell production is impaired. The cell number decreases but the cells are larger and more fragile. The MCV would rise.

$$\text{Mean cell haemoglobin (MCH)} = \frac{\text{haemoglobin (g/l)}}{\text{red cell count/l}}$$

$$= \frac{150 \text{g}}{5 \times 10^{12}}$$

$$= 30 \times 10^{-12} \text{ g}$$

$$= 30 \text{ picograms (pg)}$$

This is the average amount of haemoglobin in each red blood cell.

$$\text{Mean cell haemoglobin concentration (MCHC)} = \frac{\text{haemoglobin (g/l)}}{\text{hct}}$$

$$= \frac{150}{0.45}$$

$$= 330 \text{ g per litre of red cells}$$

This value represents the extent to which red blood cells are packed with haemoglobin. This value would be reduced in iron deficiency, for example.

Nature and metabolic activity

The mature erythrocyte is shaped like a flexible, biconcave disc (diameter $7 \, \mu m$) (Fig. 3.9A). Its two major intracellular constituents, other than water, are the oxygen-transporting protein haemoglobin and the enzyme carbonic anhydrase (see Ch. 7).

Although the erythrocyte has no mitochondria it can manufacture ATP by the process of anaerobic glycolysis (see Ch. 10) using enzymes of the cytosol, which generate ATP from glucose. Energy, in the form of ATP, is needed to maintain cell structure and normal conditions inside the cell.

Fate

Eventually, the erythrocyte pays the price for its relatively unsophisticated metabolism, defects occur in the membrane which are not repaired, swelling occurs and the cells become less flexible. As a result, cells are more likely to get stuck in tight places, particularly in

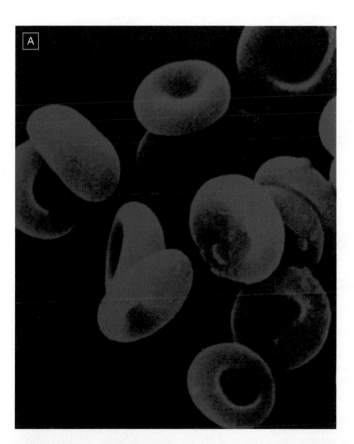

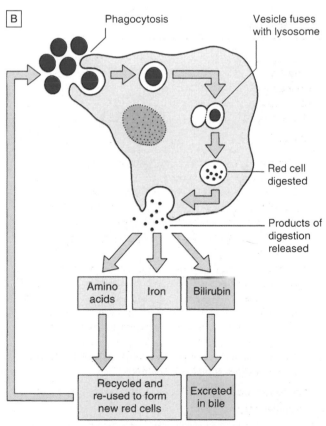

Figure 3.9 A, Colour-enhanced scanning electron micrograph showing detailed structure of RBCs. (After Thibodeau & Patton 2000, with permission of Elsevier.) B, Fate of red cells and their constituents.

the capillaries and pulp of the spleen, and to be phagocytosed by macrophages (see Ch. 16). On average, the life span of a red cell is 120 days.

The cells that have been engulfed by the macrophages are digested by them, and the products are either recycled and re-used (for example amino acids and iron) or excreted (bilirubin) (Fig. 3.9B) (see Chs 10 and 16).

Recycling of iron

This process is very efficient. Only 1 to 2 mg of iron are lost from the body each day (from cells lost from the lining of the gut and from the skin). Yet about 20 mg are released daily from the breakdown of red cells. Iron in blood binds to a specific plasma (transport) protein, transferrin. This ensures that iron is targeted to the tissues most in need of it; for example, membrane receptors for transferrin are present in large numbers on the immature erythrocytes in the bone marrow.

Iron is also bound to the protein ferritin and an assessment of plasma ferritin a good indicator of body iron stores.

Blood groups

Antigens and antibodies

Cells from different individuals are not exactly the same. They differ in the precise structure of some of the molecules, i.e. antigens, projecting from the cell membrane (see Ch. 1). Some molecules occur in many individuals. Others are limited to a small family group. These variations create an enormous number of different blood groups. Eight of the over 400 blood group systems known are listed in Table 3.2.

The existence of different blood groups is of no real consequence unless cells from one person are given to another, as for example in a blood transfusion. If the cells differ the recipient responds by developing an immune response: the molecules that are different (antigens) cause some white cells (lymphocytes) to proliferate and to secrete specific proteins (antibodies) targeted against the intruding cells (see Ch. 16 for details).

The first exposure to a brand new antigen elicits only a modest immune response. However, if the antigen is encountered again, the antibodies are ready and waiting, and react swiftly and powerfully to destroy the foreign cells.

Table 3.2 Several blood group systems

ABO	Lutheran
Rhesus	Kell
MNS	Lewis
P	Duffy

First pregnancy

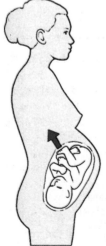

Some Rh+ cells from the baby enter the mother's circulation at birth or if a traumatic episode occurs during the pregnancy.

Antibodies develop to the Rh+ cells.

Second pregnancy

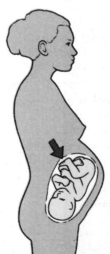

Antibodies cross the placenta and destroy some of the baby's cells.

More anti-Rhesus antibodies develop in the mother.

Third pregnancy

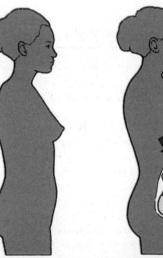

Greater immune response and greater damage to the baby's red cells.

Figure 3.10 The sequence of events occurring when a mother whose blood group is Rhesus negative bears children who are Rhesus positive.

Table 3.3 Bloods grouped according to the ABO system that can (✓) and cannot (x) be safely transferred

	Donor's blood		Recipient's blood group			
Group	Antigens present	Iso-antibodies	A	AB	B	O
A	A	Anti-B	✓	?	x	x
AB	A,B	None	x	✓	x	x
B	B	Anti-A	x	?	✓	x
O	–	Anti-A, Anti-B	?	?	?	✓

?These bloods can be mixed, if used with care. Antibodies in the donor blood will attack some of the recipient's cells, but if the volume of donor blood is small compared with the volume of the recipient's blood the effects are relatively minor.

A good example of this series of events is that of a pregnant mother who is Rhesus D negative (does not possess the Rhesus D antigen) and who carries a baby who has inherited this antigen from its father, and who is therefore Rhesus positive (Rh+). Rhesus positive cells from the baby can trigger in the mother the production of antibodies to the antigens of the Rh blood group system. These antibodies are called anti-D (anti-D immunoglobulin; see Ch. 16). This immune response in the mother can create serious difficulties for subsequent pregnancies (Fig. 3.10).

Iso-antibodies

Antibodies to the A and B antigens of the ABO system develop in the blood in many people very soon after birth. (The ABO system is the only blood group system to have iso-antibodies. All other blood groups need a sensitizing episode to induce iso-antibodies.)

It is this natural presence of these anti-A and anti-B iso-antibodies in a patient's blood that could make blood transfusion a hazardous procedure unless donated blood was previously typed and matched (Table 3.3).

Transfusion reactions

The iso-antibodies present in the recipient's plasma must be considered when attempting to cross match.

If red cell antigens encounter their corresponding antibodies, they bind to one another. This coating of antibody has several effects. It:

- makes the cells adhere to one another (agglutinate)
- activates the complement system, which breaks

Rhesus incompatibility

About one in ten babies born to Rhesus negative mothers has Rh+ blood. (If a father is Rh+ he may be heterozygous for the Rhesus D factor and the baby has a 50% chance of being Rh+. If he is homozygous the baby will certainly be Rh+. However, paternal screening is not carried out routinely.) Although the first such pregnancy usually results in a healthy baby, the antibodies that the mother may develop have potentially fatal consequences for any Rh+ babies of subsequent pregnancies when the maternal antibodies will cross the placenta and destroy fetal red blood cells. This condition is known as haemolytic disease of the newborn (HDN) and requires constant monitoring. The fetus becomes anaemic and hypoxic, and development is compromised. Brain damage and death may occur. Intrauterine exchange blood transfusion is often done to replace the Rh+ blood with Rh– and this may be repeated in the perinatal period.

In order to prevent this condition, the following measures are taken:

- Routine antenatal screening and blood grouping of all pregnant women.
- When a woman is found to be Rh– she is screened at regular intervals during pregnancy for Rh antibodies.
- A sample of cord blood is taken at birth to confirm the baby's blood group. If Rh+, the mother is given a standard injection of anti-D immunoglobulin which destroys circulating Rh+ antigens, preventing them from activating the immune system. Timing is critical and anti-D must be given within 72 hours of birth, or following any other potentially sensitizing episode, e.g. bleeding or abortion. Otherwise subsequent pregnancies would be jeopardized.
- It is important to note that not all cases of HDN are due to problems associated with the Rh antigen; other blood types can be involved.

As a result of routine antenatal screening and prompt administration of anti-D immunoglobulin, HDN is now uncommon in the West.

Before a patient receives a transfusion of blood products it is essential to avoid possible transfusion reactions.

Automated testing procedures are used to perform an antibody screen of the patient's serum while ABO and Rhesus blood groups are determined. Great care must be taken to avoid the more mundane clerical errors which might mismatch recipient and donor.

Donor blood (1 unit = 470 ml) is rarely used directly in transfusion. It is normally split into various components, e.g. red cell concentrates, platelet concentrates etc., which can be used separately. In this way only those components specifically required by the patient are infused and the risk of adverse reaction to another blood component is minimized.

open (lyses) the cell (see Ch. 16)
• singles out the cells for attack by macrophages.

The consequences of these reactions can be life-threatening if a large number of red cells are affected. In particular, the sudden rupture of cells (haemolysis) by the complement system releases intracellular consti-tuents, such as haemoglobin and potassium, into the plasma. The haemoglobin released passes through the urinary filter (see Ch. 8) into the urine and together with other released constituents can cause 'renal failure.

Raised potassium levels can detrimentally affect the functioning of nerve and muscle cells including the heart (see Ch. 14). In addition, products of digestion released by activated macrophages reduce blood pressure and add to the overall shock to body systems. It is important to stress that severe reactions to transfusion, while rare, are usually the result not of inadequacies in laboratory testing procedures but of clerical errors or failures to correctly identify a patient. Important checks for the correct cross matching of blood must be made at the patient's bedside.

LEUCOCYTES

Significance

The leucocytes (white blood cells) form a tiny part (5%) of the population of defence cells scattered throughout the tissues of the body.

Defence cells are divided into two groups:

• lymphocytes
• phagocytic cells (granulocytes and macrophages).

Both groups work together to protect the body against invasion by foreign cells and molecules. Lymphocytes identify the invaders and phagocytic cells engulf and dispose of them (see Ch. 16 for details).

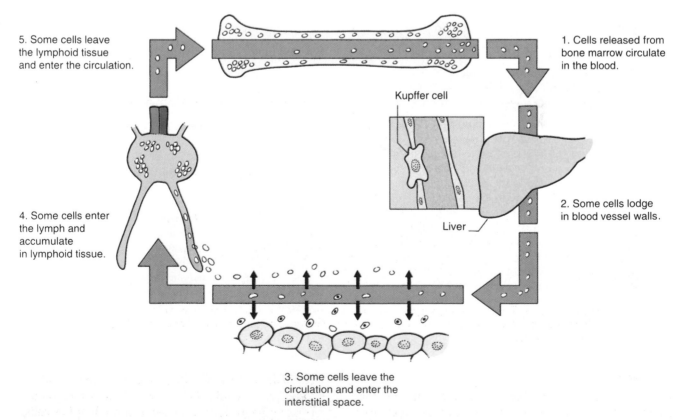

5. Some cells leave the lymphoid tissue and enter the circulation.

1. Cells released from bone marrow circulate in the blood.

Kupffer cell

2. Some cells lodge in blood vessel walls.

Liver

4. Some cells enter the lymph and accumulate in lymphoid tissue.

3. Some cells leave the circulation and enter the interstitial space.

Figure 3.11 The various fates of defence cells released from the bone marrow.

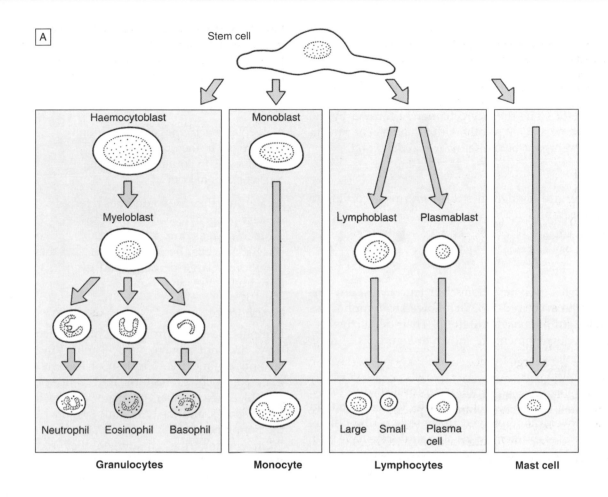

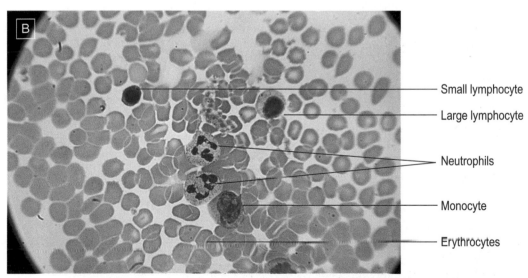

Figure 3.12 A, The different types of leucocyte and their development from stem cells. (After McDonald et al 1988, with permission of Elsevier.) B, Photomicrograph of blood cells including selected leucocytes.

Origins

Defence cells develop from stem cells in the bone marrow. Once they have left the marrow they may (Fig. 3.11):

- circulate in the blood (then known as leucocytes)
- lodge in the walls of blood vessels in some organs (macrophages lodged in the liver are Kupffer cells; see Ch. 10)

- enter the interstitial space
- pass into the lymph
- accumulate in some organs and tissues (lymphocytes in lymphoid tissue).

The cells present in blood (leucocytes: $4–11 \times 10^9$/litre) thus include some defence cells newly formed by the bone marrow as well as others that have spent time in tissues and organs before returning to the blood.

Types

Leucocytes are divided into three groups according to their appearance:

- granulocytes
- monocytes
- lymphocytes.

Granulocytes (polymorphonuclear leucocytes) are normally in the majority (42–82%) followed by lymphocytes (20–45%) and monocytes (2–10%). Their distinctive features and development are shown in Figure 3.12A & B.

Granulocytes

Granulocytes have a granular appearance due to the presence of many vesicles. These vesicles contain different chemicals involved in the role of the cells in defence. Three different types of granulocyte have been distinguished on the basis of their reaction with different histochemical stains. Most counting of white cell numbers, however, is now done automatically by cell counters rather than by looking at stained cells on a microscope slide. This has the added advantage of speed and also avoids manual handling of blood.

The granulocytes are:

- neutrophils
- basophils
- eosinophils.

Neutrophils (40–70% of total white cell population) are the first phagocytic cells to be called into action in large numbers in response to injury or bacterial invasion. They move from blood to tissue where they spend most of their relatively short life span (4–5 days). They destroy microorganisms by phagocytosis. Bacterial infection would be expected to induce an increase in neutrophil numbers. The pus that collects at a wound consists mostly of dead neutrophils.

Basophils secrete chemicals important to the process of inflammation – histamine which dilates small blood vessels and heparin which is an anticoagulant (see below).

Eosinophils also phagocytose inflammatory chemicals and produce chemicals that kill parasitic worms.

Monocytes

Monocytes are the circulating precursors of macrophages. Some monocytes lodge in the walls of blood vessels and develop there into active macrophages (fixed macrophages, such as Kupffer cells of the liver, littoral cells of the spleen). Others are attracted into the tissues and are transformed into active cells whose characteristics vary according to the tissue in which they are found, such as:

- alveolar macrophages of the lungs
- microglia in the brain
- histiocytes in connective tissue
- osteoclasts in bone.

As a group, they are sometimes referred to as the mononuclear phagocyte system (MPS).

Macrophages are large, highly active, long-lived phagocytic cells. Because of their size they are able to engulf very large particles, and even intact cells, such as red cells.

Lymphocytes

Lymphocytes differ from most other leucocytes in that they are not phagocytic. Their function is the recognition and identification of foreign or abnormal material, such as bacteria and cancerous cells (see Ch. 16). Large numbers circulate between the blood, the tissue spaces, and the lymphatic system. Many lodge in the lymph nodes.

On encountering an antigen they recognize, they undergo transformation in structure and activity, and are stimulated to reproduce in large numbers. They manufacture and secrete substances, such as antibodies, which attach to the antigen and begin the process of its destruction and disposal. Their life spans vary. Some survive for many years.

PLATELETS

Platelets, also known as thrombocytes, are tiny cellular fragments whose main function is sealing off leaks in blood vessels.

Origin and nature

Platelets are derived from the same pool of pluripotent stem cells in the bone marrow as the other cellular constituents of blood. Platelets consist of budded-off fragments of the megakaryocytes which in turn developed from bone marrow stem cells (Fig. 3.13). They secrete and produce a variety of chemicals (Table 3.4), and have a life span of around 10 days. Constant production is necessary in health.

Circulation and fate

After leaving the bone marrow, platelets tend to lodge in the spleen for a few days before circulating freely in the bloodstream. There are normally about 150 to

Significance of a differential white blood cell count

Leucocytosis – an increase in the total number of white blood cells (WBCs) – is a normal response to invading microorganisms and tissue destruction. As it is known that specific types of WBCs increase in certain disease conditions, a *differential count* may be ordered as an aid to diagnosis. For example:

- in acute infections, such as appendicitis and pneumonia, and following tissue destruction, as in myocardial infarction, the neutrophils increase rapidly (neutrophil leucocytosis)
- in chronic infections and diseases, such as measles, mumps, pertussis and infectious hepatitis, lymphocytes increase (lymphocytosis)
- the number of monocytes is increased in protozoal infections such as malaria (monocytosis)
- the eosinophil count rises in allergic reactions and with parasitic invasion of the body (eosinophilia).

The WBC count returns to normal when the infection is controlled, or initiating factor disposed of.

Note that all the above are normal reactions. However, leucocytosis is also a feature of leukaemia or cancer of the bone marrow.

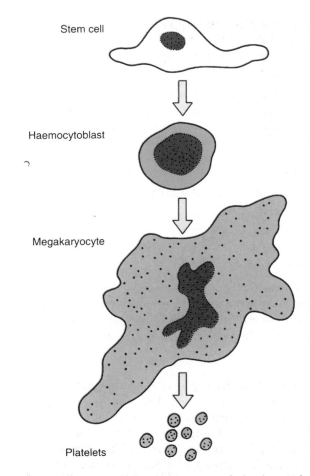

Figure 3.13 Stages in the development of platelets. (After McDonald et al 1988, with permission of Elsevier.)

400×10^9/litre. They are attracted to sites of blood vessel injury, and one of their roles is to clump together (agglutinate) and so 'plug the gap', preventing blood loss. They also produce pro-factors which contribute to the process of clotting (see below), and growth factors and inhibitors required for tissue repair.

PLASMA

Blood cells and platelets are suspended in plasma (Table 3.5). Apart from the plasma proteins and substances which bind to them, such as calcium, the concentrations of substances present in plasma are almost the same as those in the interstitial fluid.

Plasma proteins

Nature and functions

The number of different proteins present in blood is very large and their functions are diverse (Table 3.6). They have important roles in transport, blood clotting and immune defence.

Note that there is no single normal value for the level of any of the various plasma components frequently measured in laboratories. Instead the test result will be

Table 3.4 Some of the substances produced by platelets

Substance	Function
Serotonin (5HT)	Vasoconstriction
Adenosine diphosphate (ADP)	Promotes platelet aggregation
Thromboxane	Vasoconstriction and platelet aggregation
Pro-coagulants	Promotes coagulation
Platelet-derived growth factor	Stimulates wound healing

Table 3.5 Composition of plasma

Water	92% by weight
Protein	60–90 g/litre
Nutrients	e.g. glucose, lipid
Waste	e.g. urea, creatinine
Gases	e.g. carbon dioxide
Hormones	e.g. insulin, cortisol
Electrolytes	sodium, potassium, bicarbonate

White blood cell disorders

There are a number of diseases associated with disorders of the white blood cells and the following are examples.

In *leukaemia* (cancer of the blood) there is an excessive proliferation of leucocytes. Many cells remain immature (at the blast stage) and are therefore unable to perform their normal role in body defence. This renders the individual very susceptible to infection and system dysfunction as the circulating leukaemic cells infiltrate organs and tissues and impose an imbalance. The proliferation of white cells also reduces the production of red cells and platelets to the extent that patients with leukaemia are anaemic and have a tendency to bleed.

Treatment is directed towards suppressing the abnormal cell production and preventing complications. Radiation therapy or chemotherapy is often the treatment of choice followed by bone marrow transplantation.

In *leukopenia* there is a marked reduction in the number of circulating WBCs. As the most significant reduction is usually in the neutrophils, it may also be known as *neutropenia* or *agranulocytosis*.

Neutropenia is a consequence of bone marrow depression often caused by the toxic effects of drugs in people with a sensitivity or idiosyncrasy. The most frequently implicated drugs include sulphonamides, chlorpromazine, thiouracil derivatives and gold salts. It may also be an integral part of aplastic anaemia as a consequence of radiation or anti-cancer drug therapy, or associated with typhoid fever, malaria or any overwhelming infection. It may also be due to excessive destruction of neutrophils by the spleen (hypersplenism).

Treatment is directed towards identifying the cause, removing or treating it and keeping the patient free from infection in a controlled environment. A gradual increase in neutrophil numbers can be expected in 2 to 3 weeks providing the bone marrow is able to perform its normal function.

---

compared to an acceptable *range* of values. The range itself will be influenced by factors such as the age or gender of the patient.

Sources

Plasma proteins come from two main sources:

- most are synthesized and secreted by the liver
- some are produced and secreted by lymphocytes (immunoglobulins, which are antibodies; see Ch. 16).

A small proportion of the total are proteins specifically manufactured and secreted by other cells, such as hormones secreted by endocrine cells. Others are incidental constituents of plasma released from injured or dead cells. An increased concentration of these in plasma can indicate injury to a particular tissue. For example, in myocardial infarction the blood concentrations of the enzymes creatine kinase and aspartate aminotransferase (AST) are usually increased. The levels of the proteins troponin and myoglobin will also be raised.

HAEMOSTASIS

OVERVIEW

The functions of the blood in transport, communication and defence depend upon its free circulation as a liquid

Table 3.6 A selection of plasma proteins

Name	Function(s)	Concentration	
		g/l	mg/l
Albumin	Transport (fatty acids, bilirubin etc.) Contributes most to oncotic pressure (see Ch. 6)	40	
Transferrin	Transports iron	2	
Transcobalamin	Transports vitamin B_{12}	–	–
Transcortin	Transports cortisol (see Ch. 11)	–	–
Fibrinogen		2–4	
Prothrombin	Coagulation		100–150
Factor V			10
Factor VIII			0.5
Angiotensinogen	Precursor of peptide hormone	–	–
Plasminogen	Precursor of enzyme (see below at 'Fibrinolysis')		

between different organs and tissues. Should any part of the circulatory system develop a leak through injury or weakness, there is a grave threat to the body as a whole.

If a leak develops, several protective measures act to curb the loss of blood from the body.

These include:

- constriction of the blood vessels
- formation of a platelet plug
- formation of fibrin (coagulation).

Conversely, however, should any of these processes be triggered inappropriately, the normal circulation of blood to the tissues will cease. A delicate balance exists therefore between the factors that maintain the flow and fluidity of blood *within* the vessels of the circulation and the mechanisms that prevent its loss *from* the circulation. For example, in stroke (cerebrovascular accident) the failure of blood supply which results in damage to brain cells can be caused either by haemorrhage or occlusion (clot formation) in a cerebral blood vessel.

Sequence of events

When a leak occurs, the loss of blood is curbed first by:

- constriction of the injured blood vessels
- accumulation of platelets at the leak point.

These events narrow and plug the vessels. Simultaneously, blood at the site of injury begins to be converted from a fluid into a gel by the conversion of a soluble protein fibrinogen into an insoluble thread network of fibrin strands. With time the injury is repaired and then the gelled clot is liquefied by the breakdown of fibrin (fibrinolysis) and circulation is restored.

VASCULAR REACTIONS TO INJURY

If a blood vessel is cut, the immediate response is contraction of the smooth muscle in the vessel wall (see Chs 6 and 19). Contraction narrows and may even block off the vessel, reducing blood flow locally and restricting blood loss. The degree and duration of the constriction is related to the extent of the injury. A clean cut is sealed less well by this means than one that involves more trauma, probably because there is less release of vasoactive chemicals (see Chs 6 and 12) from the cut tissues, and less stimulation of nerve and muscle fibres.

PLATELETS (THROMBOCYTES)

Adhesion

When injury occurs to a blood vessel, such that the endothelial cells (Fig. 3.14) are traumatized or underlying tissues consisting of collagen are exposed, platelets adhere to the injured cells and tissues. The platelet plug is also capable of contracting and thus pulling the walls of the damaged vessel together. Platelets seal off any tiny gaps that may appear in the endothelial lining of the blood vessels. This is

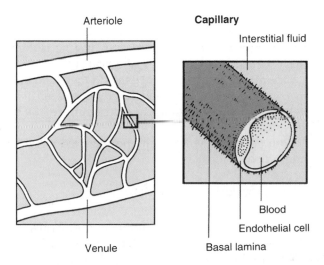

Figure 3.14 Capillary – structure.

Labels: Arteriole, **Capillary**, Interstitial fluid, Blood, Endothelial cell, Basal lamina, Venule

---

Bleeding from injured vessels

Bleeding may be external and observable or internal and hidden.

The observable differences between arterial, venous and capillary bleeding reflect the structure and function of the particular vessels and the pressure within them.

In arterial bleeding, bright red oxygenated blood spurts out with each wave of arterial distension as the heart pumps blood around the body. Because of high pressure within arteries, blood loss may be considerable and is potentially fatal.

Deoxygenated venous blood, which is bluish in colour, flows more evenly from damaged vessels because it is at a much lower pressure.

Capillary bleeding is characterized by oozing and is reddish in colour.

Haemostasis can be achieved by appropriate first-aid treatment, which facilitates the body's defence mechanisms. When a vessel is injured, these mechanisms are triggered to prevent undue blood loss and include reflex vasoconstriction, formation of haemostatic plug and blood coagulation (see main text). Initial first-aid treatment is the same for all types of bleeding: direct, firm pressure over the injury until haemostasis is achieved or, when major vessels are involved, surgical intervention to tie off or repair the injured vessels (see Ch. 19).

particularly important in the blood capillaries (which consist entirely of endothelial cells; see Ch. 6). Small gaps occur all the time and platelets act as the main protection against these spontaneously occurring leaks.

Release of chemicals

The adhesion of platelets to one another and to other surfaces triggers the release of a variety of chemicals stored within their vesicles (Table 3.4). These have a number of different functions. Some:

- promote adhesion of platelets
- contract smooth muscle in the blood vessels
- participate in coagulation.

Aggregation of platelets at the site of injury creates a temporary plug. This is most effective in sealing small vessels. Coagulation may follow, enhanced by platelet factors, and a firmer seal is formed (see below).

Abnormalities

If the number of platelets in blood is much lower than normal (thrombocytopenia) there is an increased tendency for bleeding to occur spontaneously, particularly from smaller blood vessels. When injury occurs, haemostasis is also less effective. Thrombocytopenia can result from:

- bone marrow deficiencies
- accumulation of platelets in the spleen in splenomegaly
- an autoimmune disorder (the platelets are destroyed by the body's immune system).

COAGULATION

The blood clot

In coagulation, interlacing strands of fibrin are formed when a precursor plasma protein, fibrinogen, is exposed to the enzyme thrombin (Fig. 3.15). The meshwork of fibrin strands traps water and its dissolved constituents to form a gel, and erythrocytes, leucocytes and platelets are entrapped. This is the blood clot or thrombus. It is soft at first but then further chemical changes occur which include strengthening of the fibrin strands. Later clot retraction occurs, caused by the platelets in the clot contracting, and some fluid (serum) is squeezed out in the process. Serum contains all the constituents of plasma except those, such as fibrinogen, that have been used up in coagulation.

The clot acts as a temporary seal to the damaged vessel, and also as a scaffold for the repairs made subsequently to the vessel itself.

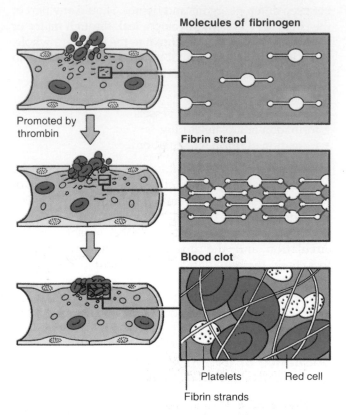

Figure 3.15 The process of coagulation and formation of a blood clot.

Formation of fibrin

The formation of fibrin from fibrinogen is triggered in one of two ways by:

- chemicals released from injured tissues (extrinsic pathway)
- contact with an abnormal surface (intrinsic pathway).

When tissue damage occurs there is usually a release of factors from the tissues (tissue thromboplastin). Blood which has escaped into the tissues will be clotting by this (extrinsic) pathway.

The intrinsic pathway is activated when blood comes in contact with a damaged internal wall of a blood vessel (e.g. exposed collagen) or the surface of a blood sample tube.

Both pathways will usually be activated when tissue injury occurs.

Clotting factors

Both the extrinsic and intrinsic pathways involve the sequential activation of a number of different factors (Fig. 3.16 and Table 3.7) and require the presence of calcium and platelet phospholipid, and other factors facilitating the process.

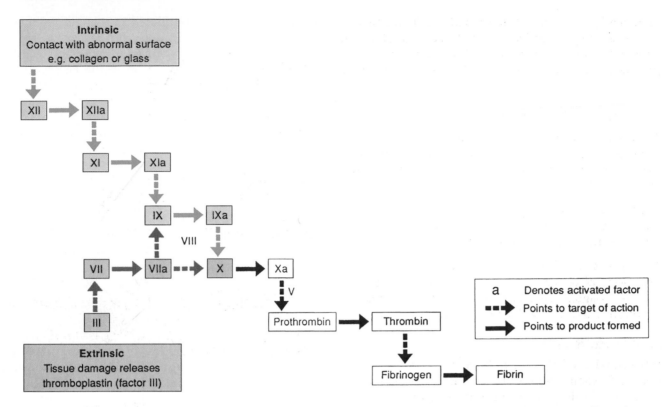

Figure 3.16 Intrinsic and extrinsic pathways of coagulation. Factors are activated in turn, resulting eventually in the formation of fibrin. Factors VIII and V are additional factors needed for coagulation to proceed.

Table 3.7 Coagulation factors

Factor	Other names commonly used
I	Fibrinogen
II	Prothrombin
III	Thromboplastin (tissue factor)
IV	Calcium ions
V	
VII	
VIII	Anti-haemophilic globulin (AHG)
IX	Christmas factor
X	
XI	
XII	Hageman factor
XIII	Fibrin-stabilizing factor

Most, but not all, of the clotting factors are proteins normally present in plasma in an inactive form. Those which are earlier in the coagulation sequence are present in low concentration (Table 3.6) and have a short life span in the blood, whereas the concentrations of prothrombin and fibrinogen are relatively high and their life span is longer. This arrangement has the benefit of allowing just a small change in the concentration of one of the earlier activated factors to bring about progressively larger effects in the later ones. In other words, the effect snowballs and very rapidly a clot forms and the flow of blood is stemmed. If the synthesis of plasma proteins is threatened, as in liver disease (see Ch. 10), deficiencies arise first in the earlier factors, preventing the process of coagulation from getting underway.

FIBRINOLYSIS

While the injured blood vessel is repaired by the growth of new cells, the clot is broken down gradually by the action of the enzyme plasmin, which breaks down fibrin (Fig. 3.17). Plasmin is formed from its precursor plasma protein, plasminogen, by the action of activators secreted chiefly by the endothelial cells of the blood vessel wall. Other endogenous plasminogen activators include urokinase, present in the kidney. This has the important effect of reducing the amount of fibrin which might otherwise be deposited in the small renal vessels. A number of fibrinolytic activators have been developed for use as 'clot-busting' drugs (see 'Fibrinolytic therapy').

In capillaries

The concentration of activating factors is especially high in capillary blood, largely because the space into which they are secreted is small. Consequently fibrin is broken down easily in capillaries. This feature in fact makes it

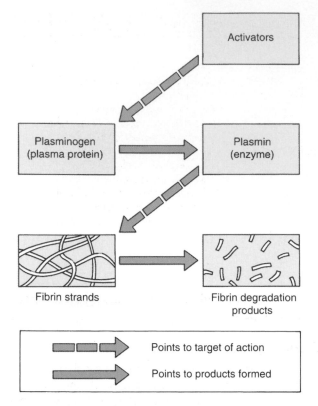

Figure 3.17 The process of fibrinolysis.

difficult for clots to form in the capillary circulation. Any fibrin that is formed is rapidly broken down. Thus the balance between the *fluid* and the *gel* forms of blood is tipped towards fluidity within the capillaries. This is important in preserving the flow of blood through these tiny vessels and thus in maintaining the supply of oxygen and nutrients to the tissues (see also 'Flow characteristics of blood' in Ch. 12).

In large blood vessels

In the largest blood vessels the situation is different. Here the plasminogen-activating factors released from

Table 3.8 Some abnormalities of haemostasis

Abnormality	Disease
Fragile blood vessels	Purpura
Lack of platelets	Thrombocytopenia
Lack of clotting factors, e.g. prothrombin factor VIII	Hypoprothrombinaemia Classic haemophilia
Thrombophilia (tendency to clot)	Deep vein thrombosis (DVT) Cerebrovascular accident (CVA) Pulmonary embolism (PE) Transient ischaemic attack (TIA)

the endothelial cells are diluted in a larger volume of blood, and fibrinolysis does not occur as easily. Consequently, clots are broken down more slowly. However, the pressure of blood in the larger arterial vessels is much higher and the flow characteristics different (see Ch. 12) and, though the chemical balance favours coagulation, the high pressures may dislodge clots forming after injury. Clots that form and then break away can form blockages (emboli) in other parts of the circulation.

ABNORMALITIES

The delicate balance achieved between keeping blood flowing and preventing its loss from the circulation can easily be tipped inappropriately in the direction of bleeding or thrombus formation by defects in any one of the component systems (Table 3.8).

It is important to stress that while it is vital that blood clots form and so prevent loss of blood from the body, inappropriate blood clotting too poses a severe health risk for many of the population. Whenever blood flows slowly or is restricted, the chances of clotting being initiated increase. Such a clot may seriously restrict the blood supply to body tissue or may break down with the release of fragments which travel and lodge in a vessel of narrow diameter, again blocking vital blood supply.

A travelling clot is known as an embolism and can lodge in tissues such as the lung or heart.

Clot formation initiated by platelets adhering to damaged endothelium is also likely in arteries damaged by fatty deposit accumulating in their inner walls (atherosclerosis). This is a leading factor in the pathogenesis of stroke and myocardial infarction.

A variety of automated tests can be used to investigate the ability of blood to clot. For example, the number of platelets can be counted. In addition different sections of the cascade process outlined in Figure 3.16 can be investigated in three laboratory tests which all measure the time taken to produce fibrin. The prothrombin time (PT) is measured by adding factor III to plasma (to initiate the extrinsic pathway), while the activated partial thromboplastin time (APPT) and thrombin (TT) tests investigate the intrinsic and common pathways and the last stage of the common pathway respectively (see Fig. 3.16).

Again it is important to stress that many of the more traditional investigations of coagulation, e.g. bleeding time, involve an unnecessary risk for laboratory staff and have been abandoned.

Many laboratory tests are also performed to assess thrombophilia – a tendency of the blood to clot or hypercoagulation. The level of fibrin degradation

Table 3.9 Anticoagulants

Name	Mode of action	Use
Heparin	Promotes action of antithrombin III*	Clinical treatment of thrombosis (by injection) Also used prophylactically Used in some blood collection tubes to prevent sample clotting
Warfarin	Reduces synthesis of factors II, VII, IX and X	Clinical prevention of thrombosis (oral)
Aspirin	Reduced platelet adhesion (see Ch. 2)	Used prophylactically to reduce thrombotic risk (oral)
Sodium citrate	Removes calcium from solution	Collection of blood for transfusion
EDTA	Binds calcium	Laboratory blood samples

* An inhibitor circulating in the blood that blocks the action of some clotting factors.

products (FDP) can be estimated, providing evidence of a clot having formed.

ANTICOAGULANTS

Anticoagulants are commonly used in two ways, to:

- prevent the coagulation of some samples of blood collected for analysis
- reduce the chance of thrombus formation in a patient.

Examples of both kinds of anticoagulant and how they work are given in Table 3.9. Some of the anticoagulants (such as EDTA) used to prevent coagulation in blood samples are harmful to the body and therefore cannot be used in patients.

Anticoagulant therapy

Anticoagulants are used to reduce the risk of thrombosis and to prevent extension of clots by disrupting the natural blood clotting mechanism. They are not fibrolytic and do not dissolve existing clots.

Heparin given by subcutaneous injection is used as a short-term anticoagulant as its action is immediate. It acts by promoting the inactivation of some clotting factors. Small doses are given to high-risk perioperative patients because it has been found to reduce the incidence of postoperative deep vein thrombosis. With these routinely small doses, there is little risk of excessive bleeding but the patient should always be carefully monitored.

Larger doses are given by continuous intravenous infusion when a thrombus has already formed, and are adjusted according to regular tests of clotting times.

If long-term anticoagulant therapy is necessary, oral drugs such as warfarin (which act to prevent the formation of some clotting factors in the liver) are used. Again the dosage is calculated according to clotting times but, as the individual dose becomes established, these tests are done less frequently. It should be noted that it takes 24 to 36 hours for warfarin to influence coagulation and its effects continue for a similar period after it has been discontinued.

There is a delicate balance between clotting and increased risk of haemorrhage, and there is a need to be constantly alert and the patient well briefed on self-monitoring and care. It is wise for the patient to

Venous thrombosis

Although risk factors are known and routine precautions are taken, venous thrombosis is still relatively common in hospitalized patients and occasionally may lead to a life-threatening pulmonary embolus. This is when a clot breaks free from the site of origin, often the deep veins of the legs, and lodges in the pulmonary vessels. It can follow a period of immobilization during the perioperative period, or bed rest during debilitating disease or after extensive trauma. It may also occur in apparently healthy individuals after periods of inactivity, e.g. long haul air flights.

Blood flow is reduced and slowed by immobility, while surgery and trauma carry a double risk because of activation of clotting factors in response to blood vessel and tissue damage.

Prevention is through early mobilization and physiotherapy, administration of anticoagulants and the use of anti-embolic stockings.

carry a Medialert card indicating the name and dose of the drug.

FIBRINOLYTIC THERAPY

Anticoagulants reduce the risk of clot formation, fibrinolytics break up a clot once it has formed. Fibrinolysis or thrombolysis has become part of the treatment of conditions where thrombi have formed causing ischaemia in the tissue supplied, e.g. myo-cardial infarction, pulmonary embolism and stroke. The more the tissue function can be preserved, the better the outcome. The drugs used include streptokinase, recombinant urokinase, and the many tPAs (tissue plasminogen activators) such as alteplase, reteplase, lanoteplase etc. The latter vary in their half-life, the longer-acting drugs having some advantages but extending the risk of bleeding.

Anyone with a current or recently healed injury would normally be unsuitable for this particular treatment.

REFERENCES AND FURTHER READING

Bain B J (ed) 1996 A beginner's guide to blood cells. Blackwell Scientific Publications, Oxford

Dacie J V, Lewis S M 2001 Practical haematology, 9th edn. Churchill Livingstone, Edinburgh
Explains techniques used in laboratory investigation of blood. Useful for reference

Higgins C 2000 Understanding laboratory investigation. Blackwell Scientific Publications, Oxford
Textbook aimed at nurses and health care professionals

Hillman R S, Finch C A 1996 Red cell manual, 7th edn. F A Davis, Philadelphia
Small paperback giving further information about red cells and their function, and the identification and management of anaemia

Kumar O, Clark P 1998 Clinical medicine, 4th edn. W B Saunders, London

Hughes-Jones N C, Wickramasinghe S N 1996 Lecture notes on haematology, 6th edn. Blackwell Scientific Publications, Oxford
Blood diseases and their treatment. Useful for information

Kelton J G, Heddle N M, Blajchman M A 1984 Blood transfusion: a conceptual approach. Churchill Livingstone, Edinburgh
Unusual format of friendly diagrams and adjacent explanatory notes conveys a lot of information in a simple way

Ludlam C (ed) 1990 Clinical haematology. Churchill Livingstone, Edinburgh
Blood diseases and their treatment. Useful for reference

McDonald G A, Paul J, Cruickshank B 1988 Atlas of haematology, 5th edn. Churchill Livingstone, Edinburgh

Rogers A W 1992 Textbook of anatomy. Churchill Livingstone, Edinburgh

Thibodeau G A, Patten K T 2000 Structure and function of the body. Mosby, Edinburgh

In practice you may be asked to consider the following:

1. A drug such as lidocaine (lignocaine) reduces the permeability of the neurone membrane to small ions. What are the clinical applications of this property?

2. What would be the effect of inhibiting acetylcholinesterase? What is the clinical application of such an effect?

3. What would be the effect of moving threshold potential further from resting membrane potential? How could this be used?

4. Why does an action potential travel in one direction only down an axon?

5. Axon diameter affects the speed of conduction. Are thicker axons quicker axons? – or not?

6. What is COMT?

7. A synapse causes a delay in transmission along a pathway. Why is this?

8. What would be the effect of a transmitter which increased the postsynaptic membrane permeability to chloride ions?

While you are sitting happily reading this text and making notes, neurones are transmitting innumerable signals, in the form of electrical impulses, from one part of your body to another. Impulses are passing continually from your eyes to your brain and from your brain, via your spinal cord, to your muscles.

Neurones have the function of detecting disturbances, converting that information into electrical impulses and then transmitting those signals faithfully, sometimes over considerable distances, to other neurones and cells. Transmission of signals between neurones, and between neurones and other cells is achieved by neurotransmitters released at synapses. This mode of transmission enables there to be the considerable flexibility in information processing and in response that characterizes our lives as human beings. Whenever you hover between two decisions, excitatory and inhibitory neurotransmitters are being used to translate the pros and cons of the situation into electrical signals, the balance of which will determine what you actually do.

Neurones develop contacts (synapses) with other neurones and with other cells during development. New contacts, but not new cells, still form once maturity is reached. As a result we continue to be able to learn new things and develop new skills throughout our lives.

STRUCTURE OF NEURONES

There are two main cell types found within nerve tissue:

- neurones, or nerve cells, which transmit electrochemical signals (nerve impulses)
- neuroglia, or glia, which insulate, nourish, support and protect neurones.

The human nervous system contains approximately 10 billion neurones and 100–500 billion neuroglia.

There are three main parts to most neurones (Fig. 4A.1):

- cell body
- dendrites
- axon.

The membrane of the cell body is receptive to stimuli from other neurones, thereby creating neuronal pathways. The cytoplasm contains a nucleus, all the usual cell organelles, as well as other structures characteristic of neurones:

- Nissl bodies, or rough endoplasmic reticulum
- neurofibrils which provide support and shape
- lipofuscin pigment which is the end product of lysosomal activity.

The branched projections extending from the cell body are known as dendrites, and they receive stimuli from the environment, the sensory organs or adjacent neurones. The axon is a single process that conducts nerve impulses to other cells.

Two of the most important structures associated with the neurones are the Schwann cells and the nodes of Ranvier (Fig. 4A.2). Schwann cells are a type of glial cell, which produce myelin and act as an insulator, thereby increasing the rate at which an impulse propagates along the axon. Schwann cells only act as an insulator on neurones of the peripheral nervous system, with the same role being taken in the central nervous system by oligodendrocytes. The nodes of Ranvier are breaks in the myelin coating where the axon is exposed to the surrounding extracellular fluid. The nodes play a critical role in the process of saltatory conduction (see later).

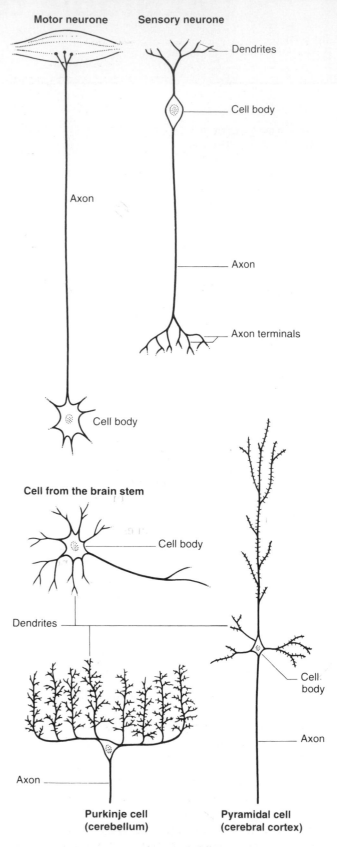

Figure 4A.1 Structure of several different types of neurone.

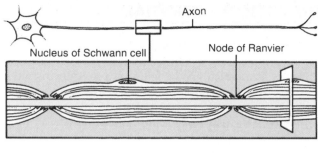

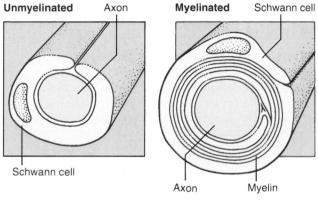

Figure 4A.2 Myelinated and unmyelinated axons.

STRUCTURAL CLASSIFICATION

Neurones can be classified in terms of their structure (Fig. 4A.1). Unipolar (and pseudounipolar) neurones have a single process extending from the cell body, e.g. sensory neurones. Bipolar neurones have one dendrite and one axon and are found in the retina, internal ear and olfactory mucosa. Multipolar neurones have several dendrites and one axon, and most neurones in the brain and spinal cord are of this type, e.g. motor neurones.

FUNCTIONAL CLASSIFICATION

Neurones can also be classified with respect to their function.

Afferent neurones (sensory neurones) carry impulses towards the central nervous system (CNS). There are four main types of afferent neurones:

- somatic neurones carry impulses from the skin, skeletal muscles and joints (general) and the retina and internal ear (special)
- visceral neurones carry impulses from the internal organs (general) and the tongue and olfactory mucosa (special).

Efferent neurones (motor neurones) carry impulses away from the CNS. There are three main types:

- general somatic carry impulses to most skeletal muscles
- visceral carry impulses to the internal organs (general) and the tongue and olfactory mucosa (special).

Interneurones are located within the central nervous system and carry impulses from one neurone to another. It is by using these interneurones that the central nervous system is able to set up such complex neuronal pathways or circuitry.

THE NERVE IMPULSE

ION CHANNELS

One of the many uses for the proteins in the body is as ion channels in the cellular membrane. What makes the ion channels in nerve cells (and muscle cells) different is that they are able to respond to stimuli. Stimulation of these ion channels in the nerve cell membrane causes them to open, thereby creating a channel for ionic flow.

MEMBRANE POTENTIALS

The voltage difference across the membrane of a neuronal cell can be measured in the following way. One microelectrode is inserted outside the cell, with a second inside the cell, and both are connected to a voltmeter. The voltage difference recorded would be in the range 5–100 mV. The net charge inside the cell is negative with respect to the outside of the cell, and it varies with the state the cell is in:

- resting (resting potential)
- active, excited state (action potential) where charge is reversed, and the inside is positive with respect to the outside.

RESTING MEMBRANE POTENTIAL

The resting potential of the cell membrane is –40 to –90 mV (normally –70 mV). This potential difference is a result of the differing ion concentrations on each side of the membrane (Table 4A.1).

It can be seen from Table 4A.1 that there are 14 times more Na^+ ions outside the cell than inside and 37 times more K^+ ions inside the cell than outside. This uneven distribution is produced by a Na^+/K^+ pump in the cell membrane (using Na^+/K^+ ATPase as a carrier) which transports 2 K^+ ions into the cell and 3 Na^+ ions out of the cell. Since the pump leads to a net negative charge

Table 4A.1 Intracellular and extracellular levels of various ions

Substance	Intracellular (mmol/l)	Extracellular (mmol/l)
Cations		
Na^+	10	140
K^+	150	4
Ca^{2+}	1	2.5
Mg^{2+}	15	1
Anions		
Cl^-	10	110
HCO_3^-	10	28
$HPO_4^{2-}/H_2PO_4^-$	50	1
SO_4^{2-}	10	0.5
Non-diffusible A^-	150	146

inside the cell it is referred to as being electrogenic. Concentration gradients also exist across the membrane and these act as a force to promote diffusion of ions, i.e. the K^+ force acts outwards and the Na^+ force acts inwards, both down their respective concentration gradients.

The diffusion is controlled by the relative permeability of the two major ions, with the membrane permeability of K^+ being 100 times that of Na^+. As K^+ ions diffuse out down the concentration a positive charge builds up on the outside, thereby blocking further diffusion. If this process were allowed to continue unchecked a state of equilibrium would be reached, since K^+ outflow would be balanced by the outside positive charge. At this point there would be no net movement of K^+ ions, with a resultant membrane potential of approximately –95 mV. The accompanying Na^+ movements would produce a membrane potential of approximately +60 mV. The underlying role of the Na^+/K^+ pump should also be acknowledged.

For any single action potential the actual number of sodium and potassium ions crossing the cell membrane is relatively small, and have no real effect on the ionic content of either the intra- or extracellular fluid. It actually takes the generation of many action potentials close together to cause the intracellular sodium to increase and the extracellular potassium to decrease. Even though nerve impulses are generated rapidly, this is a situation that does not occur because the sodium entry and potassium loss are offset by the action of the Na^+/K^+ pump.

At the resting potential of approximately –70 mV the equilibrium point has been achieved with no net movement of either Na^+ or K^+.

THE ACTION POTENTIAL

When the cell membrane is stimulated there is a resultant increase in Na^+ permeability. In most cases the stimulus is chemical in the form of a neurotransmitter released by a presynaptic neurone. However, it is also possible for an action potential to be stimulated in a variety of other ways including pain or light.

Local anaesthetics

Local anaesthetics, such as lidocaine (lignocaine) hydrochloride, bupivacaine hydrochloride and tetracaine (amethocaine) hydrochloride, alter the cell's permeability to ions, particularly sodium, which is necessary for the generation of action potentials. Local anaesthetics block voltage-gated channels and therefore inhibit the production and transmission of impulses in sensory neurones.

There are several methods of using local anaesthesia, the most common being:

- surface or topical – teething gels, lozenges for mouth ulcers
- infiltration – used for minor surgery, suturing, episiotomy during childbirth
- nerve block – used by dentists particularly for work on lower teeth
- epidural – used mainly during childbirth.

During an action potential the membrane potential changes from the resting potential mentioned above (–70 mV), up to a peak of approximately +30 mV, and back to –70 mV (Fig. 4A.3). Following membrane stimulation the aforementioned increase in Na^+ permeability results in the opening of voltage-gated Na^+ channels, thereby allowing Na^+ ions to flow down their electrochemical gradient. The movement of Na^+ ions, and therefore positive charge, into the cell results in the membrane potential shifting towards, and beyond, zero, i.e. depolarization. Depolarization peaks at +30 mV. The reason the membrane potential does not reach the +60 mV mentioned above for Na^+ is simply due to the fact that Na^+ permeability is not large enough. After a fraction of a millisecond the increased permeability to Na^+ is replaced by an increased permeability to K^+, which in turn leads to the opening of voltage-gated K^+ channels. The loss of K^+ from the cell is mirrored by the downward slope of the action potential trace, i.e. repolarization. Since the permeability to K^+ remains higher than normal for a short period of time the membrane potential in fact drops below –70 mV, i.e. hyperpolarization. At this point the Na^+/K^+ pump starts to work to restore the original ionic balance

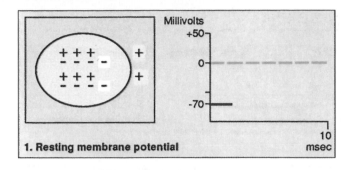

1. Resting membrane potential

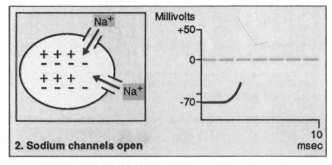

2. Sodium channels open

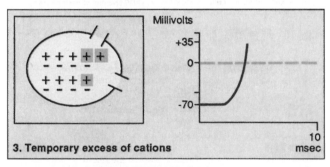

3. Temporary excess of cations

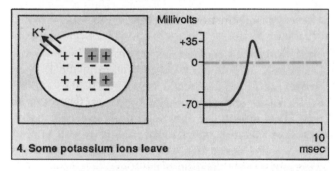

4. Some potassium ions leave

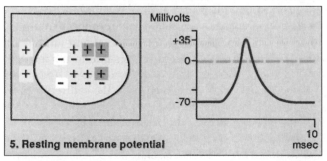

5. Resting membrane potential

Figure 4A.3 The action potential: how the voltage of a nerve cell changes as a result of the opening and closing of sodium and potassium channels.

and the membrane potential returns to the resting value of –70 mV.

The stimulus required to produce an action value must be large enough to cause a degree of depolarization such that the membrane potential crosses a given value, the threshold potential or firing level. Above this value, the rate of depolarization increases, the membrane polarity is reversed and an action potential is developed. If the stimulus is not large enough, threshold potential is not reached and no action potential occurs. Increasing the strength of the stimulus cannot increase the value of the action potential, i.e. the height of the spike. The action potential is all or nothing and this principle is described as the 'All or Nothing Law'. Threshold values carry but are of the order of –50 to –40 mV.

Propagation of action potentials

Local current flow is responsible for the transmission of the action potential to a neighbouring section of the unmyelinated cell membrane. The charges on both the inside and outside of the membrane of the active region of the membrane are the opposite of those on the neighbouring section. This results in the attraction of ions to areas of opposite charge. This triggers a depolarization of the neighbouring membrane to threshold value, followed by the generation of an action potential. This process can continue over the entire length of the neurone and the rate of conduction varies from neurone to neurone, dependent on a number of factors (see below). The conduction in the smallest diameter unmyelinated axons is approximately 0.5 ms^{-1}.

Speed

Nerve axons normally conduct impulses at rates ranging between about 1 metre/second to 100 metres/second (Table 4A.2), the speed of transmission depending on:

- temperature
- myelination
- diameter of the axon.

An increase in any of these increases the speed of transmission.

The conduction rate in myelinated axons is faster than in unmyelinated (>100 metres/second in the most heavily myelinated axons). The myelin sheath acts as an insulator, producing an approximate 5000-fold increase in resistance to ion flow. The nodes of Ranvier offer little resistance to ion diffusion (Fig. 4A.4) and since action potentials are only generated at sites where Na$^+$ and K$^+$ exchange can take place between cytoplasm and surrounding fluid, they can only be generated at the nodes of Ranvier. As a result of this, the impulse appears to jump from node to node (saltatory

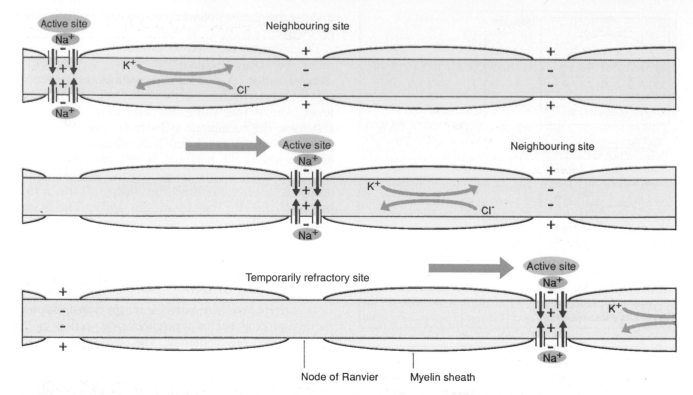

Figure 4A.4 Conduction of the nerve impulse in a myelinated axon: how the movement of anions and cations between active and inactive sites depolarizes the neighbouring axonal membrane, opens voltage-gated sodium channels and generates another action potential.

The role of axonal transport in disease

Axonal transport is used normally to move neurotransmitters between cell body and nerve endings and to carry other materials back to the cell body for recycling. However, it is also made use of by viruses and toxins. The best known of these are the herpes and rabies viruses, and the toxins produced by the organisms that cause tetanus and diphtheria.

Many people suffer from 'cold' sores on the lips and nose (herpes labialis). After the initial infection, usually early in life, the virus remains dormant within nerve cells. Certain circumstances, such as pyrexia, hot sunshine, cold winds and, less frequently, cosmetics, seem to reactivate the virus. Some people experience tenderness along the nerve before the lesions appear. The exudate from the blisters contains active viruses secreted by the nerve endings, and care should be taken not to transfer it to the eyes or to other people.

The rabies virus enters the body most commonly through wounds caused by dog bites. It is capable of travelling in both directions along nerve axons. The virus multiplies in ganglion cells of the brain and spinal cord (see Ch. 20) causing degenerative changes. The incubation period seems to depend on the distance of the bite from the appropriate ganglia. Thus, symptoms may appear after 2 months, or longer, if the bite is on the leg, or after less than 1 month if the bite is on the head. Great care should always be taken when approaching strange dogs and, if a stray or wild animal must be handled, protective clothing should be worn. The risk of infection is diminished if the bite is through clothing because much of the saliva is removed.

The bacillus *Clostridium tetani* produces a toxin that travels by axonal transport from the site of infection, giving rise to the symptoms of tetanus (lockjaw). Usually, the first symptom is pain and stiffness of the jaw muscles, progressing to rigid clamping of the jaws – hence lockjaw. Eventually severe, painful muscular spasms involve the whole body. Death may result from asphyxiation. Like rabies, the time between infection and the appearance of symptoms depends upon the time taken for the toxin to travel along the nerve axons. The bacilli, which are *anaerobic* (live without oxygen), are found in soil, particularly that which is well manured, and can survive for many years as spores, in Victorian horsehair furniture, for example, or in inadequately sterilized catgut. They enter the body via deep dirty wounds. Protection against tetanus is included in infant immunization schedules. Adults are advised to renew immunization every 10 years – even if one is not a gardener, road traffic accidents can happen to almost anyone.

Demyelination

In some diseases the myelin sheath is destroyed with the result that the nerve axon loses ability to conduct impulses quickly. Little is known about why the myelin sheath degenerates but research shows that demyelination is responsible for the symptoms of many neuropathies (-*opathy* = something is wrong but exactly what is not known).

In *multiple sclerosis*, patchy demyelination occurs within the spinal cord and brain, followed by damage to nerve fibres and the formation of plaques of scar tissue. The disease is characterized by remissions and relapses, which are unpredictable. The relapses may be very distressing for the patient. Initially, the person experiences sensations related to abnormal impulse conduction – tingling, numbness, weakness in one or both arms or legs. Visual disturbances are also common. The disease is progressive and the person eventually becomes confined to a wheelchair.

The *Guillain–Barré* syndrome develops rapidly following an often mild, pyrexial illness. Although marked demyelination of spinal nerve roots and peripheral nerves (see Ch. 20) occurs, the nerve fibre is not damaged. The myelin sheath gradually regenerates and normal function returns. The affected person suffers severe motor impairment and the muscles are very tender. It is an alarming condition due to the rapidity and severity of onset. The person requires careful nursing and much reassurance.

Symptoms of inadequate transmission of nerve impulses, such as numbness, are also experienced by some people suffering from *diabetes mellitus*. Research shows that these symptoms are caused by demyelination and axonal degeneration. When numbness affects one or both feet the risk of infection, following unfelt injury, is high. The cutting of toenails must be carried out with great care, if necessary by a chiropodist, and the feet should be inspected daily. It is advisable for the person to wear shoes that provide adequate protection. It has been known for an affected person to walk long distances with a sharp object embedded in the foot.

conduction) whereas, in fact, each node generates a new impulse in rapid succession.

Direction

The action potential generated at neighbouring sites does not reactivate that part of the membrane from which it has just come. This part of the membrane is less sensitive to stimulation (refractory). There are two reasons for this. Firstly, during the action potential, there is a phase when the voltage-gated sodium channels are either open or have just closed and cannot immediately be re-opened (sodium inactivation).

Table 4A.2 Different types of nerve fibre

Name	Speed of conduction (m/s)*	Myelination	Diameter (μm)
A α	100	Yes	15
A β	50	Yes	10
A γ	20	Yes	5
A δ	20	Yes	4
B	10	Yes	2
C	1	No	1

* Typical values.

Secondly, at the end of the action potential there is a phase when the membrane hyperpolarizes slightly, because extra potassium channels are still open. The membrane voltage is then further away from threshold and the membrane is more difficult to excite.

TRANSMISSION OF SIGNALS BETWEEN NEURONES

The transmission of signals between one neurone and the next occurs through the mediation of one or more chemical transmitters (neurotransmitters). Neurotransmitters, released from nerve endings by the action potential, diffuse across the intervening space (synapse) and then excite the next cell.

NEUROTRANSMITTERS

Synthesis and storage

Transmitters are synthesized either at the nerve endings or in the cell body of a neurone. The necessary enzymes (which are proteins) are made on the ribosomes in the cell body of the neurone and transported down the axon, where they concentrate in the axon terminals. The protein synthesis processes within the cell are set up to produce the necessary enzymes to produce the appropriate neurotransmitter for each neuronal subtype. The amount and activity of the enzymes produced in this way dictate the amount of transmitter synthesized. Other factors influencing the process include the availability of the necessary substrates and co-factors. Following synthesis, the transmitter is stored within synaptic vesicles at the axon terminals.

Those manufactured in the cell body are packaged in vesicles and transported along microtubules in the axon to the nerve endings (axonal transport) (Fig. 4A.5).

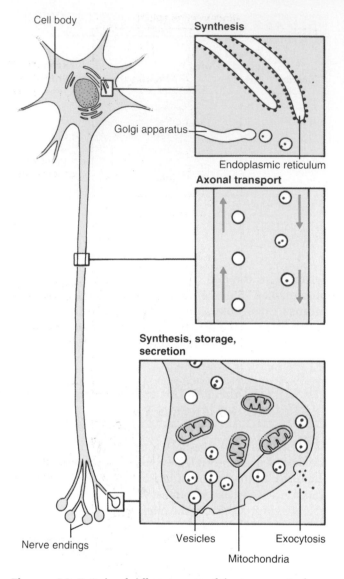

Figure 4A.5 Role of different parts of the neurone in the production, delivery and storage of neurotransmitter prior to secretion.

Much traffic occurs in both directions along the axon, as has been shown by speeded up film of neurones in culture.

Two distinctive features are apparent at the nerve endings (Fig. 4A.5):

- many tiny storage vesicles containing neurotransmitters
- an abundance of mitochondria.

Both features reveal the high degree of activity at this site.

Release

When the action potential reaches the axon terminal there is a resultant opening of the voltage-gated Ca^{2+} channels in the terminal membrane. Ca^{2+} ions diffuse in from the extracellular fluid and cause the synaptic

vesicles to fuse with the presynaptic membrane. The neurotransmitter is then released into the synaptic cleft by exocytosis.

The more action potentials arriving at the ending per second, the more transmitter is released. The amount of transmitter released depends also on the original voltage across the membrane. Transmitters secreted by other neurones nearby can alter this voltage.

SYNAPSES

ARRANGEMENT AND STRUCTURE

The nerve terminals of one neurone make contact with the dendrites and cell bodies of other neurones at junctions known as synapses. Dendrites and cell bodies are normally smothered with nerve terminals (Fig. 4A.6). A single motor neurone in the spinal cord may have about 10 000 terminals on its dendritic tree and cell body, whereas a Purkinje cell of the cerebellum (Fig. 4A.1) may be in contact with 100 000 other neurones.

> Non-depolarizing or competitive muscle relaxants used in general anaesthesia, for example tubocurarine and pancuronium, compete with acetylcholine at the receptor site, thus blocking its action.
> Anticholinesterases, such as neostigmine, reverse the effects of competitive muscle relaxants by combining with acetylcholinesterase to inhibit its action, thus allowing more acetylcholine to accumulate.

In a typical synapse the gap (synaptic cleft) between the first nerve (presynaptic neurone) and the second nerve (postsynaptic neurone) is very tiny, only about 20 nm in width (about 1/350th of the size of a red cell).

FATE OF SECRETED NEUROTRANSMITTERS

Neurotransmitters released by the presynaptic neurone diffuse into the gap. At least one of three things may happen to them subsequently. They may:

- interact with the postsynaptic membrane
- interact with the presynaptic membrane
- diffuse away and be metabolized in body fluids.

Postsynaptic membrane

At the postsynaptic membrane neurotransmitters may bind to receptor proteins (Fig. 4A.7) and activate G

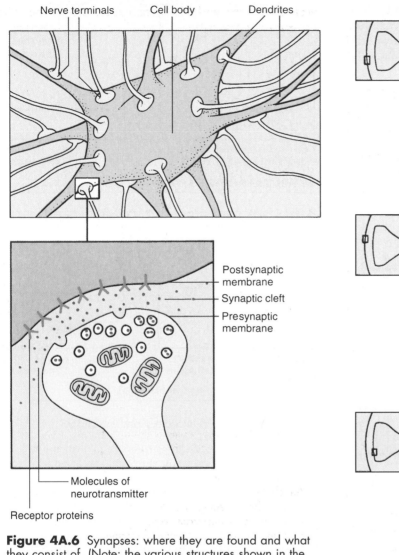

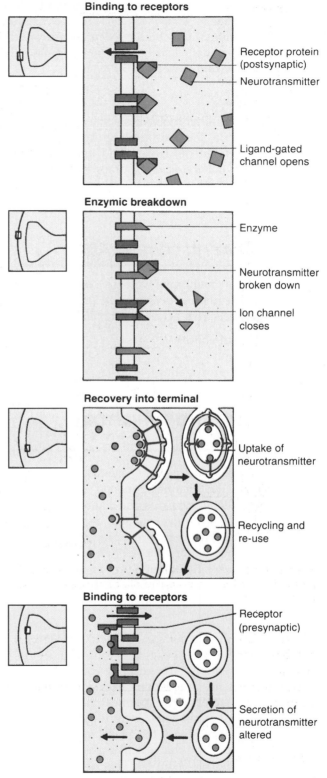

Figure 4A.6 Synapses: where they are found and what they consist of. (Note: the various structures shown in the inset are not drawn to scale. If they were the receptor proteins, for example, would be invisible.)

Figure 4A.7 Fate and action of neurotransmitters at postsynaptic (top two panels) and presynaptic (bottom two panels) membranes.

proteins in the membrane. As a result, channels (ligand-gated channels) allowing the movement of ions across the membrane open or close depending on the transmitters involved. The change in permeability alters the voltage across the postsynaptic membrane.

In some instances, enzymes in the membrane then break down the transmitter substance attached to the receptor and release the products of breakdown into the interstitial fluid. For example the enzyme acetylcholinesterase, located on the postsynaptic membrane of cholinergic synapses, splits acetylcholine into acetic acid and choline (see Ch. 5).

Presynaptic membrane

Neurotransmitter in the vicinity of the presynaptic terminal can be re-accumulated by the terminals of the presynaptic neurone, and recycled. Noradrenaline is a good example of this.

Products of transmitter metabolism such as acetic acid and choline from acetylcholine may also be taken up by a specific transport mechanism into the presynaptic terminal and be re-used in the synthesis of more acetylcholine.

Some transmitter also binds to receptors on the presynaptic terminal. These receptors regulate the function of the terminal (see Ch. 5).

Tissue fluids

Some of the transmitter molecules just leak away, out of the synapse, into the surrounding interstitial fluid. Enzymes present in the tissue fluid and blood then break them down. For example, noradrenaline escaping into the blood is broken down by the enzyme catechol-*o*-methyltransferase (COMT) (see Ch. 5).

POSTSYNAPTIC POTENTIALS

The changes in membrane voltage occurring at the postsynaptic membrane (postsynaptic potentials) differ in several respects from action potentials. They are:

- excitatory or inhibitory
- graded in size
- local (not self-propagating).

EXCITATORY AND INHIBITORY POTENTIALS

The membrane voltage may increase or decrease depending on the channels opened (Fig. 4A.8). A decrease in voltage increases the likelihood that the postsynaptic cell will fire an action potential. This change in voltage is therefore termed an excitatory postsynaptic potential or epsp. Conversely an increase in the voltage takes the voltage further away from the threshold level and makes it less likely that an action potential will be fired. This is an inhibitory postsynaptic potential or ipsp.

Ion channels

Excitatory potentials are usually caused by the transmitter–receptor interaction causing the opening of channels that increase the permeability of the cell membrane to all small ions, including sodium. This reduces the voltage across the membrane. Inhibition, however, is caused by the selective opening of either potassium or chloride channels. This may increase the voltage or simply make it more difficult for the cell to be depolarized and become excited.

Size

Postsynaptic potentials are not explosive all-or-none changes in voltage. Instead they develop and fade away

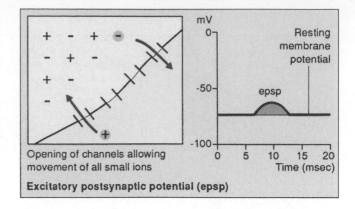

Excitatory postsynaptic potential (epsp)

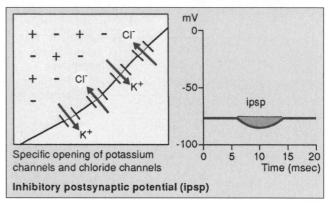

Inhibitory postsynaptic potential (ipsp)

Figure 4A.8 Basis of excitatory and inhibitory postsynaptic potentials.

relatively slowly. They may also be large or small depending on the quantity of transmitter released. If just a single action potential occurs in the presynaptic neurone then only a small quantity of transmitter is released and this results in a small postsynaptic potential. However, if a series of action potentials excite the presynaptic neurone, a series of bursts of transmitter is released from the terminal. Because postsynaptic potentials fade away relatively slowly, each succeeding pulse of transmitter may reach the membrane before it has recovered from the preceding pulse. As a result, each postsynaptic potential adds on to the previous one and a much larger total change in voltage occurs. This adding together of small changes in voltage is termed temporal summation (added over a period of time) (Fig. 4A.9A).

Location

The electrical changes produced at the postsynaptic membrane do not reproduce themselves on either side of the active site, as action potentials do. Instead, like ripples in a pond, the electrical disturbance spreads out but becomes smaller the further away it is from the initiating disturbance.

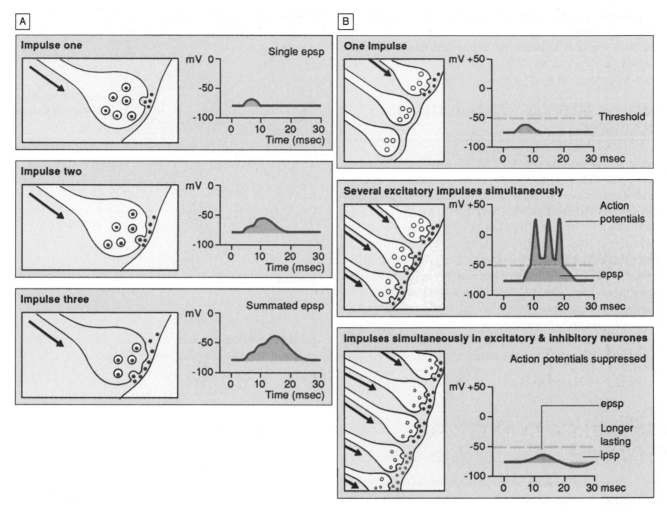

Figure 4A.9 Summation of postsynaptic potentials due to: A, a train of nerve impulses arriving at a single nerve terminal (temporal summation); B, several nerve endings being excited simultaneously (spatial summation).

FUNCTIONS OF CHEMICAL TRANSMISSION

Impulses are transmitted from one neurone to the next by chemical means so that information from different sources can be integrated and regulated before being passed on. This is how decisions, determining our experience and actions, are made within the nervous system.

INTEGRATION OF INFORMATION

An action potential will be triggered in the postsynaptic neurone if the change in voltage is sufficiently large to trigger the opening of voltage-gated sodium channels.

A single epsp is not big enough for this to happen. There must be either temporal summation or spatial summation of epsps or both.

Spatial summation occurs when a number of synapses (within a space) on the dendritic tree are active at the same time (Fig. 4A.9B). If these are excitatory synapses, then a big enough postsynaptic potential may be generated to open voltage-gated sodium channels. Once this happens one or more action potentials are produced and, as explained above, this event is self-propagating. The signal is then passed on along the axon of the postsynaptic neurone.

However, if the synapses activated are inhibitory then the postsynaptic cell will be made less excitable. If it had been firing action potentials previously then either the frequency of firing will decrease, or the cell will be silenced.

Usually postsynaptic neurones receive a blend of excitatory and inhibitory signals. How they respond depends on the balance of excitation and inhibition occurring at any time.

REGULATION OF INFORMATION TRANSFER

Some nerve endings form synapses with presynaptic nerve terminals (Fig. 4A.10). The transmitters released bind to receptors on the nerve terminals, and these alter the permeability of the membrane there. In so doing they change the effectiveness of the action potentials arriving at the terminal at releasing transmitter. In presynaptic inhibition less transmitter is released. These changes are longer lasting than postsynaptic potentials. Their usefulness lies in the fact that some inputs to the postsynaptic neurone can be selectively suppressed without affecting the sensitivity of the postsynaptic cell to other stimuli. For example, when you hold on to a hot plate that you do not want to drop, presynaptic inhibition is being used to inhibit transmission of the sensory impulses urging you to let go.

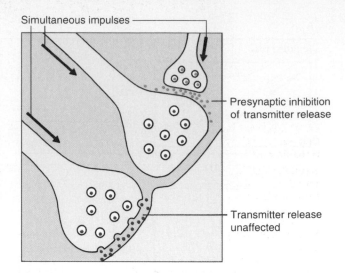

Figure 4A.10 Regulation of synaptic function.

REFERENCES AND FURTHER READING

Aidley D J 1998 The physiology of excitable cells, 4th edn. Cambridge University Press, Cambridge

Carlson N R 2000 Physiology of behavior, 7th edn. Allyn & Bacon, Boston, MA

Keynes R D, Aidley D J 2001 Nerve and muscle, 3rd edn. Cambridge University Press, Cambridge

McGeown J G 2002 Master medicine: Physiology, 2nd edn. Churchill Livingstone, Edinburgh

Matthews G G 1998 Cellular physiology of nerve and muscle, 3rd edn. Blackwell Scientific Publications, Oxford

In practice you may be asked to consider the following:

1. Why is muscle fatigue painful?

2. Why does cardiac muscle, in the normal heart, not suffer fatigue?

3. Muscle response to stretch is contraction. How is it that the bladder can fill without ejecting its contents?

4. The myocardium is made up of separate cells. How is synchronized contraction achieved in the myocardium?

5. Digoxin indirectly increases intracellular calcium ion concentration by decreasing calcium extrusion. How is this action used clinically?

6. You are lifting a heavy patient. Does this require isometric or isotonic contraction of your arm muscles? What is the difference? Which has the higher energy requirement?

7. What is tetanus? Fortunately, normal cardiac muscle does not exhibit tetanus. Why not?

8. A patient who has myasthenia gravis is prescribed neostigmine. What is myasthenia gravis? What is neostigmine? How does it work?

Almost all cells can alter their shape by contraction of specific intracellular proteins. This enables the cell to move. White cells, for example, creep along blood vessels in an amoeba-like way, and find their way through capillary walls into the interstitial fluid. Other cells, such as those lining the respiratory tract, possess cilia that are driven to and fro. But in muscle cells this ability to contract dominates cell activity. The forces developed are harnessed in various ways: activity in gastrointestinal muscle mixes and propels food and digestive secretions; contraction of cardiac muscle drives blood around the circulation; contraction and relaxation of skeletal muscle enables us to walk, write, speak and laugh.

There are three different types of muscle (Fig. 4B.1):

- smooth
- cardiac
- skeletal.

Contraction of muscle is caused by the interaction of two proteins – actin and myosin. The interaction of

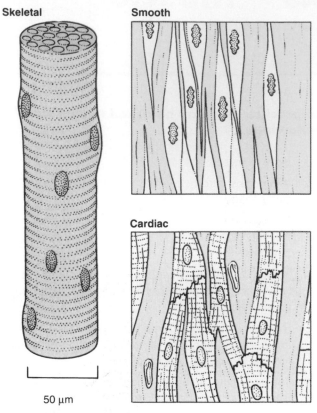

Skeletal   **Smooth**

Cardiac

50 μm

Figure 4B.1 The three main types of muscle: skeletal, smooth and cardiac. All three are drawn approximately to scale. Skeletal muscle fibres are very long. Consequently only a short section of a single fibre is shown.

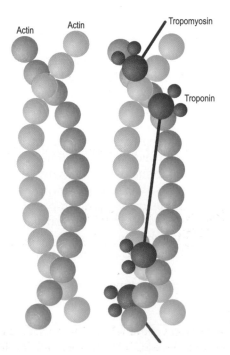

Actin   Actin   Tropomyosin

Troponin

Figure 4B.2 Filaments. (After Davies et al 2001, with permission of Elsevier.)

these two proteins is caused by intracellular calcium levels, which, in turn, is controlled by stimuli on the muscle cells. This stimulus can be neural, hormonal or inherent. The three types of muscle differ, however, in their structure, method of excitation and other properties, according to the roles each plays within the body.

BASIC MECHANISM OF CONTRACTION

The protein molecules are arranged to form thin filaments (actin) and thick filaments (myosin) (Fig. 4B.2). Actin and myosin have a natural affinity, with the myosin heads attracted to sites on the actin molecules, thereby forming crossbridges. A bond forms, the crossbridge bends and the thick filament is pulled along the thin filament. ATP binds to the myosin head and is split by myosin-ATPase (Fig. 4B.3). As a result, energy is released, the bond is broken and the myosin head swings to a new position and the cycle is then repeated. The bonds between actin and myosin form and break, again and again, the thick filaments are pulled along the thin filaments, and tension in the muscle develops. Actin and myosin have to be free to associate. In the relaxed state their association is prevented by the influence of other proteins which are controlled by calcium.

CONTROL BY CALCIUM

Calcium ions carry two positive charges and therefore can bind to negatively charged groups, such as those found on protein molecules. The proteins that regulate the interaction of actin and myosin have binding sites for calcium. When calcium is attached to these sites, changes occur allowing actin and myosin to interact and produce contraction.

The amount of calcium that binds, and therefore the degree of contraction produced, depends on the concentration of calcium in the cytoplasm (sarcoplasm in muscle cells). The greater the calcium concentration, the greater the number of binding sites occupied by calcium ions. Consequently, the number of bonds formed between actin and myosin, and the degree of contraction, increases. If calcium concentration falls fewer bonds are made and contraction decreases (Fig. 4B.4).

The concentration of unbound (free) calcium in the cytoplasm of relaxed muscle cells (0.0001 mmol/l) is 20 000 times less than that outside (2 mmol/l). Intracellular concentration is affected by the amount of calcium:

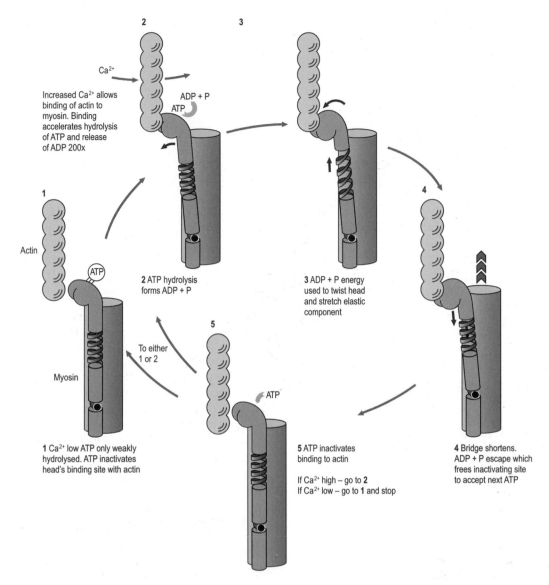

Figure 4B.3 The crossbridge cycle and the reactions which provide its energy. (After Davies et al 2001, with permission of Elsevier.)

Within the figure:

Increased Ca²⁺ allows binding of actin to myosin. Binding accelerates hydrolysis of ATP and release of ADP 200x

2 ATP hydrolysis forms ADP + P

3 ADP + P energy used to twist head and stretch elastic component

1 Ca²⁺ low ATP only weakly hydrolysed. ATP inactivates head's binding site with actin

To either 1 or 2

5 ATP inactivates binding to actin

If Ca²⁺ high – go to **2**
If Ca²⁺ low – go to **1** and stop

4 Bridge shortens. ADP + P escape which frees inactivating site to accept next ATP

Actin

Myosin

ADP + P

ATP

Ca²⁺

- entering the cell from the extracellular fluid
- released from intracellular stores.

Both of these depend on pumps, carriers and channels governing the movement of calcium from one place to another (Fig. 4B.5).

The entry of calcium into the cell, and its release from compartments inside the cell where it is present at high concentrations, such as the endoplasmic reticulum (sarcoplasmic reticulum in muscle cells), is achieved by the transitory opening of calcium channels that simply allow calcium to diffuse into the sarcoplasm. On the other hand, removing the calcium from the sarcoplasm requires assistance, as it has to be moved from a region of low to high concentration. Carriers are present both in the cell membrane (sodium–calcium exchangers) and

in membranes of the sarcoplasmic reticulum (calcium pumps).

ISOTONIC AND ISOMETRIC CONTRACTION

Muscle contraction can be

- isotonic
- isometric.

Isotonic contraction occurs where the muscle is able to shorten. The muscle length is reduced but the tension remains the same, i.e. 'isotonic'. This is compared with isometric contraction where the muscle cannot shorten,

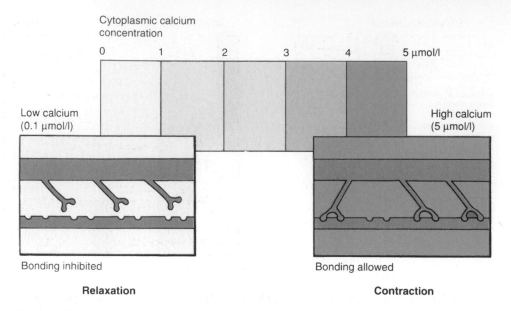

Figure 4B.4 Cytoplasmic calcium concentration and muscle contraction.

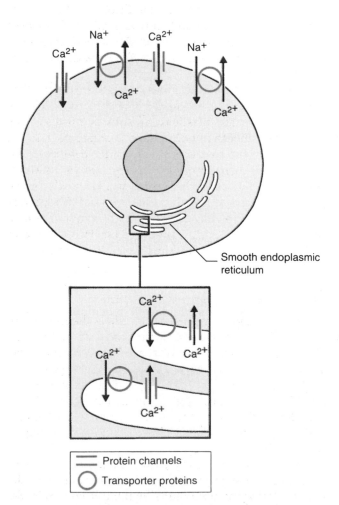

Figure 4B.5 Calcium movement into and out of the cytoplasm: ion channels allow calcium into the cytoplasm (sarcoplasm); transporter proteins eject calcium from it.

either because it is tethered at each end or because it is part of a closed chamber, e.g. a ventricle in the heart. In an isometric contraction the length remains the same – isometric – but the tension is increased. The energy and oxygen required for isometric contraction is much greater than for isotonic contraction (see Ch. 6).

SMOOTH MUSCLE

Smooth muscle is present in blood vessels, the gastrointestinal tract, the bile duct, the gall bladder, the uterus and fallopian tubes, the urinary bladder and ureters, and the bronchioles.

STRUCTURE

Smooth muscle is the least complex of the three types of muscle. The cells are small (50 to 700 μm in length), spindle-shaped and relatively featureless (Fig. 4B.6). They are linked to one another by gap junctions, which allow electrical impulses to spread from one cell to the next. Actin and myosin filaments are scattered throughout the cell, and the sarcoplasmic reticulum is sparse.

HOW CONTRACTION IS TRIGGERED

Most smooth muscle cells are spontaneously active, therefore no external stimuli are required to cause contraction. Instead the cells contract and relax regularly in response to their own internal mechanism

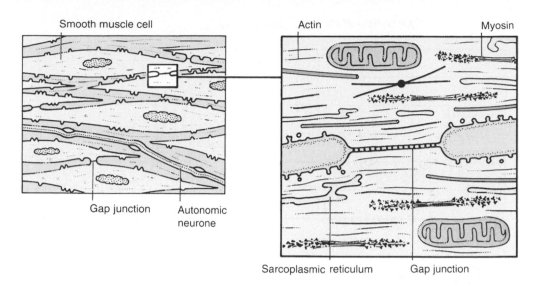

Figure 4B.6 Structure of smooth muscle cells. (After Williams et al 1989, with permission of Elsevier.)

of excitation. External stimuli can make the contractions stronger or weaker but they do not initiate contraction.

Spontaneous excitation

Contractions are triggered regularly as a result of a regular cycle of depolarization and repolarization of the cell membrane (slow wave) (Fig. 4B.7). The slow wave is caused by the regular opening and closing of ion channels in the cell membrane in a set sequence. At particular phases of this cycle, action potentials are triggered. These open calcium channels in the cell membrane and calcium flows into the cell, triggering contraction.

Role of calcium

Within the cell, calcium binds to calmodulin, and this complex promotes the bonding of actin and myosin, leading to contraction. The activity of the calcium pumps in the cell membrane is increased, calcium is pumped out of the cell, the intracellular calcium concentration falls, calcium detaches from calmodulin and the actin/myosin interaction is inhibited, leading to relaxation. This cycle is repeated regularly, contraction occurring each time there is a burst of action potentials (Fig. 4B.7).

FACTORS AFFECTING CONTRACTION

Stretch

If smooth muscle is stretched abruptly it responds by contracting. This response is said to be myogenic in that it originates within the muscle. Stretch is thought to depolarize the muscle and thus to excite it. Responses like this have been described in the smooth muscle of the gastrointestinal tract and in the smooth muscle of blood vessels.

If, however, the stretch is maintained, it is found that after an initial contraction the muscle 'gives'. This is referred to as the plasticity of smooth muscle. This property of smooth muscle is seen in organs such as the bladder, and the stomach. It allows the volume of the contents of these organs to vary greatly without substantially affecting the tension in their walls, or the pressure developed within the organ. Without this property, the stretch caused by filling would stimulate the muscle to contract, resulting either in resistance to further expansion or in premature expulsion of the contents.

Neural and hormonal control

Neurotransmitters and hormones affect the number of action potentials generated per cycle of activity by changing the excitability of the cell membrane. Some substances, such as acetylcholine, acting on the muscle of the gastrointestinal tract, depolarize the membrane making it more excitable. More action potentials are fired per cycle of activity, more calcium enters the cell, and consequently the resulting contraction is bigger (Fig. 4B.7).

Other substances, such as adrenaline acting on β_2 adrenergic receptors of gastrointestinal muscle, hyperpolarize the membrane, making it less excitable. Fewer action potentials are triggered (or even none if the effect is strong) and contractions become weaker or disappear (Fig. 4B.7).

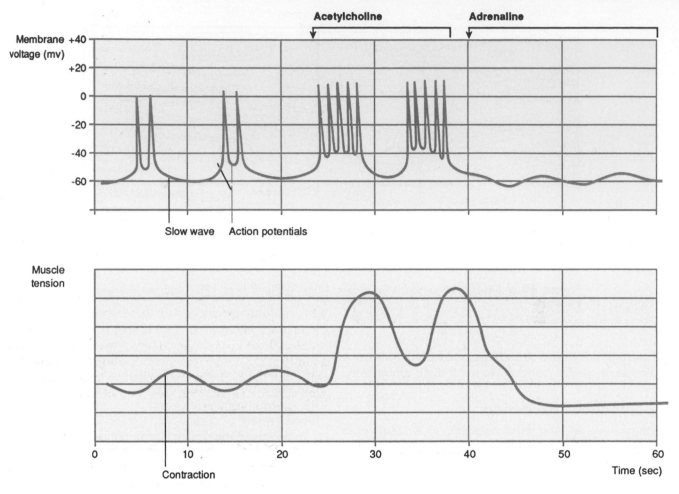

Figure 4B.7 The regular cycle of depolarization and repolarization (slow wave) characteristic of most smooth muscle cells. The slow wave triggers action potentials (top panel) that excite muscle contraction (bottom panel). Acetylcholine stimulates the muscle whereas adrenaline inhibits it.

INNERVATION OF SMOOTH MUSCLE

The nerve fibres that release transmitter onto the cells are interspersed between the muscle cells. The branching nerve fibres have swellings along their length (varicosities) from which transmitter is released (Fig. 4B.6). Once released, the transmitter diffuses over quite a wide area influencing any muscle cells in the vicinity. The membrane receptors to which the transmitters bind are distributed all over the muscle membrane. Blood-borne hormones reach their receptors by diffusing through the interstitial fluid.

COORDINATION OF ACTIVITY

Because of the gap junctions linking adjacent cells, if one smooth muscle cell is excited spontaneously or by the action of locally released neurotransmitter, the adjacent cell is also activated. The activity of neighbouring cells is thus co-opted and coordinated and cells work together as if they were a single unit (a syncytium).

MULTIUNIT SMOOTH MUSCLE

Multiunit smooth muscle is slightly different from the smooth muscle (single-unit or visceral muscle) described so far. One place in which multiunit muscle is found is the iris of the eye. Gap junctions are sparse in this form of smooth muscle. Consequently, excitation does not spread easily through the tissue. Also the cells are not spontaneously active. Instead, contraction is mainly controlled by the autonomic nerves with which it is richly innervated (see Ch. 5). In this respect, multiunit smooth muscle is more like skeletal muscle.

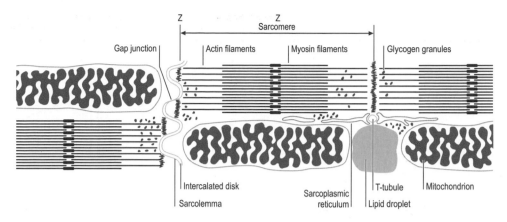

Figure 4B.8 The ultrastructure of cardiac muscle. (After Davies et al 2001, with permission of Elsevier.)

CARDIAC MUSCLE

The myocardium consists of two types of cells:

- contractile (atrial and ventricular muscle)
- conducting tissue (SA node, AV node, bundles of His, Purkinje cells) (see Ch. 6).

CONTRACTILE CELLS

Structure

The structure of the cardiac contractile cells is very different from smooth muscle (Fig. 4B.8). It has two distinctive features – intercalated discs and striations. Intercalated discs are specialized structures linking cells. They make up an interwoven network of cells, with gap junctions present. As a result, electrical events spread easily from cell to cell, as they do in smooth muscle. This means that cardiac muscle cells work as a unit, i.e. a functional syncytium. The cells appear striped (striated), with thick and thin filaments arranged in an orderly manner, interleaved and arranged in groups, which are divided by the 'Z line' (sarcomeres). This arrangement is repeated (Fig. 4B.9), leading to bands of light and dark, i.e.

- no overlap ('I (isotropic) band')
- thick/thin overlap ('A (anisotropic) band').

(Isotropic – allowing the same amount of light to pass through (as the background), i.e. 'light' band; anisotropic – not allowing the same amount of light to pass through, i.e. 'dark' band.)

Other features

Contractile cells have many mitochondria, lying between the myofibrils that generate the ATP that powers the contraction. The sarcoplasmic reticulum, which is more extensive than that in smooth muscle, is an important store of intracellular calcium. It is interlaced between the myofibrils. The T-tubules form an invaginated cell membrane, dipping deeply into the cell interior to form long narrow tubes, and are responsible for the transmission of the excitatory impulses into the cell.

How contraction is triggered

Cardiac muscle, like smooth muscle, contracts and relaxes regularly. But, unlike smooth muscle, the control of excitation lies not with the contractile cells but with the conducting tissue. The conducting tissue generates action potentials, which are transmitted to the muscle cells and act as the pacemakers for the muscle cells.

Cardiac action potential

When cardiac muscle cells are excited, they generate an action potential that is conducted along the cell membrane and carried deep into the interior along the membrane forming the T-tubules. The action potential is strikingly different from that recorded in nerve axons. It lasts about 100 times longer and it has a plateau (Fig. 4B.10). However, the first part, the rapid depolarization and reversal of membrane voltage, is similar in form and basis to that in nerve axons. It is caused by the opening of voltage-gated sodium channels. The plateau that follows is caused by the opening of voltage-gated calcium channels. Because these stay open for quite a time, the membrane voltage cannot return to its unexcited state very quickly. Eventually, however, the original potential is restored as these channels close.

The long plateau is important. It is longer than the time taken for the muscle to complete a contraction and,

Muscle cell

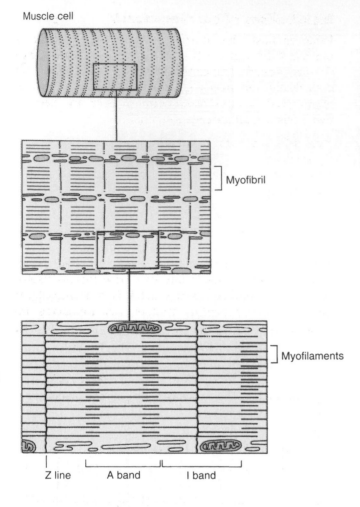

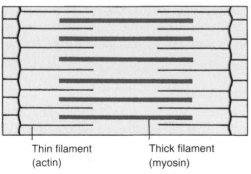

Figure 4B.9 Basic structure of striated (i.e. striped) muscle: organization of filaments and fibrils within a muscle fibre (cell) giving rise to its striped appearance.

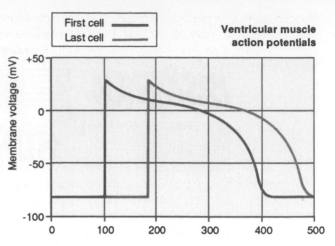

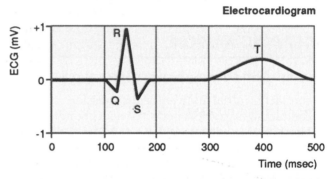

Figure 4B.10 The shape of the cardiac action potential (top panel). Two separate action potentials are shown, one from the first muscle cell in the ventricle to be excited, and the other from the last cell. The action potentials from the rest of the muscle occur between these two (shaded area). Clearly during the periods 100–180 msec and 300–500 msec there is a lot of electrical disturbance as one after the other the cells depolarize and repolarize. These two periods of electrical activity are picked up in the electrocardiogram (ECG) as the QRS and T waves respectively (bottom panel).

Role of calcium

Calcium channels open during an action potential, allowing calcium to enter the cell from the extracellular fluid. The action potential is transmitted down the T-tubule, thereby stimulating the sarcoplasmic reticulum. This produces calcium release from the sarcoplasmic reticulum. Since calcium comes from two sources there is a shorter time to contraction. Calcium binds to troponin that is attached to tropomyosin (on actin filaments). The troponin/tropomyosin complex inhibits the actin/myosin interaction. When calcium binds to troponin the troponin/tropomyosin complex is displaced, allowing the myosin heads to bind to actin. When the calcium levels fall, the inhibitory effect of the troponin/

since the cells remain refractory during this time, the next contraction cannot be stimulated. Cardiac contractions are therefore clearly separated single events. In comparison, skeletal muscle, without the electrical plateau, will respond to a second stimulus near the end of the first contraction; the effect is then a sustained contraction. Sustained contraction of the heart muscle would be fatal.

tropomyosin complex is restored. This occurs more quickly than in smooth muscle because calcium is pumped back into the sarcoplasm as well as being transported out of the cell.

Factors affecting contraction

Stretch

In striated muscle, the strength of contraction depends upon the extent to which the muscle is stretched. If the muscle is pulled to a greater length, the same stimulus produces a bigger force of contraction. This property of striated muscle is referred to in Chapter 6 in relation to the Frank–Starling mechanism. The reason for this behaviour is not fully understood. It has been suggested to be due to the degree of overlap of the actin and myosin filaments, which changes as the muscle is stretched, and the number of crossbridges which can therefore be formed. A more recent theory is that the stretching of the filaments somehow increases the affinity of troponin–tropomyosin for calcium.

Neural and hormonal control

The bigger the increase in calcium concentration inside the cell, the bigger is the resulting contraction. The hormone adrenaline, and the neurotransmitter noradrenaline released from sympathetic nerves, both act on β_1 receptors in the cell membrane affecting the channels allowing calcium to flow into the cell when it is excited. The drug digoxin indirectly raises intracellular calcium concentration by partially inhibiting the Na^+/K^+ pump. This increases intracellular sodium concentration and, in so doing, reduces the amount of calcium extruded from the cell by sodium–calcium exchange (see Fig. 4B.5).

Innervation

Both atrial and ventricular muscle tissue are innervated by sympathetic nerve fibres, but only atrial muscle is innervated to any extent by parasympathetic fibres. There are no specific junctions between the nerve and the muscle cells. Transmitter released from the varicosities influences several muscle cells. This is similar to the arrangement in smooth muscle.

Coordination of activity

Because the cells are linked to one another by gap junctions in the intercalated discs (Fig. 4B.8), the electrical excitation of one cell spreads to neighbouring cells so that, once excited, cardiac muscle cells all contract almost simultaneously. This coordinated activity is also helped by the rapid distribution of the excitatory signal to all cells by the specialized conducting tissue (see below).

Metabolism of cardiac muscle

Whereas most other muscles in the body have spells of inactivity, the heart beats from early in embryonic life to the day of death. This continual activity is dependent on a sufficient and steady supply of ATP. The supply is guaranteed by the production of ATP by aerobic metabolism. Cardiac cells contain:

- an abundance of mitochondria to generate ATP aerobically
- myoglobin that, like haemoglobin, binds oxygen reversibly.

The fuel used by the cells is chiefly fatty acids, though glucose can be used in large amounts as well, particularly after carbohydrate-rich meals. The heart muscle, unlike skeletal muscle, metabolizes lactate. In exercise, when plasma lactate levels rise, this is a useful adaptation to reduce levels of lactate in heart muscle, at the same time providing another fuel. Ketoacids are used in starvation and uncontrolled diabetes. The

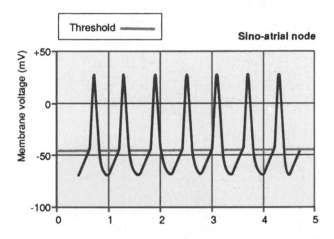

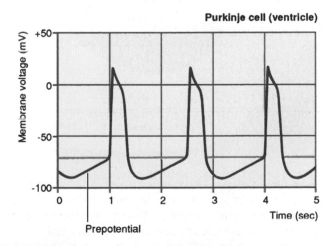

Figure 4B.11 Electrical activity recorded from two different types of cell in the heart (sino-atrial node cell and Purkinje cell) when each is allowed to depolarize and repolarize at its own pace.

supply of fuels and oxygen is guaranteed by a very rich network of blood vessels (see Ch. 12). If the flow of blood to a part of the heart muscle is reduced so that the tissue is deprived of oxygen, the consequences are more serious than in skeletal muscle because the capacity of cardiac cells to generate ATP anaerobically is much more limited.

CONDUCTING CELLS

Conducting cells generate impulses that excite cardiac muscle and set heart rate. They carry the primary signal that is generated in the sino-atrial (SA) node (the pacemaker). The impulses are generated spontaneously. An action potential fires when the voltage drops below threshold (Fig. 4B.11). The conducting tissue is spontaneously active. The impulse frequency of the SA node is higher than the other cells, therefore the SA node sets the pace.

Neural and hormonal control

The slow depolarization (prepotential) occurring just ahead of the action potential (Fig. 4B.11) is believed to be caused by a decrease in the permeability of the membrane to potassium and an increase in permeability to sodium and calcium. The slope of this prepotential is affected by noradrenaline from the sympathetic nerve terminals, and acetylcholine from the parasympathetic fibres. Noradrenaline, acting on β_1 receptors, increases the flow of sodium and calcium into the cell and speeds up the rate of depolarization. Threshold is reached more speedily and so it takes less time for an action potential to be fired. Repolarization also occurs more quickly and as a result the number of impulses generated per minute increases.

Acetylcholine, in contrast, promotes the opening of potassium channels in the membrane. This restrains depolarization and so it takes longer for the voltage to reach threshold. Consequently heart rate decreases.

SKELETAL MUSCLE

The amount of skeletal muscle tissue in the body is considerable (normally 40–50% of the body weight in an adult).

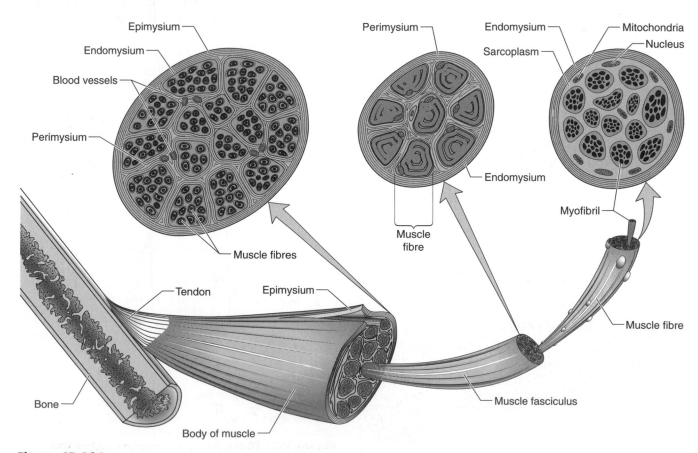

Figure 4B.12A

STRUCTURE

Skeletal muscle is made up of exceedingly long cells, which are a fusion of many cell units end to end. This structure forms long multinucleated fibres (Fig. 4B.1), with the ends anchored in the tendon, which, in turn, is firmly attached to the skeleton. There are no cross connections and no gap junctions. Skeletal muscle is striated in appearance and also possesses a T-tubule system. It has an extensive network of sarcoplasmic reticulum, which stores and releases calcium. Like cardiac muscle, skeletal muscle fibres are striated in appearance (Fig. 4B.12).

HOW CONTRACTION IS TRIGGERED

Skeletal muscle fibres do not normally contract unless stimulated by nerve impulses. When excited, an action potential is generated by the muscle membrane (sarcolemma), conducted up and down the fibre, as well as being carried down the T-tubules. The opening of Na$^+$ channels causes a muscle action potential.

Muscle action potential

The muscle action potential is similar to that in nerve fibres. It is caused by the opening of voltage-gated sodium channels. Voltage-gated sodium/calcium channels are not involved. The muscle action potential therefore does not have a plateau and it lasts for only a short time (2–4 msec).

Role of calcium

The muscle action potential causes the release of calcium from the sarcoplasmic reticulum. Little or no calcium enters from the extracellular fluid. Just as in cardiac muscle, calcium binds to the troponin/tropomyosin complex and the process continues as for cardiac muscle.

FACTORS AFFECTING CONTRACTION

Stretch

Like cardiac muscle, if the length at which skeletal muscle is held is varied, the force of contraction developed varies too. The basis of this is believed to be

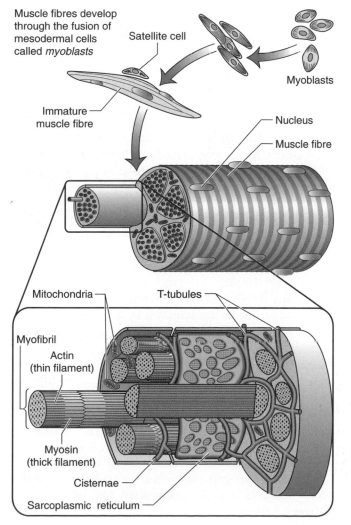

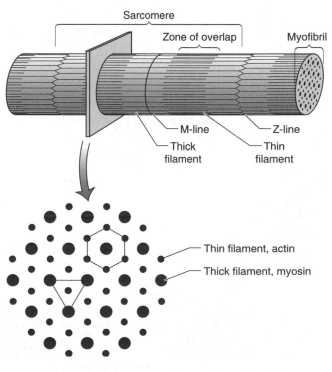

Figure 4B.12B The structure of normal muscle. (After Sambrook et al 2001, with permission of Elsevier.)

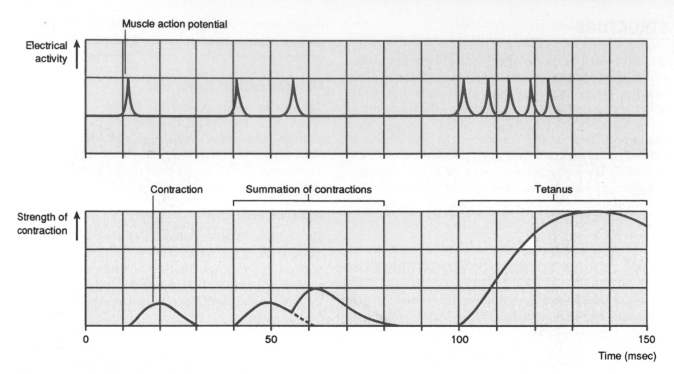

Figure 4B.13 The relationship between electrical and contractile events in skeletal muscle. The contractile process outlasts the duration of the action potential. Consequently, another contraction can begin before the first one has finished, resulting in a much bigger overall contraction.

the same as in cardiac muscle. The relaxed length of skeletal muscle fibres in the body has been shown to be their optimum length for the development of force.

Neural control: frequency of action potentials

The duration of the muscle action potential is very much shorter than the duration of the contractile events that are triggered by it (Fig. 4B.13). Consequently, it is possible for a second action potential to be generated in the muscle membrane long before the muscle fibre has completed its cycle of contraction and relaxation. As a result, more calcium is released from the sarcoplasmic reticulum to add to that remaining from the previous impulse and a second contraction is added on top of the first (summation). If a whole series of impulses excite the fibre, the contractions are added on top of one another so swiftly that a smooth and very strong contraction results (tetanus) (see 'Cardiac muscle' section).

INNERVATION

Organization

Skeletal muscle cells are innervated by motor neurones of the somatic nervous system. The nerve terminals form specific contacts with the fibres at a region known as the motor end-plate (Fig. 4B.14). In the adult there is just one end-plate per muscle fibre, and this is usually situated at about the midpoint of the fibre.

However, one nerve axon branches to form several endings, so that one motor neurone in fact innervates not just one fibre but a group of fibres (Fig. 4B.14). The group may be large (e.g. about 2000 fibres in calf muscles) or small (about 10 fibres in muscles of the eyeball). The motor neurone plus all the muscle fibres it innervates is termed a motor unit.

The force developed by a muscle, such as the biceps, depends on the size of the motor units activated. Small forces are developed by activating the small motor units. Larger forces are achieved by activating the large motor units as well (recruitment).

Neuromuscular junction

The junction between the nerve terminal and the skeletal muscle fibre is intricate in structure. The nerve terminal sits in a recess in the muscle cell (Fig. 4B.14). Beneath the nerve terminal, the muscle cell membrane is thrown into folds. The gap between the nerve and the muscle cell (50 to 100 nm – about 1 million times smaller than the gap between the two letter l's of the word 'cell') is a little larger than that at synapses between nerves.

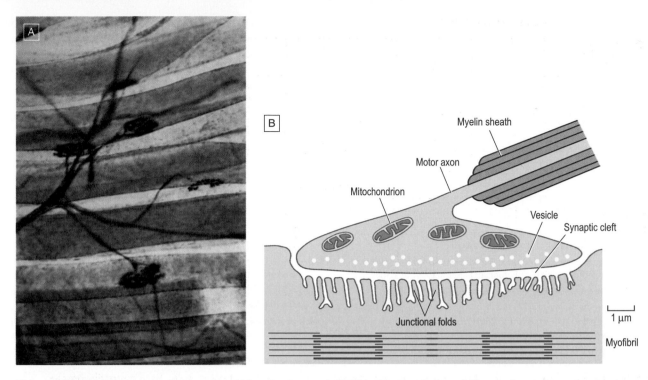

Figure 4B.14 Neuromuscular junction. (After Davies et al 2001, with permission of Elsevier.)

When a single nerve impulse arrives at the terminal it triggers the release of acetylcholine from about 200 to 300 vesicles. The acetylcholine diffuses across the synapse and binds to nicotinic receptors in the membrane. When activated, these receptors increase the permeability of the membrane to sodium and potassium ions, thus depolarizing the membrane. This depolarization is termed the end-plate potential.

End-plate potential

In character, the end-plate potential (epp) resembles an epsp in a nerve cell (see Ch. 4A).

It:

- lasts longer than an action potential
- can be summated
- fades away on either side of the end-plate.

But the epp differs from an epsp in that it is normally always big enough to generate an action potential in the muscle membrane on either side of the end-plate. One action potential in the nerve terminal therefore normally always gives rise to one action potential in the muscle fibre.

Acetylcholinesterase is present at the end-plate. Consequently acetylcholine is swiftly broken down as in other cholinergic synapses. If this enzyme is inhibited by an anticholinesterase, such as neostigmine, the end-plate potential increases and lasts for longer. This drug has been used to treat myasthenia gravis, a condition in which there is a shortage of functional nicotinic receptors at the end-plate.

Effects of denervation

If the nerves to skeletal muscle are severed, as they may be as a result of an accident, the nerve terminals degenerate, and changes occur in the muscle. These include:

- hypersensitivity to acetylcholine
- atrophy (wasting) and eventual loss of the muscle fibres.

If a group of muscles is paralysed but the antagonists (opposing muscle group) are still functioning, then contraction deformities may occur. For example, 'claw hand' in untreated ulnar paralysis.

Hypersensitivity

When nerve terminals degenerate and the concentration of acetylcholine at the end-plate decreases, the muscle fibre responds by increasing the number of receptors inserted into the muscle membrane (upregulation – see Ch. 11). Consequently, the muscle fibre becomes very responsive (hypersensitive) to small amounts of transmitter. Whereas in a normal muscle fibre the receptors are restricted to the end-plate, in a denervated muscle fibre they are inserted all over the membrane. This probably increases the chances of the cell being brought under the control of the regrowing nerve fibre.

Atrophy

At least two reasons have been suggested for the atrophy of skeletal muscle cells as a result of denervation:

- lack of use
- loss of growth factors secreted by the nerve terminals.

Muscles that are exercised can grow larger (hypertrophy), whereas inactivity results in wasting (atrophy). This may be due to the direct effects of activity of the muscle cells or may be due to factors released from the nerve. If the muscle is re-innervated within a few months through the regrowth of axons, or the sprouting of adjacent motor neurones, then the muscle also regrows.

REFERENCES AND FURTHER READING

Aidley D J 1998 The physiology of excitable cells, 4th edn. Cambridge University Press, Cambridge

Alberts B, Johnson A, Lewis J, Raff M, Roberts K, Walter P 2002 Molecular biology of the cell. Garland Science, New York

Berne R M 2002 Cardiovascular physiology, 8th edn. Mosby, St Louis

Davies A, Blakeley A G H, Kidd C 2001 Human physiology. Churchill Livingstone, Edinburgh

Imai S 1999 Muscle physiology and biochemistry. Kluwer Academic Publishers, Dordrecht

Jones D A, Round J M 1990 Skeletal muscle in health and disease: a workbook of muscle physiology. Manchester University Press, Manchester

Junqueira L C, Carneiro J, Kelley R O 1998 Basic histology, 9th edn. Appleton & Lange, East Norwalk, CT

Keynes R D, Aidley J 2001 Nerve and muscle, 3rd edn. Cambridge University Press, Cambridge

Matthews G G 1998 Cellular physiology of nerve and muscle, 3rd edn. Blackwell Scientific Publications, Oxford

Sambrook P, Schrieber L, Taylor T, Ellis A 2001 The musculoskeletal system: basic science and clinical conditions. Churchill Livingstone, Edinburgh

Stone R J, Stone J A 1999 Atlas of skeletal muscles. McGraw-Hill, New York

Williams P L, Warwick R, Dyson M, Bannister L H 1989 Gray's Anatomy. Churchill Livingstone, Edinburgh

5 The autonomic nervous system

In practice you may be asked to consider the following:

1. You are taking someone's pulse. You can feel the rate rise as you are counting. Which autonomic division have you stimulated?

2. The room where you are is cold. Your patient's hands are cold and the skin is pale. Which receptors are responsible for the skin vasoconstriction?

3. Sympathetic stimulation of the adrenal medulla causes the release of which neurohormones?

4. A patient has myasthenia gravis. Neostigmine helps the condition, but causes autonomic 'side' effects. What autonomic effects can it produce and how could they, in turn, be treated?

5. Why is it necessary to use tropicamide or a similar drug when an ophthalmoscope is used?

6. Tropicamide is a short-acting substance, but how could it be reversed if necessary?

7. A patient with a history of asthma has been prescribed an adrenoceptor blocker. A β_1 selective blocker is required. Why?

8. The catecholamines can produce vasoconstriction and vasodilation. How is this achieved?

9. The thought of food can produce a flow of saliva even before you eat it. Which division, which transmitter, which receptor site type and which target tissues?

10. Urinary retention may be caused by stress or fear. Please explain.

The nervous system can be thought of as two parts:

- somatic
- autonomic.

The somatic nervous system is concerned with activities which are conscious and voluntary, and which are part of the interaction with the external environment. It monitors external events and enables the body to interact with and influence those events. The somatic nervous system is described in detail in Section 2 of this book.

The autonomic nervous system (ANS) has sensory signals usually below the level of consciousness and effects which are involuntary. It is chiefly concerned with control of the activities of the organs and tissues which maintain and regulate the internal environment. It supplies the cells of:

- the cardiovascular system (Ch. 6)
- the respiratory system (Ch. 7)
- the renal and urinary system (Ch. 8)
- the gastrointestinal system (Ch. 9)
- the liver (Ch. 10)
- the endocrine glands (Ch. 11).

Much of the internal environment is controlled by the ANS. The regulation of many homeostatic parameters such as blood pressure, blood gases and gut activity is shared by the ANS and endocrine system. However, the short-term, more immediate control is almost entirely the province of the ANS.

ORGANIZATION

The ANS is driven both directly from the higher centres in the brain and reflexly by the lower brain in response to 'body' signals. For example, the sight of blood at a road traffic accident can activate a range of autonomic responses in the bystander almost as powerfully as can the injury in the accident victim.

The 'normal' level of homeostatic regulation by ANS, however, is achieved by a series of reflexes (a reflex can be defined as 'the same stimulus always producing the same effect'). Sensory information goes via afferent pathways to the brain (or cord) to be organized by the interneurones in the brain and cord, which in turn stimulate motor activity via efferent pathways. The outline organization is shown in Figure 5.1.

AUTONOMIC SENSORY COMPONENTS

Sensory receptors are widely distributed in organs and tissues and respond to a variety of stimuli. The recep-

Table 5.1 Autonomic sensory receptors and the parameters which they monitor

Sensory receptor	Homeostatic parameter monitored
Mechanoreceptors	
baroreceptors	Blood pressure (blood vessels, atria)
stretch receptors	Stretch in gut wall, bladder and respiratory tract
Osmoreceptors	Osmotic pressure – concentration of body fluids
Chemoreceptors	Concentrations of chemicals, e.g. oxygen, carbon dioxide, H^+
Thermoreceptors	Core and surface temperature
Nociceptors	Tissue damage

tors include those in Table 5.1, shown with the aspect of internal environment which they monitor. Even this short list makes it clear how much of the internal environment depends on autonomic mechanisms.

AUTONOMIC CENTRAL AND INTEGRATING COMPONENTS

The central areas

The hypothalamus is the major central area coordinating and controlling homeostasis. Continuous streams of sensory information on all the homeostatic parameters are relayed to the hypothalamus, which can then coordinate the responses to be made. In addition to its control of the ANS, it has an important role in coordinating many of the endocrine systems, and it is at this level that many ANS and endocrine activities are integrated. It should be remembered, however, that despite its apparently powerful role, the hypothalamus is not independent. Under certain circumstances, such as the road traffic accident earlier, all its autonomic and endocrine mechanisms can be affected by stimuli from the cerebral cortex. Even in less dramatic circumstances, many of the autonomic reflexes can be inhibited by voluntary control, for example, the bladder emptying reflex shown in Figure 5.2.

Other areas with central ANS activity are the pons, medulla oblongata and cord; these are the central components of brain stem and spinal reflexes. The medulla oblongata has within it many of the 'operating' centres for ANS controlled mechanisms, such as changing heart rate, vascular capacity and gut function. The pons is the site of the upper part of the respiratory complex which also has components in the medulla oblongata (see Ch. 7). The activities of these operating centres are integrated by the hypothalamus.

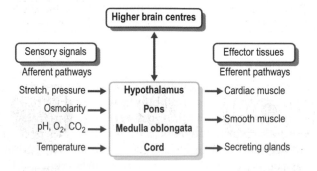

Figure 5.1 Outline organization of the autonomic nervous system.

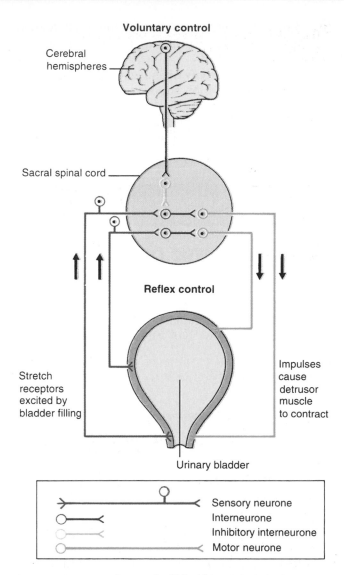

Figure 5.2 Neural control of bladder emptying.

ANS pathways and are sometimes referred to as the enteric nervous system.

AUTONOMIC MOTOR COMPONENTS

Anatomically and functionally, the motor output of the ANS can be divided into two divisions, the parasympathetic division and the sympathetic division.

The two divisions usually have opposite effects on a tissue, one excitatory and the other inhibitory. Since the pathways are always active (described as being tonically active), with a variable level of activity, the effect on the tissue will depend on the balance of activity in each division. The classical phrase describing this is that the effects of the two divisions are 'antagonistic but synergistic'. The outcome is that the body can vary tissue function according to requirement.

Of the two divisions, the parasympathetic is probably simpler than the sympathetic division. The parasympathetic system is a kind of 'in-house maintenance system', running body activities at an economical level, managing absorption and digestion of food and excretion of waste products. The sympathetic system is associated with higher levels of activity, work, exercise, excitement. The phrase associated with the sympathetic response is 'flight, fight and fright', although this suggests that the sympathetic system is active only in extreme circumstances. In fact, as with parasympathetic activity, sympathetic tonic activity goes on continuously, for example maintaining blood pressure while just standing upright.

Local interneurones

Some interneurones form a network called a plexus (pleural plexi) which is the integrating component of a local autonomic reflex. Good examples are the plexus systems found in the gastrointestinal tract (see Ch. 9).

The myenteric plexus (Auerbach's plexus) lies between the circular and longitudinal layers of muscle of the tract, and the mucosal plexus (Meissner's plexus) between the mucosa and submucosa. Sensory endings respond to local stimuli within the gut, e.g. the degree of stretch, affecting the interneurones within the plexus. These in turn affect local effector cells in the gut, such as the secretory or muscle cells. These local reflexes are an important part of the functioning of the gut and an example of mechanisms which allow local responses to be exactly matched to local conditions. These reflexes are able to function without the influence of the main

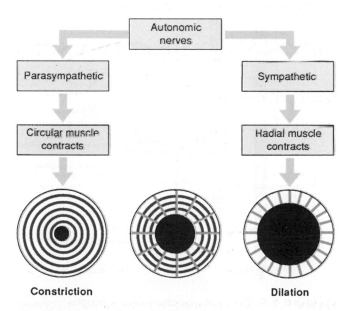

Figure 5.3 Neural control of pupil diameter.

Dual innervation and cooperative effects

Many organs such as heart, gut and bladder have both supplies; this is dual innervation. The sympathetic effect on heart rate is to increase it, the parasympathetic effect is to reduce it, the combined effect is to give a variable rate suited to requirement (see Chs 6 and 12). The response of a tissue depends on the balance of activity in each division. Heart rate can be made to increase not only by increasing sympathetic activity but also by decreasing parasympathetic activity.

Some structures are made up of two tissues, each with its own supply and each producing a different effect, the two acting in cooperation. The iris of the eye, for example, is made up of two rings of muscle, the radial and the concentric (or circular) muscles. The radial muscle has only sympathetic supply and contracts when stimulated, dilating the pupil. The concentric muscle is supplied by the parasympathetic division only and will also contract when stimulated. Contraction of this circular structure will constrict the pupil.

The cooperative effect is to manage the pupil diameter and allow light appropriate to the circumstances to enter the eye (Fig. 5.3).

Some tissues have only one supply. For example, only the sympathetic division supplies the adrenal medulla and only the parasympathetic division has control of the ciliary muscles which alter the shape, and so the focal length, of the lens of the eye.

THE PARASYMPATHETIC DIVISION OF THE ANS

PARASYMPATHETIC OUTFLOW

The central or interneurones for the efferent parasympathetic nerves lie in the brain stem and the cord. The outflow is via cranial and sacral nerves, i.e. a cranio-sacral outflow. Not all of these nerves carry

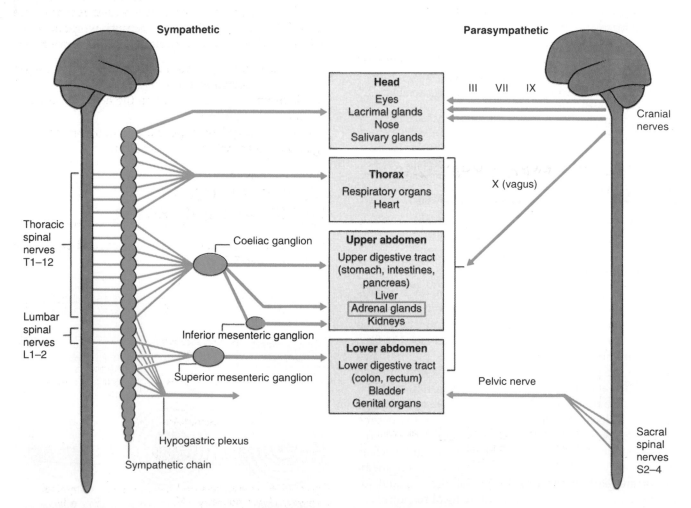

Figure 5.4 The parasympathetic and sympathetic divisions of the autonomic nervous system and the tissues they supply.

parasympathetic fibres. The head is supplied by the oculomotor (third), facial (seventh) and glosso-pharyngeal (ninth) cranial nerves, the thorax and upper abdomen by the vagus (tenth) and its branches. The second to fourth sacral nerves supply the lower gut, bladder and external genitalia (Fig. 5.4). (The spinal nerves contain nerve fibres of the somatic nervous system as well as ANS fibres).

PATHWAY STRUCTURE

Each parasympathetic efferent pathway is composed of two neurones, one presynaptic and one postsynaptic, the presynaptic long and myelinated and the postsynaptic short and unmyelinated (Fig. 5.5). At some tissues, the postsynaptic axon is so short that the synapse is almost on the tissue surface.

Although each separate pathway is constructed as in Figure 5.5, the outflow consists of numerous pathways running together as nerve tracts. In addition, each presynaptic neurone may synapse with several post-synaptic neurones. The synapse regions are located close to one another in the tracts and the presence of the group of postsynaptic cell bodies shows as a lump or small swelling known as a neural ganglion. The terminology was adapted to suit and presynaptic neurones are also known as preganglionic and the postsynaptic neurones as postganglionic neurones. Parasympathetic ganglia are close to or on the target tissue surface.

ACTIVITY IN A PARASYMPATHETIC PATHWAY

Acetylcholine is the transmitter used at both ganglionic and neuroeffector junctions in the parasympathetic division. However, different types of receptor are used at the two locations (see also Chs 2 and 4A).

CHOLINERGIC RECEPTORS

The receptors at the ganglia and the effector tissue have two types of molecular structure. Both types of site are cholinergic, i.e. worked by acetylcholine, but the different molecular structures give different responses to acetylcholine. The sites on the postsynaptic surface at the ganglion are described as nicotinic, and those on the tissue surface, at the neuroeffector junction, as muscarinic (Fig. 5.6). The receptor sites are therefore cholinergic (nicotinic) and cholinergic (muscarinic).

The adjectives 'nicotinic' and 'muscarinic' originate from the substances used in the early work to distinguish between the two types of cholinergic receptor. It was found that the postsynaptic site could also be made to work with small doses of nicotine and the tissue receptors with muscarine. Nicotine and muscarine mimicked the effects of acetylcholine at those sites and gave their names to the site type. Many subtypes of autonomic receptor have been and are still being identified; only the most commonly used are included here.

To date, five molecular types of muscarinic receptor have been identified. Three muscarinic receptor site types, M_1, M_2 and M_3, are recognized pharmacologically and central M_4 receptors have been identified.

- M_1 is excitatory, e.g. found in the gut. Activity causes gastric acid secretion and muscle contraction.
- M_2 is inhibitory and is found in the heart; the effect is to reduce heart rate.
- M_3 is excitatory. This type is found in secretory glands and activity causes secretion.

TISSUE RESPONSES TO PARASYMPATHETIC ACTIVITY

Examples of effects in the major systems and organs are shown in Table 5.2.

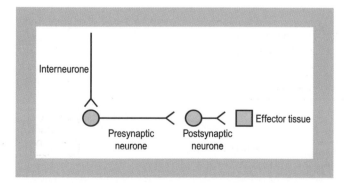

Figure 5.5 A typical parasympathetic pathway.

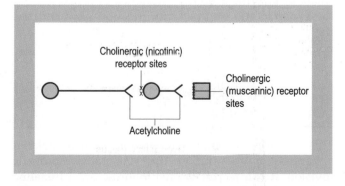

Figure 5.6 Transmitters and receptor sites in a typical parasympathetic pathway. (After Watson 1999, with permission of Elsevier.)

Table 5.2 Tissue effects produced by parasympathetic activity

System/organ	Tissue effects
Cardiovascular system	Reduced heart rate Vasodilation at tongue, salivary glands, gut, external sex organs
Gut	Increased motility, secretions
Pancreas	Increased exocrine secretion Increased insulin and glucagon release
Bladder	Contraction of bladder wall Relaxation of internal sphincter
Eye	Contraction of constrictor (circular) muscle of iris – pupil constriction Contraction of ciliary muscle – shortening and thickening of lens (near focus)

Parasympathetic ganglia are not interconnected and they are also very close to, or in some cases on the surface of, the target tissues. Parasympathetic effects can therefore be closely targeted to a tissue or organ, without other structures being affected. The urinary bladder, for example, is reflexly stimulated by parasympathetic nerves in response to distension, but the bladder can be emptied without causing simultaneous emptying of the bowel!

TRANSMITTER CATABOLISM

In order that any nerve pathway can be kept working, the transmitter, once released, must be used and then destroyed. If it is allowed to accumulate, continued stimulation would inhibit the generation of a new action potential in the postsynaptic neurone and activity in the effector tissue would be disturbed. The catabolic enzyme acetylcholinesterase is found in both the synaptic and neuroeffector junction gaps and has the effect of breaking down acetylcholine so that it can no longer act as a transmitter.

THE SYMPATHETIC DIVISION OF THE ANS

This division has many adaptations which make it apparently more complex than the parasympathetic division. It can recruit the neurohormones, adrenaline and noradrenaline, to give the sympathomedullary or sympathoadrenal effects. The receptor sites have more identified subtypes, one of which provides a negative feedback mechanism. The concentration of the transmitter or neurohormone is also more critical since the sensitivity of the receptor sites varies more.

The transmitter noradrenaline and the neurohormones adrenaline and noradrenaline have alternative names *norepinephrine* (noradrenaline) and *epinephrine* (adrenaline). The strategy, likely to be agreed for prescribing authorities in the United Kingdom, is to retain the names noradrenaline and adrenaline (Medicines Control Agency Consultation document, 2002). This text uses these names as recommended.

SYMPATHETIC OUTFLOW

The interneurones in the cord give rise to efferent pathways emerging from the cord at the thoracic and upper lumbar segments; the system therefore has a thoraco-lumbar outflow (Fig. 5.4). Like the parasympathetic outflow, each pathway is composed of two neurones, one presynaptic (preganglionic), the other postsynaptic (postganglionic).

PATHWAY STRUCTURE

The typical sympathetic pathway consists of a short, myelinated preganglionic neurone followed by a long, amyelinated postganglionic neurone (Fig. 5.7).

The nerve tracts are made up of numerous individual pathways running in tracts; therefore the groups of synapses are marked by substantial ganglia. Most of the ganglia are arranged in two chains (the bilateral sympathetic chains), one on either side of the spinal column. Some preganglionic neurones run, uninterrupted, through the spinal ganglia to synapse in the coeliac and mesenteric ganglia situated outside the chains (Fig. 5.4). Postganglionic neurones from these ganglia supply gut and bladder.

The adrenal medulla is supplied by preganglionic neurones emerging from the mid-lumbar segments.

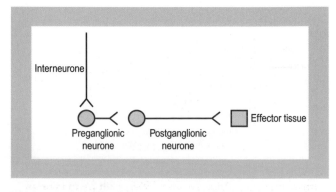

Figure 5.7 A typical sympathetic pathway.

ACTIVITY IN A SYMPATHETIC PATHWAY

The transmitter used at the synapse in sympathetic pathways is acetylcholine; all autonomic ganglia use this transmitter. The receptor sites at sympathetic ganglia are, as with those at parasympathetic ganglia, cholinergic and nicotinic. The transmitter released by most sympathetic postganglionic neurones is noradrenaline. The receptor sites on the effector tissues are adrenergic receptors or adrenoceptors (Fig. 5.8) (see also Chs 2 and 4A).

SYMPATHOMEDULLARY EFFECT

One of the additional aspects of the sympathetic division is its ability to recruit the neurohormones of the adrenal medulla, noradrenaline and adrenaline, referred to by their chemical group name catecholamines. The adrenal medulla is supplied by sympathetic preganglionic nerves (Fig. 5.9) and stimulation causes the release of the catecholamines

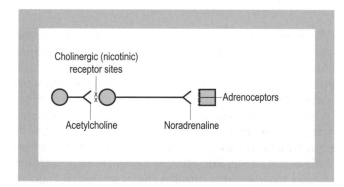

Figure 5.8 Transmitters and receptor sites in a typical sympathetic pathway. (After Watson 1999, with permission of Elsevier.)

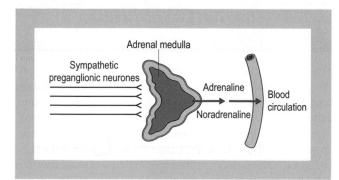

Figure 5.9 Sympathetic preganglionic supply to the adrenal medulla. (After Watson 1999, with permission of Elsevier.)

into the general circulation. They are produced in the ratio of approximately 4:1 adrenaline to noradrenaline, from the amino acid tyrosine. The last step in the series of reactions is the conversion of noradrenaline to adrenaline by the action of the enzyme phenylethanolamine-*N*-methyltransferase (PNMT).

They are rapidly distributed throughout the body and can affect any tissue which has the appropriate adrenoceptor sites. Therefore tissues with no direct sympathetic nerve supply can produce a 'sympathetic' response. Where a tissue has a sympathetic nerve supply, the circulating catecholamines will augment the effect of the noradrenaline produced by the nerve. The sympathetic/sympathomedullary response is often referred to as the fight or flight response.

ADRENOCEPTORS

Adrenoceptors are of different subtypes, α and β, and these are further subdivided into α_1 and α_2, β_1, β_2 and β_3. Each of the subtypes is capable of a different effect and the same subtype may give different effects at different tissues. Noradrenaline, for example, acting on α_1 will cause vasoconstriction at smooth muscle in an arteriole but relaxation at smooth muscle in the gut wall.

Noradrenaline and the neurohormone adrenaline, although both catecholamines, have different effects on adrenoceptors. Their effects on the receptor site types are compared below.

TISSUE EFFECTS OF ADRENALINE AND NORADRENALINE COMPARED

Adrenaline and noradrenaline share some effects but there are marked differences between the two catecholamines:

- noradrenaline has a more pronounced effect on α receptors, adrenaline on β receptors.

Adrenaline has important metabolic effects mediated through β receptors, for example mobilization of liver glycogen and gluconeogenesis, both resulting in the increased availability of glucose. Since adrenaline also suppresses insulin release, it plays an important role in the maintenance of plasma glucose (see Ch. 18). This effect assumes great importance in physical stress or injury where maintaining an adequate plasma glucose level is part of the survival strategy of the body. Details of other endocrine characteristics of adrenaline can be found in Chapter 11.

Examples of catecholamine effects in the major systems and organs are shown in Table 5.3.

Table 5.3 Tissue effects produced by sympathetic/sympathomedullary activity

System/organ	Adrenoceptor	Tissue effects	Produced by
Central or presynaptic adrenoceptors	α_2	Inhibition of further release of catecholamines (negative feedback mechanism)	Both
Cardiovascular system			
heart	β_1	Increased rate	Both
		Force of contraction	Both
blood vessels	α_1	Constriction	Noradrenaline
	β_2	Dilation	Adrenaline
	*(Cholinergic(M)	Dilation	Acetylcholine)
Bladder			
wall	β_2	Relaxation	Adrenaline
sphincter	α_1	Contraction	Both
Airways	β_2	Bronchodilation	Adrenaline
Gut	α_1, β_2	Tissue dependent	Both
Eye			
radial muscle	α_1	Contraction, pupil dilation	Both
Metabolism			
liver	β_2	Breakdown of glycogen	Adrenaline
pancreas	α_1	Insulin suppression of release	Adrenaline
adipose tissue	β_3	Lipolysis	Both

* Sympathetic cholinergic effects – see below.

SYMPATHETIC CHOLINERGIC EFFECTS

The sympathetic system has yet another modification. In some locations, for example, sweat glands and some skeletal muscle blood vessels, the sympathetic nerves release acetylcholine not noradrenaline. The receptor sites are cholinergic and muscarinic, but, despite this, the mechanism is sympathetic. The effects are production of sweat by the sweat glands and vasodilation at those particular vessels. The vasodilation is not a large effect but it may reduce afterload on the heart at the beginning of exercise (see Ch. 6).

CATABOLISM OF THE CATECHOLAMINES

The catecholamines, like acetylcholine earlier, must be broken down if sympathetic activity is to be maintained. If not taken up into storage vesicles, they are broken down by enzymes within the cells. Two main enzymes are involved. One found in the cytoplasm of most cells and at high concentrations in the liver is catechol-O-methyltransferase (COMT). COMT is also found in synaptic and neuroeffector junction gaps. The other, monoamine oxidase (MAO), also widely distributed, is bound to the mitochondria. The two together catabolize catecholamines and any other similar substance which might enter the cells.

MAO is of particular interest since it is found in the cells of the gut, where it breaks down monoamines contained in some foods. If MAO is inhibited, these substances, left intact, can act like the catecholamines and raise blood pressure in some individuals. Inhibitors of MAO (MAOI) can occasionally be used clinically as antidepressants and although the drug is aimed at inhibiting MAO in the central nervous system, it also inhibits gut MAO. The effect is to allow the absorption of food monoamines, introducing a small risk of acute hypertension. People who take MAOI drugs are warned about the possible risks from foods such as cheese and meat extracts which contain monoamines.

OTHER TRANSMITTERS USED IN THE ANS

Apart from the major transmitters, acetylcholine and noradrenaline, the list of other transmitter substances continues to grow. Many of these are mediators of non-adrenergic non-cholinergic (NANC) transmission. Neurones secreting amines (aminergic) such as dopamine and 5-hydroxytryptamine (sometimes called serotonin) have been shown to participate in autonomic activity, as do neurones secreting one of the many peptides (peptidergic). Nitric oxide (NO) can be included in the group since it is the active substance which is directly responsible for many autonomic type responses.

Some of these transmitters act as co-transmitters. An interesting example is seen in the salivary gland where acetylcholine and vasoactive inhibitory peptide (VIP) are found in the same neurones. Parasympathetic stimulation increases the flow of salivary secretions using acetylcholine at muscarinic receptors, but the vasodilation of the local blood vessels, required to provide the extra fluid for the increased saliva, is produced by VIP. In addition to its effect on the blood vessels, VIP appears to have the effect of potentiating the effect of acetylcholine on the salivary flow, increasing the amount and the duration of the flow.

The flow of saliva can be blocked by atropine (see below), i.e. it is a muscarinic effect. The local vasodilation cannot be blocked by atropine; therefore this effect must be due to some other agent, in this case, VIP.

PHARMACOLOGY

(First read Chapter 2 – 'How drugs work'.)

GENERAL POINTS

1. Drugs can be designed to alter the effects of the ANS at different sites of activity in the pathways (Fig. 5.10):

- within the neurone at the site of synthesis of the transmitter
- within the neurone at the site of storage of the transmitter

- at the site or in the mechanism of release of the transmitter
- at the receptor site
- within the mechanism of breakdown of the transmitter.

2. For either division of the ANS, tissue effects can be altered by a drug which is:

- agonistic – having the same effects or increasing the effects of the division
- antagonistic – opposing the effects of the division.

3. Selective or non-selective? As continuing work on the molecular structures and the chemistry of the reactions gives more precise information on how mechanisms work, drugs can be developed which are more specific, i.e. more accurately targeted. Drugs which are non-selective (e.g. affecting all receptor subtypes) produce many effects, some of which are unwanted or side effects. Although no drug is likely to be completely selective, the more closely targeted it is, the fewer unwanted effects it will have.

4. Blockers. A drug substance which resembles the molecular shape of the transmitter enough to be bound to the receptor site, but is not similar enough to cause activity in the site, is a site antagonist. Such a drug is commonly referred to as a site blocker.

PARASYMPATHETIC DIVISION

In clinical practice, the pharmacology of the parasympathetic division is largely limited to agonists and antagonists (blockers) of the muscarinic receptor sites. Manipulation of synthesis and release of the transmitter is possible but not applicable to practice. The ganglionic (nicotinic) site is not a routine ANS target since any drug affecting this site would affect all autonomic ganglia, i.e. all the tissues supplied by both the parasympathetic and sympathetic divisions and the adrenal medulla! Ganglion blockers, such as hexamethonium and mecamylamine, are available but are very rarely used. They do have antihypertensive effects achieved mainly by blocking the sympathetic effects at arterioles but, as can be imagined, their unwanted effects are widespread and make them unsuitable for clinical practice.

A drug which is an agonist at muscarinic sites imitates the parasympathetic nervous system and can be described as parasympathomimetic or cholinomimetic. It has cholinergic (muscarinic) effects. Drugs such as these are sometimes used to increase motility in the gut (bethanechol) or the bladder

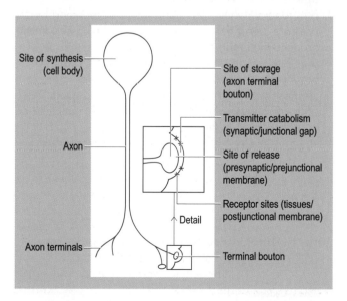

Figure 5.10 Potential sites of drug activity in autonomic pathways.

Site of synthesis (cell body)

Axon

Axon terminals

Detail

Site of storage (axon terminal bouton)

Transmitter catabolism (synaptic/junctional gap)

Site of release (presynaptic/prejunctional membrane)

Receptor sites (tissues/postjunctional membrane)

Terminal bouton

(carbachol), although both are non-selective, producing unwanted effects in addition to the effect required.

Parasympathetic antagonists are usually employed at muscarinic sites and would be called antimuscarinic or anticholinergic (muscarinic) drugs or simply muscarinic blockers. Such a drug is atropine. This substance has a long history, being familiar in folklore long before its actions were understood. The original use of atropine was as an eye cosmetic. The plant from which it was extracted has the name belladonna – beautiful lady. When the extract was used as eye drops it produced pupil dilation, an effect thought to be attractive. (It also blurred the vision, an effect obviously thought to be less important!)

Atropine was used in the early investigative work on the ANS and the classical definition of a muscarinic site is 'one which can be blocked by atropine'. Atropine is non-selective, giving (depending on the dose) a wide range of effects. It still has a number of applications. Atropine can be used clinically to dilate the pupil, but it is a long-acting drug and has given way to shorter-acting drugs such as homatropine or tropicamide. It is also used in the preparatory stages before surgery since it has the useful effects of reducing airway secretions, at the same time protecting the heart against bradycardia during surgery.

As specific site types became known, drugs which were more site specific were developed. The antagonist pirenzepine, for example, is specific for the M_1 sites which control acid production in the stomach and can be used to reduce acid production without affecting the other muscarinic sites such as those in the heart or bladder. (Pirenzepine is only one of the means by which acid production can be reduced; for other pharmacological alternatives see Ch. 9.) Ipratropium is also a blocker with its main effects on M_1 receptors. Its use, however, is in the airways where it can be used to relieve bronchospasm.

SYMPATHETIC/SYMPATHOMEDULLARY SYSTEM

Pharmacology of the sympathetic/sympathomedullary system is again mainly applied to the tissue receptors. The exceptions to this are antihypertensives, such as clonidine and methyl DOPA, acting on presynaptic α_2 sites to reduce the amount of noradrenaline produced. MAOIs (monoamine oxidase inhibitors) increase the amount of noradrenaline available in storage, but are used for their activity in the central nervous system as antidepressants.

Much commoner are the many drugs that have been developed to act at tissue level. Drugs which imitate the sympathetic nervous system are sympathomimetic drugs, or sympathetic agonists. They may be non-selective, acting at all adrenoceptors, or they may be selective, acting at one or more of the subtypes. The non-selective drugs may produce many unwanted effects, because of the wide range of the sympathetic and sympathomedullary systems. As with other drugs, the general rule is that the more specific a sympathomimetic is, the fewer the 'side effects'. An important selective agonist is salbutamol, a β_2 agonist used as a bronchodilator in asthma. Although no drug is totally selective, salbutamol can affect the β_2 sites in the airways without greatly affecting β_1 sites in the heart, so avoiding raising heart rate excessively.

Antagonists or blockers are similarly either non-selective or relatively site specific. β blockers can reduce both heart rate and contractility, so reducing cardiac workload. Since cardiac output is also reduced, β blockers are commonly used as antihypertensive agents. Those which are non-selective, such as propranolol, while they are effective in reducing blood pressure, carry the risk that they will block sympathetic bronchodilation in the airways, increasing the risk of precipitating an attack in someone who is prone to asthma. In that case it would be much safer to use a cardioselective antagonist, metoprolol or atenolol, i.e. one which was specific for β_1 in the heart with little or no effect on β_2 in the airways.

REFERENCES AND FURTHER READING

Dodd J, Role L W 1991 The autonomic nervous system. In: Kandel E R, Schwartz J H, Jessel T M. Principles of neural science, 3rd edn. Prentice Hall, London

Ganong W F 2001 Review of medical physiology, 20th edn. McGraw-Hill Education, Philadelphia

Kruk Z L, Pycock C J 1993 Neurotransmitters and drugs, 3rd edn. Chapman and Hall, London

Rang H P, Dale M M, Ritter J M 1995 Pharmacology, 3rd edn. Churchill Livingstone, Edinburgh (ANS pharmacology in Chapters 5, 6 and 7)

Shepherd G M 1994 Neurobiology, 3rd edn. Oxford University Press, Oxford

Watson R 1999 Essential science for nursing students. Baillière Tindall, London

In practice you may be asked to consider the following:

1. A patient who is prescribed a β blocker gets out of bed rather quickly and falls to the floor. Why?

2. A dentist complains that, by the end of a day in surgery her ankles are swollen, especially in hot weather. Why? In the morning, however, the swelling has gone. Why?

3. A patient is to have an ECG. She is nervous and wants to know what will happen, what the results are likely to look like and, of course, what they mean.

4. You are asked by a patient 'I have found on the web that this drug reduces afterload, what does that mean?'.

5. One of your colleagues has noticed that her heart sometimes 'misses a beat'. Can you explain?

6. A patient has suffered from poorly controlled (diastolic) hypertension for some time. He has now been found to have reduced cardiac output. Is the reduction likely to be in stroke volume, heart rate, both or neither?

7. An athlete (distance runner) has a low resting heart rate. Please explain.

8. On a cold day, your fingers are pale. Why?

9. A school student visiting your unit has asked you, 'If there are no valves at the entrances to the atria, what controls the flow of blood into them, or does it flow in continuously?'.

10. One of your patients has noticed that when he lies down, his heart rate is reduced. When he stands up, the rate rises. Explain.

WHY HAVE A CIRCULATORY SYSTEM?

Cells need a supply of water, oxygen, nutrients and regulatory chemicals. They also need a means of exporting the material they manufacture and the waste produced. All the substances exchanged are water soluble or capable of being transported in water; therefore, theoretically they could travel through the body fluids by simple diffusion and concentration gradients. However, if one imagines the passage of oxygen from the air to the extremities of a large animal such as a human, the process of diffusion over such a distance would be impossibly slow. Evolution gave rise to the development of an efficient circulatory system which rapidly transports material almost all the way and allows the distance over which materials must travel by diffusion to be kept at a minimum. This is usually only the very short distance between a capillary and a tissue cell membrane, where another transport system takes over. Proof of the efficiency of the system is seen clinically when the diffusion distance is increased abnormally. In pulmonary oedema, the fluid collecting in the lung tissue widens the gap between the alveolar gas exchange membranes and the red cell. Gas, particularly oxygen, takes longer to travel between the two and oxygen uptake by blood is impaired. Carbon dioxide excretion is also less efficient and the clinical evidence is the breathlessness of the subject.

HOW IT WORKS

The circulatory system consists of a highly sophisticated pump (the heart), which develops the head of pressure which drives the transport fluid (blood) along the circulatory route (the blood vessel network). The all-important part of the system designed to allow exchange between circulating blood and the tissue cells is the permeable capillary network, which allows the fluid carrying the dissolved substances to move in and out. The forces controlling the rate and direction of movement are the hydrostatic pressure developed by the heart, the osmotic pressure due to substances dissolved in blood and other body fluids, and the degree of permeability of the capillary vessel.

THE PRINCIPLES OF EXCHANGE

Since the whole purpose of the circulatory system is to allow tissues to exchange material when required and at the rate required, the principles underlying the process of exchange are important. If a fault develops, it can lead to damage, or even death of the tissue, if not corrected.

The physical conditions at the capillary bed are central to the exchange. All the mechanisms which control the activities of the cardiovascular system, and many of those controlling other systems such as the kidneys, are aimed at providing the correct conditions in the capillary beds to meet the requirements of the tissue to be met. The details of the mechanisms which allow the conditions to be achieved are considered later (see Ch. 12).

Note that in this chapter, pressure values are quoted in mmHg.

$$1 \text{ mmHg} \approx 0.1333 \text{ kilopascals (kPa)}$$

or

$$7.5 \text{ mmHg} \approx 1 \text{ kPa}$$

The route through the circulation

The route through the circulation is shown in Figure 6.1.

The components

- heart
- vessels.

HEART STRUCTURE

The heart is about the size of a clenched fist and lies in the thorax (Fig. 6.2A & B) beneath the sternum of the rib cage. The heart consists largely of muscle tissue (see Ch. 4B at 'Cardiac muscle') and has four chambers (Fig. 6.3A & B):

- two atria which receive blood from the veins
- two ventricles which pump blood out into the arteries.

Valves guard the entry and exit points of the ventricles (Fig. 6.3B).

TISSUE LAYERS

The walls of the heart consist of three layers:

- pericardium
- myocardium
- endocardium.

Pericardium

This outer part of the heart consists of a double layer of epithelium (serous pericardium) and some connective tissue. A tiny amount of fluid secreted by the epithelial cells is present between the two layers. This lubricates the layers and allows them to move easily over one another. Surrounding the heart as a whole and

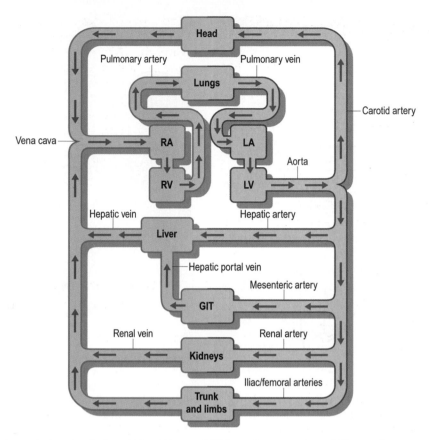

Figure 6.1 The route through the circulation. (After Watson 1999, with permission of Elsevier.)

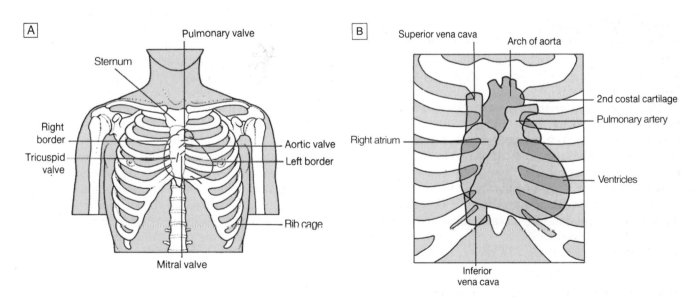

Figure 6.2 A, Position of the heart in the thorax. B, Chambers and vessels in relation to the rib cage. (After Rogers 1992, with permission of Elsevier.)

anchored to the diaphragm is the fibrous pericardium which supports the heart and prevents it distending too much due to rapid filling or overfilling. Its attachment to the diaphragm means that the apex of the heart is relatively fixed. Therefore, when the ventricles contract, the heart is pulled towards the apex, expanding the atria. This reduces the pressure in the atria and makes filling easier.

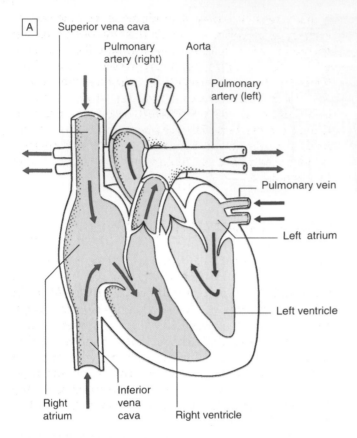

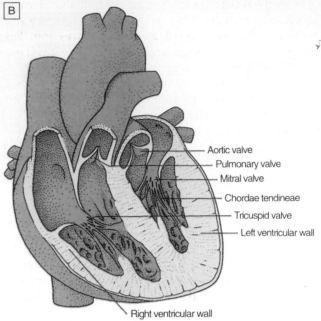

Figure 6.3 A, Chambers and vessels of the heart. Deoxygenated blood (blue) is pumped by the right heart to the lungs. Oxygenated blood (red) from the lungs is pumped by the left heart to the rest of the body. B, Valves of the heart. (Part B: After Rogers 1992, with permission of Elsevier.)

The connective tissue between the pericardium and the myocardium contains blood vessels, nerves and autonomic ganglia.

Myocardium

The myocardium consists of muscle cells and forms the bulk of the wall of each of the chambers. The myocardium of the left ventricle is much thicker than that of the right and can develop much greater pressures when it contracts.

Some muscle cells are specialized in a way that makes them behave more like nerves than muscle cells. They generate and transmit impulses causing the heart to contract. These cells include:

• sino-atrial node cells
• atrioventricular node cells
• Purkinje fibres of the bundle of His and the ventricles.

Endocardium

The innermost layer consists of connective tissue, blood vessels, and nerves, covered by a layer of endothelial cells continuous with the endothelial lining of the blood vessels.

CHAMBERS

Blood entering the right atrium from the venae cavae (Fig. 6.3A) is moved from there into the right ventricle, and from the right ventricle into the pulmonary circulation. The blood picks up oxygen and releases carbon dioxide as it passes through the lungs before returning to the left atrium in the pulmonary veins. It is moved from the left atrium to the left ventricle and is then ejected from the heart into the aorta.

The fibrous skeleton of the heart is a tough fibrotendinous ring with the atria on one side and the ventricles on the other. There are four openings in this band of tissue, all guarded by valves, one between each atrium and ventricle, and one at each exit point from the ventricles into the pulmonary artery and aorta.

The wall (septum) separating the right and left sides of the heart normally prevents blood passing directly from one side to the other.

VALVES

Atrioventricular (AV) valves

The flaps of connective tissue which form the valves between the atria and the ventricles on the left and right sides of the heart are the bicuspid (mitral) and tricuspid valves respectively (Fig. 6.3B). When the ventricle contracts, the pressure of the blood forces the flaps (cusps) of the valves together, closing off the opening so that blood is prevented from re-entering the atria. The ends of the cusps of the valves are attached by cords, chordae tendineae, to the papillary muscles which project from the wall of the ventricle. The papillary muscles contract when the ventricle wall contracts, tightening the cords and helping to prevent the flaps of the valves from being pushed right through into the atria when the ventricles contract.

Arterial valves

The valves guarding the exits from the left and right ventricles (aortic and pulmonary valves), also connective tissue flaps, are called 'semilunar' because of their shape. Unlike the AV valves the flaps of the arterial valves are not tethered by cords of connective tissue.

VENOUS ENTRANCES

The openings between the veins and the atria on both sides of the heart are not guarded by valves. Consequently some blood can be forced backwards into the veins, as well as forward into the ventricles when the atria contract.

EXCITATION

The impulses making the heart contract normally originate in the sino-atrial node (SA node) and are conducted from there to the ventricles. The electrical activity of the heart is recorded routinely as an electrocardiogram (ECG). For a detailed account of ECG methods and data interpretation, see 'References and further reading' at the end of this chapter. An outline trace of the electrical events and the resulting mechanical effects is shown at Figure 6.6.

PACEMAKER CELLS

All the specialized cells of the heart (SA node, AV node and Purkinje fibres) can generate impulses sponta-neously, and rhythmically. The cells of the SA node have the highest intrinsic frequency of discharge (normally 110 impulses per minute) and therefore dominate the other cells, such as those in the ventricles which fire off more slowly (about 40 impulses per minute). The SA node acts as the pacemaker of the heart (see Ch. 4B).

In abnormal states, cells other than the pacemaker can discharge spontaneously, producing an ectopic focus. If it discharges once only, it produces an ectopic beat or extra-systole. This is a beat close to the one preceding and followed by a longer interval, described by those who experience it as 'my heart missed a beat'. If the focus discharges repeatedly, it disturbs the normal rhythm and disorganizes contraction. It may set up a local abnormal pathway which produces repeated firing from the focus. This may be a cause of fibrillation, rapid and disorganized contractions. Atrial fibrillation is relatively harmless, ventricular fibrillation is fatal unless treated.

CONDUCTION OF THE IMPULSE

The impulses generated by the cells of the SA node are carried across the right atrium, to the left atrium (causing both of these to contract) and to the AV node (Fig. 6.4). The impulses travel relatively slowly through the AV node (AV nodal delay) and are then carried along a bundle of Purkinje fibres (bundle of His) running downwards in the wall between the two ventricles. The bundle splits into two, a left and right bundle, each of which conducts the impulse to the Purkinje fibres of the ventricle, exciting the cardiac muscle cells to contract.

Throughout this conducting system, and within the cardiac muscle, the impulses are carried from cell to cell via gap junctions which allow the rapid spread of depolarization and the muscle to act as an organized unit, described as a functional syncitium (see Ch. 4B). Because the Purkinje fibres are able to conduct the impulse rapidly (2–4 metres per second) and are widely

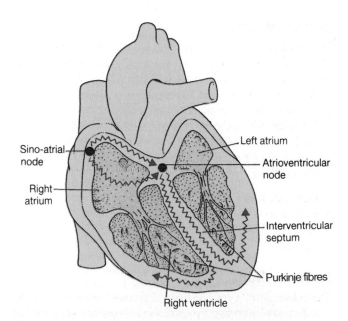

Figure 6.4 Origin and path of conduction of cardiac impulses. (After Rogers 1992, with permission of Elsevier.)

distributed, all the muscle cells in each ventricle are excited within about 0.1 of a second, giving rapid compression of the blood within the ventricle from all sides.

THE HEART AS A PUMP

The heart is a four chambered pump (Fig. 6.5).

THE CARDIAC CYCLE

The events which make up the cycle of filling, ejection and refilling are called 'the cardiac cycle'. A description can begin at any point in the cycle, but it is convenient to start when the heart is completely relaxed at total diastole. A complete cycle takes about 1 second at a resting rate of 60 beats per minute. If the rate is greatly increased, rest time between contractions will be reduced and the time for filling the chambers will be less. In addition, some parts of the myocardium are only perfused during the diastolic period when flow is possible in the coronary vessels there (see Ch. 12 at 'Specialized circulations').

Total diastole

All chambers relaxed, pressure is low in all chambers, and blood flows into the right atrium from the great veins and into the left atrium from the pulmonary circuit. The left and right atrioventricular (AV) valves are open and blood flows through the open valves into the ventricles. Arterial blood pressure recorded at this point, with the heart completely relaxed, would be *diastolic pressure*.

Emergency – cardiac arrest

A nurse is returning home when a man in front of her suddenly collapses. She quickly examines him: his face is grey and pouring with sweat; he does not appear to be breathing; and there is no carotid pulse. She diagnoses that the man has suffered a cardiac arrest and proceeds with the resuscitation measures she has learned and practised in her hospital.

What has happened to the man? What does cardiac arrest mean?

The fact that the nurse cannot feel a pulse does not mean that the heart has given up completely, that there is no electrical activity. What it does mean is that the heart has ceased to pump blood around the body.

In cardiac arrest there are two basic arrhythmias that can cause death (although others may precede these or have a profound effect on cardiac output). These arrhythmias are *asystole* and *ventricular fibrillation*. The nurse in the scenario above does not know which of these has occurred; she is only aware that the victim has no effective cardiac output. By performing external cardiac massage she is attempting to provide such an output.

Within a few minutes, however, the ambulance arrives, the patient is attached to a cardiac monitor and it is possible to see what electrical activity is going on in his heart. Asystole shows as a straight line on the monitor screen, and is the result of a loss of electrical activity within the heart muscle. Ventricular fibrillation results from excessive, uncontrolled electrical activity, and shows as an irregular, bizarre tracing on the screen. Electrical activity within the myocardium is so uncoordinated that no effective pumping of the heart occurs. (During heart surgery, theatre staff can observe a heart that is in ventricular fibrillation; they describe it as quivering or trembling.)

Asystole is treated by cardiac stimulant drugs and external cardiac massage (together with the provision of air or oxygen by whatever means are available). The *sympathomimetic* drug adrenaline (epinephrine) is used to counteract asystole. It increases the rate and strength of each heart contraction. Early in the resuscitation procedure, adrenaline can be injected directly into the myocardium through the chest wall. Once an intravenous line has been established, it may be given intravenously in combination with external cardiac massage, which 'flushes' the drug through the veins towards the heart.

Adrenaline may cause ventricular fibrilliation and the student may wonder what advantage there is in precipitating the patient from one form of arrest into another. However, ventricular fibrillation can often be reversed with a direct current electric shock from a machine called a defibrillator. The monitor would show ventricular fibrillation followed by a 1 or 2 second pause immediately after shock, then, hopefully, normal rhythm resumes as the sino-atrial node takes over as pacemaker.

Calcium chloride is also a cardiac stimulant and is usually given intravenously, although it may be given directly into the myocardium. It excites the heart muscle, strengthens contractility and, like adrenaline, may enhance defibrillation by lowering the heart's defibrillation threshold. Calcium chloride is therefore used in cases of asystole with the intention of bringing about some electrical activity to the heart.

Lidocaine (lignocaine), unlike the previous two drugs, is given when the heart muscle is over-excitable. It has a membrane stabilizing action, reducing the passage of ions through the nerve membrane, thus reducing its excitability. Lidocaine (lignocaine) is used in cardiac arrest situations where defibrillation leads repeatedly to yet more ventricular fibrillation. By reducing the heart's excitability it is hoped that a further DC shock will convert its rhythm to normal.

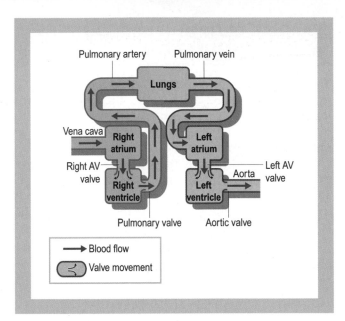

Figure 6.5 The heart as a four chambered pump. (After Watson 1999, with permission of Elsevier.)

Atrial systole

The atria contract, their capacity is reduced and the pressure inside rises. Blood moves under pressure from the atria through the open AV valves completing the filling of the ventricles. About 75% of ventricular filling is completed before the atria contract. The contribution of atrial systole to ventricular filling becomes more important when heart rate is increased, for example in exercise. The volume in the chambers at the end of filling, i.e. at the end of (ventricular) diastole is *end-diastolic volume*.

Ventricular systole

The ventricles begin to contract, ventricular capacity is reduced and pressure inside increases. When ventricular pressure rises above the pressure in the atria, which have by this time begun to relax again, the AV valves close. The flaps balloon back slightly into the atria but do not leak because they are tethered by the cords of tissue attached to the papillary muscles in the walls of the ventricles. The papillary muscles contract at the same time as the ventricles, tightening the cords and ensuring that any backflow of blood into the atria is prevented. For a brief period, the ventricles are closed chambers; this is the *isovolumetric stage of ventricular systole*.

The ventricles continue to contract and, because the volume cannot change, pressure rises steeply until the pressure inside the ventricle is above the pressure outside in the vessel. At that point, the semilunar valves open like swing doors when pushed, and blood is ejected from the ventricles. This is *stroke volume*, being

ejected at *ejection pressure* during *ventricular systole*. Blood is ejected faster than it can flow away into the arteries and it has to be accommodated by stretching the arterial walls. Arterial pressure recorded at this point would be *systolic pressure*.

Ventricular diastole

The pump now has to be refilled. The ventricles begin to relax, they enlarge and pressure is reduced.

When pressure is below that in the vessels outside, the semilunar valves close again, pushed closed by the higher pressure in the vessels on the outside of the heart. The ventricles are again closed chambers with the AV valves still closed and the semilunar valves having just closed. This is the *isovolumetric stage of ventricular diastole*. The atria have been in diastole since early in ventricular systole and being filled from the veins. Atrial pressure has been rising and when the pressure is greater than that in the relaxed and relatively empty ventricles, the AV valves open. Blood flows through to the ventricles and the cycle begins again.

Figure 6.6 shows the electrical events in the heart, the resulting mechanical effects, and the pressure changes which make up the cardiac cycle.

RIGHT ATRIAL AND CENTRAL VENOUS PRESSURE DURING THE CARDIAC CYCLE

The pressure changes occurring in the right atrium during the cycle are transferred to the veins.

As there are no valves between the atria and the veins, variation in pressure occurs in the veins near to the heart such as the jugular vein.

There are two main pressure waves, 'A' and 'V', with a smaller 'c' wave (Fig. 6.6):

- 'A' is due to atrial contraction. Atrial systole causes some backflow into the great veins and raises central venous pressure.
- 'c' occurs as the ventricle contracts, causing the bulging of the AV valves into the atria.
- 'V' is due to an increase in pressure caused by atrial filling during and just after the beginning of ventricular systole. The pressure is reduced immediately on the opening of the AV valves.

HEART SOUNDS

The two most clearly heard sounds made by the heart when it beats are sometimes described as *lubb – dup*, *lubb – dup*. When the pressure rises rapidly in ventricular systole, the closure of the AV valves and

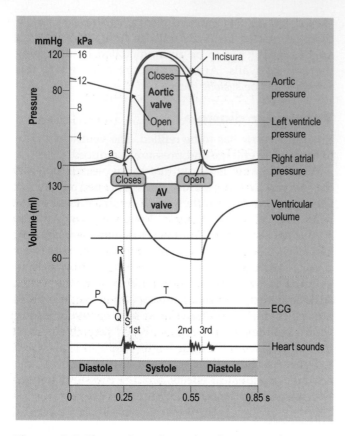

Figure 6.6 Electrical, mechanical and pressure changes in a cardiac cycle. (After Pocock & Richards 1999 Human physiology: the basis of medicine. Reprinted by permission of Oxford University Press.)

their ballooning back into the atria, cause turbulence heard as *lubb*. The sharper sound *dup* is the sound of the semilunar valves closing.

Two other sounds (third and fourth sounds) can be detected instrumentally, but are difficult to identify without training and experience.

VOLUMES

In a resting individual, just prior to ejection there are about 120 to 130 ml of blood in the ventricles (end-diastolic volume). At each beat, when the ventricle contracts, about 70 to 80 ml of this blood is ejected (stroke volume), so that 50 to 60 ml remain (end-systolic volume or cardiac reserve). If the heart is stimulated to contract more forcibly, by increased sympathetic nerve activity, for example, more blood is ejected, stroke volume is increased and cardiac reserve is reduced.

Stroke volume, expressed as a fraction of end-diastolic volume, is called the ejection fraction. Clinically expressed as a decimal fraction, it is normally about 0.66 at rest. It is a valuable indirect indicator of the effectiveness of cardiac contractility.

CARDIAC OUTPUT (PUMP OUTPUT) AND ITS REGULATION

The heart is the pump which provides the head of hydrostatic pressure driving the circulatory system. Pump output, i.e. cardiac output, is therefore directly related to arterial blood pressure (ABP) and an important determinant of overall blood pressure (BP).

Cardiac output (CO) is the amount of blood ejected from the heart per minute. In an adult at rest it averages about 5 litres, but the actual value is related to body size. CO equals the product of the heart rate (HR) (about 70 beats per minute) and the stroke volume (SV) (about 70 ml).

$$\text{CO (ml/min)} = \text{HR/min} \times \text{SV ml}$$
$$\text{CO (ml/min)} = 70/\text{min} \times 70 \text{ ml}$$
$$= 5 \text{ litres } (4900 \text{ ml})$$

A change in either heart rate or stroke volume will produce a change in CO with a resulting change in BP.

In fact, CO is continually being altered to achieve the changes in BP required for daily activities. Moving from a lying to a standing position reduces CO by about 20% (see Fig. 6.9), excitement can increase CO by 25% and heavy exercise may increase it by four times.

In healthy individuals heart rate can range from 60 to 90 beats per minute at rest to a normal maximum of about 180, as, for example, in physical activity.

Stroke volume ranges between 70 and 120 ml. Cardiac output can therefore be adjusted between 5 litres per minute at rest to a maximum of over 20 litres per minute. By physical training some people achieve higher values as a result of a larger, more muscular heart and a larger SV. This allows them to reach a high CO without increasing heart rate to the level at which its filling periods are curtailed. Many athletes show evidence of this larger SV in their low resting heart rate. Excessive enlargement of the heart muscle (cardiac hypertrophy), however, stiffens the chamber walls, reduces their contractile efficiency and reduces cardiac output.

HEART RATE

The heart is excited to contract by impulses generated spontaneously by cells of the SA node. The activity of these cells is influenced by neurotransmitters and hormones.

The SA node is innervated by both parasympathetic (vagus nerve) and sympathetic nerves (cardiac nerve). Parasympathetic nerves release acetylcholine which affects muscarinic (M_2) receptors (see Ch. 5). This

In certain cardiac conditions, such as sinus bradycardia, or complete heart block where no impulses from the SA node get through to the ventricles, the patient's pulse falls to as low as 40 beats per minute. If drugs fail to help, the condition can be overcome by the insertion under local anaesthetic of an artificial pacemaker, a battery driven device which stimulates the ventricles at a set rate nearer to that of a healthy heart – about 70 beats per minute. The battery will need to be changed about every 2 years. As the device is situated just under the skin, this may easily be achieved.

makes the cells less excitable and the heart rate decreases. Sympathetic fibres release noradrenaline which affects β_1 adrenoceptors, making the cells more excitable, and the heart rate increases. At rest, the influence of the parasympathetic fibres is dominant. Consequently resting heart rate (approximately 70/minute) is below the natural firing rate of the SA node (110/minute).

The neurohormones, noradrenaline and adrenaline, are both released by the adrenal medulla in response to sympathetic stimulation. Both affect β_1 adrenoceptors in the nodes and myocardium and increase heart rate and contractility, noradrenaline being more effective here than adrenaline. In circumstances such as emotional excitement and increased physical activity, activity in the sympathetic fibres increases and that in the parasympathetic fibres decreases to give a net increase in heart rate. The effects of circulating noradrenaline and adrenaline augment this (see Ch. 12 at 'Heart rate'). The thyroid hormones increase the sensitivity of the cells to noradrenaline and adrenaline and have an augmenting effect. The increased resting heart rate (tachycardia) associated with overactivity in the thyroid gland is so familiar as to be almost a diagnostic sign.

A substance which affects heart rate is said to have a chronotropic effect, positive if heart rate is increased, negative if the rate is decreased; e.g. acetylcholine has a negative chronotropic effect.

Many factors change heart rate, most changes occurring as responses to a requirement to alter blood pressure (see Ch. 12). Some, however, arise from other sources, e.g. the effect of breathing on heart rate. Sinus arrhythmia is a normal phenomenon, although it is most easily seen in small children. Heart rate increases on breathing in and decreases on breathing out, sometimes with about 30 beats difference. The effect is produced by decreasing and increasing parasympathetic discharge, due partly to the effect of pulmonary stretch receptors and partly to a central effect.

STROKE VOLUME

Stroke volume can be varied in two ways:

- extrinsically (nerves and hormones)
- intrinsically (Frank–Starling mechanism).

Stroke volume is also affected by preload and afterload.

Extrinsic control

Sympathetic nerves, releasing noradrenaline, richly innervate the atria and the ventricles. Parasympathetic innervation is sparse and largely restricted to the atria. When sympathetic activity increases, contractility increases, each beat of the heart is stronger and more blood is expelled per beat. In other words the stroke volume increases. This extra volume is drawn from end-systolic volume, ejection fraction is increased and cardiac reserve reduced. Sympathetic activity also stimulates the adrenal medulla, releasing the circulating catecholamines. These augment the sympathetic effect on the heart by increasing the force of contraction and the heart rate.

Noradrenaline and adrenaline act on receptors which control channels in the cell membrane regulating the entry of calcium. This affects both the electrical

Calcium-channel blockers

People with cardiac disorders are prescribed a variety of drugs, all of which have different actions on the structures of the heart. The calcium-channel blockers interfere with the movement of calcium ions through calcium channels in cell membranes. The cells chiefly affected are those of the myocardium, the specialized conducting system and vascular smooth muscle. Thus, the actual contractility of the myocardium may be reduced, the electrical impulses in the conducting system may be depressed, and the tone of the coronary and systemic vessels may be reduced.

Calcium-channel blockers differ in their ability to bring about these changes. Nifedipine, for example, which is used to relieve angina pectoris (*angina* means 'pain'; *pectoris*, 'of the chest'), a symptom of heart disease not a disease in itself, chiefly relaxes vascular smooth muscle and so dilates coronary arteries. Thus, the blood supply to the myocardium is increased and pain relieved. Peripheral vessels are also dilated, so flushing of the skin and headache may be experienced. Verapamil, which is also used to relieve angina, decreases the contractility of the myocardium and influences the AV and sinus nodes as well as dilating coronary and peripheral vessels. Therefore verapamil has a wider use than nifedipine because it can be used to correct cardiac arrhythmias.

excitation of the cell and the intracellular concentration of calcium required for muscle contraction (see Ch. 4B).

Substances which affect contractility are described as inotropic. Those which increase contractility are positive inotropes, for example adrenaline itself, calcium ions, thyroxine, caffeine. Those which decrease contractility are negative inotropes. Some drugs used in treating cardiac conditions, such as the calcium antagonists nicardipine and verapamil, act on calcium channels and are used as negative inotropes.

Intrinsic control

Stroke volume is also affected by the degree to which the ventricles are filled during diastole. The greater the filling, the greater the end-diastolic pressure and the greater is the degree to which the muscle fibres are stretched. In the late nineteenth century, Otto Frank had demonstrated that frog heart muscle responded to stretching by contracting more strongly. This property was quantified by Starling (1912) using an isolated dog heart preparation and the Frank–Starling mechanism was formulated. This mechanism has been fundamental to the modern understanding of the workings of the cardiovascular system.

PRELOAD

The filling pressure which stretches the muscle fibres, causing them to contract, is called preload (Fig. 6.7). Preload is directly related to the volume per unit time of blood filling the heart, i.e. venous return (see below). The function of the mechanism is to ensure that the output of the two pumps, the left and right hearts, are matched.

If the output from the right ventricle increases, the pressure in the pulmonary circuit increases. This in turn

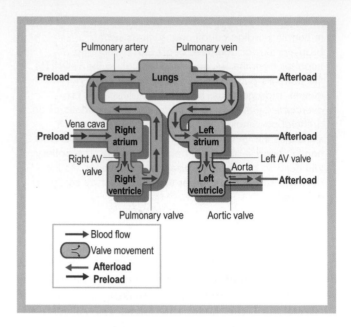

Figure 6.8 The principles of preload and afterload in the right and left hearts. (After Watson 1999, with permission of Elsevier.)

increases the filling of the left heart, whose fibres are more stretched and contract more strongly. The left output is greater, i.e. matched to that of the right heart (approximately on individual beats and accurately matched over a number of beats) (Fig. 6.8).

The Frank–Starling mechanism copes with changes in venous return, i.e. the volume of blood returning to the right atrium via the great veins. The volume itself is not the important factor; in a closed system it is, after all, only the volume coming out at the left ventricle. The important factor is the pressure of the returning blood in the central veins, i.e. central venous pressure. This affects the filling of the chambers and, in turn, is a major determinant of stroke volume.

There is a limit, however, to the capacity of the mechanism. If the heart is constantly overfilled, i.e. if preload is consistently high, the heart becomes dilated and less effective as a pump. This is the case in right heart failure, where the volume entering the heart cannot be adequately cleared, central venous pressure increases and exacerbates the problem by increasing preload on a heart already struggling. Clinical management would include reducing preload, possibly by the use of a diuretic drug.

VENOUS RETURN

Venous return is the blood returning to the right atrium via the great veins. This returning blood will be used to fill the heart ready for the next ejection; therefore

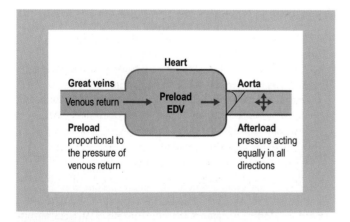

Figure 6.7 The principles of cardiac preload and afterload, showing the heart as a single chamber. EDV, end-diastolic volume. (After Watson 1999, with permission of Elsevier.)

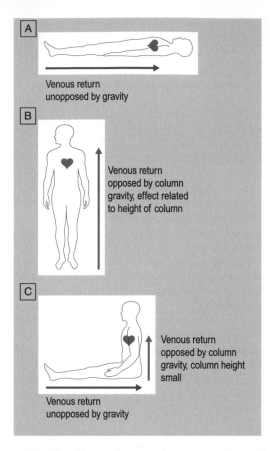

Figure 6.9 The effects of posture on venous return. (After Watson 1999, with permission of Elsevier.)

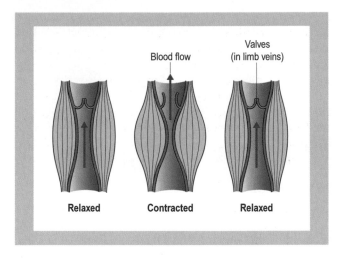

Figure 6.10 The muscle pump. (After Watson 1999, with permission of Elsevier.)

cardiac output is greatly dependent on venous return. Many factors affect venous return and it is likely to be variable. Constantly changing heart rate provides indirect evidence of this, since heart rate is used to compensate for changes (particularly short-term changes) in stroke volume (see Ch. 12 at 'Baroreceptor reflexes').

Factors that affect venous return include posture, pumps and pressures.

Posture

Standing up poses a problem for the circulatory system. Blood must return to the heart from the lower body for a distance of perhaps over a metre. Hydrostatic pressure in veins is low, the driving force is much reduced and the effect of gravity is to oppose the upward flow of blood to the heart. If cardiac output is measured immediately on standing, it can be found to be reduced by about 20%. It may even be reduced enough to make the subject feel dizzy for a few seconds (Fig. 6.9).

Venous return is very good when lying down, but in the upright position it has to be assisted by mechanisms which include muscle and respiratory/abdominal

pumps, changing venous tone and the inward pressure gradient produced during atrial diastole.

Muscle pump

As skeletal muscles contract, pressure on the veins running through them is increased, forcing blood up through the veins. When the muscles relax venous pressure drops, but the blood, which would otherwise drop back down the vessel, recedes only as far as the nearest of the valves which are found in limb veins. The lower pressure allows the vein to refill and the next muscle contraction pushes this blood further up the vessel (Fig. 6.10).

This step-by-step movement of blood up the veins happens most forcibly in physical activity, but the continuous rhythmic contractions of the posture muscles, as they keep the body upright, contribute to venous return.

Respiratory/abdominal pump

This is the rhythmic pumping action produced by breathing in and out.

At inspiration, the thoracic cavity enlarges and consequently pressure here is lowered. In the abdominal compartment, pressure is raised as the diaphragm is lowered and abdominal wall muscles are tightened. Since blood will move from higher to lower pressure, blood moves from the abdominal compartment to the lower pressure thoracic compartment.

At expiration, thoracic pressure is raised and blood in the thoracic veins moves to the area of nearest low pressure, which is the right atrium, thereby increasing venous return. The lower pressure now in the abdominal compartment allows blood to flow in from the lower limbs, ready for the next inspiratory stroke of the pump (Fig. 6.11).

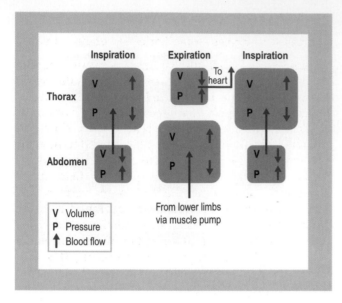

Figure 6.11 The respiratory/abdominal pump. (After Watson 1999, with permission of Elsevier.)

Venous tone

About 60% of the total blood volume is held in the veins and venules. Veins are capable of constricting or dilating and therefore changing the pressure of the blood they contain. The effect is to increase or decrease the pressure of the blood flowing back to the heart, i.e. central venous pressure, and therefore change venous return (the mechanisms involved are considered in Ch. 12).

Atrial inward pressure gradient

When atrial diastole is in progress, the pressure of blood in the atria is lower than that in the veins entering. This favourable gradient is further improved at the point in the cycle where the ventricles begin to contract. They are attached at the apex by a fibrous connection which pulls all the chambers down including the atria. This has the effect of sucking blood into the atrial cavity and increasing the filling of the atria and, via the still open AV valves, the ventricles. Atrial systole then completes ventricular filling.

AFTERLOAD

Stroke volume is ejected from the left ventricle into the aorta where there is already blood at a pressure of perhaps 60 to 80 mmHg, i.e. diastolic pressure. The pressure generated by the ventricle at systole must be enough to overcome the pressure in the vessel outside in order that the semilunar valve can be opened and stroke volume can be expelled. The higher the pressure

Angina pectoris

Narrowing of the coronary arteries by the disease process atherosclerosis can lead to a characteristic symptom, the pain of *angina pectoris*. Here, exertion such as climbing stairs can cause severe 'crushing' central chest pain and referred pain down the left arm. When the individual is resting, blood flow through the coronary arteries is adequate to meet the heart muscle's demands for oxygen and nutrients. During activity, however, those demands increase beyond the level that can be supplied by the narrowed coronary circulation. Pain then results, caused by substances, such as bradykinin, histamine and serotonin, produced from the ischaemic tissues.

To reduce demands on the heart, the patient is advised to restrict activity to that which does not bring on chest pain. How might stopping smoking and losing weight also help?

Glyceryl trinitrate is a drug commonly and effectively used in the treatment of angina. It brings about a generalized peripheral vasodilation by relaxing the smooth muscle of the systemic venous system, so reducing preload. This decreases venous return to the heart, and so reduces the output of the left ventricle.

outside, the harder the heart must work to open the valve and eject the volume. The pressure outside keeping the valve closed can be called afterload.

- The higher the diastolic pressure, the greater the afterload.
- The ventricle must generate about half as much pressure again before afterload can be overcome; therefore if diastolic pressure is 80 mmHg, systolic pressure must be about 120 mmHg.
- High diastolic pressure, i.e. high afterload, increases the workload of the heart. When the ventricle is closed, the muscle is contracting without being able to shorten (see Ch. 4B), i.e. in isometric contraction. Isometric contraction has a higher oxygen demand than isotonic contraction when the muscle is able to shorten, and the longer the muscle has to spend in the isometric phase, the greater the oxygen requirement.

Two rules:

1. The higher preload is, the greater systolic pressure is likely to be – see Frank–Starling mechanism.
2. The higher the afterload is, the harder the heart must work to achieve ejection; therefore a rise in diastolic pressure causes a rise in systolic pressure in a healthy heart.

BLOOD VESSELS

Angiogenesis, the formation of blood vessel, is controlled by a complex array of growth factors and growth inhibitors now becoming better understood (see Ch. 19 at 'Wounds and wound healing'). The information is being used in many clinical fields including provision of better wound care and advancing the treatment of tumours by limiting their blood supply.

VESSELS IN THE CIRCULATION

Blood flows from the heart to the tissues and then back to the heart in vessels which make up the systemic circulation (Fig. 6.12).

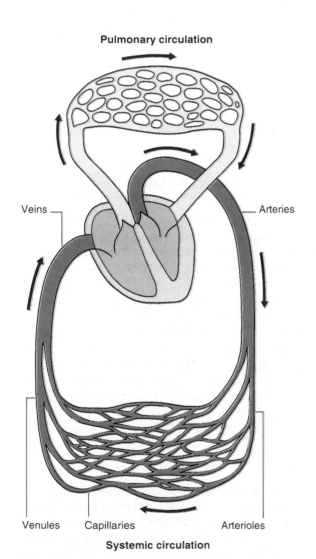

Figure 6.12 The systemic circulation.

They run in the following order:

arteries → arterioles → capillaries → venules → veins

Throughout the vascular system, the relative number of vessels affects both pressure and flow rate. Single arteries lead into a larger number of smaller arteries, which in turn supply many arterioles and even more capillaries. The effect is to progressively step down the pressure from the high ejection pressure and to slow the flow rate until the conditions are suitable for exchange at the capillary bed. The capillaries lead in to successively smaller numbers of larger venules and veins until the great veins are reached. Pressure continues to drop with increasing vein size and distance from the pump, but, as the number of vessels coming after the capillaries progressively decreases, flow rate increases, so that venous return is large and fairly rapid even if the pressure is low.

VESSEL STRUCTURE

The walls of blood vessels, capillaries excepted, consist of three layers of tissue:

- intima
- media
- adventitia.

The *inner layer* (intima) consists of endothelium together with a variable amount of connective tissue. Capillaries consist of this layer alone. The endothelial layer secretes a number of vasoactive substances, such as nitric oxide (see Ch. 12). It also acts as a barrier to the passage of larger molecules such as the plasma proteins.

The *middle layer* (media) is composed of smooth muscle cells along with some elastin, and collagen. The muscle is innervated by motor nerve fibres, most of which are part of the sympathetic nervous system (see Ch. 5). This layer is responsible for the contractility of the vessel.

The *outer layer* (adventitia) consists of collagen and elastin. Some vessels, such as veins, are also innervated by sensory neurones.

The cells of the blood vessels receive a supply of nutrients and oxygen from the blood which passes through them. This is sufficient for the smaller vessels but is supplemented by a network of tiny vessels (vasovasorum) in the adventitial layer of the larger ones.

The several types of blood vessel differ from one another in the contribution made by each of the three constituent layers to the wall as a whole (Fig. 6.13). All carry blood, but the differences in structure are related to differences in the additional functions of each type of vessel.

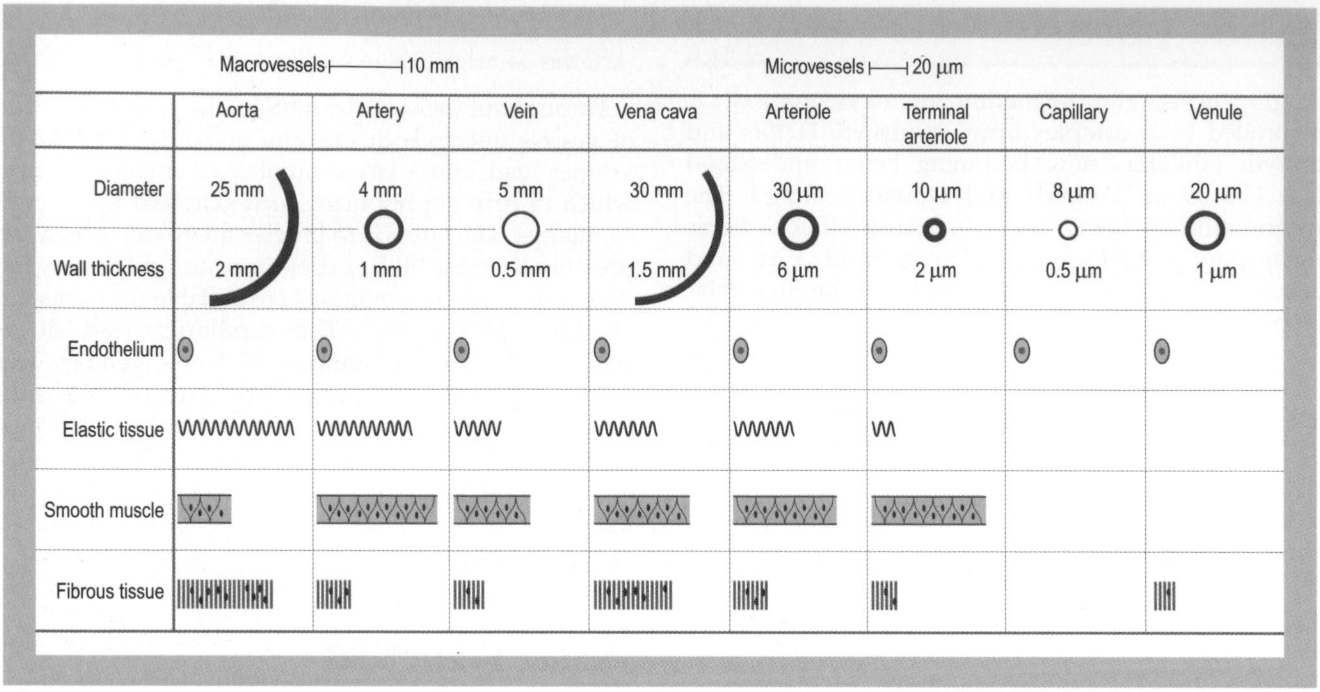

Figure 6.13 Internal diameter, wall thickness and relative amounts of the principal components of the various blood vessels that compose the circulatory system. (After Berne & Levy 1993, with permission of Elsevier.)

ARTERIES – THE PRESSURE VESSELS

The arteries distribute blood to the tissues. The largest, those exposed to the highest and most pulsatile pressure near the heart, are sometimes called the pressure vessels. The larger arteries have smooth muscle and elastic tissue (elastin), the smaller have proportionately more smooth muscle and less elastin. All have collagen which supports the vessel and stops it being overstretched.

Contraction of the muscle reduces the internal diameter of the vessel (vasoconstriction), whereas relaxation increases the internal diameter (vasodilation). Usually the muscle is in a state of partial contraction.

This is the characteristic of smooth muscle called tone. Tone can be either increased or decreased by the action of a wide variety of substances including neurotransmitters, hormones and local factors. Such substances are termed vasoactive. Examples are listed in Table 6.1 (see also Ch. 12).

ELASTIC ARTERIES AND ELASTIC RECOIL

Elastin, some in the media and some in the adventitial layer, has an important role, particularly in the largest of

Table 6.1 Examples of vasoactive substances

Substance	Action	
	Constrictor	Dilator
Neurotransmitters		
Noradrenaline	α_1	–
Acetylcholine	–	✓
Substance P	–	✓
Hormones		
Adrenaline	α_1	β_2
Angiotensin	✓	–
Progesterone	–	✓
VIP	–	✓
Local hormones		
Serotonin (5HT)	✓	–
Bradykinin	–	✓
Histamine	–	✓
Prostaglandins	series F	series E
Local factors		
Carbon dioxide*	–	✓
Hydrogen ions*	–	✓
Hypoxia*	–	✓
Potassium	–	✓

VIP, vasoactive inhibitory peptide; 5HT, 5-hydroxytryptamine.
* Constrictor in pulmonary vessels.

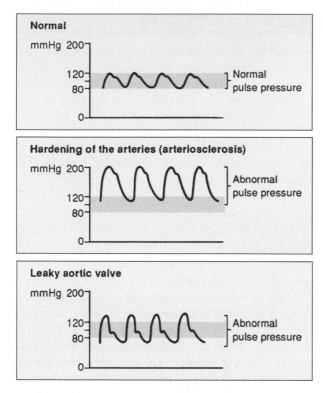

Figure 6.14 Pulsatile arterial pressure, normal and abnormal. (After Guyton 1986, with permission of Elsevier.)

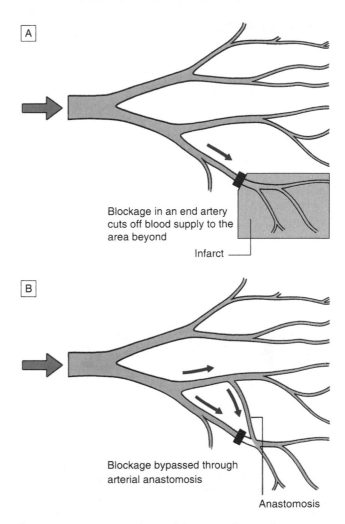

Figure 6.15 A, Branching of the arterial tree, showing blockage in an end artery. B, Blockage bypassed by arterial anastomosis.

the arteries. Because of the large elastin component, the vessels are able to stretch at systole when the pressure is at its highest. The vessel walls will then recoil and raise pressure at diastole. This helps to maintain a high driving pressure and causes the fluctuations in blood pressure, to which these vessels would otherwise be subjected, to be damped. When arteries harden with age, less damping occurs and the fluctuations in arterial pressure are much larger (Fig. 6.14).

MUSCULAR ARTERIES

Some medium-sized arteries have a thick middle layer with a large proportion of smooth muscle. The muscle, however, is not normally used to regulate flow, but, instead acts as a support, stopping collapse of the vessel if it were to be sharply bent, e.g. at the knee.

ARRANGEMENT

The arteries branch, much like a tree, and, in some organs and tissues, 'end arteries' act as a single supply to a discrete area of tissue (Fig. 6.15A). Should there be an obstruction to flow then the tissue supplied by the blocked end artery will be starved of vital supplies, and

the cells will die. Such an area is an infarct. This can occur in any tissue but is of great significance when in the heart, the brain and the kidneys.

ARTERIAL ANASTOMOSES (ARTERIAL SHUNTS)

In some sites, however, there are linking vessels (anastomoses) between different arteries (Fig. 6.15B). In this case, a blockage in one artery does not necessarily lead to cell death because the anastomoses may allow the blockage to be bypassed.

When arteries become narrowed with age, and by disease, all arteries in the body are affected, but the deterioration has more serious consequences in organs such as the heart and the brain because there are fewer anastomoses.

ARTERIAL PULSE

When the pressure in the aorta rises and falls at each beat of the heart, pressure increases and decreases almost simultaneously throughout the arterial part of the circulation. This rise and fall in pressure is sensed as the arterial pulse. Several features of the pulse provide important information about the circulation:

- number of pulsations per minute (heart rate)
- irregularities in rhythm (information about the pattern of electrical excitation)
- strength (clues about cardiac output)
- character or form of the pulse (may suggest leaky or narrowed valves).

Even the 'feel' of the arteries themselves (whether they are sinewy or soft) provides useful information. With advancing age arteries stiffen.

ARTERIOLES – THE RESISTANCE VESSELS

RESISTANCE

In the smallest arteries, the arterioles, the internal diameter of the vessel is small in comparison with the thickness of the muscle layer. Consequently, small changes in muscle contraction have a large effect on the size of the vessel and thus on the flow of blood (Fig. 6.16). Contraction of the muscle will increase resistance and reduce blood flow (see Ch. 12). Conversely, relaxation dilates the vessels and increases the flow of blood. By increasing resistance in one part of the circulation and decreasing it in another, blood will flow to the area of least resistance, i.e. it will be redirected. Since there is not enough blood to fill every available blood vessel, arterioles have an important role in the distribution of blood, supplying tissues according to demand.

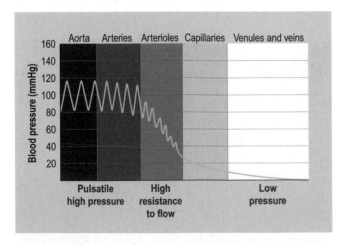

Figure 6.16 The effect on pressure of resistance to flow.

TERMINAL ARTERIOLES

These are the vessels immediately before the capillary beds. They can constrict to the point where flow to those capillaries ceases, i.e. the tap has been turned off; they can therefore regulate the number of capillaries actively perfusing a tissue. The term 'pre-capillary sphincter' has been used in the past to describe the structure carrying out this function, but only a few tissues, e.g. the mesentery, actually have sphincters.

CAPILLARIES – THE EXCHANGE VESSELS

Capillaries are the smallest of the blood vessels, consisting of only a single layer of cells. They are short and have an extremely narrow bore, some so narrow that red blood cells can only go through by deforming (see Ch. 12). They are so numerous that the distance between cells and capillaries is very short and in some circulations, e.g. the coronary circuit, the capillary density (the number of capillaries per unit area) is so high that each cell is likely to be adjacent to a capillary.

They form a vessel network between the arterioles and the venules (Fig. 6.17) and are the site at which the all-important exchange of substances occurs between the blood and the tissue fluid surrounding the cells. Some limited exchange takes place in small pre-capillary arterioles and some post-capillary venules. For

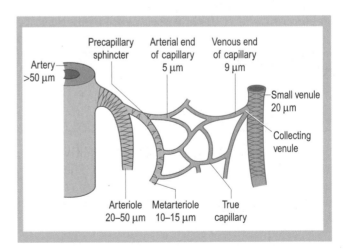

Figure 6.17 The microcirculation. Arterioles give rise to metarterioles, which give rise to capillaries. The capillaries drain via short collecting venules to the venules. The walls of the arteries, arterioles and small venules contain relatively large amounts of smooth muscle. There are scattered smooth muscle cells in the walls of the metarterioles, and the openings of the capillaries are guarded by pre-capillary sphincters. The diameters of the various vessels are also shown. (After Ganong 1995.)

a detailed account of the mechanisms regulating exchange see Chapter 12.

STRUCTURE AND PERMEABILITY

Capillary walls consist of a single layer of endothelial cells on a basement membrane. They have only occasional strands of smooth muscle (Fig. 6.18).

Capillaries differ in:

- the nature and extent of the basement membrane
- the presence and size of 'pores' in, and between, the endothelial cells

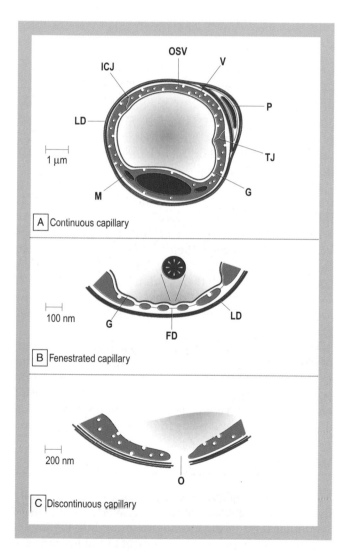

Figure 6.18 Sketches of the capillary wall in transverse section, based on electron micrographs. FD, fenestral diaphragm; inset shows fenestral diaphragm *en face*; G, glycocalyx; ICJ, intercellular junction; LD, lamina densa of basal lamina; M, mitochondrion; O, open intercellular gap; OSV, open surface vesicle; P, pericyte; TJ, tight junction; V, vesicle. Scale only approximate. (After Levick, An introduction to cardiovascular physiology, 3rd edn (Arnold 2000). Reprinted by permission.)

- the degree to which endocytosis and exocytosis occur.

They are the barrier between blood and tissue fluid, and determine which blood constituents are able to pass easily from the blood into the tissue fluid, and which cannot. Capillary permeability varies according to structure. Their wall structure can be described as:

- sinusoidal or discontinuous
- fenestrated
- continuous.

At the 'very permeable' end of the permeability range are the sinusoidal or discontinuous capillaries, sometimes referred to as 'sinusoids'. These are found in the liver, spleen and bone marrow. They have very little basement membrane and are very permeable to all the constituents of plasma including plasma proteins. Sinusoids of the spleen and bone marrow have gaps between the cells large enough to permit the passage of blood cells.

Fenestrated (*fenestra* – window) capillaries are found in tissue involved in fluid exchange, e.g. renal glomeruli, gut mucosa and endocrine and exocrine glands.

Continuous capillaries vary in permeability but, as a group, they are the least permeable to fluid. The membrane is penetrated by clefts protected by strands of membrane particles through which the fluid must make its way. Where there are no breaks in the membrane, this is referred to as a 'tight junction'.

At the 'least permeable' end of the range, capillaries in the brain have very low permeability to fluid. They lack pores and, in addition, adjacent cells are linked very closely by tight junctions. The cerebral capillaries permit easy movement only of very small molecules such as oxygen, water and carbon dioxide, and restrict the passage of small ions such as K^+ and H^+. This unusual selectivity led researchers to coin the term 'blood–brain barrier', to emphasize its distinctiveness (see Ch. 12 at 'Specialized circulations').

ARRANGEMENT

Capillaries form a network of interconnected vessels between the arterioles and the venules.

Many capillary beds are not in constant use. They may be open when the smooth muscle of the arterioles (and, if present, the pre-capillary sphincter) immediately preceding the bed is relaxed, or closed or partially closed when the smooth muscle is contracted. This allows the perfusion of the tissue to be geared to the activity in the tissue. In skeletal muscle at rest, for example, most blood bypasses much of the capillary bed (Fig. 6.19A). When muscles are active, however, the

Inactive tissue

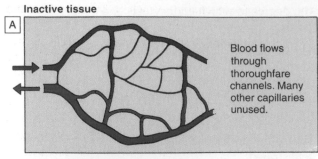

Blood flows through thoroughfare channels. Many other capillaries unused.

Active tissue e.g. exercising muscle

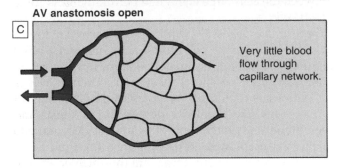

Blood flows through all capillaries.

AV anastomosis open

Very little blood flow through capillary network.

Figure 6.19 Blood flow in inactive tissue (A), in active tissue (B), and with AV anastomosis open (C).

smooth muscle in the arterioles at the opening of the capillaries relaxes and blood flows through more of the capillary bed (Fig. 6.19B). The smooth muscle activity is regulated by neural or hormonal effects or by the effects of locally acting chemicals, e.g. carbon dioxide or hydrogen ion (see Ch. 12).

ARTERIOVENOUS ANASTOMOSES (AV SHUNTS)

AV shunts are vessels which run directly from arteriole to venule. This is a structural modification used to make it possible for blood to bypass the capillary bed completely (Fig. 6.19C). They have smooth muscle in their walls, supplied by sympathetic nerve fibres and with adrenoceptors which can use the circulating catecholamines. AV shunts are found in skeletal muscle and skin circulations and in the latter case are part of the temperature regulating system (see Ch. 12 at 'Specialized circulations').

VEINS AND VENULES – THE CAPACITY VESSELS

As well as just conveying blood back to the heart, veins and venules are distensible vessels which can stretch to accommodate extra blood – hence the description 'capacity vessels'. They are able to accommodate an increase in blood volume without much rise in pressure and make it possible for the volume of blood in the circulation to change without seriously threatening the overall pressures in the system.

Veins and venules increase in diameter and decrease in number as they near the heart; therefore the flow rate increases as blood nears the heart, but the pressure is progressively reduced. Pressure in small veins is about 10 to 15 mmHg and only about 2 to 3 mmHg in the great veins.

Veins and venules are very thin walled by comparison with the arterial vessels. Of the three layers of tissue present in the wall, the outer adventitial layer, consisting largely of collagen fibres, is the most prominent. The walls have smooth muscle allowing them to be constricted or dilated; therefore there is some degree of control over the capacity.

Like that of the arterioles, the smooth muscle is innervated by sympathetic nerve fibres, and is influenced by vasoactive substances. However, unlike arterioles, the contraction of the muscle in venous vessels tends to reduce their tendency to stretch rather than significantly narrowing them. When there is constriction, although there is an increase in pressure, it cannot be compared with the increase achieved by arteriolar constriction and it has little effect on the resistance to flow.

Venoconstriction does contribute to the maintenance of blood pressure, however; if blood volume falls, as for example in haemorrhage, reflex venoconstriction occurs. This displaces some of the large volume of blood held in the venous reservoir into the arterial side of the circulation and helps to maintain blood pressure.

VALVES

Many of the small and medium-sized veins, especially those in the limbs, have valves. These consist of pairs of semilunar flaps of the intima projecting into the lumen (Fig. 6.10). They prevent backflow of blood towards the capillaries and are important in the maintenance of venous return when standing.

VENOUS PULSE

Venous pulses differ from arterial pulses in that they are very small and cannot normally be felt. Light pressure of the fingers over a vein will compress it and obstruct blood flow. Observation of the veins, however, can be useful. When a person is sitting upright, pressure in the veins of the neck, such as the jugular, is less than that at heart level because of the effect of gravity. In normal circumstances, the veins of the neck do not appear distended. However, if venous pressure is abnormally increased, for example if cardiac function is poor, or if the volume of fluid in the circulation is excessive, then the veins distend, and the ripple of the jugular venous pulse will be seen quite clearly.

VENOUS PRESSURE

Pressure in small veins is about 10 to 15 mmHg and only about 2 to 3 mmHg in the great veins. This low pressure in small veins is an important factor in the return of fluid in the capillary beds (see Ch. 12). In large veins, pressure is high enough to allow blood to enter the atrium but not enough to flood the chamber. The low pressure has clinical significance when an entry to a central vein has to be made, for example for an infusion line. The entry must be made with the head below the horizontal so that the vessels are engorged; this way blood may flow out but air cannot flow in.

REGULATION OF BLOOD FLOW

The degree of vasoconstriction or vasodilation depends on the balance of factors, neural, hormonal and local, acting on the smooth muscle at any given time. Control is coordinated by the hypothalamus and mediated through the brain stem and the autonomic nervous system. In some regions, regulation by sympathetic and parasympathetic activity is under the control of higher brain centres.

A number of hormones are vasoactive and local factors such as metabolites are used to regulate perfusion.

Details are to be found in Chapter 12.

LYMPHATIC SYSTEM

LYMPHATIC DRAINAGE

The volume of fluid leaving blood vessels is always more than can be recovered by them. The difference is drained into the lymphatic vessels which run close to the vascular system throughout the tissues. Although both the vascular and lymphatic systems act as fluid distribution systems, there are marked differences in

structure, in the mechanics by which they function and the fluids which they carry.

The small lymphatic vessels which are within tissues and close to the capillaries are closed ended like the fingers of a glove. These run via the lymph nodes into larger and larger lymphatic vessels ending at the large ducts in the thoracic region. Here the lymphatic fluid is emptied into the great veins. Since there is no pump action of the heart driving lymph, the hydrostatic pressure is lower even than that in tissue. Flow is achieved by the milking movements of muscle near the lymphatic vessels, by the rapid emptying into the subclavian veins and, probably to the largest extent, by the rhythmic contractions of the walls of the large ducts (Fig. 6.20).

The smallest lymphatic vessels are very permeable and allow the entry of large protein molecules, particularly in the area of the liver. The movement of protein into lymph is substantial and may amount daily to about a third of the total circulating plasma protein. The effect of the protein content is to give lymph an osmotic pressure which, although lower than that of blood, is higher than that of tissue fluid. The combination of a hydrostatic pressure lower than in tissue fluid, and a colloid osmotic pressure which is higher, makes lymphatic drainage highly effective. In an adult, about 3 litres of fluid is exchanged daily and an obstruction in a lymphatic vessel rapidly leads to tissue swelling around the site.

Lymph is derived from tissue fluid which enters the lymphatic vessels, and is therefore very similar to tissue fluid as far as the concentrations of electrolytes and small solutes are concerned. It contains clotting factors, however, and will clot on standing. Protein content varies according to the site and, as above, contains about 60 g of protein per litre near the liver (compared with plasma which contains 60 to 90 g/l) but only about 20 g/l in skeletal muscle. Near the gut, lymph absorbs fats via the lacteals and may have a distinct milky appearance after a fatty meal.

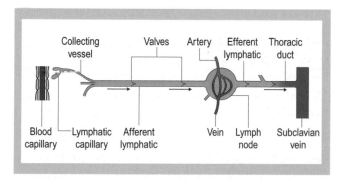

Figure 6.20 The principal features of the organization of the lymphatic system. (After Pocock & Richards 1999 Human physiology: the basis of medicine. Reprinted by permission of Oxford University Press.)

REFERENCES AND FURTHER READING

Aaronson P I, Ward J, Weiner C M, Schulman S P, Gill G S 1999 The cardiovascular system at a glance. Blackwell Science, London

Bennett D H 2002 Cardiac arrhythmias – practical notes on interpretation and treatment, 6th edn. Hodder Arnold, London

Berne R M, Levy M N 2000 Cardiovascular physiology, 8th edn. Mosby, St Louis

Clancy J, McVicar A J 1995 Physiology and anatomy – a homeostatic approach. Edward Arnold, London

Davies A, Blakeley A G H, Kidd C, McGeown J G (eds) 2001 Human physiology. Churchill Livingstone, Edinburgh

Ganong W F 2001 Review of medical physiology, 20th edn. McGraw-Hill Education, Philadelphia

Guyton A C 1986 Textbook of medical physiology. Saunders, Philadelphia

Guyton A C, Hall J E 2001 Guyton and Hall Pocket Companion to Textbook of medical physiology. Saunders, Philadelphia

Houghton A R, Gray D 1997 Making sense of the ECG: a hands-on guide. Oxford University Press, Oxford

Jordan D, Marshall J (eds) 1995 Cardiovascular regulation. Portland Press, London

Levick J R 2000 An introduction to cardiovascular physiology. Arnold, London

Pocock G, Richards C D 1999 Human physiology: the basis of medicine. Oxford University Press, Oxford

Rogers A W 1992 Textbook of anatomy. Churchill Livingstone, Edinburgh

Watson R 1999 Essential science for nursing students. Baillière Tindall, London

7 The respiratory system

In practice you may be asked to consider the following:

1. A patient has had extensive facial trauma due to a road traffic accident. The damage affects the nasal area. Which of the following is NOT a function of the nose?
   (a) detecting smells
   (b) warming of incoming air
   (c) gas exchange
   (d) filtering incoming air.

2. What is the main function of the epiglottis?

3. A patient has been admitted to Accident and Emergency after traumatic pneumothorax and collapse of the right lung. What is normally found between the visceral and parietal layers of the pleura and how does it prevent lung collapse in normal circumstances?

4. What is the residual volume of the lungs? (Please give definition and typical value.)

5. During respiratory function tests, a subject's tidal volume was found to be higher than the normal resting value. What is the tidal volume? What would be a typical resting value? Why might the subject's tidal volume have been raised?

6. A preterm infant is at higher respiratory risk because of reduced levels of surfactant. Where is the surfactant and what does it do?

7. Which of these statements is/are true:
   (a) it normally requires little effort to inflate the lungs
   (b) the internal intercostal muscles may be used in forced expiration
   (c) the diaphragm is not involved in ventilation
   (d) the elastic recoil of the lungs is very important in expiration.

8. Breathlessness is characteristic of pulmonary oedema. Why is it important that the barrier between alveolar air and blood in the pulmonary capillaries is thin? How is the barrier affected in pulmonary oedema?

9. What are the main receptors (sensors) involved in controlling respiration? Where are they? What are they sensitive to?

10. Consider the following disease states and, in each case, work out both what the effect(s) on the

functioning of the respiratory system will be and what responses the body might make to try to overcome this effect:

(a) chronic bronchitis – the lining of the larger bronchi becomes greatly thickened, usually following prolonged irritation of this lining

(b) emphysema – destruction of alveolar walls occurs, leading to large air spaces developing in the lungs

(c) pneumonia – inflammation of the lung, often with a lot of inflammatory fluid present in the alveoli

(d) asthma – the airways go into muscular spasm (e.g. as a result of an allergic reaction), causing them to be greatly narrowed.

Most cells in the human body need oxygen (O_2) to survive and to carry out their functions. As cells work, they use up O_2 and produce carbon dioxide (CO_2) as a waste product that must be eliminated (excreted).

The term respiration refers to the processes by which O_2 is transported to and used by the cells and CO_2 is produced and eliminated (Fig. 7.1). This complicated task is achieved by the cooperative work of:

• the respiratory system
• red cells in the blood
• the circulatory system.

This chapter describes firstly the respiratory system and the respiratory process and secondly how O_2 and CO_2 are transported in the blood. The circulatory system is dealt with in detail in Chapters 6 and 12.

The oxygenation of the blood and the elimination of carbon dioxide from the body is termed external respiration. The use of O_2 by cells and their production of CO_2, sometimes described as internal or cellular respiration, is covered in Chapters 1 and 10.

THE RESPIRATORY PROCESS AND RESPIRATORY SYSTEM

The main components of the respiratory system (Fig. 7.2) are the:

• airways (nose, pharynx, larynx, trachea, bronchi)
• lungs.

Closely related to and very important in the functioning of the respiratory system are the:

• thoracic cage (ribs, sternum and thoracic spine) and respiratory muscles
• pulmonary circulation.

These structures cooperate in the respiratory process, which can be subdivided into three parts (Fig. 7.3):

• ventilation of the lungs with air
• gas exchange between air and blood
• perfusion of the lungs with blood.

Each of these is vital for the efficient uptake of O_2 into the body and for the elimination of CO_2.

VENTILATION

The first step in the respiratory process is ventilation – that is, getting air into and out of the lungs. When we breathe, air is alternately sucked into (inspiration) and blown out of (expiration) the lungs. This process is powered by the respiratory muscles, which are stimulated by nervous signals generated in the brain. Ventilation can feel effortless or laboured depending on the stiffness of the respiratory system and on the narrowness of the airways.

AIRWAYS

The passages that conduct air into and out of the lungs (the airways) consist of a series of branching tubes which become progressively narrower, shorter and more numerous as they go deeper into the lungs (Figs 7.2, 7.4A & B).

Air is breathed in through the mouth and nose and passes through the pharynx and larynx before entering the trachea. During its passage through these upper parts of the respiratory tract, the air is filtered, warmed and moistened. The membranes of these cavities possess a rich blood supply and can produce copious mucous secretions to trap any impurities. These chambers are also intimately involved in the functions of smell and speech.

At the entrance to the trachea and oesophagus there is a small mobile flap of cartilage called the epiglottis that blocks the trachea during swallowing to prevent food entering the trachea (see below).

The trachea is the tube that runs down from the pharynx through the neck into the chest; it is about 10 cm long, about 1.8 cm in diameter and is made of connective tissue and smooth muscle. It is held open by C-shaped rings of strong cartilage. Like most of the respiratory tract below it, it is lined with ciliated epithelium which can transport mucus and trapped particles upwards to the epiglottis for swallowing (see below).

The trachea divides within the chest into right and left main (or primary) bronchi. The right bronchus is slightly larger and more vertical than the left (due to the presence of the heart on the left side of the chest); hence, it is the right main bronchus that is more likely to become obstructed by an inhaled foreign body. These bronchi divide into the smaller secondary (or lobar) and

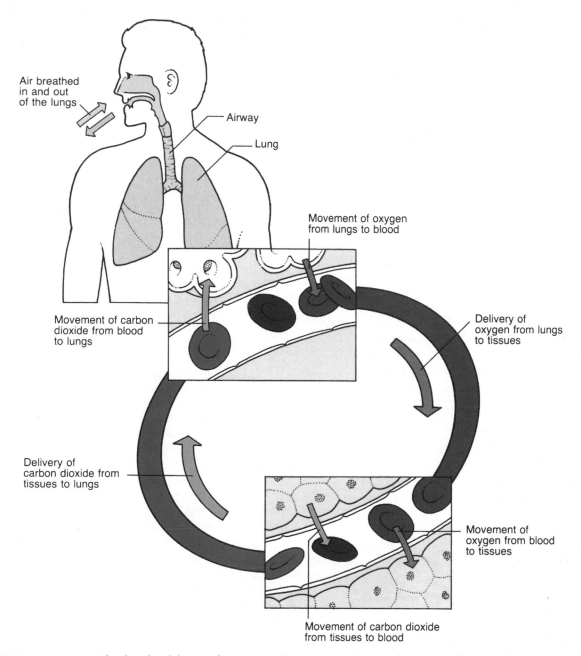

Air breathed in and out of the lungs

Airway

Lung

Movement of oxygen from lungs to blood

Movement of carbon dioxide from blood to lungs

Delivery of oxygen from lungs to tissues

Delivery of carbon dioxide from tissues to lungs

Movement of oxygen from blood to tissues

Movement of carbon dioxide from tissues to blood

Figure 7.1 Processes involved in the delivery of oxygen to the tissues and in the elimination of carbon dioxide.

then tertiary (or segmental) bronchi; all these bronchi are also held open by incomplete rings of cartilage (Fig. 7.4A).

This branching continues down to the terminal bronchioles, which are the smallest airways without alveoli (Fig. 7.4B). Note that the airways down to this point in the respiratory tract take no part in gas exchange and serve only to conduct air into and out of those parts of the tract in which gas exchange can occur. They are thus collectively referred to as the anatomic dead space and together contain about 150 ml of air.

The terminal bronchioles divide into respiratory bronchioles which have occasional alveoli budding from their walls. These eventually come to form alveolar ducts which are completely lined with tiny distensible sacs that are known as alveoli (singular: alveolus). These are the principal site of gas exchange between air and blood (Fig. 7.4B).

Respiratory epithelium

The airways are lined internally by a ciliated layer of cells, the respiratory epithelium (Fig. 7.4C). Glands

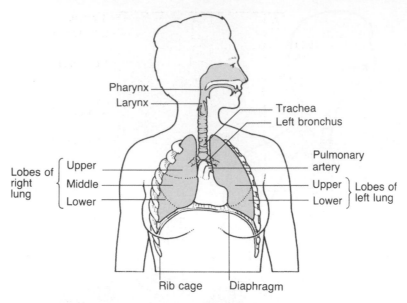

Figure 7.2 Parts of the respiratory system.

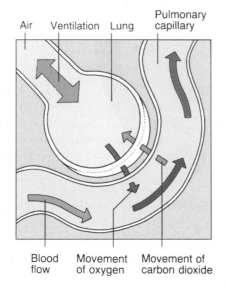

Figure 7.3 Processes involved in external respiration, gas exchange and perfusion.

under the epithelial surface and goblet cells of the epithelium itself secrete mucus, which coats the inner surface of the airways and traps inhaled particles. The cilia drive these secretions away from the alveoli, up and out of the airways into the throat, or pharynx, where they are swallowed. Each day, about 100 ml of mucus are secreted and moved upwards at a rate of 1 to 2 cm/hour. In the lower parts of the respiratory tract, closer to the alveoli, Clara cells are also found in the epithelium. They absorb fluid and may help to prevent the tiny alveoli from becoming filled with secretions and tissue fluid.

Tobacco smoke not only stimulates more mucus secretion but can destroy the ciliary epithelium. This means that smokers have more mucus to clear from their airways but have a reduced mechanism for doing so. They – and the people around them – are very conscious of the smokers' productive cough.

Swallowing

Swallowing is an almost completely reflex process. It has three stages:

- oral
- pharyngeal
- oesophageal.

Several muscles are involved and their contraction is coordinated by a cluster of cells (swallowing centre) close to the respiratory centres in the medulla oblongata of the brain stem. When swallowing occurs, breathing is normally interrupted. The motor neurones controlling the muscles involved in swallowing form part of cranial nerves IX, X and XII.

Oral stage

The oral stage is usually initiated voluntarily but may be a reflex triggered by the presence of substances in the mouth. The masticated food is formed into a bolus by the lips, cheek muscles and tongue and positioned on the back of the tongue. Contraction of several muscles including those of the tongue forces the bolus back into the oropharynx (the part of the pharynx behind the oral cavity). The pressure developed in the process can be as great as 75 mmHg (10 kPa).

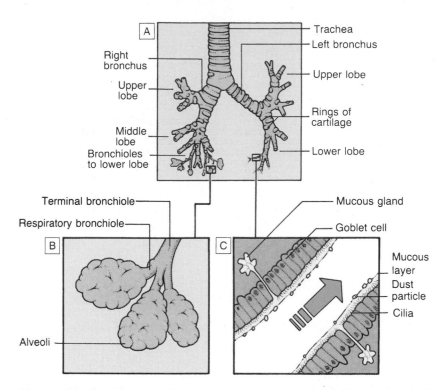

Figure 7.4 Bronchial tree (A), terminal airways and alveoli (B) and lining of the airways (C).

Pharyngeal stage

From the pharyngeal stage onwards, swallowing is entirely reflex. Once the process has been triggered it cannot be interrupted voluntarily. The reflex is triggered by irritation of receptors at the back of the oral cavity and involves propulsive movements as well as those that seal off all exits other than the oesophagus.

Reflex excitation

The presence of food at the back of the mouth excites sensory receptors around the entrance to the pharynx, on the soft palate, tonsils, epiglottis, base of the tongue and the posterior wall of the pharynx. These receptors excite the cells in the swallowing centre of the medulla oblongata. The swallowing centre controls the contraction of several pharyngeal muscles and inhibits the cricopharyngeus muscle, which forms part of the upper oesophageal sphincter. A stimulus of some kind is needed to evoke these responses, even if it is only the presence of saliva at the back of the mouth. Without this, swallowing is very difficult, if not impossible.

Sealing off other exits

The bolus of food is propelled through the pharynx into the oesophagus with some force and speed (up to 20 m.p.h.). As there are two other exits from the pharynx, there is a risk of food being forced either up into the nose or down into the larynx (Fig. 7.5).

Normally, this does not happen. The exit into the nose is sealed off by the elevation of the soft palate, caused by contraction of the levator and tensor palati muscles. Contraction of these muscles also opens the auditory tubes (Eustachian tubes), which is why swallowing helps to relieve the discomfort felt in the ears by air travellers on landing and take-off.

The laryngeal exit is avoided (Fig. 7.5) by:

- pulling the larynx upwards and forwards under cover of the tongue
- diversion of the bolus away from the laryngeal opening by the epiglottis
- bringing together of the vocal folds (closure of the glottis).

Oesophageal stage

Once the bolus has entered the oesophagus, it is carried along by a wave of peristalsis controlled by the 'swallowing centre' in the medulla oblongata. Secondary waves of peristalsis are triggered by irritation of the oesophagus by any food particles left behind. A food bolus takes several seconds to reach the stomach, whereas liquids travel much more quickly, aided by the effect of gravity if someone is sitting upright.

Impairment of swallowing

Swallowing may be impaired for a number of different reasons. For example, damage to the swallowing centre

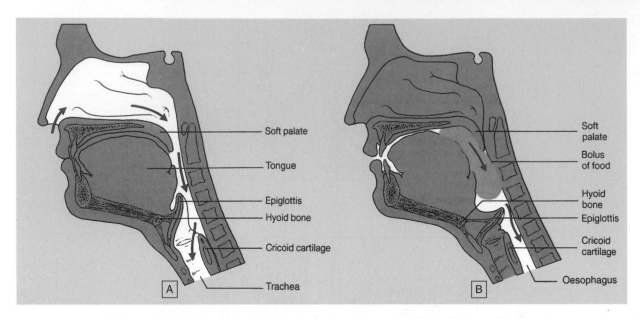

Figure 7.5 Position of structures in the mouth and throat during breathing (A) and swallowing (B). (After Rogers 1992, with permission of Elsevier.)

Choking

Normally, only air is drawn into the respiratory system, as the entrance to the airways is protected during the act of swallowing by the epiglottis, which closes off the larynx. However, we have all choked on something that has suddenly 'gone down the wrong way'. The offending item is usually coughed up and then swallowed, as it should have been in the first place.

Occasionally, an object that is accidentally inhaled is large enough to obstruct the airway and completely cut off air supply. If it is not removed, the person will become unconscious, collapse and may die from asphyxiation in a few minutes. Emergency action must be taken immediately.

A sharp blow on the victim's back may loosen the object by force. Small children can be turned upside down first as gravity may help to remove the obstruction. An alternative and increasingly recommended method is the use the Heimlich manoeuvre (or Heimlich abdominal thrust), which uses the person's own lungs as an air pump to propel the object out with the force from a sudden increase in air pressure.

To perform the Heimlich manoeuvre, the first-aider stands behind with arms high around the victim's waist, making a fist against the upper abdomen and quickly and firmly thrusting the fist upwards towards the diaphragm. The compression causes a sudden rise in air pressure within the lungs, which, if sufficient, may dislodge the obstructing object upwards and out of the windpipe.

may cause partial or complete paralysis, resulting in an inability to swallow. If paralysis occurs in the pharyngeal area, food may pass into the trachea and nasal cavities. If the sphincter at the oesophageal opening remains relaxed during breathing, air is drawn into the oesophagus during inspiration. If the swallowing reflex is absent (e.g. in an unconscious patient or during general anaesthesia) food or water may be inhaled into the lungs, resulting in choking and possible airway obstruction, lung collapse and pneumonia.

LUNGS

The lungs are located in the thoracic cavity. They are held in place only by their attachment to the left and right bronchi. The space that lies between the two lungs, which contains the heart, the thymus gland, most of the oesophagus, lymph nodes and many large blood vessels, is known as the mediastinum.

The lungs are composed of millions of alveoli. Each alveolus is roughly 0.3 mm in diameter (which is less than the size of a full stop). The alveoli are bounded by elastic connective tissue and are covered on their outer surface by pulmonary capillaries.

Pleural epithelium

Each lung is completely covered externally by a single layer of flat epithelial cells, the visceral pleura. This layer doubles back on itself at the point of entry of the main bronchus into the lung and then lines the internal surfaces of the structures surrounding the lungs (chest wall, diaphragm and organs of the mediastinum), thus

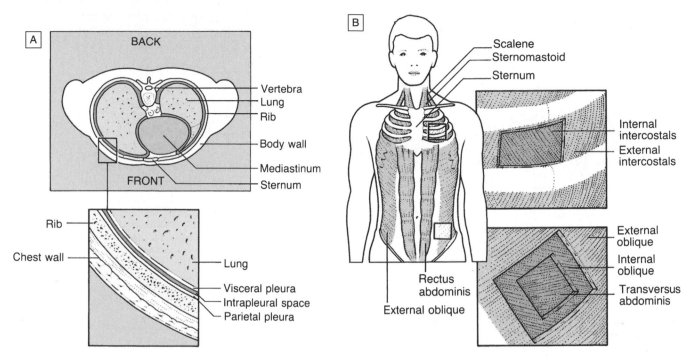

Figure 7.6 The thorax and associated structures. A, Cross-section of the thorax showing the pleurae. B, Rib cage and muscles. The enlarged insets show the different layers of muscle.

Pleurisy is an inflammation of a part of the pleural epithelium. In dry pleurisy every breath can be quite painful as the inflamed layers rub against rather than glide over the opposing surfaces. People with painful pleurisy try to reduce their pain by taking small shallow breaths and may also restrict chest movement by holding or splinting the painful area with their hands.

forming the parietal pleura. Hence, each lung is separately enveloped by a double layer of pleural epithelium (Fig. 7.6A). Between these two layers is a very narrow cavity – the intrapleural space or pleural cavity – which contains a small amount of a serous (watery) fluid. This pleural fluid acts both to keep the two layers of the pleura close together (just as a film of water causes two glass slides to stick together) and as a lubricant which allows the lungs to expand and deflate inside the chest with very little frictional resistance, thus minimizing the effort required to achieve an adequate level of ventilation.

THE EVENTS OF VENTILATION

Inspiration

Air only flows from a region of high pressure to one of low pressure and thus the aim of the inspiratory process is to create a pressure within the thoracic (chest) cavity that is below the pressure of the external atmosphere so that air is drawn into the lungs. This is achieved by increasing the volume of the thoracic cavity, which in turn causes the lungs to expand (due to the strong adherence between the two layers of the pleura) and thus air is drawn into the lungs.

Inspiration is thus an active process and the respiratory muscles (Fig. 7.6B) chiefly involved in it include:

- diaphragm
- external intercostal muscles
- scalene and sternomastoid muscles (accessory muscles).

The most important of these is the diaphragm, a sheet of muscle separating the thoracic cavity above from the abdominal cavity below and which bulges into the thoracic cavity at its base. The edge of this sheet is anchored to the lower ribs (Fig. 7.7). The increase in the volume of the chest cavity required for successful inspiration is brought about mainly by the diaphragm contracting and pulling down – this pushes the abdominal organs down and increases the vertical dimension of the thorax. At rest, movement of the diaphragm alone is usually sufficient to provide an adequate level of inspiration to meet the body's gas exchange needs. If more forceful inspiration is needed, the diaphragm contracts more vigorously and the external intercostal muscles contract and pull the ribs

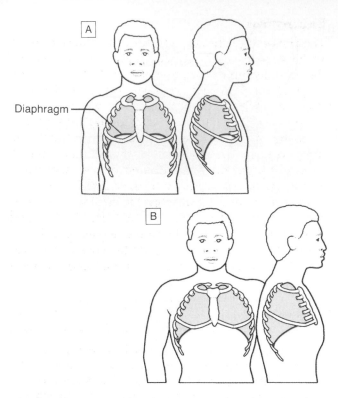

Figure 7.7 Dimensions of the thorax during breathing. A, At the end of a gentle expiration. B, After a deep inspiration. (After Wilson 1987, with permission of Elsevier.)

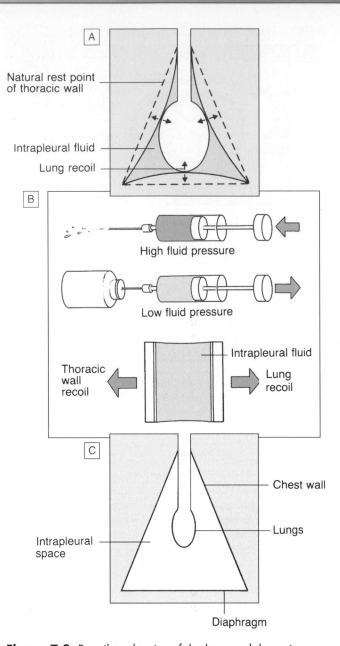

Figure 7.8 Recoil tendencies of the lung and thoracic wall: A, act one against the other so long as pleural fluid holds the two together; consequently the lungs cannot collapse, and the chest wall and diaphragm are pulled away from their natural rest points; B, create a sub-atmospheric intrapleural pressure; C, cause lung collapse and thoracic expansion if a large amount of air enters the intrapleural space (pneumothorax).

up and out (rather like lifting up the handle of a bucket), thus increasing the cross-sectional area of the chest and also increasing the volume of the chest cavity (Fig. 7.7). In situations where a still greater inspiratory effort is required (e.g. severe exercise; lung disease where gas exchange capability is greatly reduced), the accessory muscles of inspiration can be used to aid expansion of the chest: the scalene muscles lift the first two ribs, and the sternomastoids raise the sternum.

Note that, firstly, the pressure within the pleural cavity is always less than atmospheric pressure (this is possible because the cavity is sealed off both from the atmosphere outside the body and from the air in the alveoli) as the two layers of the pleura are being pulled in opposite directions – the lungs tending to recoil to a smaller size (see below), the chest wall tending to expand (Fig. 7.8A & B). Secondly, the variations in pressure within the thoracic cavity required to provide an adequate level of ventilation are not very large – a change of only some 0.3% in this pressure is sufficient to meet resting ventilatory requirements, e.g. intrathoracic pressure changes from 760 mmHg at rest to 758 mmHg during inspiration. Thirdly, if the chest wall is stabbed or, more likely, if the lung tissue is torn, the intrapleural space may then be opened to air from the lungs or the

The fluctuation in intrapleural pressure between each expiration and inspiration can be seen reflected in the steady rise and fall of the fluid level within the tube of an underwater seal chest drainage set.

Pneumothorax

A pneumothorax may occur because of damage either to the chest wall or to part of the surface of the lung. The degree of breathlessness depends upon the suddenness of onset and the size of the pneumothorax.

The consequences of a pneumothorax depend upon the type:

- in an *open pneumothorax*, air is drawn into the pleural space through the area of damage, such as a wound in the chest wall or a tear in the visceral pleura. In other words, air is 'breathed' in via the abnormal opening with each inspiration and, once the pneumothorax is established, blown out again with each expiration. The air that occupies the pleural space obviously contributes nothing to gas exchange. Instead, it interferes with inflation of the lungs and creates breathing problems.

  Because the pressure within the pleural space eventually equilibrates with atmospheric pressure (with small fluctuations during respiration), there is nothing to hold the lung in its normal position tightly against the chest wall. The stretched elastic fibres recoil and the lung deflates and collapses. It cannot reinflate until the injured area closes over and air is either removed by pleural aspiration or is absorbed naturally from the pleural cavity.

- In a *closed pneumothorax*, air is sucked out of the lung into the intrapleural space through a tear in the lung tissue, which then seals over, and the lung collapses with the loss of the normal negative pressure. In time, as the air in the intrapleural space is gradually absorbed, the lung will reinflate to its normal shape and size.

- In a *valvular pneumothorax*, a type of closed pneumothorax, the small injury in the pleura acts as a one-way valve allowing air to be drawn into the intrapleural space but with no way of escape during expiration. If the air tries to escape, the increased intrapleural pressure forces the edges of the damaged area to collapse together and block the flow of air (like the valve on a bicycle tyre). The result is that each breath adds to the air volume and pressure within the intrapleural space. The increase in volume and pressure not only causes the affected lung to collapse but also pushes the mediastinal structures towards the opposite chest wall (mediastinal shift), compressing the other lung as well. The consequences of this type of pneumothorax are very grave and, unless treated, the patient may suffocate.

atmosphere, resulting in a pneumothorax which usually results in lung collapse and consequent respiratory difficulties (Fig. 7.8C).

Expiration

The aim of the expiratory process is to create a pressure within the thoracic cavity that is above the pressure of the external atmosphere so that air is forced out of the lungs along a pressure gradient. This is achieved by decreasing the volume of the thoracic cavity.

However, in contrast to inspiration, expiration is normally an entirely passive process. This is because the lungs contain a great deal of elastic tissue that is stretched when the lungs expand during inspiration. The lungs return passively to their initial volume by recoil of this elastic tissue when the inspiratory muscles rest, so forcing air out. (This passive recoil is also aided by the surface tension in the fluid lining the alveoli – see below.) When expiration needs to be more forcible (e.g. during exercise, blowing up a balloon) or more

Out of breath

Normally, we are not conscious of the work that our respiratory muscles do except when we are 'out of breath' after exercise when the natural tendency is to remain still so that no further demands for O_2 are made and we can concentrate on 'getting our breath back'. The work of the respiratory muscles becomes obvious when we are 'breathing hard' (e.g. the sternomastoid muscles may be seen contracted in the neck) and we instinctively want to loosen any tight clothing so that respiratory muscle movement is not restricted.

Patients who are very breathless because of a respiratory problem react in exactly the same way. They do not want to be moved unnecessarily and they need to have the freedom to use their muscles to capacity.

Because so many muscles, thoracic as well as abdominal, are involved in the work of respiration, patients who need to make a consistently increased respiratory effort can quickly become tired. Also, any local injury can disrupt the normal smooth pattern of breathing because of the associated pain. Following thoracic or upper abdominal surgery, for example, where the surgical incision is in or very close to respiratory muscles, patients naturally attempt to control pain and discomfort by minimizing respiratory muscle movement. The very shallow respirations that result, along with their natural reluctance to cough, are counterproductive – mucous secretions remain in the lungs and form a potential site for infection. Various strategies can be used to help patients contract their muscles properly in order to breathe deeply and cough effectively; e.g. analgesics given before breathing exercises work by reducing the perception of pain. The patient's wound can be supported on either side or a pillow can be used to control tension on the wound edges – only the wounded area is splinted so that the healthy surrounding muscle can contract and move normally.

controlled (playing a wind instrument or speaking), muscular effort is required and then expiration becomes an active process). The most powerful of the muscles used are those of the abdominal wall (Fig. 7.6B):

- rectus abdominis
- internal and external oblique muscles
- transversus abdominis.

Contraction of these muscles increases intra-abdominal pressure and pushes the diaphragm upwards. Also, internal intercostal muscles act to pull the ribs down and inwards (rather like the handle of a bucket going down). Both these actions cause a decrease in the thoracic volume and thus assist expiration.

FACTORS AFFECTING VENTILATION

Three factors affect the process of ventilation:

- compliance
- airway resistance
- surface tension of the alveolar fluid.

Compliance

Compliance refers to how much effort is required to expand the chest wall and inflate the lungs. In health, the effort required to expand the lungs in gentle breathing is very small since the lungs and associated structures easily yield to (or comply with) the forces acting on them; for example, a normal breath requires only a tenth of the pressure required to blow up a balloon. Thus, the compliance (volume change per unit of effort) of the lungs and chest wall is said to be high. An important contributor to this usual state of high compliance is a substance known as surfactant – see below.

If the respiratory system becomes stiffer, as it does in old age, often due to the accumulation of pollutant materials in the lung tissue, compliance is reduced. Compliance is also reduced in some respiratory disorders (e.g. pulmonary oedema – fluid is present in the tissue spaces and inside some of the alveoli, causing the normally soft lung tissue to be much firmer; e.g. disorders that produce scarring of the lung, such as tuberculosis). Whatever the precise cause, reduced compliance always means that a greater effort is consistently required to expand the lungs to any particular extent.

Conversely, in some diseases, the lung tissue is more rather than less compliant. In emphysema, for example, there is loss of lung tissue. As there is less tissue present to be stretched, inflation requires less effort. However, the power of elastic recoil of the lungs is also reduced by the loss of lung tissue. Consequently, expiration may require muscle power even when breathing at rest.

Airway resistance

Airway resistance is the resistance posed to airflow by the walls of the airways. This is normally low, and thus the pressure required to move air through the airways is also usually very small.

The diameter of the airways is very important in determining how easily air flows into and out of the lungs: the wider the airways are, the easier it is for air to flow (Fig. 7.9); if they are narrowed (e.g. through inflammation or the accumulation of secretions), then airflow is more difficult.

The size of all but the larger airways (those stiffened by cartilage) changes appreciably during the breathing cycle. When we breathe in, the airways as well as the alveoli expand, making airflow progressively easier. When we breathe out, however, the airways get narrower and the resistance to the flow of air increases. In a forced expiration, the smallest airways close completely and trap air in the alveoli. If the airways are already narrowed because of disease, such as bronchitis, closure occurs sooner and more air is trapped (i.e. the residual volume increases; see below – 'Lung volumes').

Airways close prematurely in emphysema, a condition where there is loss of lung tissue. Patients often find it easier to exhale through pursed lips. This prolongs expiratory time and maintains pressure in the airways, which helps to keep the small airways open.

The diameter of the airways is also affected by contraction and relaxation of the smooth muscle in their walls. Bronchodilator stimuli (e.g. activity in sympathetic nerves, adrenaline, CO_2) relax this smooth muscle while bronchoconstrictor stimuli (e.g. activity in parasympathetic nerves, histamine) cause it to contract. Certain drugs can be used therapeutically to bring about a change in airway diameter – e.g. the β_2 adrenergic drug salbutamol in the treatment of asthma.

As the smallest airways are very small in diameter, it might be assumed that these make the greatest contribution to the resistance to airflow. However, because they are so numerous, they, in fact, collectively offer less resistance to airflow than the trachea and bronchi (Fig. 7.10). At least 50% of the total resistance to airflow is normally contributed by the upper airways – mouth, nose and pharynx.

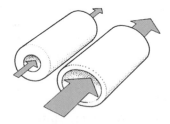

Figure 7.9 Airflow through the airways is affected by airway size.

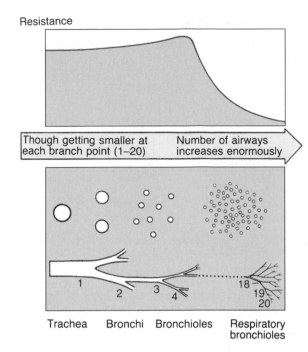

Resistance

Though getting smaller at each branch point (1–20)

Number of airways increases enormously

Trachea Bronchi Bronchioles Respiratory bronchioles

Figure 7.10 The resistance to airflow offered by different sections of the airways. (Adapted from West 1990, based on Pedley et al 1970 and Weibel 1963, with permission.)

Surface tension of alveolar fluid

Surface tension is caused by forces of attraction between molecules in a liquid, which make the molecules on the surface hold tightly together and resist being spread out. This is the force which holds the two layers of the pleura together.

In the lung, the surface of the alveoli in contact with the air is lined with a watery liquid to permit gas exchange (see below). This liquid layer alone would cause the alveoli to collapse due to its surface tension. However, some of the alveolar cells secrete a material called a surfactant which is a mixture of substances (chiefly lipids) and acts like a detergent. This dramatically lowers the surface tension of the fluid lining the alveoli and prevents such collapse. (Surfactants associate with the water molecules in the fluid layer and weaken the attraction between them.)

The reduction in surface tension brought about by the surfactant is one reason for the normally high compliance of the lungs and it also helps to prevent fluid being sucked into the alveoli from the interstitial space.

Since normally the lungs have high compliance and low airway resistance, the energy expenditure associated with normal breathing is low. If, however, something occurs to lower lung compliance (e.g. presence of scar tissue in the lung, lack of surfactant) and/or to raise airway resistance (e.g. inflammatory

The first breath

The moment of birth is not just a special moment emotionally but a crucial one physiologically. In going from the mother's womb to the outside world, the baby's respiratory system must undergo a tremendous adaptation to make the transition from the fluid intrauterine environment to the air outside (see Ch. 31).

Even in a healthy, full-term baby, that first breath is not an easy one. Before birth, fluid fills the respiratory passageways and the alveoli are collapsed. At birth, air must replace this fluid and the alveoli must expand to be able to take part in gas exchange. The baby must make a tremendous effort to replace the fluid with air and to inflate the alveoli. Surfactant plays a vital role in the success of this transition and, most importantly, helps to make each subsequent breath a little easier.

Because the surfactant is not formed by the growing fetus until the last few weeks before birth, infants who are born prematurely often develop breathing problems. The lack of surfactant means that some of the alveoli remain collapsed (atelectasis), as they were in fetal life, and others open stiffly and only with some difficulty (reduced compliance) when the baby first tries to breathe as well as with each subsequent breath.

Because fluid passes easily into the alveoli from the capillaries (transudation of fluid) when the level of surfactant is low, alveolar space within the baby's lungs is also reduced. These clinical problems, when present, form the infant respiratory distress syndrome.

Respiratory difficulty increases with the degree of prematurity. Often some assistance with ventilation is necessary until the baby reaches the normal gestational age at which sufficient surfactant is produced. Once this is present, the lungs easily expand with each breath and ventilation becomes normal.

Adult respiratory distress syndrome
Surfactant deficiency can also occur in adults when changes develop inside the lungs similar to those in infants with low surfactant. Adult respiratory distress syndrome can occur following severe shock, trauma or massive blood transfusion. These patients, who are very ill, develop increasing respiratory distress with rapid, shallow, ineffectual breathing, and many, like the infants, require some assistance with ventilation.

swelling of the airway mucous membrane), then the effort required to maintain an adequate respiratory effort can become considerable.

LUNG VOLUMES

The volume of air breathed in and out and the number of breaths taken per minute vary between people according to age, sex, build and activity. The pattern of

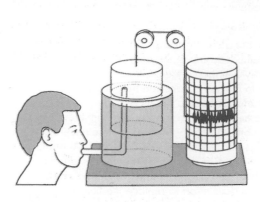
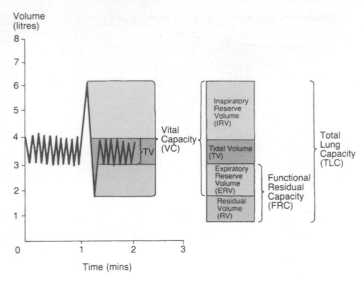

Figure 7.11 Measurement of lung volumes by spirometry. This classical instrument demonstrates the principle of the method. A cylinder of air is inverted into a water reservoir which forms a seal. As air is breathed in and out, the cylinder rises and falls, its movements being transferred as a pen trace to a chart on a slowly revolving drum. The pattern of results is shown above. This same pattern is produced by many more modern instruments.

breathing in any individual can be recorded using a spirometer (literally breath-meter). Various lung volumes can be measured and can be used to assess respiratory function (Fig. 7.11).

Typically, at rest, about 500 ml of air are inspired and expired with each breath (tidal volume) and the frequency of breathing is about 10 to 15 breaths per minute. In ordinary gentle breathing, about 2 litres of air remain in the lungs at the end of expiration (functional residual capacity). With maximum effort, the lungs can be expanded to hold between 4 and 6 litres of air (total lung capacity); most, but not all, of this volume can be expelled. The maximum volume that can be expelled starting from a maximal inspiration is known as the vital capacity, but note that, after such a maximum expiration, about 1 litre of air still remains trapped in the lungs (residual volume). This arises because the sub-atmospheric intrapleural pressure keeps the alveoli slightly inflated and some air also remains in the non-collapsible airways (anatomic dead-space).

Many respiratory disorders will affect the performance of the respiratory system and thus alter one or more of these lung volumes recorded by spirometry, e.g. pulmonary fibrosis, which reduces the ability of the lungs to expand, reduces vital capacity. Clinical measurement of the various lung capacities can be of great value in diagnosis.

Factors that may affect vital capacity include:

- age, sex and build
- position of person during measurement
- strength of respiratory muscles
- distensibility of lungs and chest cage.

Assessment of airflow

There are two commonly used measurements to assess airflow through a patient's respiratory system and both of these can be of great value clinically:

- *PEFR* 'peak flow': the maximum rate of airflow that can be achieved when expiring as hard and as quickly as possible, starting from fully inflated lungs, is known as the peak expiratory flow rate

Peak flow

In conditions such as asthma where the bronchioles are narrowed (i.e. in bronchospasm), measurements of peak expiratory flow rate (PEFR) can provide an objective measurement of the severity of bronchiolar constriction and give an early indication of the onset of an asthma attack. When mild bronchospasm occurs a fall in the PEFR occurs even before breathlessness becomes evident, so it is a helpful early warning measure and can alert someone in good time to the need to take prescribed bronchodilators and/or to seek medical help before the bronchospasm gets worse.

Peak flow measurements are also used to assess the effect and, therefore, the effectiveness of a particular type of bronchodilator or a particular course of bronchodilator drugs. To do this, PEFR is measured before and after the drug is administered.

(PEFR). It is measured using a simple instrument (peak flow meter) that registers the maximum airflow achieved during a breath. In health, PEFR ranges from 400 to 600 litres/minute.

- FEV_1 and FEV_3: the proportion of the vital capacity that can be expelled from the lungs in 1 and then 3 seconds, again while breathing out as quickly as possible. In health, at least 80% can be expelled in the first second and about 100% by the third. This measurement is the forced expiratory volume and is abbreviated to FEV_1 and FEV_3 for 1 and 3 seconds, respectively.

If the airways are narrowed, as in asthma, both PEFR and FEV will be lower than normal (Fig. 7.12).

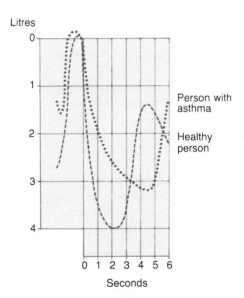

Figure 7.12 Forced expiratory volume (FEV) measured by spirometry in two adult men, one of whom has asthma. Each man filled his lungs to capacity and then at 0 seconds breathed out as hard and fast as he could. (Data courtesy of D. E. Evans.)

GAS EXCHANGE

Following ventilation of the alveoli with fresh air, the next step in the respiratory process is the transfer of gases between the air in the alveoli (alveolar air) and the blood in the pulmonary capillaries.

Partial pressures of gases

The composition of air containing a mixture of gases can be described in two ways:

- per cent composition
- partial pressures of the constituent gases (kPa).

'Partial pressure' is an equivalent term to 'concentration' that is used when considering gases and it indicates the part of the total pressure being exerted by a mixture of gases that is due to any one gas in the mixture.

For example, if overall atmospheric pressure is 100 kPa and O_2 makes up 21% of air, then 21% of the total pressure of the atmosphere is due to O_2. Thus, the part of the pressure due to O_2 (partial pressure of O_2, or PO_2) is equal to:

$$21/100 \ (21\%) \times 100 \ kPa = 21 \ kPa$$

Alveolar air

The air inside the alveoli is not the same in composition as that in the atmosphere (Table 7.1). The differences arise because alveolar air has gained water from the moist epithelia lining the respiratory tract and picked up CO_2 and lost O_2 within the alveoli. The composition of alveolar air obviously changes during the breathing cycle as fresh air is drawn into the lungs and some alveolar air is expelled. In gentle breathing these changes are not dramatic because the volume of fresh air added at each breath (tidal volume – about 500 ml) is small compared with the volume of air already in the lungs (functional residual capacity – about 2 litres).

Table 7.1 Composition of air

	Dry atmosphere		Alveolar air (37°C)	
	%	**kPa***	**%**	**kPa***
Oxygen	21	21	13.2	13.2
Carbon dioxide	0.04	0.04	5.3	5.3
Nitrogen†	79	79	75.2	75.2
Water vapour	‡	‡	6.3	6.3

* Assuming barometric pressure is 100 kPa.

† Includes <1% rare gases (argon, helium etc.).

‡ Amount of moisture in atmosphere depends on humidity and temperature. If moisture is present, percentage of other constituents will then be correspondingly decreased.

Alveolar–capillary barrier

The alveolar air is separated from the blood in the pulmonary capillaries by a very thin barrier, often referred to as the respiratory membrane (Fig. 7.13). This membrane is only 0.5 μm in thickness and consists of four parts:

- the fluid lining the inner surface of the alveoli
- a single layer of alveolar cells (alveolar epithelium)
- the interstitial space
- the capillary endothelium.

The alveolar epithelium is remarkable for its extensiveness – if all the 300 million alveoli were spread out to form a single sheet, it would have a total surface area of about 85 square metres. Capillaries of the pulmonary circulation cover about 60% of this surface.

Transfer of oxygen and carbon dioxide

Both O_2 and CO_2 move between blood in the pulmonary capillaries and alveolar air by simple diffusion (Fig. 7.14). This diffusion is a passive process and will occur only from a region of high partial pressure to one of low partial pressure.

Although the blood coming to the lungs already has some O_2 in it, the partial pressure of O_2 in this blood (5.3 kPa) is less than that in the alveolar air (13.2 kPa). Hence, there is net transfer of O_2 from alveolar air to pulmonary capillary blood. Conversely, the partial pressure of CO_2 in the pulmonary capillary blood (6 kPa) is greater than that in the alveolar air (5.3 kPa) and so diffusion of CO_2 occurs from the blood to the alveolar air.

It can be seen that the partial pressure gradient for CO_2 is much less steep than that for O_2, yet equilibration of both gases across the respiratory membrane occurs

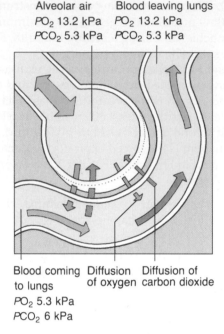

Alveolar air
PO_2 13.2 kPa
PCO_2 5.3 kPa

Blood leaving lungs
PO_2 13.2 kPa
PCO_2 5.3 kPa

Blood coming to lungs
PO_2 5.3 kPa
PCO_2 6 kPa

Diffusion of oxygen   Diffusion of carbon dioxide

Figure 7.14 Gas transfer between alveolar air and blood. The gases in the blood leaving the lungs are in equilibrium with air in the alveoli.

very quickly. (It takes less than a second for blood to pass through the pulmonary capillary network and only 0.25 second to reach equilibrium.) This is explained by the fact that CO_2 is much more soluble in water than is O_2 and thus it can equilibrate very quickly even if there is only a small partial pressure gradient.

Factors affecting transfer of oxygen and carbon dioxide

The rate at which the gases are transferred between alveolar air and pulmonary capillary blood depends upon:

- the differences in partial pressures of the gases
- the distance between the alveolar air and the blood (thickness of the respiratory membrane)
- the total surface area available for gas exchange.

Alterations in any of these factors will result in a change in the rate of gas exchange across the respiratory membrane.

For example:

- Anything that increases the thickness of the respiratory membrane will slow down the rate of transfer because the gradient for movement is made less steep. Thus, in pulmonary oedema, the interstitial space becomes congested with fluid and some may even accumulate in the alveoli. The distance that the gases have to diffuse is thus

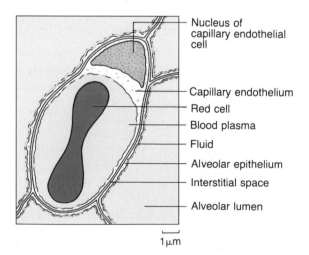

Nucleus of capillary endothelial cell

Capillary endothelium
Red cell
Blood plasma
Fluid
Alveolar epithelium
Interstitial space
Alveolar lumen

1 μm

Figure 7.13 Cross-section of a piece of lung tissue showing alveoli, a single pulmonary capillary and the alveolar–capillary barrier.

The bends

Although the most abundant gas in alveolar air is nitrogen, its concentration in body fluids is relatively low because it is not very soluble in aqueous fluids. If the pressure of nitrogen is increased, however, more of the gas is forced into solution. In divers working a long way below the surface of the sea, the weight of the water increases the pressures of the gases breathed and nitrogen dissolves in larger amounts in body fluids and body fat (nitrogen is especially soluble in fatty substances).

If a diver ascends from the depths very quickly, nitrogen is released so rapidly from the fat stores into the blood that bubbles of gas form in the body fluids, similar to the effect of opening a bottle of fizzy drink. These nitrogen bubbles in blood vessels may obstruct blood flow, causing ischaemic damage, pain, perhaps even death.

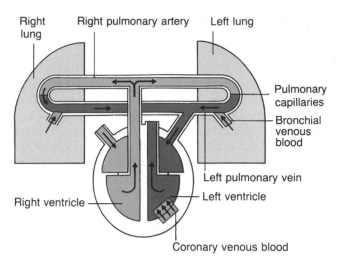

Figure 7.15 The heart and the pulmonary circulation. Oxygenated blood is delivered to the left heart via the pulmonary veins. Note that the airways received their own blood supply (bronchial circulation) and that a little deoxygenated blood from the bronchial and coronary veins mixes with the oxygenated blood. Note also that only one pulmonary vein is shown entering the left atrium. In fact there are four.

increased, transfer is slowed, and equilibrium may not be achieved before the blood leaves the lungs. Consequently, the blood may not become fully oxygenated. (Note that an increase in the diffusion distance affects the diffusion of O_2 more than that of CO_2 since CO_2 diffuses much more quickly and easily because of its greater solubility.) (See also Ch. 12 at 'Pulmonary circulation'.)

- In emphysema, the total surface area available for gas exchange is decreased and there may not be sufficient area to meet the body's gas exchange needs, leading to both inadequate oxygenation of the blood and retention of CO_2.

PERFUSION

The amount of O_2 taken up into the body and the amount of CO_2 that can be eliminated from it depend not only on the ventilation of the lungs and the efficiency of gas exchange but also on the quantity of blood passing through the lungs (perfusion).

PULMONARY CIRCULATION

The human cardiovascular system is a closed double circulatory system – i.e. the blood is contained within the blood vessels and there are apparently two separate systems of blood vessels within it. These are: the pulmonary circulation (concerned *only* with carrying the blood to and from the lungs for the purposes of gas exchange) and the systemic circulation (concerned *only* with the supply of oxygen and nutrients to the tissues of

the body and the removal of waste materials from these tissues). These two circulations are anatomically quite separate from each other (after birth), but blood passes from one to the other in a defined and ordered manner, i.e. they are in series with one another (see Ch. 12).

In the pulmonary circulation, blood is pumped from the right side of the heart (right ventricle) via the pulmonary trunk and pulmonary arteries to the pulmonary capillaries where gas exchange occurs. The blood then passes to the left side of the heart (left atrium) via the pulmonary veins (Fig. 7.15).

Blood flow and pressure

The pulmonary circulation thus has a very large blood flow: the entire output of the right side of the heart passes through it. As the output of the right and left sides of the heart is the same, the blood flow through the pulmonary circulation is the same as the cardiac output (see Ch. 6), ranging between 5 litres/minute in a resting person to 25 litres/minute at the limits of physical exertion.

Blood pressures in the pulmonary circulation are characteristically low: pulmonary arterial pressure is only 24/8 mmHg as compared with 120/80 mmHg in the systemic circulation (see Ch. 12). This pressure is sufficient, however, to take the blood to all parts of the lungs. Also, pulmonary capillary pressure is lower than systemic capillary pressure (10 mmHg and about 24 mmHg, respectively), which ensures that the amount of tissue fluid formed in the lungs is relatively small, thus avoiding the potentially very serious problem of pulmonary oedema. About 20 ml of excess tissue fluid normally forms each hour in the lungs, but this is removed by the pulmonary lymph vessels.

However, if the hydrostatic pressure of the blood in the pulmonary capillaries increases acutely (e.g. failure of the left side of the heart), the amount of tissue fluid formed increases greatly. If the pulmonary lymph vessels cannot drain this increased amount of tissue fluid, fluid accumulates in the interstitial space and eventually is forced into the alveoli. Pulmonary oedema may well then develop, and will both restrict ventilation of the lungs (by decreasing the compliance of the lungs) and impair gas exchange (by increasing the thickness of the respiratory membrane).

Reservoir function

The pulmonary arterial vessels are unusually thin-walled, making them much more distensible than other arteries (e.g. the systemic arteries). This structural feature is related to the fact that the pulmonary circulation depends on being a low pressure system. If pulmonary arterial pressure increases, the vessels distend (rather like veins do in the systemic circulation) and the volume of blood contained in them increases. The pulmonary circulation can thus act as a blood reservoir and, indeed, normally contains about one litre of blood. Like systemic vessels, the small amount of smooth muscle in the walls of the pulmonary vessels is innervated by sympathetic nerves. However, these nerves do not regulate the flow of blood through the lungs as they do in other parts of the circulatory system; rather, as with systemic veins, their function appears to be to stiffen the vessels. Changes in the capacity of the vessels to hold blood will alter the size of the pulmonary reservoir.

Vasodilator effect of oxygen

The pulmonary circulation is the only place in the body where arteriolar smooth muscle dilates if there is an abundance of O_2 close by and constricts if there is a deficiency. In all other circulations, a lack of O_2 in the tissues promotes vasodilation, which increases the amount of O_2 to those tissues (see Ch. 12). This distinctive response of the pulmonary arterioles is useful. If the concentration of O_2 in some alveoli is lower than average because of poor ventilation, the pulmonary arterioles supplying that part of the lung tissue constrict. This reduces the blood supply to that area and allows more blood to flow through other parts of the lung that have a higher O_2 concentration.

VENTILATION–PERFUSION BALANCE

For optimal gas exchange between alveolar air and blood, perfusion and ventilation should be matched in

---

Chronic obstructive airways disease

Chronic bronchitis, emphysema and some forms of asthma can all be described as types of chronic obstructive airways disease (COAD). COAD is a permanent and incurable condition in which the primary respiratory difficulty is with exhalation of air. Although asthma is generally characterized by intermittent and reversible episodes of bronchospasm, it may eventually develop into chronic bronchitis, emphysema, or both. Although the pathology of chronic bronchitis and emphysema is quite distinct, the two conditions are often found together with different degrees of severity.

The major feature of chronic bronchitis is excess mucus production from enlarged mucous glands in the bronchioles and bronchi. The mucus clogs up and partially blocks the already oedematous airways, increasing airway resistance and the work of breathing. This is often especially noticeable during expiration as the small soft airways become occluded more easily then, trapping air behind them. The reduction in ventilation with the retention of alveolar air produces a low alveolar PO_2 which is reflected in a low plasma PO_2. Again, because of the retention of air, the PCO_2 is often increased in both alveoli and plasma.

In emphysema (from the Greek, meaning bodily inflation), the walls of many of the alveoli have been destroyed and the remaining alveoli are abnormally large. This reduces not only the alveolar surface but also the pulmonary capillary bed. Because the total area over which gas exchange takes place is much reduced, breathlessness, driven by the increase in PCO_2, is one of the main features of emphysema.

As the tissue destruction also involves the elastic tissue in the lungs, the elastic recoil that assists in making normal expiration a passive rather than active process is lost also and expiration becomes more difficult. Again, air is trapped in the distorted, distended alveoli with a resultant increase in the amount of air left in the lungs after expiration (residual volume).

The priority is to help these patients to breathe more easily, perhaps by finding the most comfortable position and teaching breathing techniques. Difficulty with breathing often causes anxiety and a physiotherapist or nurse may help by teaching the patient to relax tense muscles to allow easier breathing.

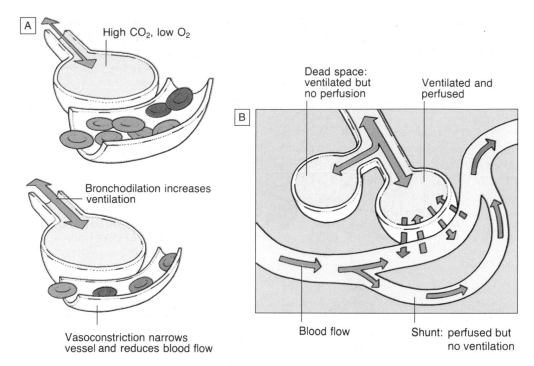

Figure 7.16 Matching ventilation and perfusion. A, The unit above is underventilated and overperfused, but the effects of low O_2 and high CO_2 on the blood vessels and bronchioles bring about a better match between ventilation and perfusion (unit below). B, How gross imbalances create dead space and shunts.

all parts of the lungs. If they are not, there will be surplus ventilation and/or perfusion.

Regional differences in ventilation and perfusion do, however, exist even in health. At least two mechanisms normally help to match up ventilation and perfusion locally so that gas transfer occurs as efficiently as possible (Fig. 7.16A):

- O_2 regulates local blood flow (as described above)
- CO_2 regulates local ventilation: the smooth muscle of the bronchioles relaxes in response to a build-up of CO_2. If ventilation of some alveoli is poor, the concentration of CO_2 increases locally and causes bronchodilation. This eases the flow of air into those alveoli and improves ventilation.

Dead space

Those parts of the respiratory system that do not take any part in gas exchange are collectively referred to as the dead space of the system. This dead space is subdivided into:

- anatomic dead space – the airways down to the level of the terminal bronchioles which can take no part in gas exchange due to their wall structures; they together contain about 150 ml of air – see above
- physiologic dead space (parts of the respiratory system in which gas exchange can occur but in which at any particular time, for a variety of reasons,

gas exchange does not occur – e.g. alveoli that are ventilated but not perfused with blood (Fig. 7.16B).

In health, the physiologic dead space volume is almost zero and thus the total dead space volume is nearly the same as the anatomic dead space volume. But, in disease, the physiologic dead space can increase significantly (e.g. if there are underperfused alveoli), causing a great increase in the overall dead space volume, and giving rise to a situation in which much of the inspired air is not available for gas exchange. Also, if blood passes from the right side of the heart to the left side without coming into contact with ventilated alveoli, it cannot pick up O_2 or offload CO_2. A bypass route of this kind is termed a shunt (Fig. 7.16B) and can occur in pneumonia because areas of consolidation in the lung may be perfused but not ventilated.

TRANSPORT OF OXYGEN AND CARBON DIOXIDE IN THE BLOOD

The transport of gases between the lungs and body tissues is accomplished by the blood. Very large quantities of O_2 and CO_2 are carried safely and efficiently in the blood: O_2 is carried principally within the red cells of the blood (erythrocytes) whilst CO_2 is carried in three different ways (see below), including

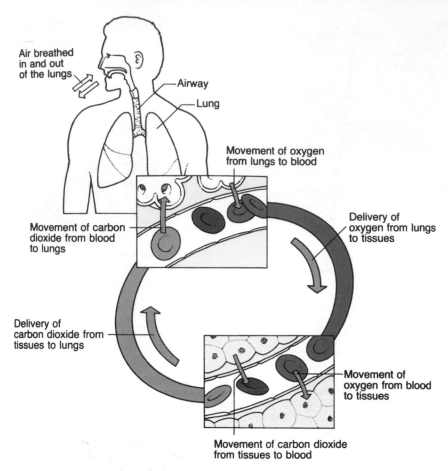

Figure 7.17 Transport of oxygen and carbon dioxide between the lungs and the tissues.

some in the red blood cells (Fig. 7.17). The single most important constituent of the red blood cell is haemo-globin, which is a complex and highly specialized molecule that plays a vital role in the transport of both O_2 and CO_2.

OXYGEN TRANSPORT

O_2 is transported in the blood in two ways:

- dissolved in the plasma (1.5%)
- associated with haemoglobin (oxyhaemoglobin; 98.5%).

The amounts of O_2 and CO_2 present in arterial and venous blood are shown in Table 7.2. O_2 is not very soluble in water and so only a little can be carried dissolved in plasma.

HAEMOGLOBIN

Haemoglobin is a complex molecule that has both protein (globin) and non-protein (haem) parts

Table 7.2 Oxygen and carbon dioxide in blood* (ml/litre)

	Arterial blood	Venous blood†
Oxygen		
– dissolved	3	1.2
– oxyhaemoglobin	195	150
Carbon dioxide		
– dissolved	26	30
– carbonic acid	‡	‡
– carbamino compounds	26	34
– hydrogen carbonate	438	463

* Assuming a haemoglobin concentration of 150 grams/litre.

† Composition of the mixture of venous blood entering the heart (mixed venous blood).

‡ Very tiny amount.

(Fig. 7.18). The globin component consists of four protein chains, two of each of two different types: two alpha (α) and two beta (β) chains. Associated with each of these chains is a haem unit; in the centre of each haem

Each gram of haemoglobin should, when fully saturated, carry 1.39 ml of O_2. If someone has a blood haemoglobin concentration of 15 g/100 ml, the maximum amount of O_2 that could be carried in blood (discounting the tiny amount in solution) is 20.8 ml per 100 ml.

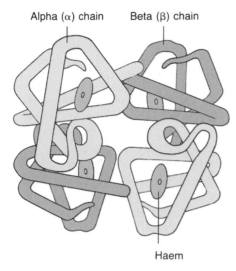

Alpha (α) chain   Beta (β) chain

Haem

Figure 7.18 Component parts of a single molecule of haemoglobin.

unit is one ion of iron (Fe^{2+}), which is crucial in the binding of O_2. Thus, one molecule of haemoglobin has four haem groups and four iron ions.

The four protein chains (or subunits) are held together by weak chemical bonds between their constituent amino acids but it is important to appreciate that the shapes and relative positions of the subunits can change according to the surrounding conditions (e.g. pH, PCO_2, temperature). These changes alter the ability of the molecule to bind O_2 and are thus very important in the function of haemoglobin as a gas transport molecule.

As each molecule of haemoglobin contains four ions of iron, and each iron ion can bind one molecule of O_2, each molecule of haemoglobin can carry up to four molecules of O_2. When all four O_2 binding sites are occupied, haemoglobin is said to be fully saturated with O_2. (If one, two or three binding sites are occupied, haemoglobin is said to be partially saturated.) The compound then formed is known as oxyhaemoglobin, which is bright red in colour, in contrast to de-oxygenated haemoglobin, which is blue/purple. It is the change from oxyhaemoglobin to deoxyhaemo-globin that brings about the colour change that is observed as blood passes from arteries through the systemic capillary beds to veins.

Different forms of haemoglobin

The main form of haemoglobin found in the red blood cells of the adult is that described above and is known as haemoglobin A. There are other forms of haemo-globin known, some normal and some abnormal:

- Haemoglobin F (fetal haemoglobin) is the form of haemoglobin that predominates normally in the red cells of the fetus. It has a different protein composition to haemoglobin A and is thus able to pick up oxygen at lower concentrations than would be typical at the lungs, i.e. from the maternal circulation, and distribute it to the tissues of the fetus. This property of haemoglobin F is clearly crucial to the successful development of the fetus.

- In some cases, one or more of the protein chains of haemoglobin are produced with an error in them – e.g. an inherited mutant allele causes an abnormal protein chain to be synthesized. Many such abnormal haemoglobins are known: some are totally harmless, but others are so different in properties

Carbon monoxide poisoning

Carbon monoxide (CO) binds to haemoglobin in the same way as O_2, except that haemoglobin binds CO much more strongly – the affinity of haemoglobin for CO is about 250 times as great as that for O_2. This means that when CO is inhaled, some haemoglobin that should combine with O_2 combines instead with CO. Only a relatively small amount of the gas needs to be breathed for appreciable amounts of carboxyhaemoglobin to be formed in the blood and thus to significantly reduce the amount of haemoglobin available for O_2 transport.

CO, though it occurs at very low levels naturally, is found in several present-day situations in significant amounts: e.g. it may be formed by an ordinary gas fire that is not burning correctly or is inadequately ventilated; it is present in car exhaust fumes and cigarette smoke – as much as 16% of the total haemoglobin of smokers can be bound to CO.

CO poisoning is particularly dangerous because it can go unnoticed, both externally and internally. If sufficient amounts of CO are breathed for a prolonged time, the person concerned will suffer progressive O_2 deficiency while maintaining apparently rosy features (since carboxyhaemoglobin is bright red). The situation may not be identified clinically, either, because routine blood gases tests measure only dissolved O_2 and not that bound to haemoglobin. Similarly, the lack of O_2 bound to haemoglobin is not detected by the chemoreceptors, breathing is not stimulated, and the individual experiences no discomfort. It is not uncommon for CO poisoning to have a fatal outcome.

from normal haemoglobin that the transport of O_2 is impaired, e.g. the haemoglobin present in sickle cell anaemia patients – HbS. HbS precipitates when oxygen concentration is low, stiffening the red cells and preventing the axial or single line flow necessary for capillary beds.

- In other cases, the protein chains of haemoglobin are entirely normal in structure but are not produced in the right amounts, e.g. reduced or even completely absent synthesis of the alpha or beta chains. This group of disorders is termed the thalassaemias.

Haemoglobin can also be subject to interference from various environmental agents and such interference can affect its function:

- Carbon monoxide binds very strongly to the O_2 binding site and forms carboxyhaemoglobin, which is bright red. This obviously prevents O_2 binding to haemoglobin and thus reduces the capacity of the molecule to carry O_2. Carbon monoxide poisoning can be very serious – see box on page 135.
- Some drugs (e.g. sulphonamides) and chemicals (e.g. nitrites) can convert the iron into a form that can no longer bind O_2, thus forming methaemoglobin, which is very dark in colour. Small amounts exist in blood normally, but large amounts will obviously seriously compromise O_2 transport.

OXYGEN–HAEMOGLOBIN DISSOCIATION CURVE

The shape of the curve and its significance

The amount of O_2 bound to haemoglobin depends on many different factors, the most important of which is the PO_2 of the blood. At a low PO_2, most of the O_2 binding sites on haemoglobin are empty. At higher values of PO_2, the vacant sites become filled, until eventually all are occupied with O_2.

The relationship between the amount of O_2 bound to haemoglobin and the PO_2 is not a linear one, but, rather, is sigmoid ('S'-shaped) in form (Fig. 7.19). This occurs as a result of the interactions between the protein subunits of haemoglobin and the effect this has on the binding of O_2 to the haem groups (see above).

This sigmoidal relationship between PO_2 and the degree of saturation of the haemoglobin molecule has important consequences for both the uptake of O_2 in the lungs and its delivery to the tissues:

- At a PO_2 of 13.2 kPa (similar to that of the blood leaving the lungs), haemoglobin is completely saturated with O_2. Therefore, blood leaving the lungs is normally fully oxygenated.
- PO_2 has to fall substantially before the amount of O_2 bound to haemoglobin is much reduced. This ensures that virtually all the O_2 remains bound to haemoglobin during its transfer from the lungs to the tissues.
- At a PO_2 below about 5.3 kPa, the saturation of haemoglobin changes dramatically for only a small change in PO_2. As tissue PO_2 may be as low as 1.5 to 2.5 kPa, a great deal of O_2 can thus be released to active tissues.

It should also be noted that, because haemoglobin is fully saturated with O_2 at a PO_2 of 13.2 kPa, any further increase in PO_2 cannot increase the amount of O_2 carried by haemoglobin. Consequently, a part of the lung having a high PO_2 (e.g. 18.2 kPa) because of over-ventilation cannot compensate for another area that is badly ventilated and has a low PO_2 (e.g. 8.2 kPa). Thus, in respiratory disease in which ventilation to parts of the lungs is impaired, incomplete oxygenation of the blood will always occur.

Modifying factors

Several other factors also influence the saturation of haemoglobin with O_2, making it either easier or more difficult for O_2 to bind at any given PO_2. These include:

- PCO_2
- H^+ concentration
- temperature
- 2,3-biphosphoglycerate (2,3-BPG) concentration (sometimes 2,3-diphosphoglycerate (2,3-DPG)).

An increase in the value of any of these causes a decrease in the saturation of haemoglobin with O_2, whereas a decrease increases O_2 saturation (Fig. 7.19). These facts also have important practical consequences: PCO_2, H^+ concentration and temperature are all slightly higher in the tissues than in the lungs; thus the release

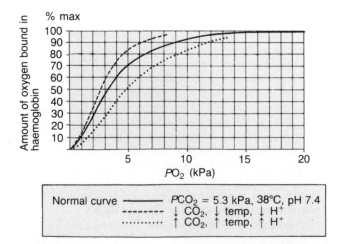

Figure 7.19 Amount of oxygen carried by haemoglobin at different pressures of oxygen and under different conditions (oxygen–haemoglobin dissociation curves).

of O_2 in the tissues and its binding to haemoglobin in the lungs is facilitated by the variations in these factors.

2,3-BPG is formed in tissues (including the red cell) as a product of metabolism in the absence of oxygen (anaerobic metabolism). The increased release of oxygen from oxyhaemoglobin in the presence of higher levels of 2,3-BPG is thus a further mechanism by which tissues in which there is a lack of oxygen can be supplied with more oxygen.

The amount of 2,3-BPG decreases gradually in blood stored for transfusion. Older blood may therefore not be as good at releasing O_2 as fresh blood.

CARBON DIOXIDE TRANSPORT

The amounts of CO_2 present in arterial and venous blood are shown in Table 7.2. CO_2 is carried in the bloodstream in three different ways:

- dissolved in the plasma – about 7%
- combined with proteins (carbamino compounds, e.g. carbaminohaemoglobin) – about 23%
- as hydrogen carbonate ions (HCO_3^-) – about 70%.

COMBINATION WITH PROTEINS

CO_2 can react chemically with certain side chain groups of the amino acids that make up proteins and thus be transported in the blood in this way.

e.g. CO_2 + haemoglobin → carbaminohaemoglobin

CARBONIC ACID/HYDROGEN CARBONATE SYSTEM

This is the major means of CO_2 transport.

In a two-stage reaction, CO_2 is converted to hydrogen carbonate ions as follows:

- CO_2 reacts with water to form carbonic acid:

$$CO_2 + H_2O \rightarrow H_2CO_3$$

- carbonic acid then dissociates to form H^+ and HCO_3^-:

$$H_2CO_3 \rightarrow H^+ + HCO_3^-$$

These reactions occur throughout the body, not just in the blood. However, the process occurs very efficiently in the red cells for several reasons (Fig. 7.20):

- Red cells contain the enzyme carbonic anhydrase, which greatly increases the rate of the reaction between CO_2 and H_2O.
- Deoxyhaemoglobin, formed when O_2 is released to the tissues, acts as a buffer (see Ch. 13) and picks up much of the H^+ formed in the second part of this reaction. This causes more carbonic acid to dissociate and thus more to be formed from CO_2 and H_2O. Thus, the net effect is the production of a great deal of HCO_3^- from CO_2.
- HCO_3^- does not accumulate in the red cell but passes out into the plasma in exchange for chloride. (The chloride ions are also negatively charged and move into the red cell to maintain the electrical state of the red cell membrane.) Thus, there is not a rise in

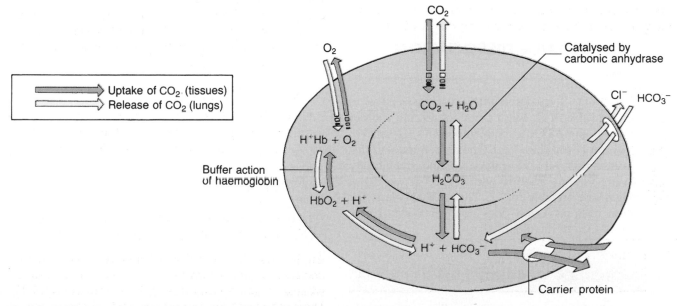

Figure 7.20 The red cell and carbon dioxide. As blood passes through the tissues (purple arrows), hydrogen carbonate is formed from CO_2, and O_2 is released from haemoglobin. As blood passes through the lungs (yellow arrows), hydrogen ions released from haemoglobin combine with hydrogen carbonate to form CO_2.

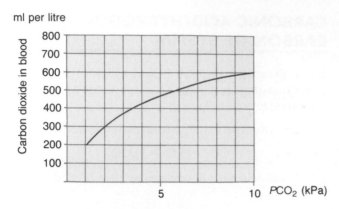

Figure 7.21 Amount of carbon dioxide carried in blood at different pressure of CO_2 (CO_2 dissociation curve).

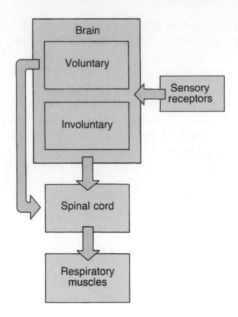

Figure 7.22 Control of the respiratory muscles.

the concentration of HCO_3^- inside the red cell, which would tend to inhibit the formation of further HCO_3^-.

All these processes are reversible. In the tissues, where the PCO_2 is high, the bias is towards the formation of HCO_3^-; in the lungs, however, where the PCO_2 is low (due to CO_2 continually being lost in the expired air), HCO_3^- is converted back into CO_2, via carbonic acid. Also, oxygenation of haemoglobin in the lungs causes the H^+ ions that had been bound to it in the tissues to be released. These combine with HCO_3^- to form carbonic acid again, and this in turn yields CO_2 and H_2O.

Hence, overall, there is a net conversion of CO_2 to HCO_3^- in the tissues and a net conversion in the opposite direction in the lungs so that CO_2 is efficiently and safely transported from tissues to lungs for elimination.

CARBON DIOXIDE DISSOCIATION CURVE

The amount of CO_2 carried in blood increases almost in proportion to the PCO_2 but it does not reach a state of saturation. If the PCO_2 is high, more CO_2 is carried, almost without limit (Fig. 7.21). One consequence of this is that overventilated and underventilated alveoli may compensate for one another with respect to CO_2 in a way that is not possible for O_2. Thus, an imbalance of ventilation and perfusion does not necessarily cause retention of CO_2 in the blood.

CONTROL OF RESPIRATION

The control of respiration is principally a neural process, and is complex, involving both voluntary and involuntary components (Figs 7.22 and 7.23). Most of the time, respiration is controlled by the involuntary components to produce the regular inspiration/expiration breathing cycle that proceeds subconsciously. But, for activities such as speaking, singing or playing some musical instruments, respiration has to be voluntarily (consciously) controlled. This voluntary control of respiration can override the involuntary controls to some extent, though not completely – e.g. you cannot hold your breath to a degree where you endanger your health.

As in other systems, the basic principle in the control of respiration is one of negative feedback, and there are three main elements involved:

- sensors – gather information from a variety of sources
- control units (voluntary and involuntary; in the brain) – analyse the information from the sensors and initiate the appropriate response(s)
- effectors – produce the required change.

There are many different sensor systems involved in normal involuntary respiratory control, the most important being sensors that respond to chemicals (chemoreceptors). The chemoreceptors involved in respiratory control respond to changes in O_2, CO_2 and H^+ levels in the blood.

The medullary or central chemoreceptors in the brain sense changes in PCO_2 and H^+ concentration in the cerebrospinal fluid surrounding the brain. There are no receptors which respond to hypoxia in the brain. Cerebrospinal fluid is relatively unbuffered because of its low protein concentration; therefore the central

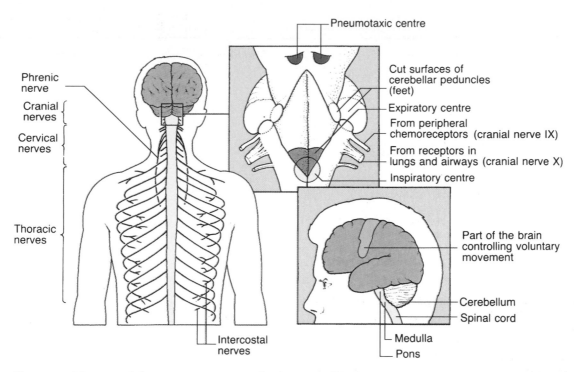

Figure 7.23 Parts of the nervous system involved in controlling breathing: brain, brain stem, spinal cord and nerves. The enlarged inset shows the position of the respiratory centres in the medulla and pons of the brain stem as viewed from behind (the cerebellum, which sits on top of this, is not shown).

chemoreceptors are very rapidly alerted to changes in H^+ concentration.

The arterial or peripheral chemoreceptors found in the aortic and carotid 'bodies' (small areas of tissue in the aorta and common carotid arteries – major arteries very close to the heart) detect changes in arterial PO_2, PCO_2 and H^+ levels.

Clearly, an increased PCO_2 and/or H^+ level or a significantly decreased PO_2 in arterial blood will bring about an increased respiratory effort, whilst the opposite changes in these parameters will bring about a reduction in this effort. The overall result of the operation of this control system, whatever the precise nature of the change in PO_2, PCO_2 and/or H^+ level, is thus that a response is produced that returns the values of these parameters to within the normal homeostatic range, thus ensuring the person's well-being.

Normally, the PO_2 of arterial blood is about 12.7 kPa in a young adult, though it can range from 11.3 to 13.3 kPa. The arterial chemoreceptors are not stimulated much until the PO_2 in the blood falls below 8 kPa. Consequently, under ordinary conditions, when the PO_2 is around 13 kPa, the PO_2 of the blood is not an important factor in the control of breathing; it only becomes important below 8 kPa. It is significant that it is at a PO_2 of about 8 to 9 kPa that oxyhaemoglobin begins to lose appreciable amounts of O_2 (see Fig. 7.19).

- PCO_2 is the parameter that normally regulates respiration – even a small change in the PCO_2 value will bring about an appropriate marked change in respiratory activity.

It is important to note that the arterial chemoreceptors monitor the PO_2 of interstitial fluid, which is related to the PO_2 of blood and not to the total O_2 content. The total O_2 content depends on the number of red cells and their content of haemoglobin. Consequently, the chemoreceptors are not stimulated in anaemia or in carbon monoxide poisoning (see carbon monoxide poisoning; p. 135). In both cases, arterial blood PO_2 is normal although the total amount of O_2 carried in blood is reduced.

Where an individual has chronically elevated PCO_2, for example in some cases of COAD, the central chemoreceptors become adapted to this and no longer respond to CO_2 as a stimulus. Breathing becomes increasingly dependent on 'peripheral hypoxic drive' and the PO_2 in the arteries. Great care must be taken if this person is to be given oxygen, since there is a risk that if the hypoxic drive is removed, breathing will stop until PO_2 is again low enough to re-establish the drive.

Table 7.3 Sensory receptors involved in the control of breathing

Type	Location		Stimulus	Effect on breathing
(A) Within the respiratory system				
Irritant receptor	Airway epithelium	Nose Trachea and bronchi Bronchioles	Inhaled particles and vapours	Sneeze Cough Increased rate and depth
Stretch receptors	Airway smooth muscle		Inflation	Slowed down
J receptors	Alveolar wall		Interstitial oedema Pulmonary emboli	Rapid and shallow
Muscle spindles (see Chs 4B and 25)	Respiratory muscles (e.g. diaphragm, intercostals)		Elongation of the muscles	Made smoother and more efficient
(B) Elsewhere Chemoreceptors (see Chs 5 and 13)	Carotid artery Aorta Brain (medulla)		$\uparrow CO_2$ $\downarrow O_2$ } in blood $\uparrow H^+$ $\uparrow H^+$ in CSF	Increased rate and depth

Other sensors include stretch receptors in the lung: these modify the respiratory process in response to the degree of stretching of the lungs – increased stretching causes a reduction in the respiratory rate by increasing the time taken for expiration, whilst decreased stretching stimulates inspiratory muscle activity.

There are also receptors which lie in airway cells, the nose, nasopharynx, larynx and trachea which are stimulated by noxious gases, cigarette smoke, inhaled dusts and cold air. Stimulation of these receptors produces reflex constriction of the airways (which is thought to be important in asthma). A summary of these various receptors is given in Table 7.3.

The control units in the brain that are responsible for involuntary control are located in the medulla oblongata and the pons of the brain stem and are known as the respiratory centres (Fig. 7.23; see also Ch. 5). They are part of a number of centres in these parts of the brain that are involved in the regulation of many important physiological processes, such as the heart rate and the regulation of blood pressure. It is to these respiratory centres that the information from the various sensory receptors of the respiratory system passes. The medullary rhythmicity centre, which includes separate inspiratory and expiratory areas,

controls the basic rhythm of respiration – typically an inspiration of about 2 seconds and an expiration of about 3 seconds. Note that the inspiratory centre is active in both quiet and forced respiration, whilst the expiratory centre is active only in forced respiration; this is because expiration during quiet respiration is achieved passively – see above. The pneumotaxic centre and the apneustic area coordinate the transition between inspiration and expiration and thus help to determine the size and duration of each breath. Voluntary control of respiration is initiated in the cerebral cortex (Fig. 7.23 and Ch. 20).

All these control units bring about changes in respiration by modifying the activities of the muscles involved in the respiratory process (i.e. the effectors of this system).

The cough reflex is triggered by stimulation of sensory receptors in the lining of the airways. A cough is not always a symptom of disorder – most of us cough several times every day. A cough is a natural defence mechanism designed to clear the airways of irritants such as dust and excess mucus.

Respiratory disease and the environment

With every breath, we inhale not only air but also dust and other pollutants, such as car exhaust fumes, which may cause or contribute to respiratory disease. In addition, some people increase their exposure to lung irritants by smoking, while others may work in environments with particularly high levels of irritant substances (such as dust from coke, iron foundry pollutants and asbestos). Both smoking and occupational exposure to dust and pollution have been linked to increased risk for chronic obstructive airways disease (COAD; see p. 132). The home as well as the work environment may affect respiratory health, with old, poorly maintained housing, which is often damp and cold, identified as particularly unhealthy.

Dust or smoke that gets into the lungs stimulates mucus secretion, which is normally cleared by the action of the cilia. However, the irritants coat the cilia so that they can no longer beat normally, and the cells eventually die. The presence of the irritants and the excess mucus causes inflammation and narrowing of the airways and also provides a site for potential infection.

Cigarette smoke also contains carbon monoxide, which binds to haemoglobin (see 'Carbon monoxide poisoning' box, p. 135) as well as other chemicals that cause further bronchoconstriction. Eventually, the airways become permanently narrowed by the formation of fibrous tissue as inflammation persists (chronic bronchitis). Moreover, the prolonged irritation slowly destroys alveolar tissue, thus reducing the lung area for gas exchange (emphysema).

Once the alveoli have been destroyed, they cannot be repaired, but removing the source of irritation (by stopping smoking or even changing jobs) can at least prevent further damage. Giving up smoking is not so easy, though, and requires an understanding attitude. In many cases, smoking can be considered a true addiction and withdrawal symptoms can be quite distressing. Success depends on a number of factors, including the will and determination of the smoker and the availability of social and family support.

The best strategy, of course, is to decrease the risk of lung disease as much as possible by avoiding exposure to environmental irritants in the first place: use protective equipment at work and DON'T SMOKE.

REFERENCES AND FURTHER READING

Boore J R P, Champion R, Ferguson M C (eds) 1987 Nursing the physically ill adult. Churchill Livingstone, Edinburgh

Pedley T J, Schroter R C, Sudlow M F 1970 The prediction of pressure drop and variation of resistance within the human bronchial airways. Respiratory Physiology 9: 387–405

Rogers A W 1992 Textbook of anatomy. Churchill Livingstone, Edinburgh

Staub N C 1991 Basic respiratory physiology. Churchill Livingstone, Edinburgh
Very useful textbook for further study of human respiration. Includes questions and answers and provides lists of further reading

Tortora G J, Grabowski S R 2000 Principles of anatomy and physiology, 9th edn. John Wiley, New York

Watson J E, Royle J R 1987 Watson's Medical–surgical nursing and related physiology, 3rd edn. Baillière Tindall, London, ch 16

Weibel E R 1963 Morphometry of the human lung. Springer Verlag, Berlin, p 111

West J B 1990 Respiratory physiology – the essentials, 4th edn. Williams & Wilkins, Baltimore
Concise textbook, explaining respiratory function in more detail. Includes questions and answers and further reading

West J B 1992 Pulmonary pathophysiology – the essentials, 4th edn.. Williams & Wilkins, Baltimore
Companion to West 1990. Describes lung function tests, what happens to respiratory function in respiratory diseases, and the principles involved in oxygen therapy and mechanical ventilation

Whipp B J (ed) 1987 The control of breathing in man. Manchester University Press, Manchester

Wilson K J W 1987 Ross & Wilson Anatomy and physiology in health and illness, 6th edn. Churchill Livingstone, Edinburgh, p 119

The renal and urinary system

In practice you may be asked to consider the following:

1. What is the approximate normal adult urinary output per 24 hours?

2. Daily intake of fluid is very variable. Which hormones regulate the renal output of water?

3. Oliguria is common following surgery. Why is this and what can be done to minimize the effect?

4. What is the renal response to hypoxia? What evidence could be found for the effect?

5. A patient has been prescribed an ACEI. What is this? How does it work? What are the effects?

6. How is glomerular pressure maintained in spite of the large volume of fluid filtered at the glomerular capsule?

7. A patient prescribed a diuretic complains that it causes palpitations. Please explain.

8. An elderly man who has benign prostatic hypertrophy has been prescribed a selective α (alpha) adrenoceptor blocker. How does this work? Why can it cause postural hypotension? How does it help the effects of prostatic hypertrophy?

9. Why is there such a large percentage reabsorption of fluid from the proximal tubule?

10. Glycosuria and polyuria appear when plasma glucose is above about 10 mmol/l. Please explain.

The functions of the renal system include regulation of the composition of body fluids and some aspects of the regulation of pressure. In doing so, the kidney filters about 150 litres daily and concentrates the urine produced to about 1.5 litres per day. As well as these primary regulatory functions, the kidney produces the hormone erythropoietin which controls red cell numbers, it is responsible for the production of 1,25-dihydroxycholecalciferol, important in calcium balance and bone maintenance, and produces the enzyme renin which, via aldosterone, affects sodium and potassium concentrations.

The urine formed continually by the kidneys collects in the distensible urinary bladder. This is emptied periodically under the control of the autonomic and somatic nervous systems.

STRUCTURE

There are two kidneys, each weighing about 140 g, situated at the back of the abdomen (Fig. 8.1). Urine passes from the kidneys, through the ureters, to the urinary bladder. Each kidney is made up of about 1 million tiny tubes (nephrons) which are richly supplied with blood, and which empty into a smaller number of collecting ducts.

NEPHRONS

Each nephron consists of a long tube, closed at one end and open at the other, made up of four sections (Fig. 8.2A):

• Bowman's capsule
• proximal convoluted tubule
• loop of Henle
• distal convoluted tubule.

Arrangement

The tubule is twisted into a characteristic shape crucial to its function (Fig. 8.2A). Part of the distal convoluted tubule, the macula densa, lies near to Bowman's capsule of the same tubule (Fig. 8.2B). The macula densa, together with adjacent granular cells of the afferent arteriole, is termed the juxtaglomerular apparatus.

Bowman's capsules and convoluted tubules lie nearer to the surface of the kidney than the loops of Henle. These loops dip inwards and converge down towards the centre of the kidney. If you slice a kidney in half you will see that the appearance of the outer part (cortex) where the convoluted tubules and Bowman's capsules are, differs from the inner section (medulla), occupied by the loops of Henle (Fig. 8.3A).

Types

All the nephrons have the same constituent parts but they do differ. Those with Bowman's capsules in the outer cortex have very short loops of Henle which do not extend very far into the medulla. Others, with Bowman's capsules sited close to the medulla, juxta-medullary nephrons, have long loops (Fig. 8.3B). The juxtamedullary nephrons are central to the process of water recovery and the concentration of urine (see below).

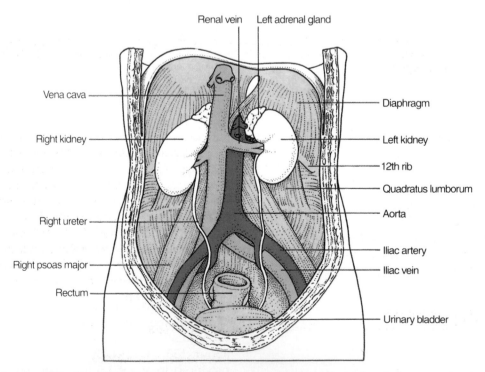

Figure 8.1 Position of the kidneys, ureters and urinary bladder in the abdomen and pelvis. (From Rogers 1992, with permission of Elsevier.)

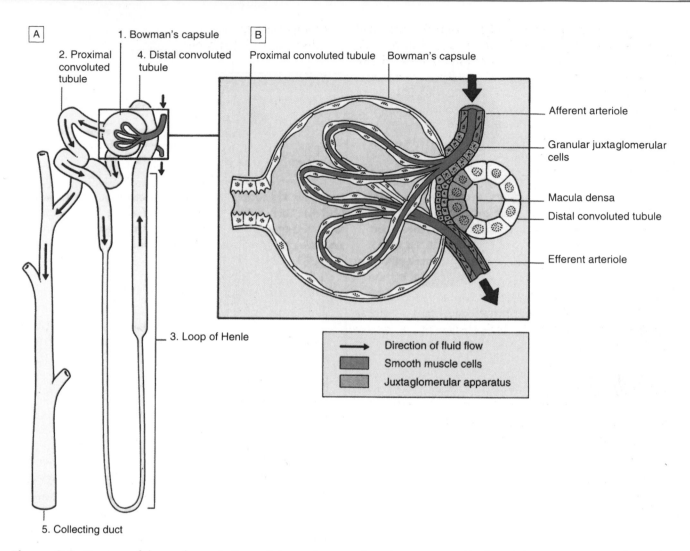

Figure 8.2 Structure of the nephron. A, Parts of the nephron numbered in sequence (1–4) and their arrangement alongside a collecting duct (5). B, The arrangement of Bowman's capsule and the region of the distal convoluted tubule which together make up the juxtaglomerular apparatus.

COLLECTING DUCTS, PELVIS AND URETERS

Fluid from several nephrons flows into the collecting ducts. These empty into large drainage vessels (calyces) at the papillae of the medullary pyramids. Urine flows from the calyces via the pelvis of the kidney into the ureter. The whole of each kidney is enclosed by a capsule of connective tissue (renal capsule).

RENAL BLOOD VESSELS

Arteries

Within each kidney the renal artery branches to form several interlobar arteries, which divide the medulla into sections (medullary pyramids) and carry the blood to the boundary between the medulla and the cortex (Fig. 8.4). At this point each interlobar artery gives rise to arcuate arteries that run along the border between the medulla and the cortex. From these, small interlobular arteries carry the blood up into the cortex. Branching off the interlobular arteries at multiple points are tiny vessels, the afferent arterioles, each of which supplies blood to a tuft of capillaries (glomerular capillaries) lodged within the expanded end of the nephron (Bowman's capsule).

Capillaries

Glomerular capillaries

The glomerular capillaries fit into Bowman's capsule rather like a hand inserted into an incubator, or isolation

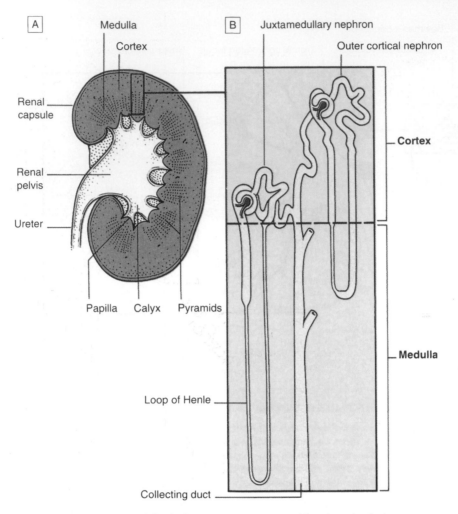

Figure 8.3 Structure of the kidney. A, Structures visible when the kidney is cut in half. B, Types of nephron and their position within the kidney.

Observing for renal trauma

A major problem facing medical and nursing staff when assessing a severely injured patient admitted to the Accident & Emergency Department is missing less obvious trauma in the face of multiple, clearly visible injuries. For example, following a road traffic accident where the patient has fractures to both legs and several ribs, and lacerations to the face and chest, it may be easy to overlook internal injuries with few external signs – such as to the spleen and kidneys.

Where a kidney is damaged, bleeding may occur into the surrounding tissue causing, perhaps, bruising, distension and loin pain. In such a situation, the renal pain may be a dull ache, and overlooked by the patient (and carers) in the face of much more acute pain from, say, broken bones. Severe trauma may cause the kidney to tear away from its major blood vessels so that haemorrhage is massive, and death can swiftly ensue. (Recollect what proportion of the cardiac output goes to the kidneys.)

Damage within the renal capsule may lead to visible haematuria (blood in the urine) and the trauma nurse may be asked to collect serial specimens of urine.
(If the patient does not, or cannot, pass urine he may be catheterized in order to obtain a specimen for examination. Catheterization should not be carried out if damage to the urethra is suspected.)

The reason for obtaining serial specimens of urine where kidney damage is suspected is as follows. The first specimen obtained may be negative to blood, either from naked eye inspection or on testing using reagent strips. However, that first specimen consists of urine that may have been present in the bladder for some time. Damage to one of the kidneys may result in a small flow of blood which, at first, occupies the kidney pelvis and ureter. A second specimen of urine may subsequently reveal visible haematuria, as bleeding from the kidney reaches the bladder and is drained by the urinary catheter.

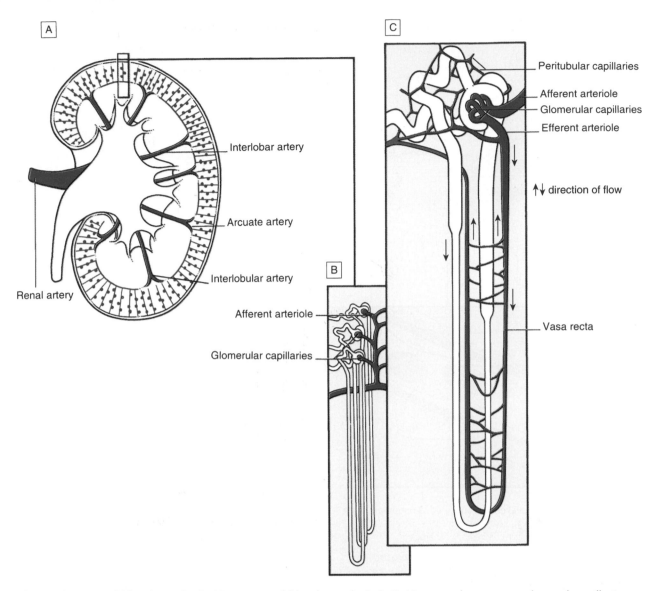

Figure 8.4 Renal blood supply. A, Major arterial blood vessels. B & C, Microcirculation: arterioles and capillaries.

chamber, through a glove. The indented part of Bowman's capsule (the glove of the incubator in the analogy) is wrapped around the glomerular capillaries (the hand). The two together form the glomerulus (Fig. 8.5A). The indented layer of Bowman's capsule consists of distinctive cells (podocytes). These have many 'feet' (podos in Greek means foot) that make contact with the basement membrane of the endothelial cells of the capillary wall (Fig. 8.5B). Fluid filtered from the capillaries passes across the endothelial cell layer, then the basement membrane and finally through gaps between the 'feet' of the podocytes, into the space inside Bowman's capsule itself (equivalent to the interior of the incubator in the analogy).

Peritubular capillaries

Blood leaves the glomerulus through a vessel which has the structure of an arteriole and is termed the efferent arteriole. This gives rise to another set of capillaries, peritubular capillaries, which surround the convoluted tubules (Fig. 8.4C).

The juxtamedullary nephrons, which have long loops of Henle, have a specialized arrangement of peritubular vessels known as the vasa recta (Fig. 8.4C). These vessels do not branch very much. Instead they extend straight down into the medulla, following the line of the loop of Henle. Near the tip of the loop they double back towards the cortex, again following the route taken by the tubule. This arrangement of loop, collecting tubules and vasa

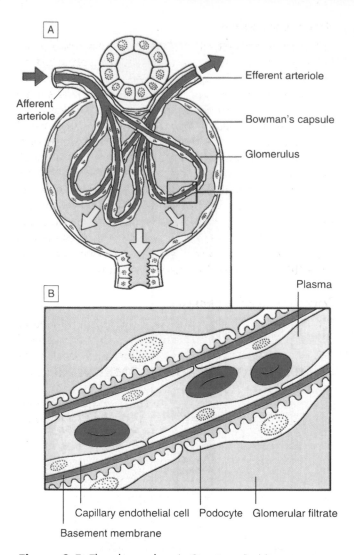

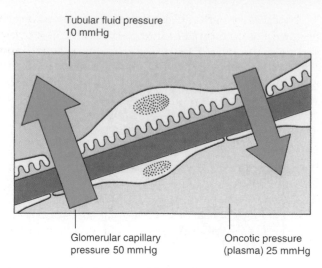

Figure 8.6 The balance of forces determining glomerular filtration.

Figure 8.5 The glomerulus. A, Structure. B, Microstructure of the glomerular filter.

those involved in the formation of tissue fluid elsewhere in the body. However, the barrier consists of the capillary wall and basement membrane plus the podocytes (Fig. 8.5B). It is practically impermeable to plasma proteins. The blood flow to the kidneys is considerable (1200 ml/min) and capillary pressures are high. Consequently, the volume of fluid filtered is large (120 ml/min). The filtration fraction is approximately 10% (whole blood) or 20% (plasma).

HYDROSTATIC AND ONCOTIC PRESSURES

The forces that are involved in the filtration of fluid by the kidneys (Fig. 8.6) are:

- the difference in hydrostatic pressure between the fluid in the glomerular capillary and the back pressure of the fluid within Bowman's capsule
- the oncotic pressure of the plasma, created by plasma proteins and the glomerular barrier.

The distinctive feature about the balance of forces in the kidney is the high hydrostatic pressure within the glomerular capillaries (45–50 mmHg).

Glomerular capillary pressure

The glomerular capillary pressure is the highest normally present in any capillary bed in the body. As such, it normally exceeds the oncotic pressure of the plasma at *all points* of the glomerular capillaries, not just at the 'arterial' end as in other capillaries (see Ch. 6). Consequently, under normal circumstances, some fluid is driven out of the plasma across the glomerular wall and none is drawn back in.

recta forms the structural basis for the water recovery system which allows the production of concentrated urine (see below at 'Control: conserving water').

Veins

From the peritubular capillaries, interlobular veins carry the blood back to arcuate veins, interlobar veins and then the renal vein, along the same route, in reverse, as the arteries.

HOW FLUID IS FILTERED

The first step in the formation of urine is glomerular filtration, the formation of a filtrate of plasma. This filtrate contains all the constituents of plasma except the plasma proteins. The processes involved are the same as

The uniquely high capillary pressure is caused by the resistance offered by the efferent arterioles. The driving pressure for filtration is affected by constriction and dilation of the efferent arterioles as well as the afferent arterioles. Both sets of vessels are innervated by sympathetic nerves and are influenced by hormones such as angiotensin and adrenaline.

Afferent arteriole

If the afferent arteriole constricts, the hydrostatic pressure in the capillaries decreases and the rate of fluid filtration decreases also. This happens if there is a reflex increase in the activity of the sympathetic nerves innervating the vessels, as in haemorrhage (see Ch. 12).

Control of efferent arteriole

The driving pressure is also affected by the ease with which blood is able to leave the glomerulus, which depends on the degree of dilation or constriction of the efferent arteriole. If this vessel constricts, the pressure of blood upstream in the glomerulus increases, and glomerular filtration rate (GFR) will also increase.

If both afferent and efferent arterioles constrict simultaneously then glomerular capillary pressure, and GFR, may not change.

Autoregulation

Filtration is very closely linked to capillary perfusion. While the main pressure fluctuations are controlled by the autonomic effects on the afferent and efferent arterioles, local control is also very important. The renal circulation has very highly developed autoregulation. The mechanism may be myogenic, i.e. the response of muscle when stretched is to contract (see Ch. 4B) or it may be due to locally produced vasoactive agents such as nitric oxide (see Ch. 12). It is more likely that no single mechanism is responsible. The effect is that when pressure rises inside the vessel, the smooth muscle relaxes, lowering the pressure and removing the stimulus; it then contracts, raising the pressure again. The changes are small and the overall effect is smoothing of the local perfusion pressure.

Tubular fluid pressure

The hydrostatic pressure of the fluid within Bowman's capsule (tubular fluid pressure) is normally around 10 mmHg. This acts as back pressure and counteracts the pressure in the capillaries so that the net hydrostatic pressure is actually 35 to 40 mmHg. If the flow of tubular fluid through the nephrons, the collecting ducts and ureters is obstructed in any way, tubular pressure rises and the rate of filtration decreases.

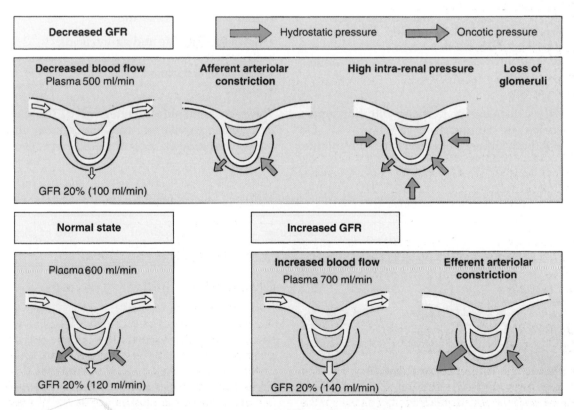

Figure 8.7 The factors decreasing and increasing glomerular filtration rate (GFR).

Observing for renal failure

Urine production relies on an adequate pressure of blood within the renal arteries. A fall in blood pressure, if severe or sufficiently prolonged, may cause damage to renal tissue, and the patient suffers acute renal failure. This condition can be fatal but, if treated swiftly, is reversible. Swift treatment relies on nursing observations of blood pressure and urine output, which can inform medical staff that renal failure is likely. Steps are then taken to prevent it.

Patients following major surgery, myocardial infarction or severe burns, for example, have frequent observations made of their pulse and blood pressure. A prolonged systolic pressure below about 60 to 70 mmHg would be regarded as possibly heralding acute renal failure. In such cases, urine output would be measured hourly; daily totals of fluid balance are insufficient. Such a severely ill patient will probably be catheterized, perhaps for the sole reason of assessing urine formation. Special collecting chambers are available, which attach to the catheter tubing and measure small amounts of urine.

Swift treatment to improve a patient's blood pressure should result in an improvement in urine output. Such treatment might include a blood transfusion to restore blood volume following severe haemorrhage. In some cases of heart failure, drugs such as dobutamine may be given intravenously to improve cardiac performance and therefore renal blood flow.

Following surgery, a brief period of oliguria (reduced urine output) is to be expected. Where blood pressure is maintained, and blood volume restored, this period of oliguria should not exceed 2 to 3 hours.

Factors which increase or decrease filtration across the glomerulus are summarized in Figure 8.7. On average, GFR (both kidneys together) is 120 ml/minute. It varies with body size and so is slightly smaller in women (110 ml/min) than in men (125 ml/min).

COMPOSITION OF THE GLOMERULAR FILTRATE

The composition of the filtered fluid depends on the permeability of the barrier layers separating the blood from the tubular fluid. The barrier allows free movement of small water-soluble molecules but restricts the passage of molecules and particles of the size of the plasma proteins and bigger. Thus the glomerular filtrate contains all the constituents of plasma with the exception of most plasma proteins. A little protein does get through, just as some escapes into the tissue space in other capillary beds, but the amounts are not large. If the permeability of the barrier increases, as in the *nephrotic syndrome*, the glomerular filtrate contains appreciable amounts of protein which then appears in the urine (proteinuria).

HOW VITAL CONSTITUENTS OF THE FILTRATE ARE RECOVERED

The second step in the formation of urine is the recovery of constituents of the filtrate that must be retained within the body. These are:

- nutrients (glucose and amino acids)
- electrolytes (sodium, potassium, chloride etc.)
- hydrogen carbonate
- water.

These constituents are returned to the blood in the peritubular capillaries from the tubular fluid in the convoluted tubules, loop of Henle and collecting ducts.

Table 8.1 Approximate composition of the tubular fluid at different sites along the nephron

		Glomerular filtrate	End of proximal convoluted tubule	End of distal convoluted tubule
Albumin	g/l	0.2	0.0	0.0
Glucose		5	0.5	0.0
Amino acids		2	0.2	0.0
Sodium (Na$^+$)	mmol/l	135	135	40–135
Potassium (K$^+$)		4	4	4–40
Chloride (Cl$^-$)		115	135	35–135
Hydrogen carbonate (HCO$_3^-$)		25	6	1–10
Osmotic pressure	mosmol/kgH$_2$O	300	300	80–300
Fluid flow rate	ml/min	120	40	5–10

NUTRIENTS: GLUCOSE AND AMINO ACIDS

If the composition of the glomerular filtrate is compared with the composition of fluid at the end of the proximal convoluted tubule (PCT) (Table 8.1) it can be seen that almost all of the glucose and the amino acids filtered at the glomerulus have been removed by the time the fluid reaches the end of the PCT. Normally, only minute quantities of these substances, undetectable by routine clinical methods, are lost in the urine. They are recovered by carrier-mediated transport. The transport mechanisms are very similar to those described for the absorption of glucose and amino acids in the small intestine (see Ch. 9).

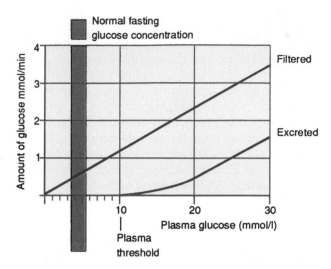

Figure 8.8 Urinary losses of glucose in humans at different plasma glucose concentrations. At high glucose concentrations (>20 mmol/l) the difference between the amount of glucose filtered and that excreted is the maximum the tubules can absorb (Tm). (After Emslie-Smith et al 1988.)

The diabetic patient

Glycosuria is one of the signs of diabetes mellitus. Lack of effective insulin production by the pancreas (see Ch. 18) means that glucose in the blood cannot be utilized by all tissues. Plasma glucose levels consequently rise until the renal threshold is reached and exceeded – glycosuria then occurs. This can happen suddenly in youngsters (mostly boys) or occur more gradually in, principally, middle-aged or elderly, overweight women. This is an extremely simplified summary of events.

The osmotic force of high levels of glucose excreted in urine leads to polyuria – excessive urine volumes. Reabsorption of water from the tubules is diminished because of the osmotic pull of glucose in the glomerular filtrate. Increased water, as well as glucose, enters the collecting tubules and is eventually excreted as urine. This loss of water from the body leads to dehydration. Reduced blood volume is balanced by withdrawal of fluid from the interstitial compartment into the blood, which in turn leads to movement of water from body cells into the interstitial compartment. In other words, there is a shift of water out of the cells into the bloodstream and then into the urine.

One of the first signs of diabetes mellitus in a young child might be excessive drinking to counteract an intense thirst (the osmoreceptors in the thirst centre being stimulated by an increase in the osmolarity of blood passing through it). Parents may then notice increased visits to the toilet. A child may even start bedwetting at night, having previously outgrown this, because of the increased urine production.

Urine is tested for glucose by reagent strips that change colour according to the level of glucose present. Incidentally, one of the earliest tests for diabetes was tasting a sufferer's urine for sugar, or leaving a container of the urine outside, where it attracted bees because of its sweetness.

There is an upper limit to the amounts that can be transported by the cells, the transport maximum (Tm). If they are presented with too much glucose or amino acids, some is not recovered, and substantial losses of these substances occur in the urine (glycosuria and amino-aciduria). The amount of glucose lost (excreted) in the urine at different plasma concentrations of glucose is shown in Figure 8.8. At normal fasting concentrations of plasma glucose (3.5–5.5 mmol/l), urinary glucose is virtually undetectable. Above 10 mmol/l appreciable amounts of glucose begin to appear, and the urinary output increases in proportion to the increase in plasma glucose concentration.

The plasma concentration of glucose at which the increase in output begins (Fig. 8.8) is the plasma or renal threshold. As nephrons, like people, are not identical, some reach their maximum absorptive capacity for glucose before others. So, at first, just a trickle of glucose appears in the urine before most nephrons are overloaded.

ELECTROLYTES (SODIUM, POTASSIUM, CHLORIDE, CALCIUM)

About 70% of the electrolytes filtered at the glomerulus are returned to the blood in the peritubular capillaries surrounding the proximal convoluted tubule. Most of the remainder is recovered into the blood by distal parts of the nephron and peritubular capillaries. The amounts of electrolytes recovered and excreted are adjusted according to need.

Proximal convoluted tubule

From Table 8.1, it can be seen that the concentrations of sodium, potassium and chloride are almost the same at the end of the proximal convoluted tubule (PCT) as they were in the glomerular filtrate. However, the volume of fluid emerging from the proximal convoluted tubules (~40 ml/min) is much less than the volume entering them at the glomerulus (~120 ml/min). Thus about 70% of the electrolytes that were filtered at the glomerulus have in fact been removed from the tubular fluid by the end of the PCT.

Mechanisms

Some of the ways in which the electrolytes are returned to the blood include (Fig. 8.9):

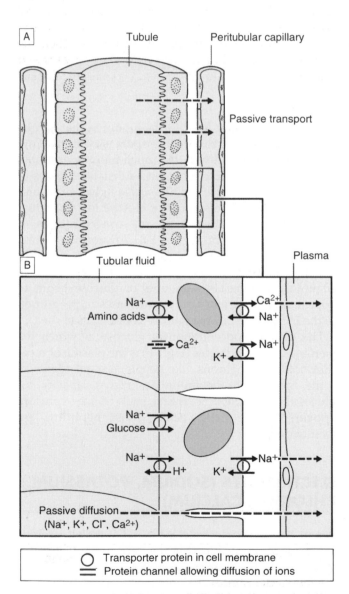

Figure 8.9 Ways in which electrolytes are absorbed into the blood from the tubular fluid by cells of the proximal convoluted tubule.

- passive transport (either by diffusion or swept along with the water absorbed by osmosis)
- carrier-mediated transport.

Control

Most of this absorption is not under hormonal control. In that sense it is unregulated and is therefore often referred to as obligatory. However, reabsorption and filtration must be matched. If filtration rate is high, some solute would be lost if Tm were to be exceeded; if filtration rate is low, the reabsorption might be excessive. The two are matched by tubulo-glomerular feedback. The mechanism is unclear but it may be that if the filtration fraction is high, the osmotic pressure of the blood in the peritubular capillaries will be high and this may increase fluid (and solute) recovery from the tubule. It has also been proposed that the filtered sodium, by affecting the cells of the macula densa (see below) and causing the release of renin, will adjust the tone of the afferent and efferent arterioles and so filtration rate. The recovery of calcium is influenced by a variety of factors including the hormones parathyroid hormone and calcitonin (see Ch. 14) and the concentration of phosphate in the tubular fluid.

Distal convoluted tubule

In Table 8.1, it can be seen that the composition of the tubular fluid at the end of the distal convoluted tubule (DCT) varies. The fluid here may be hypotonic (osmotic pressure less than plasma) or isotonic (osmotic pressure equal to plasma). This part of the nephron adjusts the amounts of sodium, potassium, water, and acid and base that are recovered or excreted, and so helps to maintain normal water, electrolyte and acid–base balance within the body (Ch. 14). Some of the processes involved in electrolyte transport here are summarized in Figure 8.10.

Control

The absorption of sodium by the distal convoluted tubule is increased by the steroid hormone aldosterone (see Chs 11 and 12). Aldosterone stimulates the synthesis of some of the transporter proteins that carry sodium. If aldosterone secretion increases, the recovery of sodium chloride is gradually enhanced over several hours. This allows the excretion of these electrolytes to be adjusted, for example, according to long-term variations in the dietary intake of sodium. Aldosterone also increases the urinary excretion of potassium.

The kidney and systemic blood pressure management

Aldosterone has an important role in the regulation of blood pressure as part of the renin–angiotensin–

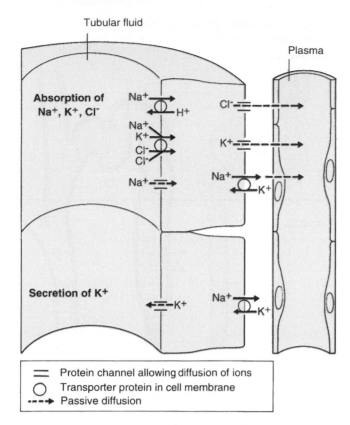

Figure 8.10 Absorption and secretion of electrolytes by cells of the distal convoluted tubule.

aldosterone mechanism. This mechanism regulates intravascular volume, one of the major areas of pressure management. Details of this mechanism and of the renal regulation of intravascular volume are given in Chapter 12.

Other parts of the nephron

Substantial amounts of sodium, potassium and chloride (25% of that filtered) are absorbed into the blood from the loop of Henle. Small amounts of electrolytes are also recovered by the collecting ducts (Table 8.2). Potassium differs from sodium in that some is added to the tubular fluid by cells of the distal convoluted tubules. Thus the

Table 8.2 Amounts of sodium recovered by different parts of the nephron (as % filtered load)

	%
Proximal convoluted tubule	66
Loop of Henle	25
Distal convoluted tubule	4
Collecting duct	4
Total	>99%

amount of potassium excreted per day (150 mmol) is as large as the amount of sodium excreted (also about 150 mmol), even though there is much more sodium than potassium in the glomerular filtrate (see Table 8.1). This high urinary excretion of potassium is needed to balance the high dietary intake of potassium (see Ch. 15).

HYDROGEN CARBONATE (HCO$_3^-$)

HCO$_3^-$ is, like the electrolytes, recovered by both the proximal and distal convoluted tubules, but the extent to which it is recovered depends on the acid–base status of the body (see Ch. 13). If the extracellular fluid (ECF) is more acid than normal, then all the hydrogen carbonate filtered at the glomerulus is recovered, and none is excreted in the urine. However, if the extracellular fluid is more alkaline than normal, then the tubular recovery of hydrogen carbonate decreases and some is excreted in the urine, making the urine alkaline.

Mechanism

The absorption of hydrogen carbonate relies on the presence of the enzyme carbonic anhydrase both within and on the luminal surface of the tubular cells. As in red

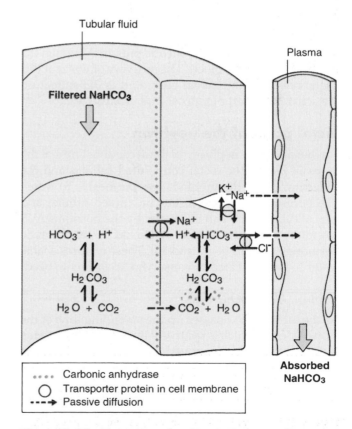

Figure 8.11 Absorption of sodium hydrogen carbonate from the tubular fluid into the blood.

blood cells (see Ch. 3) it catalyses the reversible conversion of CO_2 and H_2O into carbonic acid. Hydrogen carbonate in the tubular fluid combines with H^+ ions, which are transported into the tubular fluid in exchange for sodium, to form carbonic acid (Fig. 8.11). Carbonic acid is rapidly converted into CO_2 and H_2O. CO_2 diffuses easily into the tubular cells and is used to re-form HCO_3^-, which is transported out of the cells into the interstitial fluid surrounding the peritubular capillaries.

Control

The recovery of hydrogen carbonate is not under hormonal control. It is regulated simply by the concentrations of carbon dioxide and H^+ ions inside and outside the kidney cells. These depend, in turn, upon the acid–base status of the body as a whole (see Ch. 13).

WATER

Throughout the nephron, the absorption of water is driven entirely by osmosis.

Proximal convoluted tubule

Seventy per cent of the water filtered at the glomerulus is recovered here. The balance of hydrostatic and oncotic pressures in the peritubular capillaries (low hydrostatic pressure, high oncotic pressure) favours the return of fluid to the blood. The recovery of water at this site is not under hormonal control; it is dependent on the active transport of glucose and electrolytes.

Distal parts of the nephron

Further along the nephron, in the ascending limbs of the loops of Henle, the distal convoluted tubules and the collecting ducts, the tubule is less permeable to water. The permeability of the distal convoluted tubules and the collecting ducts can be altered by the hormone AVP (arginine vasopressin) also called ADH (antidiuretic hormone) (see Chs 11, 12 and 14). These features enable water to be eliminated or conserved according to need.

Control: eliminating water

As the tubular fluid passes up the ascending limb of the loop of Henle, which is relatively impermeable to water, sodium chloride is removed and the fluid becomes dilute (Fig. 8.12), becoming hypotonic in the cortical segment. When the distal tubules and the collecting ducts are impermeable to water, water is not absorbed here even though a substantial difference of osmotic pressure exists between the tubular fluid and the plasma. Under these conditions, large amounts of dilute urine would be formed (900 to 1500 ml/h). Massive

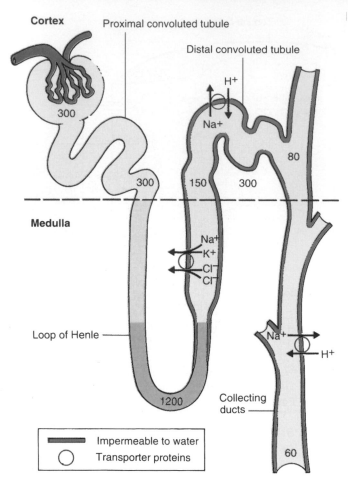

Figure 8.12 Eliminating water: formation of a dilute urine when the walls of the distal tubule are impermeable to water. The numbers and orange shading indicate how the osmotic pressure of the tubular fluid changes along the nephron and collecting duct.

urinary flows of this kind occur in disease in the condition known as diabetes insipidus in which the hormone AVP/ADH is either absent or ineffective.

Control: conserving water

AVP/ADH increases the permeability of the distal convoluted tubules and the collecting ducts to water, and thus allows water to be conserved. The volume of urine excreted can be reduced to a minimum of 18 ml/hour by concentrating the fluid. As a result it becomes hypertonic. The power of the kidneys to achieve this is due to the distinctive arrangement and characteristics of the loop of Henle in the long loop or juxtamedullary nephron. It creates a difference in osmotic pressure between the interstitial fluid of the cortex and that of the medulla. Whereas the osmotic pressure of the cortex is similar to that of the plasma, at the tip of the medulla it may be four to five times as great (Fig. 8.13). The way in which this difference in osmotic pressure is developed is explained later.

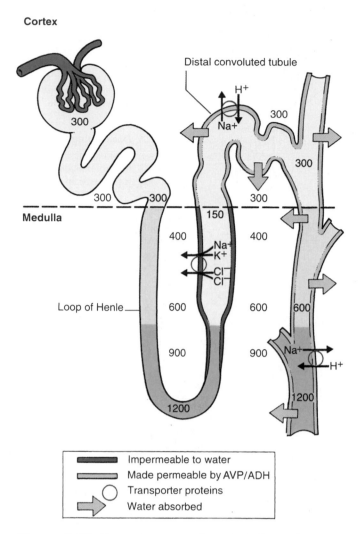

Cortex

Distal convoluted tubule

Medulla

Loop of Henle

300
300
300 300
300
300
H+
Na+
150
400 400
Na+
K+
Cl-
Cl-
600 600 600
900 900 Na+
H+
1200
1200

Impermeable to water
Made permeable by AVP/ADH
Transporter proteins
Water absorbed

Figure 8.13 Conserving water: formation of a concentrated urine when the walls of the distal tubule are made permeable to water by the action of the hormone AVP/ADH. The numbers and orange shading indicate how the osmotic pressure of the tubular fluid changes as it passes along the nephron and collecting duct.

The collecting ducts through which the tubular fluid passes are thus surrounded by an environment which becomes increasingly more concentrated as the papillae are approached. If the walls of the collecting duct are impermeable to water, the tubular fluid tracking through the collecting duct remains the same as when it left the distal convoluted tubule (Fig. 8.12). However, if the walls are made permeable by AVP/ADH, then water in the tubular fluid is drawn by osmosis into the hypertonic environment of the medullary interstitium, and moves from there into the blood in the vasa recta. The tubular fluid is gradually concentrated. A maximally concentrated urine will have an osmotic pressure similar to that of the interstitial fluid at the tips of the loops of Henle (1200 mosmol/kgH$_2$O – about four times that of blood plasma).

Loop of Henle

This consists of two limbs, descending and ascending (Fig. 8.14A). Fluid leaving the proximal convoluted tubule enters the descending limb and flows down and then up into the ascending limb. The flow of fluid in the two limbs of the loop of Henle is thus in opposite directions (*countercurrent*).

Creating hypertonicity

Cells of the ascending loop of Henle actively transport sodium and chloride from the tubular fluid out into the interstitium. The upper ascending limb is impermeable to water; therefore the ions leave unaccompanied by water. Chloride and sodium diffuse through the interstitium. Some enters the fluid in the descending limb of the loop. The direction of fluid flow sweeps the ions down towards the tip of the loop. When the tubular fluid rounds the bend and flows back towards the cortex some of the sodium and chloride in it is picked up again by the transporter proteins in the cells of the ascending limb and ejected once more into the interstitium. Thus, sodium and chloride get recycled and trapped in the loop and the medullary interstitium. In this way the concentration of sodium and chloride build up towards the tip and it is this which chiefly creates the difference in osmotic pressure between the cortex and the medulla.

Role of the vasa recta

If the blood capillaries supplying the loop of Henle formed a network similar to that around the convoluted tubules, then much of the sodium and chloride transported out of the ascending limb would simply diffuse into the capillaries and be swept away in the bloodstream. Consequently, few ions would be trapped in the medulla and the difference in osmotic pressure between the cortex and medulla would be much less.

However, the capillaries follow the loop around. Consequently, although the blood flowing in the descending limbs of the vasa recta gains sodium and chloride from the interstitium (Fig. 8.14B), that passing up the ascending limbs loses most of it again back into the medullary interstitium. Hence sodium chloride and other solutes tend to be retained in the medulla rather than washed away.

The amount of sodium chloride and other solutes retained in the medulla depends on the rate of flow of blood through the vasa recta. If flow increases, more is lost and the difference in concentration between the cortex and the medulla decreases. Consequently tubular fluid passing through the collecting ducts cannot be concentrated to the same extent and a less concentrated urine is formed. Conversely, if blood flow decreases, as it does under the action of AVP/ADH, which causes vasoconstriction of the vasa recta, the concentrating power of the kidney increases.

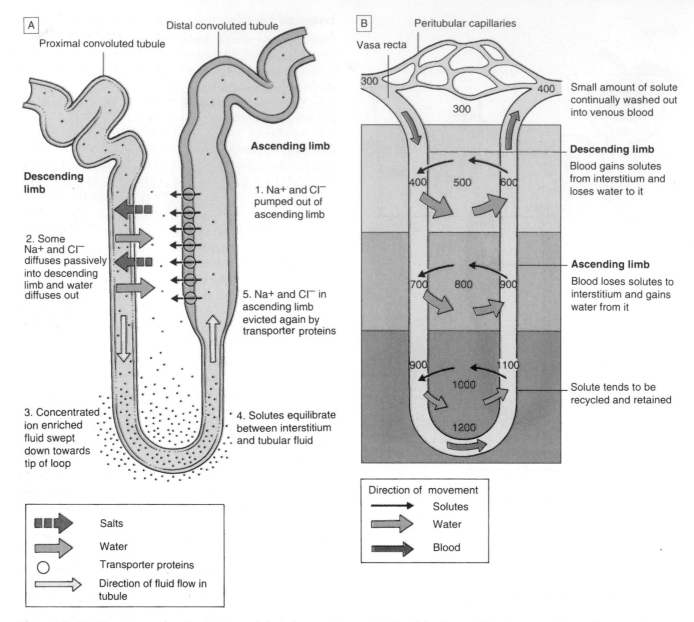

A

Proximal convoluted tubule

Distal convoluted tubule

Descending limb

Ascending limb

1. Na+ and Cl⁻ pumped out of ascending limb

2. Some Na+ and Cl⁻ diffuses passively into descending limb and water diffuses out

5. Na+ and Cl⁻ in ascending limb evicted again by transporter proteins

3. Concentrated ion enriched fluid swept down towards tip of loop

4. Solutes equilibrate between interstitium and tubular fluid

Salts

Water

Transporter proteins

Direction of fluid flow in tubule

B

Peritubular capillaries

Vasa recta

300   400

300

Small amount of solute continually washed out into venous blood

Descending limb
Blood gains solutes from interstitium and loses water to it

400 500 600

Ascending limb
Blood loses solutes to interstitium and gains water from it

700 800 900

Solute tends to be recycled and retained

900 1100

1000

1200

Direction of movement

Solutes

Water

Blood

Figure 8.14 Creating and maintaining medullary hypertonicity. A, Role of the loop of Henle in recycling sodium and chloride and accumulating them in the medullary interstitium. B, Role of the vasa recta in minimizing losses of sodium and chloride from the medullary interstitium. Numbers indicate the osmotic pressure of the interstitial fluid and the blood plasma at different levels.

HOW WASTE SUBSTANCES ARE ELIMINATED

The waste substances that the kidneys eliminate are water soluble. Most get into the tubular fluid simply by being filtered at the glomerulus (Fig. 8.15). In addition to this a few substances are transported from the blood into the tubular fluid by carrier proteins in the tubular cells.

FILTRATION

Any substance dissolved in plasma, which is smaller in size than the plasma proteins and which does not bind to them, will pass through the glomerular filter into the tubular fluid. Its fate thereafter depends on the tubular epithelium and the characteristics of the substance concerned, such as its:

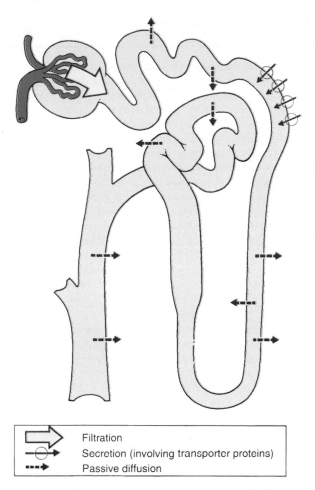

⇨	Filtration
⊖→	Secretion (involving transporter proteins)
---►	Passive diffusion

Figure 8.15 Elimination of waste materials by filtration and secretion. The amount finally excreted depends on the extent to which waste substances are absorbed by passive diffusion through the walls of the tubules.

- ability to bind to carrier proteins in the membrane of the tubular cells
- molecular size and liposolubility.

Tubular cell selectivity

The carrier proteins transporting substances across cell membranes are usually highly selective for specific molecules. The carrier that transports glucose, for example, does not transport mannitol, a carbohydrate molecule of similar size but differing in structure. In this way the tubular cells are able to selectively recover key molecules whilst rejecting others.

Molecular size and liposolubility

The permeability of the tubular epithelium to water-soluble molecules is much less than that of the glomerular filter. Thus some molecules, such as creatinine (a breakdown product of muscle metabolism), get trapped in the tubular fluid because their

molecular size stops them from passing easily through the epithelium. They stay in the tubular fluid and their concentration increases progressively as water and other constituents of the glomerular filtrate are gradually absorbed.

Water-soluble molecules which *can* leak out of the tubular fluid back into the blood are either tiny enough to pass through the water-filled channels that do exist in the cell membranes and at the junctions between cells, or they are soluble to some extent in lipids and can simply diffuse across the cell membrane. In both cases, the driving force for absorption is the difference in concentration of the substance between the tubular fluid and the blood plasma, i.e. the concentration gradient.

Concentration differences develop as fluid is absorbed by the mechanisms described previously. Consequently, if a molecule can get through the epithelium it will be absorbed passively. A good example of this is urea, a waste product of protein metabolism (see Chs 9 and 10).

Urea

Urea is absorbed passively by diffusion from the tubular fluid, but its absorption is only partial because the tubular epithelium is not fully permeable to it. The extent to which it is retained in the tubular fluid, and therefore excreted, depends on the rate of flow of fluid through the different parts of the nephron. Urea contributes significantly to the osmotic pressure in the renal medulla. As water is removed from the collecting tubule under the influence of AVP, the concentration of urea in the tubule rises until it is greater than that in the interstitial fluid surrounding the loop and tubules. It moves with the concentration gradient into the interstitial space, raising the osmotic pressure further. The effect is to withdraw even more water from the collecting tubule and further concentrate the urine. AVP has the added property of increasing the permeability of the tubular walls to urea as well as to water, so facilitating the effect.

Liposoluble molecules

Liposoluble molecules, such as steroid hormones, tend to be carried in blood, bound to plasma proteins. They are therefore not filtered to the same extent as other constituents of the plasma. The small amounts that are freely dissolved in plasma, and which therefore get through into the tubular fluid, are largely absorbed back into the blood by passive diffusion. Consequently liposoluble molecules tend to be retained in the blood and are not excreted to any great extent in the urine. They can be eliminated from the body but only once they have been converted into a more water-soluble form, usually by the liver (see Ch. 10).

Renal dialysis

When renal failure occurs, whether in its acute or chronic form, and for whatever reason, the normal functions of the kidney diminish or disappear. Substances, such as urea, potassium and water, that are usually excreted are retained in the circulation. Some of these can be especially dangerous; excessive potassium, for example, will lead to cardiac arrhythmias.

Renal dialysis replaces normal kidney function by ridding the body of excess water, electrolytes and waste products. Dialysis may be a temporary measure, maintaining the person's blood chemistry within acceptable limits until kidney function returns, or it may be permanent (or at least long term, until a renal transplant is available).

There are two main types of dialysis:

- haemodialysis
- peritoneal dialysis.

In the UK about 60% of patients on dialysis have haemodialysis and about 40% peritoneal dialysis – most patients can have either kind. It is common for patients to begin one therapy and then switch to the other. The physiological principles are the same for each.

Haemodialysis is perhaps most familiar to the general public for its use of kidney machines. Blood flows along a cannula in a vein in the patient's arm, passes through the kidney machine where it is filtered of its harmful contents, and returns to the patient via a second vein. Inside the machine, the blood passes along one side of a sterile, semipermeable membrane (that is, a membrane that permits the passage of certain substances only). On the other side of this membrane flows the dialysate. This is a sterile fluid containing carefully controlled levels of electrolytes. For example, it contains very little, if any, potassium. Potassium therefore diffuses across the membrane from the patient's blood where its level is high. Other substances that can cross the membrane, such as urea and creatinine, do the same.

You may wonder what effect the blood's osmotic pull has. Since plasma proteins cannot cross the membrane, why doesn't water flow from the dialysate into the blood? To counteract this osmotic attraction, the dialysate is made hypertonic by the addition of extra glucose. Water flow is therefore usually from the patient to the dialysate. The patient's blood chemistry is carefully monitored, and frequency and length of haemodialysis (and sometimes constituency of dialysate) will be calculated from the results.

Haemodialysis is expensive, not just in equipment but in its need for specially trained nurses. Peritoneal dialysis avoids the need for expensive equipment, though it too demands careful nursing care. Here, dialysing fluid is run into the peritoneal cavity through a sterile catheter, the peritoneum acting as a semipermeable membrane. Unwanted substances diffuse across the peritoneum from the patient's blood until, after the required time, the dialysate is run out again.

Some patients with long-term renal failure can use dialysis within a comparatively normal lifestyle by the use of continuous ambulatory peritoneal dialysis (CAPD). The dialysate is contained within a sterile 2-litre plastic bag, which, for the first part of the procedure, is elevated (either hanging from a drip stand or worn around the upper part of the body) so that the fluid runs in under gravity. After approximately 4 hours, the now empty bag is lowered to below the level of the abdomen. It can be strapped to the side of the bed or to the patient's leg if he wishes to be active. The fluid can now flow out without the sterile circuit being broken, and with as little disturbance to the patient's life as possible.

Most patients on dialysis need medication. Commonly prescribed drugs are calcium carbonate and aluminium hydroxide to prevent a build-up of phosphate, which combines with calcium to damage the blood vessels. Resonium is given if there is a danger of a high blood potassium level.

This is a very brief introduction to a complex subject. You may wish to read more detailed texts.

SECRETION

In addition to the non-specific ways of eliminating waste materials just described, cells at the end of the proximal convoluted tubule are able to transfer some selected compounds *from* the peritubular blood into the tubular fluid. This involves transporter proteins in the membranes of the tubular cells carrying the molecules across the cell membranes. These transporter proteins can handle a variety of different molecules including endogenous substances like some organic acids and drugs such as penicillin (see Ch. 2).

HORMONE PRODUCTION BY THE KIDNEY

The hormone erythropoietin is produced from the cells of the juxtaglomerular apparatus and the peritubular endothelium in response to hypoxia. It has the effect of stimulating the production of the red cell precursors by bone marrow stem cells and the release of reticulocytes from the bone marrow holding pool (see Ch. 3).

Although not a hormone, cholecalciferol or vitamin D is the precursor of a number of substances which act

Diuretics

Any substance which increases urine flow rate is termed a diuretic.

Drugs that are given to increase the loss of fluid from the body work by inhibiting the recovery of one or more electrolytes, usually sodium, chloride or hydrogen carbonate. Different drugs affect different processes (Table 8.3).

Thiazides and related compounds are moderately potent diuretics, they inhibit sodium resabsorption at the beginning of the distal convoluted tubule. They act within 1–2 hours of oral administration and most have a duration of action of 12–24 hours. These diuretics are usually administered early in the day, so as not to interfere with sleep. These drugs are used in the management of hypertension.

Loop diuretics such as furosemide (frusemide) inhibit reabsorption from the ascending limb of the loop of Henle in the renal tubule and are powerful diuretics. Loop diuretics are used in patients with pulmonary oedema due to ventricular failure and can also be used in patients with long-standing heart failure. After intravenous administration, these drugs have their peak effect within 30 minutes.

Potassium-sparing diuretics: research has shown that many patients on diuretics do not need potassium supplements and potassium-sparing diuretics are available. Spironolactone is a potassium-sparing diuretic and potentiates thiazide or loop diuretics by antagonizing aldosterone.

Osmotic diuretics are prescribed only rarely. They are used to reduce pressure rapidly within fluid-filled cavities. They work by exerting osmotic pressure within the tubular fluid. Mannitol is used to reduce cerebral oedema.

Alcohol is a diuretic. It inhibits the secretion of AVP/ADH and thus promotes the loss of water. There is evidence that caffeine acts as a diuretic too by increasing GFR. Patients who complain of troublesome urgency and frequency of voiding should therefore be encouraged to reduce their alcohol and caffeine intake.

like hormones. Cholecalciferol is converted in the liver to 25-hydroxycholecalciferol which is further converted in the kidney to the active form of vitamin D, 1,25-dihydroxycholecalciferol. This has the effect of increasing the production of calcium binding proteins in the gut and so increasing the absorption of calcium. Its effects on bone are complex (see Ch. 14) but the result is the facilitation of bone remodelling.

STORAGE AND EVACUATION OF URINE

Urine is formed continuously by the kidneys and passes through the ureters to the urinary bladder, where it is stored. Evacuation of the bladder via the urethra is controlled by the autonomic and somatic nervous systems.

Table 8.3 Types of diuretic agent and their actions

Type	Generic example	Action
Loop diuretics*	Furosemide (frusemide)	Inhibit chloride pump in upper ascending limb of loop of Henle
Thiazide diuretics*	Bendrofluazide	Inhibit sodium uptake in cortical diluting segment (distal tubule)
Potassium sparing diuretics	Spironolactone	Competitive aldosterone antagonist
Distal diuretics (aldosterone independent)	Amiloride	Block sodium channels in distal nephron
Combined diuretics*	Amiloride plus hydrochlorothiazide Spironolactone plus hydroflumethiazide	Prevent sodium uptake in more than one site
Osmotic diuretics	Mannitol	Filtered but not reabsorbed by tubule, osmotic effect
Not used as general diuretic, only used in specialist practice
Carbonic anhydrase inhibitors	Acetazolamide	Inhibit enzyme which produces carbon dioxide and water. Used in treatment of glaucoma; otherwise special use only as diuretic

*These diuretics increase the urinary loss of potassium.

Where a small stone (calculus) is produced in the renal system, and then passes down the ureter, extreme pain is caused when the sharp edges of the stone scratch the smooth lining of the ureter, and its muscle wall goes into spasm. Passage of the stone is aided by the patient drinking copious amounts of fluid and by the prescription of effective analgesia, such as pethidine, or the anti-inflammatory drug diclofenac. Larger stones formed in the renal pelvis curiously cause far less pain, because they are much too big to move.

URETERS

Urine passes to the pelvis of each kidney and is then carried via the two ureters to the bladder (Fig. 8.16). Both the ureter and the bladder are lined by an epithelium which is highly impermeable to water. Thus the osmotic pressure of urine remains the same within the ureters and the bladder even if it is different from that of the blood. The ureters, like the bladder, possess smooth muscle (see Ch. 4B) in their walls. Regular

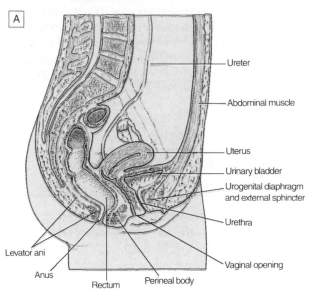

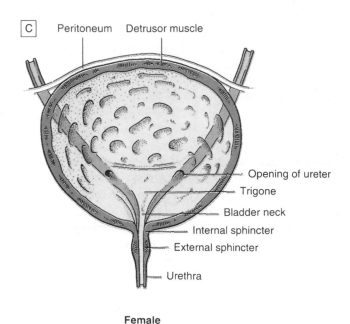

Female

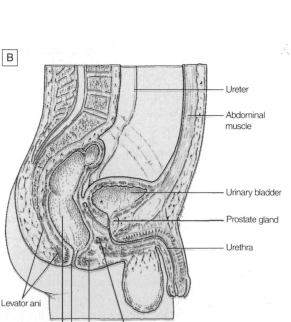

Figure 8.16 Position and structure of the bladder, ureters and urethra in men and women. A, Arrangement of pelvic structures in women. B, Arrangement of pelvic structures in men. C, Structure of the bladder (Parts A & B from Rogers 1992, with permission of Elsevier.)

contractions of this muscle move the urine along the ureters into the bladder in spurts.

The ureters enter the bladder at an oblique angle. When the bladder muscle contracts and the pressure of fluid inside it increases, the openings of the ureters are compressed by the bladder wall and backflow of the urine is prevented.

BLADDER

Filling

The bladder, which consists of detrusor smooth muscle, distends as urine flows into it, but the pressure inside it does not increase very much at first (Fig. 8.17). The maximum volume of fluid that a normal bladder can hold when fully distended varies between people. One student taking part in an experimental project produced almost a litre of urine at one sitting, but this is rather unusual except in cases of chronic urinary retention. Usually, the maximum volume that can be held in the bladder without too much discomfort is about 0.5 litres.

Sphincters

The neck of the bladder, which is connected to the urethra, has three distinct layers of smooth muscle. The first of these, which is really an extension of the detrusor muscle of the bladder, acts as the internal sphincter (Fig. 8.16C). The muscle of the bladder and the sphincter is innervated by autonomic nerves, both sympathetic and parasympathetic. The urethra (longer in men than in women) (see Ch. 30) passes through the urogenital diaphragm in the pelvic floor. Muscle associated with the diaphragm acts as a sphincter (the external sphincter). This muscle is striated (see Ch. 4B) and is innervated by somatic nerves (pudendal).

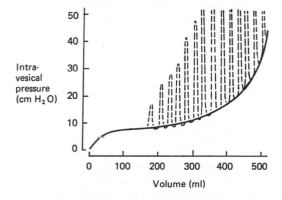

Figure 8.17 Pressure inside the bladder as it fills. The dotted lines represent the temporary increases in pressure caused by reflex contraction of the muscle of the bladder in response to stretch caused by filling. If micturition does not occur the bladder accommodates to the new volume, adaptation occurs and the intra-vesical pressure falls. (From Emslie-Smith et al 1988, with permission of Elsevier.)

Control

The passage of urine (micturition) is controlled by both involuntary and voluntary mechanisms (Fig. 8.18).

Involuntary control

Stretch receptors in the wall of the bladder are stimulated as the bladder distends. Via a spinal reflex they cause the smooth muscle of the bladder to contract. This increases the pressure within the bladder and opens the internal sphincter. As urine passes into the urethra, sensory receptors there sense the flow of urine and add to the reflex excitation of the bladder.

Both divisions of the autonomic nervous system control the bladder (see Ch. 5). Parasympathetic fibres running in the pelvic nerves supply the bladder wall and the internal involuntary sphincter. The effect of parasympathetic activity is contraction of the bladder wall and relaxation of the sphincter. The contraction is normally enough to raise the pressure inside the

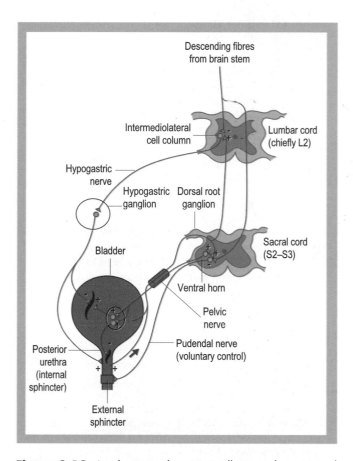

Figure 8.18 A schematic drawing to illustrate the principal nervous pathways that control micturition. Micturition is inhibited by activity in the hypogastric (sympathetic) nerves and pudendal nerves. It is facilitated by activity in the pelvic (parasympathetic) nerves. (After Pocock & Richards 1999 Human physiology: the basis of medicine. Reprinted by permission of Oxford University Press.)

bladder to expel the contents through the open sphincter.

Sympathetic fibres run in the hypogastric nerves to the wall and internal sphincter and stimulation inhibits contraction of the wall but excites contraction of the sphincter. In other words, micturition is a parasympathetic event.

Voluntary control

If it is not possible to get to a toilet, bladder emptying is prevented by voluntary contraction of the external sphincter. If this is maintained for long enough the reflex contraction of the bladder muscles wanes. More urine flows into the bladder, which distends further, until impulses from sensory receptors reflexly stimulate the smooth muscle again (Fig. 8.17). This cycle may be repeated several times before micturition occurs. When it does happen, the flow of urine through the urethra considerably strengthens the reflex contraction of the bladder by exciting sensory receptors there. In this way contraction is maintained until the bladder is emptied.

Abdominal pressure

Emptying of the bladder is also assisted by the pressure exerted by simultaneous contraction of the abdominal muscles. Sometimes an increase in abdominal pressure when coughing or lifting provokes a transient loss of urine (stress incontinence). This is more common in women than in men probably because the muscles of the pelvic floor are differently arranged and do not offer quite the same support, particularly if they have been weakened through childbirth.

TESTS AND MEASUREMENT OF BLADDER FUNCTION

Abnormalities in voiding, i.e. outflow obstruction or incontinence problems, can be diagnosed with the aid of urodynamic testing of the bladder.

Urinary retention

Hyperplasia of the prostate gland occurs in many men in middle and old age. The prostate gland surrounds the urethra as it leaves the bladder neck (Fig. 8.16B) and, as glandular tissue increases, compresses and 'kinks' the urethra. At first, micturition is more hesitant, the individual observing a poor stream and 'end dribbling'. Frequency of micturition, even at night (nocturia), follows and the person may experience incontinence. Eventually, if the condition is not treated, retention will occur. This may be acute, with severe pain, or chronic, with overflow.

Even when retention has occurred, the bladder will continue to fill as the kidneys manufacture urine, and the normal bladder capacity will be exceeded. Prolonged obstruction will eventually lead to kidney damage, since urine is unable to pass down the ureters, yet is still being produced. This will lead to back pressure on the kidneys. It is important, therefore, to treat urinary retention swiftly.

Catheterization is performed aseptically, so as to avoid introducing microorganisms, and the urine drains into a sterile collecting bag. Some urologists believe that urine should be allowed to drain continuously so as to reduce back pressure on the kidneys as quickly as possible. The nurse observes and records the amount drained in order to assist the urologist to assess the potential for kidney damage. Others believe that urinary drainage should be interrupted to avoid the sudden release of pressure in the abdomen, which, it is claimed, may induce shock and haemorrhage (Watson & Royle 1987). After an initial 500 ml is drained, the catheter is clamped for 15 minutes before a further 500 ml is allowed to drain. This process is repeated until the bladder is empty.

Causes of urinary incontinence

Stress incontinence can sometimes occur when childbirth has damaged the pelvic floor muscles and the external urinary sphincter. Control is maintained unless intra-abdominal pressure suddenly increases, as occurs with coughing, sneezing or even laughter. (It is well known that prolonged, helpless laughter may lead to 'accidents' even in those with an undamaged urinary system. Stress incontinence, however, occurs with ordinary, everyday laughter. Its effect on a person's social life and self-esteem may well be imagined.)

Incontinence may occur as a result of bladder inflammation, such as cystitis, or irritation, as in tuberculosis of the bladder and bladder tumours. Here the sensory nerve endings within the bladder wall are stimulated so that frequency of micturition occurs. In the case of urinary tract infection, micturition is not only frequent but painful. Cystitis is often caused by infection with *Escherichia coli*, and is particularly prevalent in women who have commenced sexual activity. Urge incontinence can also occur due to the failure of the bladder to store urine due to high bladder pressure. Diseases such as multiple sclerosis and Parkinson's disease can affect bladder pressures.

Interestingly, certain forms of urinary retention can also cause incontinence. Prostatic hyperplasia can interfere with outflow of urine through the internal and external sphincters. Sometimes the bladder fills so as to cause great pain, and the patient is unable to pass any urine. Sometimes, however, small amounts of urine escape, causing incontinence and adding to his misery. This is called retention with overflow.

For the test, fine catheters are passed into the bladder and attached to pressure transducers. The measurement of internal pressures in the bladder as the bladder is being filled and emptied can then be recorded on a computer screen. Abdominal pressures are measured simultaneously by a fine rectal pressure line. This abdominal pressure can then be deducted from the bladder pressures recorded so the 'true' detrusor pressure in the bladder can be noted. High bladder pressures recorded could be indicative of an outflow obstruction.

Low bladder pressures could be indicative of detrusor muscle failure.

The test results have to be interpreted by expert urologists or nurse practitioners, but can be extremely helpful in diagnosis and treatment.

FLOW TEST

The urine is passed into a 'flow meter'. A funnel channels the urine down onto a spinning 'pressure' disc and this pressure is then recorded onto a graph. The amount of urine voided and the voiding time is recorded. The maximum 'flow' pressure is also recorded and interpreted as (ml per second) on the graph.

RESIDUAL SCAN

An ultrasound scan of the bladder is carried out to measure any residual urine left behind after voiding.

FREQUENCY/VOLUME CHART

It is sometimes helpful to ask patients to keep a frequency/volume chart for 2–3 days so that an indication of their output can be given. Patients measure each void, chart time and amount. This can be a simple diagnostic tool showing sequence of voids and also indicating if a patient is drinking too much or too little fluid.

TESTS AND MEASUREMENT OF RENAL FUNCTION

URINARY VOLUME

The volume of urine formed per day normally ranges between a minimum of 500 ml to about 3 litres. The lower limit is the minimum that is required to excrete the solutes that need to be eliminated each day. Above that, the volume of urine depends largely on the balance between the daily intake and losses of water. Someone who drinks a lot, whether tea or some other beverage, is bound to have to pay rather more visits to the toilet. Frequent trips to the toilet do not necessarily indicate diabetes or bladder dysfunction.

However, if someone begins to drink more than usual for no apparent reason, and needs to visit the toilet more frequently than in the past, this may indeed point to dysfunction.

Polyuria

An increase above normal in the volume of urine formed is referred to as polyuria. If the urine formed is very dilute this suggests a defect in water conservation. In the past, a simple way of finding out how dilute or concentrated the urine was, was to measure its specific gravity or relative density with a hydrometer. Values lower than 1.010 indicated a dilute urine. Nowadays it is preferable to use an osmometer, which, by measuring the osmolality, shows whether the urine is hypo-, iso- or hypertonic.

Urinary flow rate may also increase above normal if there is an increase in solute excretion. If some glucose, for example, remains unabsorbed, as it does in *diabetes mellitus*, it acts as an osmotic force counteracting the forces promoting water recovery and more water will be excreted. This in turn upsets the recovery of electrolytes and more of these are excreted also. The presence of glucose in urine can be detected by using dipsticks. These are impregnated with chemicals that react with glucose to form a coloured compound. The depth of colour gives a rough measure of glucose concentration.

Accurate reading of dipsticks

It is important to cap the dipstick container tightly following each use, as the chemicals impregnating the sticks can deteriorate and give inaccurate readings. Similarly, the expiry date on the container should be noted.

Certain dipsticks are designed to detect substances other than glucose in the urine – for example ketones, blood and albumin. Each coloured strip on the dipstick must be read at the exact time recommended on the container's label. The timing for each strip to be read may vary: 30 seconds, 60 seconds, and so on. Each time must be measured using a watch with a second hand; a rough guess is inaccurate and unprofessional. Equipment is available where the testing strip can be read automatically and a printout of test results obtained.

SMELL AND APPEARANCE OF URINE

Other observations that may provide clues as to renal function and the presence of abnormalities in other body systems include the smell and appearance of urine.

An offensive smell suggests infection. A sweetish smell may indicate the excretion of increased amounts of keto-acids as in diabetes mellitus (see Ch. 18).

Urine is normally yellowish in colour. A very dark colour may indicate the presence of large amounts of the waste product bilirubin glucuronide formed by the liver from haemoglobin (see Chs 3 and 10). A frothy urine may suggest the presence of protein.

Blood in urine (haematuria) may vary from colouring the urine pink to dark red or brown.

Brown to dark red urine may suggest 'old' or altered blood as opposed to 'fresh' bright red colouring 'frank' haematuria.

All haematuria should be reported and investigated. Patients who report painless haematuria should be investigated promptly as it may indicate cancerous growths of bladder or renal tract.

RENAL FUNCTION TESTS

More specialized measurements may sometimes be made to assess particular features of renal function, such as glomerular filtration rate by means of creatinine. Creatinine, a product of muscle metabolism, is freely filtered at the glomerulus, and then remains completely unabsorbed. The glomerular filtration rate is calculated from the amount of creatinine excreted in the urine and its concentration in the plasma. This is known as the creatinine clearance.

Renography

Renal function can also be tested by injecting the patient intravenously with chemicals whose uptake and output through the kidneys can be measured with radiography (renography).

Renography plays an important role in the investigation of the kidney and urinary tract, providing information on individual renal function and urine transport. It is relatively simple to perform, well accepted by patients and provides valuable clinical information not available from other investigations.

The substances intravenously injected are called radiopharmaceuticals and the two main ones routinely used are 99M Tc MAG3 (mercaptoaceyl triglycine), 99M Tc DTPA (diethylenetriamine penta acetic acid.

MAG3 is a very valuable imaging agent which gives superior renal images and renograms and has become the agent of choice for investigating kidney function.

Collecting specimens of urine

Nursing staff may collect different types of urine specimens for different investigations. Where a urine infection is suspected, a *mid-stream* specimen of urine will be collected or a specimen from the patient's catheter. An *early morning* specimen of urine is usually requested when it is to be examined for constituents such as urea, sodium and potassium (biochemical tests). An early morning specimen demonstrates better the kidney's ability to concentrate substances, before the day's normal fluid intake brings about dilution. (The individual may notice that the first urine passed in the morning is darker in colour than that later in the day.) Specimens should be sent to the pathology laboratory within 2 hours. Ideally, ward tests of urine using dipsticks should be carried out immediately, or readings may alter.

Creatinine clearance test

Estimation of creatinine clearance requires the collection of all urine produced by the patient over 24 hours (a 24-hour collection of urine). A specimen of venous blood will also be taken to estimate plasma creatinine levels.

Creatinine is formed in the muscle and passes via the blood into the urine. It is valuable in the estimation of renal function, in particular the glomerular filtration rate, because blood levels of creatinine remain fairly constant. In this respect it differs from urea, another end-product of metabolism, whose blood levels vary with protein intake and metabolic state.

Creatinine is filtered by the glomerulus and remains within the kidney tubules until excreted in the urine. It is not reabsorbed into the blood. Consequently, the amount of creatinine filtered per minute by the glomeruli is equal to the amount of creatinine excreted per minute in the urine. A 24-hour specimen of urine is collected so that the total daily amount of creatinine excreted may be measured and the excretion rate per minute calculated.

In some cases of renal disease, where there is disordered glomerular filtration, the amount of creatinine excreted in the urine will fall. This will be accompanied by an elevated plasma creatinine level, because the creatinine is not being excreted via the kidneys.

If any of the urine is accidentally discarded during the collection period, the test must recommence. Failure to do so would give a reduced total creatinine value, a reduced amount of creatinine clearance per minute, and hence an inaccurate glomerular filtration rate. Strict maintenance of the 24-hour collection is therefore an important nursing responsibility.

REFERENCES AND FURTHER READING

Boore J, Champion R, Ferguson M (eds) 1987 Nursing the physically ill adult. Churchill Livingstone, Edinburgh

Bradley J, Smith K 1998 Diagnostic tests in nephrology. Edward Arnold, London

De Wardener H E 1985 The kidney, 5th edn. Churchill Livingstone, Edinburgh
Comprehensive account of all aspects of the kidney in health and disease. Useful for reference and for information about clinical aspects of renal function

Emslie-Smith D, Paterson C R, Scratcherd T, Read N W (eds) 1988 Textbook of physiology, 11th edn. Churchill Livingstone, Edinburgh, p 203

Greenberg A, Cheung A K, Coffman T M, Falk R J, Jennette J C 2001 Primer on kidney disease, 3rd edn. Academic Press

Hricik D, Sedor J R, Miller T 2002 Nephrology secrets, 2nd edn. Hanley and Belfus

Lote C 1987 Principles of renal physiology, 2nd edn. Croom Helm, London
An excellent, lucidly written, concise text explaining what the kidney does as well as how it does it. Includes plenty of suggestions for further reading and some problems and answers

Pocock G, Richards C D 1999 Human physiology: the basis of medicine. Oxford University Press, Oxford

Rogers A W 1992 Textbook of anatomy. Churchill Livingstone, Edinburgh, pp 107, 110

Seldin D W, Giebisch G (eds) 1985 The kidney: physiology and pathophysiology. Raven Press, New York
Comprehensive, weighty, two volume coverage of the physiology and pathophysiology of renal function and electrolyte metabolism written for and by specialists

Tanagho E A, McAninch J W 1991 Smith's General urology, 13th edn. Appleton & Lange, East Norwalk, CT
Clinical text covering all aspects of disease of the genitourinary tract in depth. Useful for reference and for further information about the bladder and ureters

Torrens M J, Morrison J F (eds) 1987 The physiology of the lower urinary tract. Springer Verlag, Berlin-Heidelberg
Specialist book reviewing current knowledge

Valtin H 1983 Renal function mechanisms preserving fluid and solute balance in health, 2nd edn. Little Brown, Boston & Toronto
Very well-referenced, student text explaining renal mechanisms in detail and giving the experimental basis of current theory. Includes questions to think about and answers

Watson R (ed.) 1999 Essential science for nursing students. Baillière Tindall, London
A straightforward account of the basics

Watson J, Royle J 1987 Walson's Medical–surgical nursing and related physiology, 3rd edn. Baillière Tindall, London, p 926

The digestive system

In practice you may be asked to consider the following:

1. A 60-year old woman has a history of gastrointestinal ulcers. She has now been prescribed a proton pump inhibitor and wants to know how they relieve ulcer formation in the stomach and duodenum.

2. What part does pepsin play in ulcer formation?

3. The sight, sound and smell of food are important to digestion even before it reaches the mouth. What is the effect of food in the mouth upon gastric secretion and motility?

4. A patient has had a section of small intestine removed. How is the small intestine specialized for absorption?

5. What are the main differences between the surfaces of the colon and small intestine?

6. A woman has been prescribed oral vitamin B_{12}. What is the mechanism of vitamin B_{12} absorption in the terminal ileum?

7. A young patient wants to know why faeces are normally brown in colour and why his are pale and greasy.

8. Blood may be altered or fresh when found in a faecal sample. Why is the form different and what is the significance of the difference?

9. A surgical patient has a plasma albumin of 18 g/l 2 days after GI surgery (normal level 40 g/l). Should he be given a plasma expander?

10. A patient with Crohn's disease has been found to be severely hypomagnesaemic. How should this be replaced?

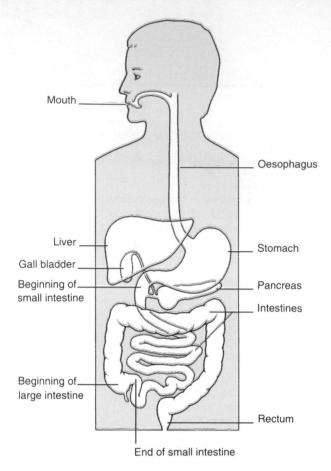

Figure 9.1 The gastrointestinal tract.

The food we eat consists of raw materials for energy-requiring and synthetic processes. Foodstuffs require to be broken down into smaller units before they can be absorbed. This breakdown is achieved by the cooperative activity of the organs of the digestive tract.

Figure 9.1 illustrates the component organs of the gastrointestinal tract, and the associated organs that are essential for the functioning of the digestive system. The system consists of the digestive tract (mouth, oesophagus, stomach and intestines) in association with the accessory digestive glands (salivary glands, pancreas and biliary system).

The overall function of the digestive system is to transfer the nutrients in food from the external environment to the internal environment where they can be distributed to the cells of the body via the circulation. Nutrients, water and salts are absorbed from digested food, and all products that cannot be absorbed are retained in the digestive tract until they are eliminated. The gastrointestinal tract is regulated, in part, by the autonomic nervous system which acts in conjunction with a variety of gastrointestinal peptides (hormones, neurocrines or paracrines).

Before reading this chapter it may be helpful to review the biochemistry of carbohydrates, proteins and fats and nutritional issues (see Ch. 15).

STRUCTURE OF THE GASTROINTESTINAL TRACT: AN OVERVIEW

The digestive tract wall consists of four structural layers (see below and Fig. 9.2). These four layers are present in all areas of the tract from the oesophagus to the anus, with some functional adaptations throughout.

GENERALIZED LAYERS OF THE GASTROINTESTINAL TRACT

- mucosa
- submucosa
- muscularis
- serosa (fibrous outer layer).

The mucosa is the innermost layer, that is, the layer nearest to the lumen of the tube, and it exhibits a great

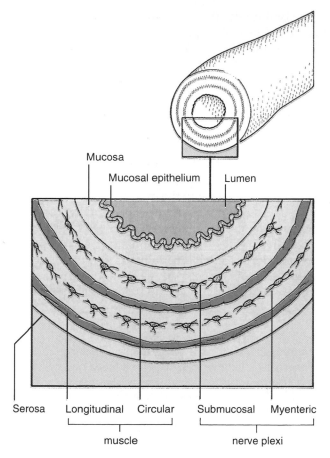

Mucosa

Mucosal epithelium   Lumen

Serosa   Longitudinal   Circular   Submucosal   Myenteric

muscle   nerve plexi

Figure 9.2 Basic structure of the wall of the digestive 'tube' (oesophagus, stomach and intestine).

BLOOD SUPPLY

The arteries supplying the abdominal organs of the digestive system are the coeliac and superior and inferior mesenteric arteries. The coeliac artery branches to give rise to the gastric, splenic and hepatic arteries that provide blood to the stomach, pancreas, spleen and liver. The mesenteric arteries supply the intestines.

Venous blood from the stomach, pancreas, spleen and liver is collected together and routed through the liver via the hepatic portal vein. Blood from the remainder of the digestive tract (oesophagus and rectum) escapes the hepatic filter and drains directly into the venous system.

NERVE SUPPLY

The digestive system is innervated almost entirely by autonomic nerves (see Ch. 5). The vagus (parasympathetic) nerve innervates all areas from the oesophagus to the mid portion of the transverse colon. The remainder of the large intestine and the rectum is innervated by the pelvic (parasympathetic) nerve.

Sympathetic nerves innervating the gastrointestinal system include the splanchnic and mesenteric nerves. Both parasympathetic and sympathetic nerves contain sensory neurones as well as motor neurones, and the majority of nerve fibres running in the vagus nerve are sensory.

deal of variation throughout the tract. Mucus stratified epithelial cells line the lumen (except in the oesophagus), and it is from this layer that all glands develop. Mucus secreting cells are situated throughout the epithelium. These cells are subjected to a tremendous amount of frictional wear and tear. The epithelial cells lie on a sheet of connective tissue called the lamina propria. Distal to this, there is a thin layer of muscle tissue called muscularis mucosa. The mucosa has throughout it patches of lymphoid tissue which serve a defensive function.

The submucosa lies distal to the mucosa, and consists of loose connective tissue which supports blood vessels, lymphatics and nerve fibres.

The muscularis layer, as its name suggests, is formed of muscle fibres. The muscle fibres in the gastrointestinal tract are referred to as smooth, involuntary, unstriated or visceral muscle fibres.

The serosa is the outermost, protective layer, formed of connective tissue and squamous epithelium.

MOTILITY (MOVEMENT IN THE GASTROINTESTINAL TRACT)

Motility refers to contraction and relaxation of the walls and sphincters of the gastrointestinal tract. Motility involves the grinding and mixing of ingested food in preparation for digestion and absorption; it then propels the food along the gastrointestinal tract. Smooth muscle in the gastrointestinal tract enables;

- contractile tone to be maintained even in the absence of food
- activity to be increased and decreased as necessary
- the tract to distend to accommodate different volumes.

The control of motility and secretion in the gastrointestinal tract is by neural, hormonal and paracrine mechanisms. The neural control is via the extrinsic nerves of the autonomic nervous system. In most instances the mediators of neural or hormonal control are peptides.

ORGANIZATION OF THE DIGESTIVE TRACT

MOUTH, PHARYNX AND OESOPHAGUS

The mouth

The mouth is divided into two parts.

The vestibule: the part between the teeth and the jaws, and the lips and cheeks. The salivary glands open here.

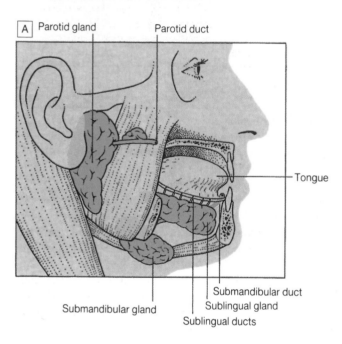

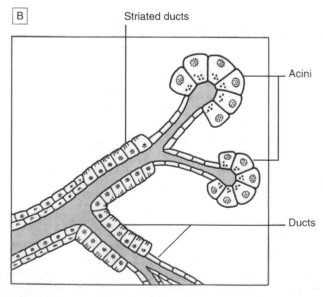

Figure 9.3 The mouth showing salivary glands. A, Position. B, Arrangement of the parotid gland. (Part A reproduced from Rogers 1992, with permission of Elsevier.)

The oral cavity: the inner area which is bounded by the teeth. The epithelium in the oral cavity is typically 15–20 layers of cells thick, and as such is adapted to the amount of friction which occurs during mastication (Fig. 9.3).

The salivary glands

There are three main pairs of salivary glands situated around the mouth, and numerous smaller glands scattered throughout the mouth. The parotid gland is the largest and lies just below the ear; its duct is about 5 cm long and enters into the mouth on the inside of the cheek. The submandibular and sublingual glands both open into the floor of the mouth (Fig. 9.3). The salivary glands are supplied by the autonomic nervous system (ANS) and the secretion of saliva is stimulated by the sight, smell or thought of food, a conditioned (or learned) reflex.

> *Dysphagia* is defined as difficulty in swallowing. Patients may be able to swallow soft foods and liquids but may be unable to take more solid foodstuffs. Dysphagia may be due to mechanical obstruction (i.e. oesophageal cancer), to dysfunction in the neuromuscular structures involved in swallowing or to diseases of the mouth, larynx and pharynx.

The pharynx

The pharynx is a muscular tube approximately 14 cm in length. Once food has been chewed and moistened the tongue rolls it into a bolus and carries it towards the oral part of the pharynx. When the bolus reaches the pharynx, swallowing begins involuntarily. The muscular wall of the pharynx constricts and pushes the food over the epiglottis (which closes the larynx), and on into the oesophagus (see also Ch. 7 at 'Swallowing').

The oesophagus

The oesophagus is a thin-walled muscular tube, about 25 cm in length, which extends from the pharynx to the stomach. It is composed of the same four layers as the bulk of the gastrointestinal tract (see Fig. 9.2). The muscular coat of the upper third is composed of skeletal muscle, the lower third smooth muscle, with a transitional zone from one to the other in between. Both skeletal and smooth muscle fibres are under the control of the vagus nerve.

There are two physiological sphincters in the oesophagus, one at either end:

- upper oesophageal sphincter (crico-pharyngeal sphincter)

Gastro-oesophageal reflux disease (GORD)

The symptoms of heartburn and acid indigestion are caused by a backflow of acidic stomach contents into the oesophagus causing sensations of burning and pressure behind the breastbone. In its simplest form GORD symptoms are mild and occur infrequently and may respond to simple non-pharmaceutical interventions, including: avoiding problem foods, stopping smoking, reducing alcohol intake or losing weight. In more severe cases acid-blocking medications (H_2 receptor antagonists) or more powerful inhibitors of stomach acid production (proton pump inhibitors) may be required to treat the symptoms.

Heartburn

A burning sensation felt at the bottom of the chest is usually referred to as heartburn. The name is misleading because the discomfort has nothing to do with the heart, but it is so called because the sensation is experienced where we imagine our hearts to be. It is caused by irritation of the oesophageal lining by regurgitated acid stomach contents. Its occurrence implies incompetence of the lower oesophageal sphincter. A common cause is herniation of the lower part of the oesophagus and part of the stomach through the diaphragm. This could be precipitated by a sharp rise in abdominal pressure, caused by straining to lift a heavy object, for example. It may also occur in pregnancy because of the displacement of various abdominal organs by the enlarged uterus and the relaxing effect of progesterone on smooth muscle. Heartburn is sometimes associated with indigestion and particular foods. It may be that the contractile tone of the sphincter muscle is inhibited by the particular blend of neural and hormonal signals evoked by the ingested food substance. For example, a fatty meal elicits increased secretion of the hormone CCK-PZ, which relaxes the sphincter.

* lower oesophageal sphincter (LOS/cardiac sphincter).

The upper oesophageal sphincter is composed of skeletal muscle. The LOS covers the distal 1–2 cm of the oesophagus. It is not anatomically distinguishable as a sphincter but pressure is normally greater in this region than in the stomach.

The movement of food through the oesophagus is by peristaltic action. Peristalsis is a coordinated wave of contraction proceeding in an orderly direction from one part of the digestive tract to the next (Fig. 9.4).

In the oesophagus, the wave of contraction is controlled by nerve impulses in the vagus and is coordinated by the swallowing centre in the medulla. The wave takes about 9 seconds to travel the length of the oesophagus.

As the peristaltic waves begin in the oesophagus, the muscle of the LOS relaxes, opening the sphincter and allowing the food bolus to enter the stomach. Should any food particles remain in the oesophagus after the first wave of peristalsis, irritation of the mucosa by the food particles evokes a secondary wave of peristalsis that helps to dislodge the remaining food particles and sweep them into the stomach.

STOMACH

Structure and function

The stomach is a dilated segment of the digestive tract located between the oesophagus and the small intestine (Fig. 9.5A & B).

The stomach is divided into several regions:

* fundus
* cardia
* body
* pylorus.

Folds, known as rugae, are present on the inner surface of the stomach. The wall structure of the stomach is similar to the rest of the gastrointestinal tract except that the stomach has an oblique muscular layer in addition to the circular and longitudinal layers in the muscularis. This additional layer facilitates distension of the stomach and storage of food.

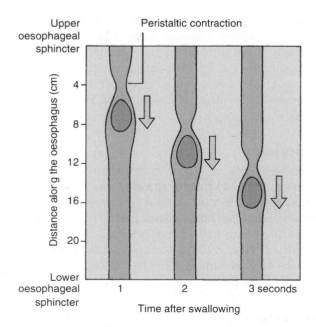

Figure 9.4 A wave of peristalsis in the oesophagus.

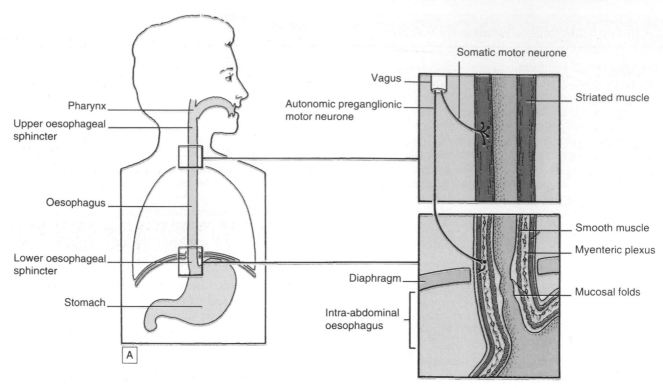

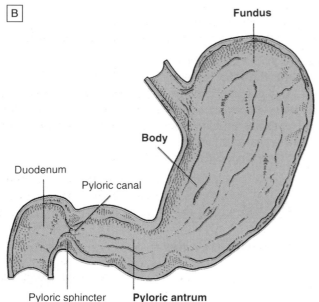

Figure 9.5 A, Location of the stomach in the gastrointestinal tract. B, Diagram of stomach.

The lining of the stomach is covered with a protective layer of columnar epithelial cells; they have tight junctions to protect the underlying tissue from the acidic gastric juices.

One of the most important functions of the stomach relates to the regulation of the rate which foodstuff enters the small intestine. The stomach is responsible for the churning and mixing of food with the gastric juices. Food passes from the stomach to the small intestine via the pyloric canal. This canal is encircled by a band of smooth muscle, the pyloric sphincter.

Mixing of food

When a meal is ingested, weak waves of muscular contraction, known as peristalsis, begin in the body of the stomach, pushing food into the antrum. Gradually these contractions become more and more intense, especially in the antrum region. This contractile activity is responsible for the churning of food material and mixing it with gastric juice. Thus, solid materials are progressively reduced to a semi-fluid material called chyme.

Emptying

About 6–10 ml of chyme are emptied into the duodenum via the pyloric sphincter each minute. The physiological function of this sphincter is to allow carefully regulated emptying of gastric contents, whilst preventing regurgitation of duodenal contents into the stomach. This is of vital importance as the lining of the stomach may be damaged by the presence of intestinal juices (including bile).

Vomiting

An account of vomiting can be found on page 299.

Peptic ulcer disease

The term 'peptic ulcer' refers to an ulcer in the lower oesophagus, stomach or duodenum, in the jejunum after surgical anastomosis to the stomach, or rarely in the ileum adjacent to a Meckěl's diverticulum. Ulcers in the stomach or duodenum may be acute or chronic; both penetrate the muscularis mucosae but the acute ulcer shows no evidence of fibrosis. Erosions do not penetrate the muscularis mucosae.

Treatment with proton pump inhibitors or H_2 receptor blockers is highly effective for both gastric and duodenal ulcers.

H_2 receptor blockers reduce gastric acid secretion by antagonizing the action of histamine. H_2 blockers compete with histamine for the H_2 receptors on the oxyntic cells. Such drugs can reduce basal and food stimulated acid by up to 90% and therefore can induce the healing of duodenal ulcers.

Proton pump inhibitors, omeprazole, and its analogues, act by blocking the activity of H^+/K^+ ATPase (the proton pump). The drug is inactive at a neutral pH, only becoming active in acid conditions. The enzyme (i.e. the pump) is irreversibly inhibited and secretion of more acid can only take place when more enzyme has been synthesized.

SMALL INTESTINE

Anatomy and structure

The small intestine is a convoluted tube extending from the pyloric sphincter to its junction with the large intestine at the ileo-caecal valve. It is approximately 6 metres long with a 3.5 cm diameter and lies in the central and lower part of the abdominal cavity. The small intestines consist of:

- duodenum (25 cm)
- jejunum (2.5 metres)
- ileum (3.5 metres).

The wall of the small intestine is composed of four layers, consistent with the remainder of the alimentary tract. However, there are three special features in the mucous membrane lining.

Features of the mucous membrane of the small intestine

- Surface area of small intestine forms a series of circular folds which increase surface area available for absorption of nutrients.
- It has a velvety appearance due to presence of fine hair-like projections called villi, each containing a lymph vessel (lacteal) and blood vessels.
- It is supplied with glands of simple, tubular type which secrete intestinal juice.

0 seconds

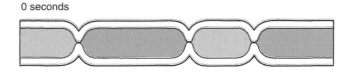

5 seconds later

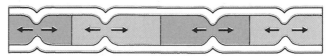

10 seconds later

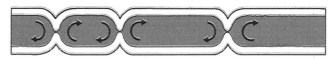

Figure 9.6 Segmentation contractions of the intestine.

The mucosa of the small intestine is simple, columnar epithelium with four major cell types:

- absorptive cells produce digestive enzymes and absorb digested food
- goblet cells produce protective mucus
- granular cells protect the intestinal epithelium from bacteria
- endocrine cells produce regulatory hormones.

The major role of the small intestine relates to digestion and absorption. The contractile activity of the intestines mixes and propels the foodstuff towards the ileum.

Movement in the small intestine

Mixing and propulsion of chyme are the primary mechanical events that take place in the small intestine. These functions are a result of segmental or peristaltic contractions, which are accomplished by the smooth muscle in the wall of the small intestine. Segmentation (Fig. 9.6) mixes the intestinal contents, and peristaltic contractions propel the intestinal contents along the digestive tract.

Motility in the small intestine is under physiological control by several factors, including stretch, autonomic nerves and circulating hormones.

LARGE INTESTINE

Structure and function

The large intestine, which is divided into several distinct sections (see below), is about 1.5 metres long and approximately 6 cm in diameter, and extends from the end of the ileum to the anus. The arrangement of the large intestine and its associated structures is shown in

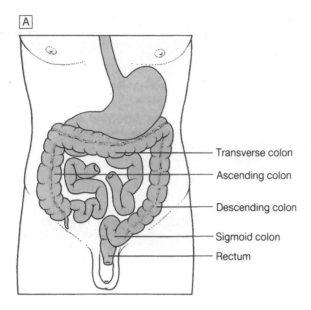

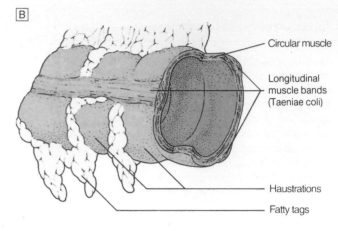

Figure 9.7 Large intestine. A, arrangement and parts. B, Structure. (From Rogers 1992, with permission of Elsevier.)

Figure 9.7A and the modifications to the general wall structure in 9.7B.

Sections of the large intestine

- caecum
- ascending colon
- transverse colon
- sigmoid colon
- rectum
- anal canal.

The main functions of the large intestine relate to the storage of faecal material and the regulation of its release into the external environment. The large intestine also absorbs water and electrolytes from chyme, producing a more solid faecal material as it passes through the colon.

Movement in the large intestine

Segmental mixing movements occur in the colon much less often than in the small intestine. Peristaltic waves are largely responsible for the movement of the semi-solid chyme along the ascending colon. Very occasionally (on average 3–4 times a day) large parts of the transverse and descending colon undergo several strong peristaltic contractions called mass peristalsis. Peristaltic waves are produced by sudden stretching (caused by bulky food residues) or by local reflexes in response to events elsewhere in the digestive tract. For example, the gastrocolic reflex is initiated by distension of the stomach following the ingestion of a meal.

Defecation

Defecation, or the passage of faeces, occurs because of the movement of food residues from the colon into the rectum, which becomes distended. This distension causes a reflex contraction of the rectal muscles which propels the contents into the anus. The exit to the rectum is guarded by two sphincters:

- internal sphincter (smooth muscle under autonomic control)
- external sphincter (striated (skeletal) muscle under somatic control).

Defecation is therefore a reflex action which can be inhibited voluntarily. The frequency of defecation, and the time of day when it is performed, is a matter of habit. In the human adult approximately 150 g of material are eliminated daily. Faeces are composed two-thirds water and one-third solid. The solids are normally undigested cellulose, bacteria, cell debris, bile pigments and some salts. The brown colour of faeces is due to the presences of the bile pigments stercobilin and urobilin (see Ch. 10) and odour is mainly related to products of bacterial fermentation.

SECRETIONS

OVERVIEW

As ingested material travels through the digestive tract, secretions are added to lubricate, liquefy and digest the food.

- Mucus, secreted all the full length of the digestive tract, lubricates the food and the lining of the tract. The mucus coats and protects the epithelial cells of the digestive tract from mechanical abrasion, from the damaging effect of acid in the stomach, and

Table 9.1 Major constituents of the digestive secretions

	Saliva	Gastric juice	Pancreatic juice	Bile	Intestinal juice
Water Electrolytes (mmol/l)	✓ Sodium (10–80) Potassium (10–40) Chloride (10–50) Hydrogen carbonate (10–40)	✓ Hydrogen ion (120) Chloride (140)	✓ Sodium (150) Hydrogen carbonate (140)	✓ Sodium (150) Chloride (100) Hydrogen carbonate (40)	✓ Sodium ⎫ Potassium ⎪ ⎬ variable* Chloride ⎪ Hydrogen ⎪ carbonate ⎭
pH	6–8	1–2	8	7–8	7–8
Enzymes	Amylase	Pepsinogens Gastric lipase	Amylase Proteases Lipases Nucleases	None	Peptidases and disaccharidases from shed epithelial cells
Glycoproteins (mucus) Other constituents	✓	✓ Intrinsic factor	A little Trypsin inhibitors	A little Bile salts	✓
Volume (ml/day)	1000	2500	1500	1000	1000

* Depends on specific site.

prevents auto-digestion of the lining by the proteolytic enzymes of the digestive tract.

- Water liquefies the food, making it more manageable to digest and absorb.
- Digestive enzymes secreted in the oral cavity, intestine, liver and pancreas break food down into smaller molecules that can be absorbed by the intestinal wall.

The major secretions of the digestive tract and their chief constituents are listed in Table 9.1.

Altogether, 7 to 8 litres of secretion are formed per day. Most are absorbed and the constituents are recycled and re-used.

SALIVA

Saliva is a mixture of secretions formed by three pairs of glands (parotid, submandibular and sublingual) together with a small number of cells scattered throughout the mouth.

Formation of saliva

The acini of the glands consist of cells that secrete either the enzyme amylase or mucus, dissolved in a solution of salts, chiefly sodium chloride. The secretion produced by the acini (primary secretion) is modified in composition as it flows through the striated ducts. Sodium and chloride are reabsorbed unaccompanied

by water so that the fluid becomes progressively more dilute.

The concentration of sodium in saliva may be as low as 5 to 10 mmol/litre. This is much lower than plasma sodium concentrate (140 mmol/litre). As flow rate increases, the concentration of sodium chloride in saliva gets closer to that in the plasma but never quite reaches it.

A variety of other substances are found in saliva in low concentrations; these mostly diffuse from blood into the saliva (see Table 9.1).

Constituents of saliva

Water makes up 90–95% of saliva, the remaining 5–10% being dissolved solutes. These include:

- ions (bicarbonate, chloride, phosphate, sodium and potassium)
- the enzyme salivary amylase
- lysozymes
- organic substances (urea, albumins and globulins)
- mucin derived from mucus-secreting cells.

Control

The salivary glands are innervated by parasympathetic and sympathetic nerves. The parasympathetic nerves are the most important in controlling secretion.

Acetylcholine, released when these nerve fibres are stimulated, provokes a large increase in salivation (see Ch. 5).

The contribution made by each pair of glands to the saliva in our mouths varies during the day and night. When a meal is eaten, it is the parotid glands that increase their secretion most of all.

GASTRIC JUICE

If the surface of the stomach is viewed with an endoscope it is seen to be pitted with numerous tiny openings. These are the openings of the tubular gastric glands.

Formation of gastric juice

At least three different cell types can be identified in the glands, each of which produces a different secretion:

- oxyntic (parietal) cells (hydrochloric acid)
- peptic (chief) cells (digestive enzymes)
- mucous cells (alkaline mucus).

Oxyntic cells are found only in the glands of the body of the stomach. Peptic cells are found here in large numbers too, although some are present also in the fundus and the antrum. Thus acid secretion, and most enzyme secretion, is localized to the body of the stomach.

The alkaline mucus clings to the surface and protects the stomach itself against the potent digestive effects of acid and enzymes.

Control

The secretory activity of the cells is controlled both by the autonomic nervous system and by hormones.

Enzyme secretion by the peptic cells is chiefly stimulated by vagal nerve fibres, whereas acid secretion is most affected by hormonal stimulants such as gastrin and histamine. The vagal nerve fibres do, however, have a small but important role in that they sensitize the cells to the other stimulants.

Histamine is released locally from mast cells. Its action on the stomach is blocked by a different class of antihistamines (H_2 receptor blockers) from those used in the relief of inflammatory responses such as the swelling caused by insect bites, and the symptoms of hay fever (H_1 receptor blockers).

The secretion of mucus is regulated by local hormones, such as prostaglandins, that are released in response to minor local injury of the mucosa.

PANCREATIC JUICE

The histological structure of the exocrine pancreas is similar in many respects to that of the salivary glands, as are some features of the secretory process.

Acute pancreatitis

Acute pancreatitis affects 10–28 per 100 000 of the population and is characterized by severe, constant upper abdominal pain which radiates to the back in 65% of cases. Nausea and vomiting are also commonly present. Acute pancreatitis is a consequence of premature activation of zymogen granules, releasing proteases which digest the pancreas and surrounding tissues. In severe cases patients can become hypoxic and develop hypovolaemic shock with oliguria. The severity of acute pancreatitis is dependent upon the balance between activity of released proteolytic enzymes and antiproteolytic enzymes.

Chronic pancreatitis

Chronic pancreatitis is a chronic inflammatory disease characterized by fibrosis and destruction of exocrine pancreatic tissue. Diabetes mellitus occurs in advanced cases as the islets of Langerhans are involved. Between 70 and 80% of cases of chronic pancreatitis relate to alcohol abuse and therefore it commonly affects middle-aged alcoholic males. Almost all present with abdominal pain. Weight loss is common and results from a combination of anorexia, avoidance of food because of postprandial pain, malabsorption and/or diabetes. In such cases alcohol avoidance is crucial in halting the progression of the disease and reducing pain.

Formation of pancreatic juice

Cells of the acini (zymogen cells) produce a secretion rich in enzymes. All the different pancreatic enzymes are manufactured by the same cells. Like other digestive enzymes, they are secreted in an inactive form, and become activated within the digestive tract. One important activator is the protein-digesting (proteolytic) enzyme trypsin. Premature activation of pancreatic enzymes is resisted by the presence of trypsin inhibitors in pancreatic juice. Centro-acinar cells and duct cells secrete an alkaline fluid rich in sodium hydrogen carbonate but free of enzymes. This is added to the primary secretion formed by the zymogen cells.

Control

Acinar and duct cells differ in their sensitivity to the following neural and hormonal stimuli:

- vagal stimulation
- cholecystokinin-pancreozymin (CCK-PZ)
- secretin.

The zymogen cells are chiefly stimulated by the vagal nerves and the hormone CCK-PZ, whereas the ducts, producing most of the fluid component of the juice, are mainly stimulated by the hormone secretin.

BILE

Bile is formed by the liver and has a dual function. It is a:

- digestive secretion
- route of excretion for waste products (such as bilirubin).

Because of its excretory function, bile is formed by the liver in large amounts all the time. In this respect it differs from other digestive secretions. Between meals, bile is diverted into the gall bladder where it is concentrated and stored.

Formation of bile

Hepatocytes secrete the organic constituents of bile, dissolved in a solution consisting mainly of sodium chloride and sodium hydrogen carbonate. This primary secretion is, like pancreatic juice, added to by an alkaline secretion formed by the ducts within the liver, which are also stimulated by secretin.

Bile salts

Bile salts, sometimes referred to as bile acids, are organic molecules involved in the digestion and absorption of fat. They are manufactured in the liver from cholesterol. Only small amounts are synthesized each day because most of the bile salts used in digestion are absorbed from the small intestine (particularly the ileum), returned to the liver and resecreted in bile (an enterohepatic circulation).

GALL BLADDER

Although a little bile trickles into the duodenum all the time between meals, most of the bile formed by the liver flows into the gall bladder. When a meal is ingested the gall bladder contracts and concentrated bile is expelled into the duodenum.

Contraction

The gall bladder distends as it fills with bile. The smooth muscle in its wall and in the ducts leading to the duodenum (cystic duct and common bile duct) contracts rhythmically. Contractions are stimulated by the hormone CCK-PZ, which also relaxes the sphincter muscle at the end of the common bile duct (sphincter of Oddi). These events are promoted by vagally mediated nervous reflexes.

Irritable bowel syndrome

Irritable bowel syndrome (IBS) is a functional bowel disorder in which abdominal pain and distension are associated with altered bowel function. Approximately 20% of the general population fulfil the diagnostic criteria for IBS and it is the commonest cause of gastrointestinal referral to secondary care settings. It is believed that the cause of IBS is multifactorial and that most patients develop symptoms in response to psychosocial factors, altered gastrointestinal motility, altered visceral sensation or lumenal factors. Most patients have a relapsing and remitting course.

INTESTINAL SECRETIONS

Intestinal secretions are not as easily measured and studied as the others because they are formed by numerous tiny glands and secretory cells throughout the intestinal tract.

Small intestine

The best characterized glands are the glands of Brunner in the upper duodenum, which form a thick alkaline mucus. Goblet cells secreting mucus are found in the epithelium throughout the rest of the small intestine. Cells in the crypts (glands) of Lieberkühn secrete a solution of sodium chloride, sodium hydrogen carbonate (sodium bicarbonate) and water. This secretion is stimulated by:

- neurotransmitters (such as vasoactive polypeptide – VIP)
- hormones (such as prostaglandins)
- bacterial toxins (such as cholera toxin).

Juice collected from the intestine contains some digestive enzymes, peptidases and disaccharidases, derived from the break-up of epithelial cells.

Large intestine

Glands secreting mucus, salts and water are also found in the large intestine. Potassium is secreted rather than sodium. Consequently significant losses of potassium can occur in diarrhoea. Factors stimulating colonic secretion include:

- bile acids
- fatty acids (from bacterial metabolism of carbohydrates)
- local hormones (prostaglandins)
- enteric nerve activity.

DIGESTION OF FOOD

OVERVIEW

Digestion is the breakdown of organic molecules into their component parts: carbohydrates into monosaccharides, proteins into amino acids, and triglycerides into fatty acids and glycerol. Digestion consists of mechanical digestion, which involves mastication and mixing of food, and chemical digestion, achieved by the secretion of digestive enzymes along the digestive tract. Digestion of large molecules into their component parts must be accomplished prior to absorption to the digestive tract.

MOUTH

Disruption of food begins in the mouth. By biting and chewing, food is moulded into malleable, well-lubricated portions (single portion = bolus), which can be swallowed. Salivary amylase is mixed into the bolus and begins the digestion of starch.

STOMACH

Amylase continues to work in the stomach despite the secretion of gastric acid which inactivates the enzyme. This is because the mixing of food with gastric juice occurs chiefly in the antrum. Most of an ingested meal collects first in the distensible body of the stomach and is stored there while small amounts are steadily supplied to the antral 'mixer'. The combined action of acid, pepsins and the mixing movements gently disrupts the plant and/or animal tissues and cells in the food and creates a partially digested suspension (chyme) of products that is slowly fed into the duodenum.

SMALL INTESTINE

Most chemical digestion of food occurs in the small intestine. Pancreatic juice is the most important of all the digestive secretions. Its variety of digestive enzymes can attack carbohydrates, proteins, fats and nucleotides and reduce them to much smaller subunits.

Carbohydrates and proteins

The digestion of carbohydrates and proteins is completed on the surface of the intestinal epithelial cells where enzymes (peptidases and disaccharidases) produce monosaccharides and amino acids from the smaller peptides and sugars.

Fats

Fats present a special digestive problem because they are not very soluble in water and tend to separate out in a mixture, as oil and vinegar do when they are left to stand. This problem is solved by the bile acids. They:

- emulsify fat
- form micelles.

Emulsification

Bile acids are partly water loving (hydrophilic) and partly fat loving (lipophilic). They can thus mix in with fat and allow a stable suspension (emulsion) of tiny fat droplets to be formed. One immediate benefit of this is that it provides a larger surface area of fat that is open to attack by pancreatic lipase.

Micelle formation

Bile acids also associate with the individual molecules generated by the action of lipase (mono- and diglycerides, and fatty acids) and form tiny aggregates of these products (micelles), which are perfectly stable in a watery environment. Other fatty molecules, such as cholesterol and the fat-soluble vitamins, are also incorporated into the micelles.

Undigested residues

Some organic dietary constituents (including dietary fibre) are resistant to chemical digestion. This applies to a variety of non-starch polysaccharides, the chief of which is cellulose. Cellulose consists entirely of glucose subunits, but these are joined together by chemical linkages that are resistant to attack by the digestive enzymes. Undigested residues and other unabsorbed constituents pass on into the large intestine.

LARGE INTESTINE

There are no digestive enzymes in the large intestine, but there is a large population of bacteria (400–4000 different types) that can metabolize food residues and other substances in a variety of ways.

Bacterial activity

The products of bacterial metabolism depend upon the types of bacteria present, which vary from one individual to another. Total numbers of bacteria vary considerably. They multiply if the supply of food residues from the small intestine increases. This happens if the amount of fibre in the diet is increased,

Constipation and laxatives

Constipation

Normal bowel habit is hard to define since the frequency with which people defecate is an individual phenomenon. When defecation takes place less frequently than an individual thinks is normal (constipation) that person will often employ laxatives in order to achieve regular defecation.

Predisposing factors to constipation can include a poor diet that is low in fibre (indigestible material largely derived from plants), low fluid intake and lack of exercise. There may also be psychological factors.

Constipation can be broken down into simple constipation and severe idiopathic constipation. Simple constipation is extremely common and does not imply underlying organic disease. It usually responds to increased dietary fibre or use of bulking agents; adequate exercise and fluid intake is also essential.

Severe idiopathic constipation occurs almost exclusively in young women. The cause is unknown but some have 'slow transit' with reduced motor activity in the colon. This condition is often resistant to treatment.

Laxatives

Laxatives work in several ways. Some are designed to increase the bulk of faeces (e.g. lactulose) by increasing the water that is retained in the large intestine. This also has the effect of softening the faeces. The laxative effect is brought about by the increased bulk of faeces in the large intestine stimulating defecation, and their softer consistency making it easier to defecate.

Other preparations directly stimulate the smooth muscle of the gastrointestinal tract, and these are called the stimulant laxatives (e.g. bisacodyl). They can be administered orally, as tablets, or rectally, in the form of a suppository. Glycerine, which softens faeces in the rectum, is also administered rectally in the form of a suppository.

Enemas are administered rectally and contain fluids that stimulate the rectum (e.g. microlette), or stimulate the rectum and also increase the water content of the faeces within it by an osmotic effect (e.g. phosphate enema).

Laxatives can become habit forming, especially if they are used indiscriminately, and, for this reason, constipation is best avoided. Attention to diet and exercise, and adequate fluid intake are usually sufficient to maintain proper bowel function.

or if proteins and carbohydrates are incompletely digested in the small intestine because of an enzyme deficiency, for example lactase. Bacterial numbers are reduced by antibiotics. Antibiotic treatment consequently alters the kinds and amounts of products generated.

Faeces

Faeces consist largely of bacteria (60% of faecal solids). Only a small proportion is actually undigested food residues. The volume of faeces produced daily depends on diet, activity and bowel habits.

ABSORPTION

OVERVIEW

Absorption involves the movement of molecules out of the digestive tract and into the circulation or into the lymphatic system. The mechanism by which absorption occurs depends upon the specific molecule in question. Molecules pass out of the digestive tract by simple diffusion, facilitated diffusion or active transport.

The epithelium lining of the inside of the digestive tract separates the contents of the gut from the interstitial fluid that is in communication with the blood and lymph capillaries of the mucosa. Substances cross the epithelium in a variety of ways: some pass through the cells (transcellularly); others pass through the junctions between the cells (paracellularly). Some simply diffuse across; others are transported across the epithelial cell membranes by carrier proteins.

Most absorption occurs in the small intestine. A small quantity of fatty substances, water and salts normally pass on into the large intestine, where most of the remaining water and salts are absorbed.

HOW SUBSTANCES ARE ABSORBED

Substances cross the epithelium by:

- passive diffusion
- carrier-mediated transport
- endocytosis and exocytosis.

Passive diffusion

If the concentration of a substance is higher within the gut lumen than it is in the fluids on the other side of the epithelial barrier, absorption will occur by passive diffusion provided the substance can get across the barrier.

However, the epithelium is normally impermeable to all molecules except those that are:

- very small and water soluble
- fat soluble.

Small water-soluble molecules pass through the junctions between cells (paracellularly), and through pores in the membranes of the epithelial cells, but cannot easily penetrate the lipid part of cell membranes.

However, fatty substances, such as fatty acids, pass through the lipid layers of the cell membranes with relative ease. Consequently large quantities of fat are absorbed passively, but only small amounts of amino acids and monosaccharides are absorbed in this way.

Carrier-mediated transport

Selected water-soluble substances, such as glucose, amino acids and calcium, that cannot cross the epithelium easily by diffusion because they are too large are assisted in their passage by carrier proteins.

Each carrier protein is able to link with only a limited group of molecules. For example, the carrier protein that transports glucose can transport the similar monosaccharide galactose, but cannot transport amino acids or calcium. There are several forms of carrier-mediated transport:

- facilitated diffusion
- active transport
- co-transport.

Facilitated diffusion

When the movement of the carrier across the membrane occurs entirely passively, driven by the difference in concentration of the transported substance (i.e. 'downhill' with the concentration gradient), the process is termed facilitated diffusion. Glucose is an example of a substance transported by facilitated diffusion.

Co-transport

If two or more different substances bind to the same carrier, but at different sites, and are transported across the membrane together, the process is termed co-transport. For example, one of the carriers that transports glucose also carries sodium. In fact sodium influences the ability of the carrier to bind to glucose. When sodium is abundant, as it is in the intestinal contents within the gut lumen, the carrier binds glucose avidly. However, when sodium is scarce, as it is inside cells, glucose is not bound as firmly. In this way the uptake of glucose into intestinal epithelial cells is normally favoured by the composition of the intestinal contents, and the release of glucose inside the epithelial cells is favoured by the low intracellular sodium concentration. This particular form of transport is termed sodium dependent co-transport.

Active transport

If movement of the carrier requires the input of energy the process is termed active transport. ATP manu-factured by cell mitochondria is usually used to power the movement of the carrier.

This form of transport moves substances 'uphill' against their natural tendency for passive diffusion. It is therefore able to create and sustain a difference in concentration, such as that of sodium, inside and outside cells.

The commonest example of this type of carrier-mediated transport is the sodium–potassium pump (Na^+/K^+ ATPase), which evicts sodium from cells, and builds up potassium inside them. The pump is present in all cells including those of the intestinal epithelium. In the intestinal epithelium it is located on the sides of the cell that face the interstitial fluid (baso-lateral membrane) and carries sodium from the cell into the interstitial fluid.

Endocytosis and exocytosis

In endocytosis, a small part of the cell membrane becomes invaginated, forming a vesicle that is drawn into the cytoplasm. Fluid and/or particles can be engulfed in this way. Exocytosis is the process in reverse: an intracellular vesicle fusing with the cell membrane and releasing its contents (see Ch. 1).

SMALL INTESTINE

Several distinctive features make the small intestine the most important site of absorption:

- large surface area available for absorption
- presence of many types of carrier proteins
- permeability of the epithelium to salts and water.

Surface area

The surface area is very large because of numerous folds and villi. This is very important for the absorption of fat. If the surface area is reduced through disease (coeliac disease), or surgery (removal of some bowel), not as much fat can be absorbed, and this results in steatorrhoea (fatty stools).

Fat absorption

Monoglycerides, fatty acids and fat-soluble vitamins enter the epithelial cells by passive diffusion. Their rate of uptake depends on the difference in concentration of fatty substances on either side of the cell membrane and the available surface area. Micelles maintain a high concentration of fatty substances in the intestinal fluid whereas intracellular proteins that bind the absorbed fats mop them up inside the epithelial cells.

Fatty acids and monoglycerides are then transferred to the endoplasmic reticulum where they are used to form new triglycerides. Tiny lipid droplets form, and a protein 'coat' is added, giving rise to small particles (chylomicrons) that are packaged into vesicles and exported from the cell by exocytosis. Chylomicrons are too large to pass through the walls of blood capillaries but can get into lymph vessels (the lacteals). Regular contractions of the villi help to 'milk' the lymphatics so that lymph is driven towards the larger vessels.

Carrier proteins

Absorption of water-soluble substances

The epithelial cells of the small intestine possess a variety of carrier proteins that facilitate the absorption of specific water-soluble substances including:

- glucose
- amino acids
- iron
- calcium
- sodium.

Amino acids and monosaccharides

There are several different carriers transporting amino acids. Each carrier transports a particular group:

- acidic
- basic
- neutral.

If one of the carriers is absent, due to a genetic defect, the absorption of some but not all amino acids is therefore reduced.

Some absorption of monosaccharides and amino acids occurs by sodium-dependent co-transport.

Carrier proteins for di- and tripeptides also exist. Complete digestion of proteins to amino acids is therefore not essential.

Calcium and iron

Calcium and iron are most easily absorbed in the upper small intestine. The intestinal contents are slightly more acid here than further down and this helps to dissolve the iron and calcium in the diet and make it more available for absorption. However, both of these elements can form insoluble complexes with other constituents of the diet, such as phytic acid, present in unrefined cereals, and phosphates. Both hinder the absorption of calcium and iron if they are present in the diet in large amounts.

Other substances

Carrier systems are also involved in the absorption of sodium, chloride, hydrogen carbonate and bile salts.

Epithelial permeability

The intestinal epithelium is more permeable to the passive diffusion of water and salts than any other epithelia in the digestive system, and the duodenum is the most permeable part of all. Water is absorbed always by osmosis, secondary usually to the absorption of solutes.

Duodenum

Water and salts diffuse relatively easily in either direction across the duodenal epithelium. This means that water and salts can be drawn into the digestive tract or be absorbed from it depending upon the concentration gradients.

If food is broken down too rapidly and many molecules of glucose and amino acids are suddenly generated from polysaccharides and polypeptides, the osmotic pressure of the intestinal contents may exceed that of the plasma and interstitial fluid, and water will be drawn into the digestive tract from the blood. This can happen if the stomach empties too quickly because of disordered function after some forms of surgery. If a lot of fluid is suddenly drawn out of the body fluids into the digestive tract, blood volume and blood

---

Lactose intolerance

Human milk contains around 200 mmol/l of lactose which is normally digested to glucose and galactose by the enzyme lactase prior to absorption. This enzyme, which is present in childhood, virtually disappears in adulthood in most of the world's population, resulting in lactose intolerance. Consequently, if milk is drunk, the lactose is not digested and remains unabsorbed in the small intestine. The effects of this are retention of water in the small intestine due to an osmotic effect exerted by the disaccharide and, when the lactose reaches the large intestine, fermentation by commensal bacteria. The retention of water in the gastrointestinal tract causes diarrhoea – the production of watery faeces. Fermentation results in the production of abnormally high levels of gas in the large intestine, which leads to distension and pain.

The outcome of lactose intolerance for the individual can range from mild inconvenience to extreme fluid and electrolyte imbalance. Dietary modification, by either cutting down on dairy products or omitting them altogether, is the only way in which the effects of this complaint can be alleviated. In some people, the enzyme lactase persists into adulthood. These are ethnic groups, including most Caucasians (e.g. north Europeans), whose ancestors were dairy farmers.

Inflammatory bowel disorders

Crohn's disease and ulcerative colitis are names for inflammatory bowel disorders, of which there are several. The distinction between these conditions is not entirely clear and the cause of such disorders is not known either. At the very least, there may be an element of autoimmunity, which leads to inflammation at various sites in the small and large intestines and affects the mucosa, submucosa and the muscle layers of the gastrointestinal tract. The person suffering from an inflammatory bowel disorder will experience recurrent bouts of diarrhoea and concomitant weight loss. Both diseases most commonly start in young adults with a second incidence peak in the seventh decade.

Best disease management depends upon a team approach involving physicians, surgeons, radiologists, nurses and dieticians. Both ulcerative colitis and Crohn's disease are lifelong conditions and have psychosocial implications; nurse counsellors and patient support groups have an important role to play in education, reassurance and coping.

Inflammatory bowel disorders cannot be cured, but treatment of symptoms is possible. Evidence of infection can be treated with antibiotics, diarrhoea can be alleviated with codeine phosphate, which reduces gastric motility, and the inflammation can be treated with steroids administered either orally or rectally. In severe cases it is necessary to hospitalize patients in order to ensure that they get adequate rest, privacy and diet. The chronic diarrhoea has consequences for the perianal region, which can become painful and excoriated. In severe cases it is necessary to intervene surgically in order to excise affected parts of bowel or to form an ileostomy. In any of the above cases, the main support required by patients with inflammatory bowel disorders is psychological – they feel embarrassed by the effects of the condition (diarrhoea) and they worry about the consequences.

Coeliac disease (gluten-sensitive enteropathy)

Coeliac disease is characterized by abnormal small intestinal mucosa which returns to normal in response to a gluten-free diet. The condition occurs worldwide but is commoner in northern Europe. The presentation of coeliac disease is highly variable, depending on the severity and extent of small bowel involvement. Some patients have diarrhoea related to malabsorption while others develop tiredness, weight loss or anaemia. On examination, features of malnutrition are common and abdominal distension may be present. The management of coeliac disease involves adherence to a gluten-free diet. This requires the exclusion of wheat, rye, barley and oats and imposes severe restrictions.

pressure fall and the patient feels faint (dumping syndrome).

Water absorption

The absorption of water is always a passive process driven by osmosis, secondary usually to the absorption of amino acids, glucose and salts. If you drink water by itself the difference in osmotic pressure between it and the interstitial fluid guarantees its absorption.

Water-soluble substances that are not absorbed can create an opposing osmotic gradient-restricting water absorption. This can happen if there is a defect in digestion (such as lactase deficiency) so that digestion products (in this case the disaccharide lactose) remain unabsorbed, or if the epithelium lacks the ability or capacity to absorb all the solutes presented to it, as is the case with a large dose of magnesium sulphate (Epsom salts). In both cases the result is diarrhoea.

LARGE INTESTINE

Sodium is absorbed in the colon by active transport, followed by chloride and water. In this way the concentration of sodium in faecal fluid is reduced to very low amounts and losses of this important ion are minimized.

Absorption of other substances occurs simply by passive diffusion depending on how easily the substance can penetrate the epithelium. Water-soluble substances do not diffuse across at all easily, whereas those that have some lipid solubility, such as some products of bacterial metabolism (fatty acids, ammonia and secondary bile acids), can do so. Usually the amounts absorbed are quite small.

OTHER SITES OF ABSORPTION

In the remainder of the tract, namely the mouth and stomach, there are no specialized forms of transport, but small amounts of various substances can be absorbed by passive diffusion. For example, the drug glyceryl trinitrate (used for the rapid relief of angina) is absorbed in the mouth from tablets placed under the tongue, and water and alcohol are absorbed in the stomach.

CONTROL AND COORDINATION OF ACTIVITY

For food to be efficiently digested and absorbed, the activities of the several parts of the digestive system need to be controlled. Control is exercised by:

- the nervous system
- gastrointestinal hormones.

These systems regulate the digestive process and coordinate activity in different parts of the digestive tract. They also regulate activity between meals and influence the growth and renewal of the tract as a whole.

MECHANISMS

Nervous system

The somatic nervous system plays only a small part in control. Its activities are limited to the control of the muscles involved in chewing and swallowing, and the control of the external anal sphincter. The autonomic nervous system controls salivary secretion and is involved in the control of all of the rest of the digestive system, from the smooth muscle of the oesophagus to the internal anal sphincter.

Sensory receptors

There are sensory receptors of various kinds throughout the digestive system. These include:

- mechanoreceptors
- chemoreceptors
- nociceptors.

Mechanoreceptors monitor the degree of distension of the tract, whereas chemoreceptors sample the gastrointestinal fluid and respond to changes in the concentrations of key constituents such as hydrogen ions and amino acids, and to osmotic pressure. Nociceptors, of which there are relatively few, respond to noxious stimuli, such as overdistension of the intestine, and ischaemia.

Reflexes

Impulses from the receptors are transmitted to the plexi (see Ch. 5). Here they influence the activity of interneurones, and motor neurones that control:

- contraction of smooth muscle
- secretion of gastric and intestinal glands
- secretion of hormones by endocrine cells.

Reflexes involving only the enteric nervous system are termed local reflexes to distinguish them from those which also involve other parts of the nervous system (extrinsic or long reflexes).

Some impulses from sensory receptors are transmitted to abdominal ganglia, the spinal cord and brain stem. These impulses are responsible for eliciting more complex reflex responses via parasympathetic and sympathetic nerve fibres. For example, distension of the stomach reflexly excites pancreatic secretion and

Neurotransmitters of the enteric nervous system
Acetylcholine
Noradrenaline
Serotonin (5-hydroxytryptamine) (5HT)
Vasoactive intestinal polypeptide (VIP)
Substance P
Somatostatin
Enkephalins
Gastrin-releasing peptide (GRP)
Neurotensin

gall bladder contraction as well as stimulating gastric activity.

Some impulses are transmitted to the cerebral cortex and create the limited awareness we have of our internal state, such as feeling 'full up' or 'bloated'.

Neurotransmitters

Many different neurotransmitters have now been identified within the enteric nervous system. Some of these substances, such as substance P, have also been found in endocrine cells of the digestive tract, and may in some circumstances be referred to as hormones if they are released into the bloodstream in appreciable amounts.

Hormones

Many gastrointestinal hormones are also involved in the control of digestive function. Occasionally in disease, tumour cells secreting one of these hormones may be found elsewhere in the digestive system, such as a gastrinoma in the pancreas.

The secretion of hormones is regulated by:

- chemical conditions within the digestive tract
- nervous reflexes
- other hormones.

REGULATION OF DIGESTION

The efficient digestion of a meal depends upon:

- the readiness of the digestive system to receive food
- optimal composition of the gastric and intestinal contents for digestion and absorption
- a transit rate which maximizes absorption and minimizes waste.

Preliminary events

When food is smelt, ingested, chewed and swallowed, chemoreceptors (taste buds in the mouth and olfactory receptors in the nose) and mechanoreceptors are stimulated. As well as exciting salivary secretion, many other parts of the digestive system are excited via the vagus nerve, including:

- stomach
- pancreas
- gall bladder.

The increase in activity is relatively small but it is important in sensitizing the system to the more potent stimuli that follow. The initial phase of digestive activity is termed cephalic because the initiating stimuli all arise from sensory receptors in the head. In some but not all people, even the thought or sight of food is an effective stimulus.

Stomach

As food accumulates in the stomach, the stomach distends and the gastric juice present is diluted by the food. Theses events trigger neural reflexes and hormone secretion which:

- promote gastric activity
- control gastric acidity (pH)
- alert organs downstream to the arrival of food.

Gastric activity

Excitation of stretch receptors (a form of mechanoreceptor) in the wall of the stomach evokes local and long reflexes (chiefly vagal), which stimulate gastric contractions and promote secretion of gastric enzymes.

Control of gastric acidity (pH)

The enzymes secreted by the stomach (pepsinogens) need an acid environment to work efficiently. When food enters the stomach the acid juice is diluted and the acidity decreases (pH increases). The acid is diluted even more if there is protein in the diet because the protein acts as a buffer and takes up some hydrogen ions. As the pH increases, G cells in the antrum of the stomach, which are sensitive to the pH of gastric juice, increase their secretion of gastrin. Gastrin stimulates the oxyntic cells to secrete acid, which progressively lowers the pH of the gastric contents. In turn, the lowered pH inhibits the secretion of gastrin. In this way the pH of the gastric contents is brought to a suitable level for the gastric enzymes to work.

The acidity of the gastric fluid is in fact greatest when there is no food in the stomach, and least immediately after a meal. Consequently, someone with a gastric ulcer is more likely to complain of discomfort during the night than during the daytime when regular small snacks may be eaten.

Alerting the ileum and colon

The presence of food in the stomach also triggers activity further along the digestive tract. For example, as well as promoting secretion by the liver and the pancreas, increased peristaltic contractions occur in the terminal ileum and the colon (gastroileal and gastrocolic reflexes). These responses are caused in part by neural reflexes, but hormones such as gastrin are likely to be involved too. Contractions of the ileum and colon help to move the food residues from previous meals further along the tract.

Small intestine

Efficient digestion of food in the small intestine depends on:

Intestinal stomas

Any artificial opening between a hollow organ and the surface of the skin is described as a stoma. A stoma of the small intestine is called an ileostomy and a stoma of the large intestine is called a colostomy. Intestinal stomas are necessary for several reasons, such as obstruction of the intestine (cancer), damage (gunshot wound) and in some inflammatory bowel diseases. Stomas can be either temporary or permanent but in either case it is necessary, for the duration of the stoma, to collect the contents of the intestine outside the body at the surface of the skin. For this purpose, specialized bags have been developed and specialist nursing advice is available to help people, and their families, adjust to having this kind of surgical procedure.

The intestinal stomas present their own particular complications. A colostomy is probably easier to manage than an ileostomy. A colostomy bag collects formed faecal material and it is sometimes possible for people with colostomies to exert some control over the expulsion of faeces. A major problem, however, is odour from the colostomy and people need to become proficient at fitting colostomy bags securely. In contrast, the product of an ileostomy is much less formed because much less water has been absorbed from the contents of the small intestine than from material in the large intestine. The contents of the small intestine still contain active proteolytic enzymes and these can harm the skin if ileostomy bags are not fitted securely and proper skin hygiene is not carried out. It is also the case that a person with an ileostomy will lose a greater amount of fluid and electrolytes than normal and this needs to be compensated for in the diet.

Dietary changes may be required of people who have intestinal stomas. It is necessary to avoid food, according to individual experience, that will cause diarrhoea as this can lead to severe fluid loss and difficulty in managing the stoma.

- the supply of enzymes and bile acids
- correct pH for enzyme activity
- appropriate delivery of chyme from the stomach.

The composition and volume of the intestinal contents are monitored by sensory receptors and endocrine cells in the wall of the intestine that respond in ways which create the right conditions.

Supply of enzymes and bile acids

Amino acids and bile acids in the intestinal contents stimulate the secretion of CCK-PZ, which stimulates the pancreas to secrete large amount of enzymes and the gall bladder to contract and expel bile through the relaxed sphincter of Oddi into the duodenum.

Control of intestinal pH

Acid chyme emptied from the stomach into the upper small intestine stimulates the production of the hormone secretin which in turn stimulates the pancreas and the liver to secrete an alkaline fluid containing bicarbonate (hydrogen carbonate). This neutralizes the gastric acid and brings the pH closer to the optimum for the pancreatic enzymes to work (about pH 7.0).

The effect of secretin on the pancreas is enhanced by CCK-PZ. Both hormones inhibit gastric emptying, thereby reducing the delivery of acid to the duodenum.

Feedback to the stomach

The delivery of chyme to the duodenum needs to be regulated so that the intestine is not overloaded. To do this, several characteristics of the intestine, in addition to acidity, are monitored:

- fat content
- osmotic pressure
- volume.

Fat is the most difficult of the nutrients to digest and absorb properly. If too much fat enters the duodenum, gastric emptying is inhibited by a hormonal mechanism. The name enterogastrone has been given to the hormonal factors involved, but their specific identity is still uncertain.

Osmotic pressure matters because it determines water movement into and out of the tissues. Too great a flow in either direction creates problems: water may be drawn out of the blood if the osmotic pressure of the intestinal contents is greater than that of plasma; or it may flood into the blood and cause cells to swell if it is much lower than plasma. Thus if the osmotic pressure of the intestinal contents deviates a lot from that of plasma, in *either* direction, gastric emptying is inhibited by a neural reflex (enterogastric reflex).

Distension of the intestine also reduces gastric emptying. Distension of the ileum, for example, evokes the ileogastric reflex. It may also decrease appetite, particularly if distension is caused by unabsorbed food residues.

Interdigestive activity

The digestive tract is not inactive in the absence of food. About 4 to 5 hours after a meal, when the stomach is 'empty', peristaltic contractions similar to those evoked by a meal occur in the stomach. These become stronger (really strong contractions are felt as 'hunger pangs') and change in character from mixing movements to those of a propulsive kind. The duodenum in turn becomes active and a band of contractile activity slowly progresses along the intestine, with activity dying away behind it. The end of the ileum is reached in about 2 hours and, as soon as it is, another wave of contractions begins in the stomach.

This complex activity is referred to as 'the interdigestive migrating contractions' or 'the migrating myoelectric complex (MMC)'. It is accompanied by increased secretion from gastrointestinal glands, the pancreas and biliary system. The control of these events is not fully understood, but it is clear that the hormone motilin is involved in stimulating muscle contraction. The role of the complex may be to 'sweep out' the gastrointestinal tract regularly, thereby discouraging bacteria from the large intestine from colonizing the small intestine as well.

REFERENCES AND FURTHER READING

Camilleri M, Choi M 1997 Review article: irritable bowel syndrome. Alimentary Pharmacology and Therapeutics 11: 3–15

Davenport H W 1982 Physiology of the digestive tract. Medical Publishers, Chicago

Heading R, Tibaldi M 1998 Oesophageal symptoms and motility disorders. Medicine 26(7): 1–6

Hobsly M 1982 Disorders of the digestive system. Edward Arnold, London

Kamm M A 1996 Inflammatory bowel disease. Martin Dunitz, London

Logan R P H, Harris A, Misiewicz J J, Baron J H 2002 ABC of the upper gastrointestinal tract. BMJ Books, London

Lundell L (ed) 1998 Guidelines for the management of symptomatic gastro-oesophageal reflux disease. Science Press, London

Rogers A W 1992 Textbook of anatomy. Churchill Livingstone, Edinburgh

Rutgeerts P, Colombel J-F et al 1995 Advances in inflammatory bowel diseases. Kluwer Academic Publishers, London

Sanford P A 1992 Digestive system physiology, 2nd edn. Edward Arnold, London

Smith G D, Watson R 2003 Gastrointestinal nursing. Blackwell Scientific, London

Smith M E, Morton D G 2001 The digestive system. Harcourt Publishers, London

10 The liver and metabolism

In practice you may be asked to consider the following:

1. If injured, can the liver regenerate?

2. The liver receives about 20% of cardiac output. Which vessels supply the liver? How is the flow regulated?

3. A patient with advanced liver disease may be very easily bruised. Why is this?

4. This patient may also experience fasting hypoglycaemia. Why is this?

5. Obstruction (e.g. in cirrhosis) to the flow of blood through the liver produces hepatic portal hypertension. Why is pressure in the portal vessel apparently more affected?

6. Interruption or obstruction to the flow of bile is likely to result in jaundice perhaps with pruritus. What has caused the symptoms?

7. A newborn baby may be slightly jaundiced (his liver is normal). What is the reason for this jaundice? Explain the method of treatment.

8. Oedema is characteristic of liver dysfunction. Why is this?

9. Spironolactone can be used to treat the oedema (and ascites) in liver dysfunction. Why that particular drug?

10. Any drug therapy requires great care, but why is there particular concern where there is liver disease?

The liver is concerned primarily with the provision and elimination of a wide variety of organic molecules such as glucose, amino acids, fatty acids, steroids, and plasma proteins, together with many waste products.

The liver is often likened to a chemical factory in that it is involved in the manufacture and processing of a wide range of substances. It cooperates with the digestive system in the supply of nutrients to the body, and complements the activity of other excretory systems in the processing and elimination of unwanted materials from the body.

Central to the function of the liver is its blood supply which supports the many different activities of the liver cells. These activities include the metabolism of carbohydrates, amino acids, fats and vitamins, and the formation of bile.

STRUCTURE AND BLOOD SUPPLY

GENERAL FEATURES

Anatomy

The liver is the largest soft organ in the body. In an adult person it weighs about 1.5 kg. It is located high in the abdomen, bounded above by the dome of the diaphragm (Fig. 10.1A & B). There are several lobes, the one on the right being the largest. The normal dark purplish-brown colour of the liver is evidence both of the richness of its circulation and of the fact that a sizeable fraction of the blood supply (70–80%) is already partially deoxygenated.

Histology

The liver is composed chiefly of one cell type (Fig. 10.2), the hepatocyte or parenchymal cell which is responsible for many of the functions of the liver (see p. 193). In addition to these cells, which form the major part of the liver tissue (80% by volume), there are a few other cell types present in smaller numbers. These include Kupffer cells, Ito cells and pit cells (see later Fig. 10.4).

> Replacement of hepatocytes by connective tissue in disordered liver function is termed fibrosis.

Kupffer cells are macrophages that engulf and dispose of bacteria, cell debris and viruses. Ito cells (also known as fat-storing cells) contain a high concentration of vitamin A and are believed to be involved in the formation of hepatic connective tissue. The function of pit cells is unclear. They may have a neuroendocrine function.

BLOOD SUPPLY

The liver has an ample blood supply (1.25–1.5 litres/ min; approximately one-fifth of the cardiac output at rest) which is derived from two sources (Fig. 10.3):

- the hepatic artery
- the hepatic portal vein.

The hepatic artery contributes only one-fifth to one-third of the supply. This blood is delivered at normal arterial pressures and is fully oxygenated. The majority of the blood supply, delivered via the portal vein, comes from the venous drainage of most of the gastrointestinal tract and is partially deoxygenated.

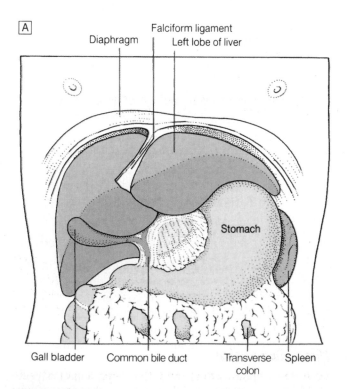

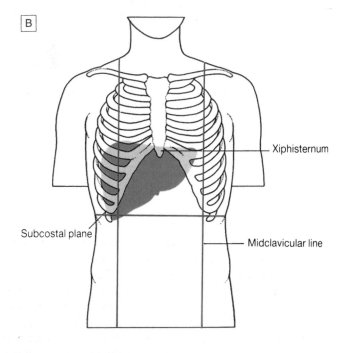

Figure 10.1 Position of the liver: A, Within the abdominal cavity. B, in relation to the rib cage. (From Rogers 1992, with permission of Elsevier.)

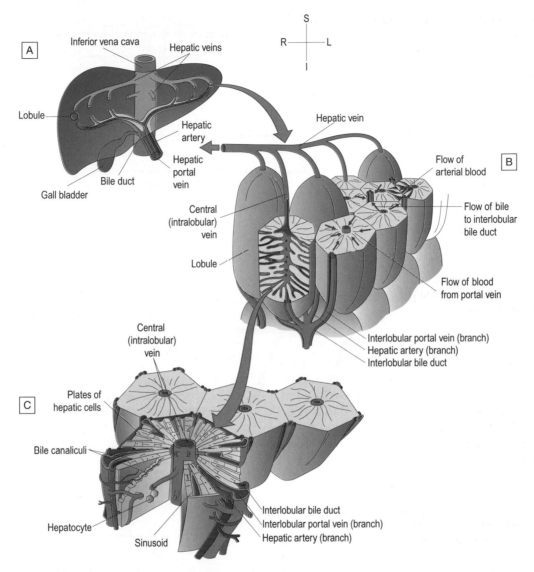

Figure 10.2 Microscopic structure of the liver. A, This diagram shows the location of liver lobules relative to the overall circulatory scheme of the liver. B and C, Enlarged views of several lobules show how blood from the hepatic portal veins and hepatic arteries flows through sinusoids and thus past plates of hepatic cells toward a central vein in each lobule. Hepatic cells form bile, which flows through bile canaliculi toward hepatic ducts that eventually drain the bile from the liver. (After Thibodeau & Patten 1993, with permission of Elsevier.)

Portal blood supply

The portal supply includes *all* the venous drainage of the gastrointestinal tract from the lower part of the oesophagus through to the end of the large intestine. Only the venous blood from the mouth, most of the oesophagus and parts of the rectum escapes the hepatic 'filter' (Fig. 10.3). There are a few linking vessels, anastomoses, between the oesophageal veins and the portal vein. If blood flow through the liver is restricted these may open up, giving rise to oesophageal varices.

Normal pressures in the hepatic portal vein are quite low (5–10 mmHg). If there is obstruction to flow through the liver, as for example in advanced cirrhosis, portal pressure rises (portal hypertension). This affects tissue fluid balance in the capillaries upstream (splanchnic capillaries) and may lead to the accumulation of large amounts of tissue fluid in the peritoneal cavity (ascites; see p. 190).

Microcirculation

Both the hepatic artery and the hepatic portal vein divide into branches which carry blood to the several lobes of the liver. Thereafter these vessels divide many

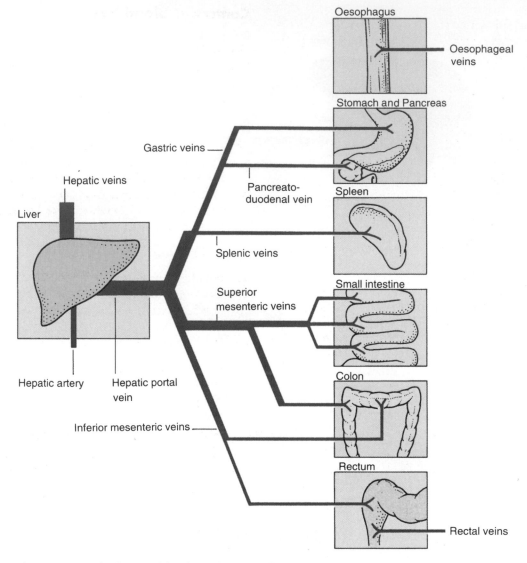

Figure 10.3 The hepatic blood supply: most of it comes straight from the digestive tract.

Ascites

Ascites is both disfiguring and distressing, leading to a grossly swollen abdomen which makes movement difficult and clothing very tight, or even impossible, to wear.

Patients with ascites feel very uncomfortable. They are, quite literally, heavier than normal due to the fluid accumulation in the abdomen. One of the main nursing observations in this condition is to establish whether or not ascites is improving or deteriorating. Since ascites represents a build-up of fluid, and that fluid is mainly water, the most accurate way of establishing whether the accumulation has increased or decreased is to weigh the patient. This may not always be possible, however, and an alternative method is to measure abdominal girth. This must be done with the patient in exactly the same position each time, using a mark somewhere on the abdomen to

position the tape measure. It is useful if several measurements can be made at one time in order to obtain an average and an accurate record kept.

Another aspect of ascites follows from the anatomy of the abdomen and thorax. The increasing size of the abdomen, and this is particularly true when the patient is lying down, restricts movement in the thorax by putting pressure on the diaphragm. Consequently, the patient with ascites has difficulty breathing and is prone to develop chest infections due to the fact that the lungs are not being properly ventilated.

Ascites is indicative of underlying disease which must be treated medically. Nursing actions revolve around caring for the distressed patient and keeping a record of fluid intake and output in addition to direct observation and reporting on the ascites.

Oesophageal varices

A varicosity is simply a part of a vein which has become dilated (stretched) and oesophageal varices are usually a sign of advanced cirrhosis of the liver. They are common in people whose livers have become severely damaged through excessive alcohol intake.

Cirrhosis is described as widespread fibrosis of the liver where functional hepatocytes are replaced by non-functional fibrous tissue. In this condition blood flow through the liver is restricted and this, in turn, increases the blood pressure within the portal circulation, which carries blood from the digestive organs to the liver. As a result of this restricted blood flow a collateral circulation which is an alternative to the normal circulation, takes place via blood vessels in the stomach and at the lower oesophagus. The collateral circulation has a higher blood pressure than normal, causing varicosities to form in the oesophagus.

A steady small loss of blood into the oesophagus can ensue, leading to anaemia, or the loss of blood can be acute and spectacular, leading to death since the varicosities can rupture, resulting in massive loss of blood and shock.

---

times again to form arterioles and venules which supply blood to a group of liver cells.

The terminal arterioles and terminal portal venules empty into capillaries, which form 'tunnels' between 'walls' of liver cells (hepatocytes) one cell thick. Liver capillaries are often referred to as sinusoids because they differ from many other capillaries in being larger and much more permeable to plasma proteins (Fig. 10.2).

The blood from the arterioles and from the portal venules mixes as it enters the sinusoids. Sphincters involved in regulating the delivery of blood to the sinusoids are present at the ends of the arterioles. By varying the amount of arterial blood the relative proportion of arterial and portal-venous blood can be altered. As the composition of the blood from these two sources differs (arterial blood is fully oxygenated, whereas portal vein blood is partially deoxygenated and contains absorbed nutrients, for example), the blood to which the hepatocytes are exposed can be varied in composition. This influences the metabolic activity of the liver cells (see below).

Veins

Sinusoids from adjacent areas of liver tissue empty into a central vein (Fig. 10.2). This in turn joins other veins to form larger and larger vessels, which ultimately form the short hepatic veins which drain blood into the inferior vena cava in the abdomen.

Control of blood flow

Portal circulation

Blood flow through the portal vein normally depends almost solely on the factors which control the blood supply to the digestive system. When a meal is being digested, the increased flow of blood to the digestive system increases the flow of blood through the hepatic portal vein to the liver. The veins entering the portal vein, and the portal vein itself, contain some smooth muscle innervated by sympathetic nerves. Contraction of this muscle stiffens the veins and alters their capacity, as it does in veins elsewhere, but has relatively little effect on the rate of blood flow (see Ch. 6).

Arterial circulation

The hepatic arterial supply is regulated independently. The arterioles are innervated by sympathetic nerves which when excited cause vasoconstriction, narrow the vessels and reduce blood flow. Blood-borne factors which influence the arterioles and regulate flow include (Table 10.1):

- hormones regulating liver metabolism
- products of cell activity
- digestive factors.

The arterial supply is vital. Without it the liver becomes susceptible to bacterial colonization. In the absence of the arterial supply, the low oxygen concentrations to which the liver is exposed favour the growth of some types of bacteria.

Capillaries

Permeability

The capillaries of the liver are unusual in that they are very permeable to plasma proteins. Under high magnification it can be seen that the endothelial cells possess clusters of pore-like structures known as sieve plates. These are believed to be the route through which plasma proteins get across the capillary wall and enter the space of Disse between the capillary and the hepatocytes (Fig. 10.4).

Table 10.1 Factors causing vasodilation of the hepatic arterioles

Hormones	Products of cell activity	Digestive factors
Adrenaline	Adenosine	Secretin
Glucagon	CO_2	Bile salts
	K^+	

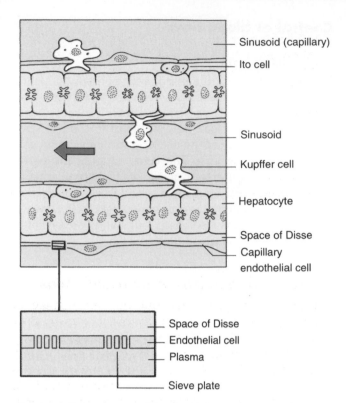

Figure 10.4 Liver capillaries and their relation to hepatocytes and other cells.

Table 10.2 Some plasma proteins manufactured by the liver

Albumin
Angiotensinogen
Factor VII
Factor IX
Factor X
Fibrinogen
Prothrombin
Transcobalamin
Transcortin
Transferrin

Because of its siting, the liver itself is at risk of infection from viruses which enter the body via the digestive system. The most common virus is hepatitis A (infectious hepatitis). It can be spread by poor personal hygiene from hands to food. Care is needed in the disposal of urine and faeces from infected patients.

Substances such as bilirubin (see Ch. 3), fatty acids and heavy metals (lead, copper) which are largely transported in blood bound to plasma proteins have very easy access to the hepatocytes. This differs from other tissues and contrasts with the capillaries of the brain (see Ch. 20). The liver 'welcomes all comers'. This enables it to fulfil its major role in the processing and disposal of waste materials. Likewise, other constituents of blood that are generally too large to cross capillary walls (such as chylomicrons; see Ch. 9) have easy access to the hepatocytes.

The traffic of proteins across the capillary wall occurs in both directions as the liver is the site of manufacture of many of the plasma proteins including albumin and a variety of the clotting factors (Table 10.2 and Ch. 3).

Activity

Endothelial cells are not simply a passive, very leaky barrier. They also play an active role in the uptake, processing and degradation of macromolecules such as proteins in the blood. They engulf these molecules by endocytosis (see Ch. 1).

Lodged at various points in the capillary wall are larger, plumper cells, Kupffer cells (Fig. 10.4). Extensions of these cells protrude both into the blood on the one side and the space of Disse on the other. The cells are phagocytic and belong to the diffuse system of macrophages found scattered throughout the body which engulf and degrade cellular debris, bacteria and viruses (see Chs 3 and 16). Kupffer cells are estimated to make up 60% of all the cells in the macrophage system. They are strategically sited as the venous blood from the digestive system, which may be carrying bacteria, viruses and foreign proteins absorbed through the digestive epithelium, must first pass through the liver before entering the rest of the circulation.

HEPATIC INNERVATION

Efferent nerves

The liver like other viscera is innervated by parasympathetic and sympathetic nerves. Nerve endings have been identified in most parts of the liver, although the density of innervation differs between one part and another.

In general, sympathetic nerves are most abundant. Adrenergic terminals are found in association with the smooth muscle of the blood vessels as well as with hepatocytes and other cells. The cholinergic innervation, by contrast, appears to be more limited.

Major functions of the efferent nerves include regulation of the hepatic circulation and the regulation of glucose metabolism.

Afferent nerves

In addition to these efferent fibres, sensory fibres have also been identified. Sensory receptors, such as baroreceptors and osmoreceptors, monitor conditions within the liver, and this information is used in the overall regulation of visceral function.

LIVER FUNCTIONS

METABOLIC ACTIVITY OF THE HEPATOCYTES

Most of the important functions of the liver are carried out by the hepatocytes. The chief histological features of these cells are shown in Figure 10.5. Liver cells are often cited as useful examples of a typical cell because they contain a balanced range of cellular organelles. This reveals the diversity of metabolic activity of these cells, which includes:

- processing of substances in the smooth endoplasmic reticulum (steroid hormones, drugs)
- synthesis of proteins for export in the rough endoplasmic reticulum (plasma proteins)
- packaging of various secretory products by the Golgi apparatus (proteins, bile salts, drugs)
- storage of substances in vesicles (glycogen, iron, vitamins).

Much of this activity is powered by the energy generated by the mitochondria.

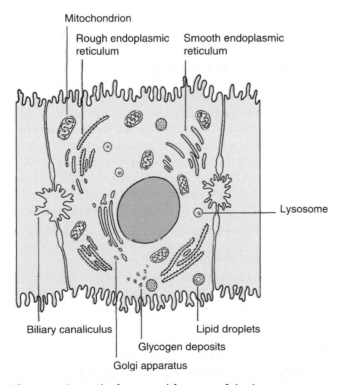

Mitochondrion

Rough endoplasmic reticulum

Smooth endoplasmic reticulum

Lysosome

Biliary canaliculus

Lipid droplets

Glycogen deposits

Golgi apparatus

Figure 10.5 Chief structural features of the hepatocyte.

Liver function tests probe different aspects of metabolic activity. For example, serum albumin is lowered when the liver is not synthesizing as much protein and the blood level of the enzyme alkaline phosphatase is raised when the secretion of this enzyme in bile in blocked.

If the liver is injured by an overdose of the drug paracetamol, it is the perivenous cells that suffer most damage.

Regional differences in metabolic bias

All the hepatocytes carry out the same range of activities. However, they differ in the bias of their activity because the cells are not all exposed to exactly the same environment. The cells, close to the supply vessels (arterioles and portal venules), are exposed to higher concentrations of oxygen and absorbed nutrients than the hepatocytes downstream closer to the central veins. Consequently the metabolic activities of the cells in the periportal regions differ in degree from those in the perivenous (or centrilobular) regions.

The activity of the cells closest to the supply vessels is biased towards the uptake, processing and metabolism of a variety of substances including monosaccharides and amino acids. Further along the sinusoid, the bias of cell activity shifts towards fat synthesis and drug metabolism (Table 10.3).

The metabolic activity of the cells is not fixed but changes with nutritional status, blood supply and hormonal balance.

Table 10.3 Metabolic bias of different hepatocytes*

Periportal	Perivenous
Uptake of – bilirubin – bile salts – glucose	Drug metabolism
Formation of – glycogen – glucose	Fat synthesis
ATP formed oxidatively†	ATP formed by glycolysis†

* All hepatocytes do the same things, but some are more active in some processes than others. This table shows what periportal and perivenous hepatocytes specialize in.
† See Chapter 15.

BILE SECRETION

The hepatocytes are linked together by specialized junctions, including tight junctions and gap junctions (see Ch. 2), to form sheets of cells, which in cross-section look like cords radiating from the central veins (Fig. 10.2). Running between adjacent cells and sealed off on either side from the interstitial space of Disse by tight junctions are tiny (1 μm in diameter) fluid-filled channels, the biliary canaliculi (little canals) (Fig. 10.2). The secretion of bile is one of the many functions of the hepatocytes. A variety of substances including bile salts (see Ch. 9) are excreted in bile. A few examples are listed in Table 10.4.

Table 10.4 Some substance excreted in bile

Type	Examples
Bile salts	Sodium glycocholate
	Sodium glycochenodeoxycholate
Endogenous waste products	Bilirubin glucuronide
	Steroid hormones
Drugs	Erythromycin
	Barbiturates
	Digitalis glycosides
Heavy metals	Lead
	Copper

In cholestasis (reduced flow of bile) substances normally excreted in bile accumulate in the body and give rise to such clinical features as itching (pruritus), caused probably by bile salts, and yellowing of the skin (jaundice) caused by bile pigments such as bilirubin.

Bile formed by the hepatocytes flows in the opposite direction to the blood, from the canaliculi nearest the central veins to the canaliculi nearest to the terminal arterioles and portal venules. From there it flows into the ducts of the biliary system. The biliary ducts lie alongside the blood vessels supplying blood to the liver sinusoids (Fig. 10.2).

The primary bile formed by the hepatocytes (canalicular bile) is modified as it flows through the ducts. An alkaline secretion of sodium hydrogen carbonate is added here and a few selected substances such as glucose are absorbed.

LIVER FUNCTIONS IN CONTEXT

Many of the general functions of the liver (Table 10.5) are shared with other parts of the body. For example,

the liver has an important role in the metabolism of carbohydrates, proteins and fats but it shares this role with other tissues, particularly skeletal muscle and adipose tissue (see Ch. 15). Similarly, the liver participates in the defence of the body against invasion by bacteria and other foreign matter through the phagocytic activity of the Kupffer cells but again it is only part of the body-wide system of macrophages (see Ch. 16). As regards specific functions, however, there are certain activities, such as the formation of urea, that are almost exclusively performed by the liver.

The several functions of the liver can for simplicity be divided into two groups:

• nutrient homeostasis
• elimination of waste and unwanted materials.

In nutrient homeostasis the liver cooperates with the digestive system, skeletal muscle, adipose tissue and the kidneys in controlling the circulating levels of nutrients such as glucose, amino acids and lipids. In the removal of waste or unwanted materials, the liver cooperates with the lungs, the kidneys and phagocytic cells throughout the body to provide a comprehensive waste disposal service. How these different tissues and organs interact will be described in two later chapters (Chs 15 and 16), but a brief mention will be made here of the major activities of the liver, in order to make clear the kind of disturbances that arise if the liver is damaged or diseased.

Nutrient homeostasis

Metabolism

Metabolism is composed of two processes which are dependent upon one another: anabolism and catabolism, which respectively build up and break down molecules in the body. These two processes work simultaneously to provide energy in the form of ATP and to facilitate the exchange of carbon between different types of molecule: carbohydrates, fats and amino acids. All the energy-using processes of the body, such as movement, are dependent upon metabolism, as are the synthetic processes whereby large molecules such as protein are made for use in muscle and other tissues.

Glycolysis and the Krebs cycle

At the centre of metabolism is the Krebs (or citric acid) cycle, a series of enzyme catalysed reactions, which is often referred to as the 'hub' of metabolism. The Krebs cycle (Fig. 10.6) completely breaks down the energy-containing molecules (substrates) that enter it and it also produces electrons for oxidative phosphorylation, which is responsible for the production of ATP. The main substrate for the Krebs cycle is glucose, which

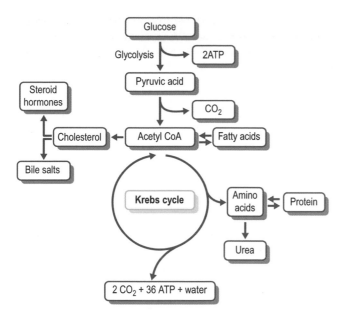

Figure 10.6 Metabolism. (After Watson 2000, with permission of Elsevier.)

enters the Krebs cycle via a metabolic pathway called glycolysis, although fatty acids, glycerol and amino acids also produce substrates for the Krebs cycle.

The sources of glucose for metabolism include carbohydrates in the diet: glucose and disaccharides, such as sucrose and lactose, which are broken down to produce glucose, and glycogen, some of which is obtained in the diet but most of which is obtained from stores in the body such as the liver and muscle. If the body requires additional glucose over and above the dietary or storage requirements, then amino acids can be used to make glucose in the process of gluco-neogenesis. Glycolysis produces pyruvic acid and two molecules of ATP. The pyruvic acid is converted to a substance called acetyl coenzyme A (acetyl CoA), losing a carbon atom in the form of carbon dioxide in the process, and this is further broken down in the Krebs cycle to produce carbon dioxide, water and 36 molecules of ATP. Acetyl CoA is also the end-product of fatty acid breakdown.

The acetyl CoA, which is a 2-carbon molecule, combines with a 4-carbon molecule (oxaloacetic acid) which is then broken down in the rest of the cycle, losing 2 carbon atoms in the process as carbon dioxide, until another 4-carbon molecule of oxaloacetic acid is produced. This 4-carbon molecule can combine with another 2-carbon molecule of acetyl Co A and the cycle continues.

Amino acids can be used to produce energy by being broken down in the Krebs cycle. Different amino acids enter this pathway at different points and intermediate molecules of the Krebs cycle can also be used to produce amino acids. Owing to the central role of the Krebs cycle in the metabolism of carbohydrate, fat and amino acids, it is possible to exchange carbon between molecules. For instance, some amino acids can be made from molecules in the Krebs cycle for subsequent use in protein synthesis and, as mentioned above, glucose can be made from some amino acids in a process called gluconeogenesis. However, fatty acids cannot be used to make glucose as the conversion of pyruvic acid to

Table 10.5 Functions of the liver

General	Specific examples
Carbohydrate metabolism	Synthesizes glucose
	Stores glucose as glycogen
	Converts galactose to glucose*
Protein and amino acid metabolism	Synthesizes and degrades many plasma proteins
	Synthesizes and degrades purines and pyrimidines
	Forms and degrades amino acids
	Forms urea and uric acid*
Fat metabolism	Synthesizes fatty acids
	Forms and secretes VLDL (very low density lipoproteins)*
	Forms ketone bodies*
	Forms bile salts from cholesterol*
Metabolism of endogenous waste	Bilirubin*
	Steroid hormones
Metabolism of xenobiotics	Alcohol
	Drugs
Phagocytosis	Bacteria, red cells
Bile secretion*	

* Functions that may be considered as exclusive to the liver as other tissues contribute so little (if at all).

acetyl CoA, where a molecule of carbon dioxide is produced, cannot be reversed.

Metabolism and injury

Metabolism in all tissues, including the liver, responds to injury by providing substrates for fighting infection and repairing tissue. Injury can be caused by trauma or by major surgery; therefore patients with metabolic disturbance may be encountered in casualty and in surgical wards. An understanding of the metabolic effects of injury will help in understanding what is happening to the trauma or surgical patient: why, for example, there is weight loss after trauma – especially muscle atrophy – and why good nutrition is essential.

Following injury there is an increase in the levels of catecholamines (adrenaline (epinephrine), and nor-adrenaline (norepinephrine)), and cortisol in the blood which have a net catabolic effect on the body. Early injury also decreases circulating levels of insulin and the net effect is to increase blood glucose level. The liver is not sensitive to insulin, but other tissues such as muscle are, and the decrease in circulating levels of insulin will also increase blood glucose levels. Blood glucose comes from glycogen stores in the liver and muscle and from protein breakdown in muscle which produces amino acids for use in gluconeogenesis, and the major effect of trauma is on body protein. At a time when large amounts of glucose are required in synthetic and repair processes, the normal synthetic processes of the body continue and the body strives to maintain a constant level of blood glucose. In due course the circulating levels of cortisol drop and the body enters a restorative phase whereby body mass and composition, which may have been adversely affected by injury and the local responses, are restored (see Ch. 19).

Storage

The liver acts as a storage site for some nutrients when these are surplus to immediate requirements. Examples are listed in Table 10.6. The synthesis of glycogen from glucose is glycogenesis.

Amino acids are used in the body to form proteins, purines and pyrimidines. Amino acids that are surplus

Table 10.6 Some nutrients stored by the liver

Vitamin A	Iron
Vitamin B	Glucose as glycogen
– riboflavin	
– niacin	
– B_6	
– folic acid	
– B_{12}	

In renal disease the excretion of urea may be inadequate because of defective kidney function (see Ch. 8). In this circumstance the danger of uraemia (raised blood urea concentration) can be avoided by reducing the amount of protein in the diet, and thus the amount of urea manufactured by the liver.

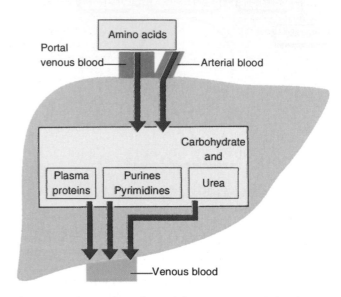

Figure 10.7 Products formed from amino acids by the liver.

to requirements are not stored in a separate protein depot but are degraded instead (deaminated) by the liver to form urea as a waste product (Fig. 10.7).

Synthesis

The liver manufactures a wide variety of substances that are used by the body. Key substances are listed in Table 10.7.

Plasma proteins including some of the clotting factors (see Ch. 3 and Table 10.2) are synthesized from amino acids. In liver disease it is the shortfall in the supply of some of the earlier factors in the clotting sequence that leads to bleeding disorders.

Large amounts of glucose (up to 250 g/day) can be formed by the liver from a variety of precursors including alanine, glycerol and lactic acid. This process is gluconeogenesis.

Triglycerides are synthesized in the liver from fatty acids and glycerol. The fat formed is normally packaged together with other lipids, such as phospholipids and cholesterol, and 'coated' with protein to form lipid-rich complexes (lipoproteins) which are secreted into the blood (see Ch. 15). The main class of plasma lipoproteins formed by the liver is VLDL (very low density lipoprotein). If the formation and secretion of VLDL

Table 10.7 Some substances produced by the liver

Type	Function	Chapter reference
Plasma proteins	Coagulation ⎫ Transport ⎭	3
	Prohormones	11
Glucose	Fuel	11, 18
Lipoproteins (chiefly VLDL)*	Lipid transport and metabolism	15
Ketone bodies	Fuel	15, 18
Bile salts (acids)	Digestive agent	9
Creatine	Precursor of creatine phosphate in muscle	4B
Urea	Waste product (affects renal function)	8
Purines ⎫ Pyrimidines ⎭	Components of DNA, RNA	1

* Very low density lipoproteins.

Bleeding disorders

The liver is responsible for the synthesis of nine of the blood clotting factors and any impairment in liver function will reduce its capacity to synthesize any of these factors. Additionally, three of the factors require the presence of vitamin K in order to be synthesized. Vitamin K, which is fat soluble, requires the presence of bile salts in the small intestine in order for it to be absorbed. Bile salts emulsify fats and form micelles which aid in the digestion and absorption of fat. In cholestasis there is a lack of bile in the intestine thus decreasing the absorption of vitamin K and consequent synthesis of some of the clotting factors.

An individual who has a tendency to excessive and prolonged bleeding due to liver disease will have to take precautions and be made aware of the possible signs. The kind of precautions that can be taken are common sense such as, in men, shaving with an electric rather than a wet razor. Additional care has to be taken, for example, when brushing teeth to avoid bleeding gums. A sign of internal bleeding may be the passing of blood in the urine (haematuria). Haematuria results from bleeding into any part of the urinary system and minor damage in a patient who has reduced blood clotting ability will lead to prolonged bleeding. This is very distressing for the patient.

A feature of the medical care of such patients will be the regular taking of blood samples for analysis of clotting times (see Ch. 3). What is being sought is a reduction in clotting time to normal, which will happen when normal liver function is restored. Where there is cholestasis, Vitamin K can also be administered by injection to help in the synthesis of clotting factors by the liver.

does not keep pace with the hepatic synthesis of triglycerides, the triglycerides accumulate giving rise to a fatty liver, as for example in liver disease in alcoholism.

Ketone bodies (aceto-acetate, beta-hydroxybutyrate and acetone) are formed from acetyl CoA which is derived from the mitochondrial oxidation of fatty acids. In starvation or in uncontrolled type 1 diabetes (see Ch. 18) large amounts of ketone bodies are formed from fat and used as an energy source.

Bile acids are synthesized in the liver from cholesterol. In humans the two major bile acids synthesized are cholic acid and chenodeoxycholic acid (Fig. 10.8). The sodium salts of these acids are sodium cholate and sodium chenodeoxycholate. These are linked (conjugated) with the amino acids glycine or taurine to give conjugated bile salts:

- sodium glycocholate
- sodium glycochenodeoxycholate
- sodium taurocholate
- sodium taurochenodeoxycholate.

The glycine conjugated sodium salts constitute the larger proportion. All these bile salts are secreted in large amounts in bile and are necessary for the digestion and absorption of fats (see Ch. 9). They are referred to as primary bile salts to distinguish them from secondary bile salts that are formed from them by the bacteria in the large intestine (Fig. 10.8).

Elimination of waste and unwanted materials

The liver has a major role in the processing and elimination of many endogenous and exogenous

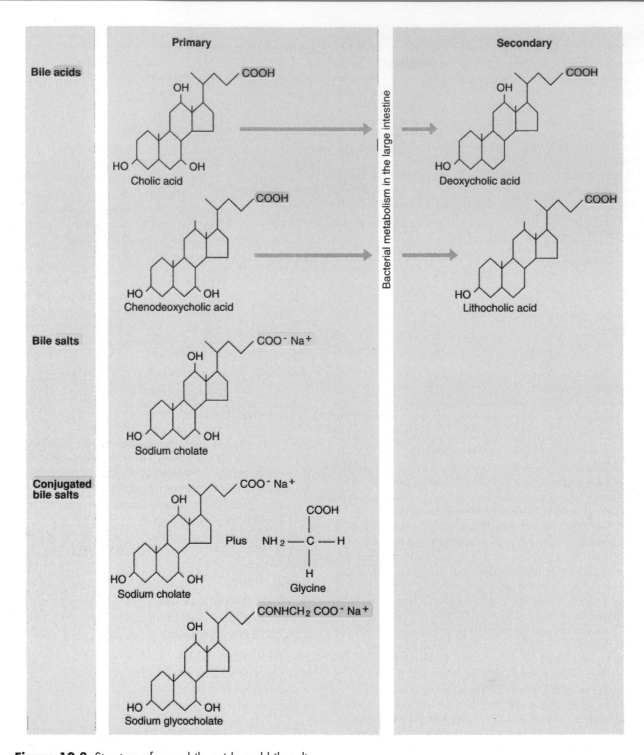

Figure 10.8 Structure of some bile acids and bile salts.

substances (Table 10.8). Some of these substances are converted into products that are secreted into the blood and then excreted in body fluids such as urine and sweat, or in expired air. Ammonia, for example, is converted into urea and excreted in the urine whereas alcohol is converted into acetaldehyde, some of which is exhaled in expired air.

Other substances, such as bilirubin (derived from the breakdown of haemoglobin; see Ch. 3) are secreted into the bile and eliminated in the faeces. If the secretion of bile by the liver is impaired or if its delivery to the gall bladder or intestine is blocked (see Ch. 9), as for example by a gall stone, then some waste products, such as bilirubin, will be dammed back into the liver

Table 10.8 Substances whose elimination from the body is assisted by the liver

Endogenous	Exogenous
Ammonia	Dietary constituents, e.g. alkaloids
Bilirubin	Drugs, e.g. antibiotics
Steroid hormones	Heavy metals, e.g. copper, lead

and spill back into the blood giving rise to various clinical features including jaundice (yellowing of the skin and mucous membranes).

LIVER FAILURE

If liver function is inadequate the consequences will include:

- a decrease in the plasma levels of manufactured products (plasma proteins, urea, glucose)
- a build-up of waste products that are normally removed (bilirubin, ammonia and steroid hormones).

If a patient with liver failure is on any medication this has to be given with great caution since the liver is the means whereby many drugs are processed and eliminated. The effect on the patient will be that drugs will cause increased side effects and their therapeutic effects will last longer. This is often taken into account by administering smaller doses.

Each of these events has its own repercussions on body function. For example, the build-up of ammonia and other waste products is associated with brain dysfunction (hepatic encephalopathy); elevated levels of steroid hormones alter cellular development and function; lowered concentrations of plasma proteins result in bleeding disorders and may contribute to tissue fluid imbalance, resulting in oedema.

In severe liver failure there may also be hypothermia as a consequence of reduced metabolic activity. Under normal conditions the extensive metabolic activity of the liver accounts for 20% of the oxygen consumed at rest which contributes a significant proportion of resting heat production.

Jaundice

Defined as a yellow discoloration of the skin and sclera (the firm outer layer of the eye), jaundice is caused by an increase in bilirubin in the blood. The source of bilirubin is the haem component of haemoglobin which is broken down when red blood cells are destroyed. The bilirubin is normally taken up by the liver and excreted in bile. If this excretory route is impaired through liver disease (*hepatocellular jaundice*) or failure of bile flow from the liver to the duodenum (*obstructive jaundice*), or if the liver is overloaded with bilirubin (as in *haemolytic jaundice*) then the skin becomes yellowed.

In severe cases of such disease the yellow discoloration is very obvious, even to the untrained eye. It is very distressing to the individual with jaundice and can be alarming for friends and family. On the other hand, it takes considerable experience to observe mild jaundice and sometimes it can be noticed only in the sclera. This is fortunate since the definition of 'yellow discoloration of the skin' only applies to those with white skins. Incidentally, this is worth bearing in mind by nurses when assessing for any condition which involves skin discoloration such as cyanosis and pallor. When caring for a patient with severe jaundice it is prudent not to express alarm at the person's appearance and to be aware that symptoms of cholestasis such as itching can be relieved by appropriate drugs. Also, yellowing of the eyes, which can be extreme in some cases and can make the patient very self-conscious, can be concealed by wearing tinted or darkened glasses.

It is possible through an understanding of the underlying physiology, for nurses to be aware of the different characteristics of the different types of jaundice. For example, in cholestasis the faeces are normally pale yellow due to the fact that stercobilin, an excretory product of bilirubin which gives faeces their characteristic colour, is reduced or absent because less bilirubin is being secreted into the intestine. Conversely, the urine may be darker than normal due to the excretion of bilirubin by the kidneys.

The signs of hepatic encephalopathy include changes in personality and intellect and also confusion, restlessness and, in severe cases, coma and convulsions. In people with liver disease, for example cirrhosis, this will be an intermitent feature of life which is precipitated by factors such as binge drinking, drug overdose, dehydration and excessive protein intake.

REFERENCES AND FURTHER READING

Arias I M, Jakoby W B, Popper H, Schachter D, Shafritz D A 1988 The liver: biology and pathobiology, 2nd edn. Raven Press, New York
Thick volume of detailed reviews written for and by hepatologists

Rogers A W 1992 Textbook of anatomy. Churchill Livingstone, Edinburgh

Sherlock S 1989 Diseases of the liver and biliary system, 8th edn. Blackwell Scientific Publications, Oxford
A very useful reference book combining authority and clarity on all aspects of liver disorder

Storer J 1988 The liver. In: Hinchliff S, Montague S (eds) Physiology for nursing practice. Baillière Tindall, London

Thibodeau G, Patten K (eds) 1993 Anatomy and physiology, 4th edn. Mosby, St Louis

Watson R (ed) 2000 Anatomy and physiology for nurses. Baillière Tindall, London

11 Endocrine systems – communication and control

In practice you may be asked to consider the following:

1. How is a target tissue identified by its hormone?

2. Many hormones cannot enter their target cells. How do they communicate with the target cell's nucleus?

3. A hormone may be circulating at adequate levels but may be ineffective. Why might this be?

4. The hypothalamus is the primary member of a number of hormone axes. Please explain.

5. A protein such as cortisol binding globulin may be measured as part of clinical assessment. What is the significance of the binding protein?

6. A patient has results which show elevated thyroid hormone levels with low TSH levels. She is thin, slightly agitated and complains about the heat in the department. She has a short-term prescription for a β blocking drug. Why? What is a possible diagnosis?

7. A young man who requires steroid therapy for an autoimmune disorder has been admitted to Accident and Emergency when he collapsed after a very minor traffic accident. He appears to be in a shocked condition. What might have caused his collapse?

8. An ambitious marathon athlete has become more and more prone to minor infections. He has been advised to reduce his training schedule so that his immune function can recover. Which hormone has been causing the problem? Why might reducing his training schedule help?

9 Phaeochromocytoma is an unusual condition characterized by episodic hypertension, tremor, headaches etc. The episodes can be brought on by coughing. What is the condition due to? What is the effect of coughing? Why are the episodes often followed by diuresis?

10. Head trauma may produce SIADH. What is that? What are the effects?

The endocrine system, with its array of hormones, affects all the tissues in the body. Many work with the nervous system to maintain homeostasis and to allow the management of stress. Although the body's size, shape and sexual characteristics are determined mainly hormonally, many of the trigger factors arise from the nervous system.

In view of the number and variety of hormones, this chapter is limited to those which demonstrate the main principles of the regulation and those whose activity contributes to selected areas of homeostasis. Other hormones are included in chapters on specific aspects of homeostasis, for example plasma glucose, and in the chapters on reproduction and development.

Simplified definitions are often misleading and this is true of those used of the endocrine system. The classic definition of a hormone as 'a chemical messenger released from one tissue, transported in blood to a target tissue whose activity it modifies' certainly describes an endocrine action, but it is worth considering some descriptions of chemical messengers which do not fit the classic definition but are relevant to the subject.

CLASSES OF CHEMICAL MESSENGER

The following words are used to describe classes of messenger:

- autocrine – acting on the cell which produced it, e.g. insulin-like growth factors (IGFs), important in body growth and in wound healing but also in the growth of some tumours
- paracrine – acting on cells close by, i.e. separated from the target cells only by tissue fluid. Insulin, glucagon and somatostatin act together in the endocrine pancreas, each affecting the release of the other

- endocrine – conforming to the classic definition in that the messenger, produced by one tissue, is carried in blood (or lymph) to a target tissue, e.g. the adrenal steroid hormones
- neuroendocrine – produced by neural tissue then released into blood to be transported to the target, e.g. oxytocin or the catecholamines.

As well as extending the list of what might be considered a hormone, the traditional list of endocrine glands, such as hypothalamus, pituitary, thyroid and so on, has had to be extended to include tissues such as kidney, gut and heart. Some hormones may only be steps in pathways which bring about the release of other hormones or agents such as the cytokines. Such is the rate of advancement in the work on cytokines, any text dealing with chemical messengers must include some reference to them.

CYTOKINES

Cytokines are chemical messengers which make up a very large and hugely complex group. They cannot strictly be defined as neurotransmitters or hormones, but they show the characteristics of messengers. They are produced by cells, act on target cells and require receptor sites. They are often named according to the first action clearly attributable to them, e.g. TNF (tumour necrosis factor), or after the cells first associated with their production, e.g. PDGF (platelet-derived growth factor). However, since each has a number of actions and may be synthesized by several different cell types, the original name may have been changed many times and the same cytokine may appear under different names in different texts. Since their effects may also vary according to their concentration and the presence of other cytokines, their influence may be everywhere but they make a short description impossible. In this text they appear principally in Chapters 16 and 19, but it should be remembered that all physiological actions are likely to involve them. As an example, Table 11.1 indicates some of the activities of one cytokine, interleukin 1 (IL-1).

The following is a summary list of some common cytokine properties.

Cytokines:

- are chemical mediators
- are low molecular weight proteins, many glycosylated
- are extremely potent
- use high affinity receptors
- show endocrine and paracrine characteristics
- may act singly or in concert
- may have different effects at different concentrations.

Table 11.1 Examples of actions of IL-1 (interleukin 1)

Blood vessels	Increased capillary permeability
Blood	Increased platelet adhesion
	Increased white cell adhesion
	Increased neutrophils
	Decreased lymphocytes
Nervous system	Increased secretion of ACTHRH
	Pyrexia
	Loss of appetite, nausea
Liver	Increased protein synthesis

Cytokines and hormones share many characteristics. Both groups act as messengers. Both groups include members with multiple actions produced by subtle differences in receptor site types. Both cytokines and hormones act in groups rather than singly and the effects may depend on the concentration present. The remainder of this chapter is mainly concerned with the properties and activities of hormones, but, in many cases, the tissue effects of a hormone will be achieved by its cytokine mediators.

GENERAL POINTS ABOUT ENDOCRINE GLANDS AND HORMONES

RELEASE AND TRANSPORT

Since a hormone is transferred directly into (usually) blood, an endocrine gland is ductless and must have a good blood supply with many capillaries. The hormone, once released, will usually be bound to a protein for transport. The binding protein might be specific to a particular hormone, for example cortisol binding globulin, or may be much more general; albumin for instance is used by a number of hormones. The bound form of the hormone is inactive; only the small unbound fraction is active. The two forms, bound and unbound, are in equilibrium, so that as the free form is used up, more is unbound to maintain the level.

REGULATION

Hormones are potent chemicals which circulate at very low and carefully regulated concentrations. When the regulation fails, the resulting endocrine disorders provide clear clinical evidence of the effects of hormone excess or deficiency.

Product regulation
Some hormones are regulated by balancing the factors which stimulate the hormone against the amount of hormone produced (or other hormones produced as a result). This is a negative feedback mechanism, 'product inhibition', and the hormone would be 'product regulated'.

Parameter regulation
Other hormones are regulated by the parameter they affect, for example plasma glucose or blood pressure. The hormone in this case would be 'parameter regulated'. The negative feedback comes, not from the concentration of the hormone, but from the state of the parameter being controlled, e.g. plasma glucose.

Although individual hormones have their own regulating systems, most will be variations on those two broad categories.

TARGET CELL RECEPTORS

The target tissue is identified by the presence of proteins which are receptor sites specific to a particular hormone and the characteristics of the hormone molecule will determine where these receptors are. Hormones, such as the steroids which are lipid soluble, or the thyroid hormones, which are small and carrying a metal atom, can penetrate the lipoprotein membrane of the target cells and have their receptors in the cytoplasm or at the nucleus. Those hormones which are not lipid soluble, for example peptides such as growth hormone and glucagon, cannot penetrate the membrane and their receptors are therefore on and within the target cell membrane.

Receptor sites are not fixed in either number or affinity. If the number or affinity increases, this is called upregulation; the target cell becomes more sensitive to the hormone and can make better use of it. Conversely, if the tissue cells are downregulated, the cells can use the hormone less well, i.e. the tissue becomes more resistant to the hormone. Downregulation is the cell's response to excess of a circulating hormone and it can have clinical implications, for example in type 2 diabetes. A feature of this condition is insulin resistance due to downregulation which can often be attributed to obesity. Glucose tolerance in these individuals can be improved if they lose weight.

SECOND MESSENGERS

Since most hormones have their effect by altering the target cell's nuclear activities, when a hormone cannot enter a cell a *second messenger* must be used, the hormone being the first messenger. The hormone binds to the membrane receptor and the combination of the two activates an otherwise inactive enzyme which then goes on to produce a substance which will act as the second messenger. One system used by a number of hormones is the activation of the enzyme adenyl cyclase which can then bring about the formation of cyclic adenosine monophosphate (cAMP) from adenosine triphosphate (ATP). Another second messenger system is diacylglycerol (DAG) and inositol triphosphate (IP_3) used by AVP/ADH at blood vessels and adrenaline at α_1 receptors. The second messenger sets in train a series of reactions culminating in the required response from the target cell. It also acts as an amplifier as a small amount of hormone will give rise to a much larger amount of second messenger.

HORMONE CATABOLISM AND EXCRETION

Hormones are metabolized mainly in the liver and are therefore dependent on the health of the liver. Where a liver is damaged, the time taken to metabolize the hormone is increased; i.e. its half-life is increased. The metabolites are excreted mainly in urine and urinalysis may be used either to identify the presence of a hormone by its metabolites or to quantitatively measure its output.

HORMONES AND THE HYPOTHALAMUS

The hypothalamus is the major regulatory area for the internal environment, acting as an interface between the two control systems, the nervous system and the endocrine system. As well as controlling the activities of the autonomic nervous system, it produces a large number of hormones involved in:

- maintenance of homeostasis
- management of stress, i.e. disturbance of homeostasis
- determination of the size, shape and sexual characteristics of the body – morphogenesis.

NEURAL CONNECTIONS

The hypothalamus receives information from many parts of the nervous system. These include receptor cells which monitor many aspects of the body's internal environment:

- pressures in the circulation
- osmotic pressure and the state of the body's fluid balance

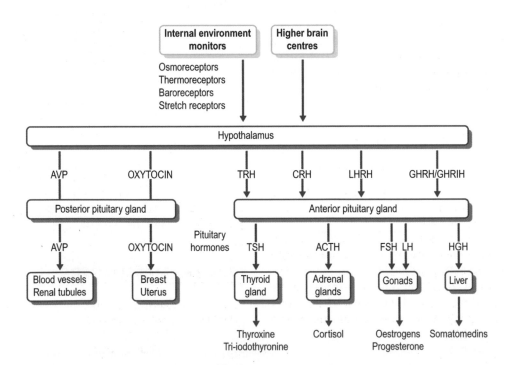

Figure 11.1 Hierarchy of hypothalamic control.

Table 11.2 Hormones of the anterior pituitary gland: their origin and actions

Cell of origin	Pituitary hormone	Actions	
		Target	Stimulatory effect
Corticotroph	Adrenocorticotrophic hormone (ACTH)	Adrenal cortex	Secretion of hormones
Gonadotroph	Follicle stimulating hormone (FSH)	Gonads	(See Chs 30 and 31)
	Luteinizing hormone (LH)	(ovaries and testes)	
Lactotroph	Prolactin	Mammary glands	Secretion of milk
Somatotroph	Human growth hormone (HGH)	Liver	Secretion of somatomedins
		All tissues	Protein synthesis
Thyrotroph	Thyroid stimulating hormone (TSH)	Thyroid gland	Growth

- composition of the body fluids, e.g. pH, electrolytes, glucose
- body temperature
- pressures in the gut, therefore the regulation of intake.

Information is also relayed from the limbic system which is concerned with appetites, emotions and desires (see Ch. 27).

The hypothalamus regulates and integrates body systems, e.g. cardiovascular, renal and respiratory, to produce an overall controlled environment. It influences many endocrine pathways and integrates these with the autonomic nervous system (ANS). It is also involved in the control of activities such as eating, drinking and sexual activity as part of the somatic nervous system (see Ch. 22).

The hierarchy of endocrine control exerted by the hypothalamus is shown in Figure 11.1. Table 11.2 lists examples of the hormones involved in the extended pathways and the body areas they affect.

HYPOTHALAMIC ENDOCRINE FUNCTION

The endocrine and neuroendocrine output to the pituitary gland is the first step in the hormonal regulation by the hypothalamus.

The hormones of the hypothalamus should properly be called neurohormones although most are simply called hormones. The cells producing the hormones are, however, neuroendocrine cells and like other cells in the brain are grouped into clusters called nuclei. The axons from these cells project to two areas near the hypothalamus (Fig. 11.2):

- median eminence
- posterior pituitary.

The nerve endings in the median eminence release the hormones which control the anterior lobe of the pituitary. The axons which end in the posterior lobe release into the bloodstream two hormones, AVP/ADH and oxytocin.

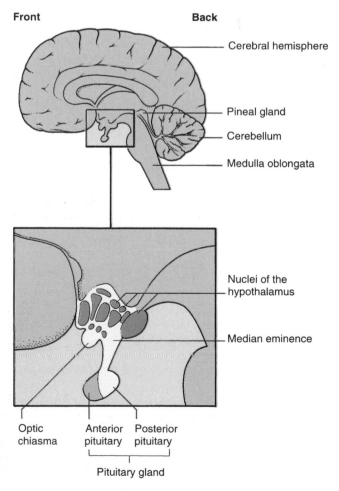

Figure 11.2 Hypothalamus and pituitary gland.

The pituitary gland or hypophysis is made up of anterior and posterior lobes; the intermediate lobe is rudimentary in humans.

The two main lobes of the pituitary gland are derived from separate embryonic tissue. The posterior lobe is neural in origin, growing down from the brain; the anterior lobe is endocrine and derived from tissue growing upwards from the roof of the mouth. The two types of tissue become associated in the embryo with the downgrowth having elongated to a stalk from which the posterior lobe is suspended.

HYPOTHALAMUS AND POSTERIOR PITUITARY LOBE

The anatomical relationship between the hypothalamus and the two pituitary lobes is different and underlies the functional difference between them.

While the link between the hypothalamus and the anterior lobe is a small portal vascular system, the link with the posterior lobe is via a nerve tract which begins in the hypothalamus and ends in the posterior lobe (the hypothalamo-hypophyseal tract) (Fig. 11.3). Two hypothalamic hormones, arginine vasopressin (AVP) (or its alternative name, antidiuretic hormone (ADH)) and oxytocin, are synthesized in the hypothalamus in the supraoptic and paraventricular nuclei as large prohormones. They travel down the axons of the nerve tract and are released into the general circulation at the posterior pituitary (Fig. 11.4).

AVP/ADH has a major role in the maintenance of fluid balance (see below) and oxytocin is concerned with reproductive function, e.g. the ejection of milk from the lactating breast (see Ch. 31).

ARGININE VASOPRESSIN (AVP)/ ANTIDIURETIC HORMONE (ADH)

AVP/ADH takes part in the maintenance of fluid balance, osmotic regulation and blood pressure. Its target tissues are the renal tubules and blood vessels (see Chs 8, 12 and 14). The effects of the hormone reflect its alternative names 'vasopressin' and 'antidiuretic hormone'. Human vasopressin contains the amino acid arginine and the word is included in the name to differentiate it from that of other species.

It is a peptide hormone unable to penetrate the target cell membrane, and therefore requires a second messenger. Unlike many hormones it travels in the unbound form, it has a rapid effect and is rapidly metabolized, i.e. it has a short half-life.

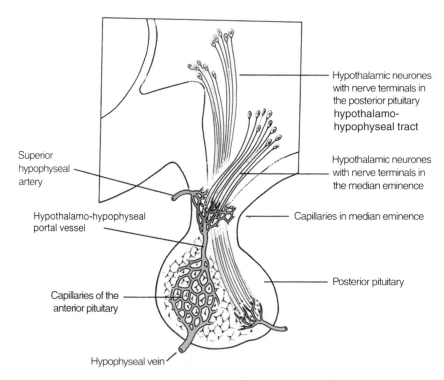

Figure 11.3 Hypothalamic neural and vascular links with the pituitary gland. (From Rogers 1992, with permission of Elsevier.)

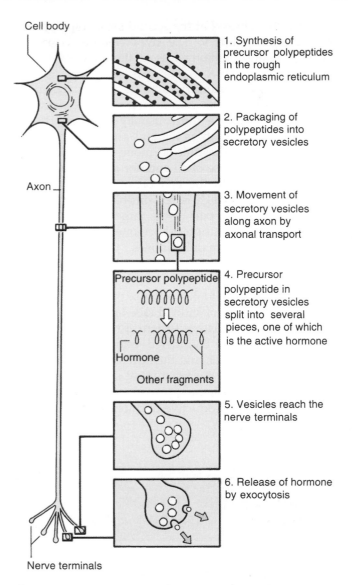

1. Synthesis of precursor polypeptides in the rough endoplasmic reticulum

2. Packaging of polypeptides into secretory vesicles

3. Movement of secretory vesicles along axon by axonal transport

4. Precursor polypeptide in secretory vesicles split into several pieces, one of which is the active hormone

5. Vesicles reach the nerve terminals

6. Release of hormone by exocytosis

Figure 11.4 Formation and secretion of neurohormones.

Actions of AVP/ADH

At the distal and collecting tubules in the nephron, the effect is to increase the reabsorption of water, which is then taken back into blood, increasing the volume and the blood (hydrostatic) pressure. The water also has a diluting effect and reduces osmotic pressure.

At higher concentrations, AVP acts as a vasoconstrictor, reducing the capacity and increasing blood pressure.

The effects on renal tubules and on blood vessels are mediated through two different types of receptor and with two different second messengers. That at renal tubules is cAMP; at blood vessels and other tissues affected by AVP/ADH, the messenger is DAG/IP$_3$.

AVP/ADH is a parameter regulated hormone, regulated by osmotic pressure and hydrostatic pressure. The two parameters are inseparable and are regulated together by a number of mechanisms of which AVP/ADH is only one (see Chs 12 and 14).

Regulation of AVP/ADH by osmotic pressure

Sensory receptors in the hypothalamus, osmoreceptors, are stimulated by a rise in osmotic pressure. These in turn stimulate the area in the hypothalamus producing AVP/ADH. The increased AVP/ADH retains water, diluting the solutes and reducing osmotic pressure. A fall in osmotic pressure has the opposite effect, resulting in the excretion of water and restoration of normal osmotic pressure (see Ch. 14).

Regulation of AVP/ADH by blood pressure

Baroreceptors located in low pressure circulations such as the pulmonary circuit are stimulated by rises in pressure. Their firing rate increases in response to the pressure rise and the effect is to inhibit the output of AVP/ADH. The amount of water reclaimed at the kidney is reduced and blood vessels are less constricted, both actions helping to reduce blood pressure. A fall in BP has the opposite effect, the increased output of AVP/ADH causing water retention and vasoconstriction and a consequent rise in pressure (see Ch. 12).

DEFICIENCY AND EXCESS OF AVP/ADH

Deficiency of AVP/ADH

This is the condition diabetes insipidus, which dramatically illustrates the actions of AVP/ADH.

The subject, unable to regulate water retention, excretes large amounts of dilute urine. As long as a source of drinking water or fluid containing water is available, the subject can usually keep pace with the large loss. However, if water is unavailable, because it cannot be retained as would be the normal response, osmotic pressure rises and blood pressure falls. Other mechanisms, e.g. tachycardia and vasoconstriction by mechanisms other than AVP/ADH compensate (see Ch. 12) to some extent, but the subject suffers extreme thirst. A water deprivation test is sometimes carried out during the diagnosis of diabetes insipidus and great care must be taken that the test is not overlong; otherwise there is a risk of damage arising out of overconcentration of body fluids. The condition is treated by replacement therapy using a synthetic AVP/ADH.

Excess AVP/ADH

This is found in a number of primary and secondary forms and is given the overall name of 'syndrome of inappropriate ADH' (SIADH). In spite of the growing use of the term AVP, 'SIADH' has remained the conventional name of this syndrome.

It can be due to primary causes such as a functioning tumour, but it is more often found in head injury or surgery, or as an unwanted effect of a large variety of drugs. These include the opiates, particularly morphine, tricyclic antidepressants and chlorpropamide.

The most obvious effect is hyponatraemia which cannot be accounted for otherwise (i.e. it must be due to dilution), inappropriate urinary concentrations and low plasma osmolarity. AVP/ADH is seldom found to be in excess if measured; in fact, a patient clearly identified as suffering from SIADH may have no detectable AVP/ADH in plasma.

The cause of the syndrome must be identified and measures taken to excrete the water load without further jeopardizing electrolyte levels.

HYPOTHALAMUS AND ANTERIOR PITUITARY LOBE

The hypothalamus secretes hormones which are transferred to the anterior pituitary via a small portal circulation, the hypothalamo-hypophyseal portal vessels. The first set of capillaries takes up the hypothalamic hormones, and these travel down the circuit to be released at the second set of capillaries in the anterior pituitary. The hypothalamic hormones either promote or inhibit release of the anterior pituitary hormones (Fig. 11.5).

The anterior pituitary acts as an intermediate endocrine stage in an axis arrangement between the hypothalamus and a third, usually endocrine tissue, sometimes referred to as the end organ. In these axis systems, the hypothalamic hormone causes the release or inhibits the release of an anterior pituitary hormone which is trophic to the end organ tissue. A trophic hormone is one which is responsible for the growth, maintenance and repair of the target tissue. In many axis systems, the trophic hormone also causes the release of the end organ hormones.

The major axes are examples of negative feedback by product.

It is convenient to look at anterior pituitary hormones not as a collection of individuals, but as members of their own axis regulatory system. To demonstrate this, three hormones are considered below, two in typical axes, the thyroid axis and the adrenocortical axis, and one other which is the less typical system controlling human growth hormone.

The gonadal/reproductive hormones are considered in Chapter 30.

THE HYPOTHALAMUS, ANTERIOR PITUITARY AND THYROID HORMONES – THE HPT AXIS

Hormones are complicated by their collection of alternative names, the following lists those applying to the

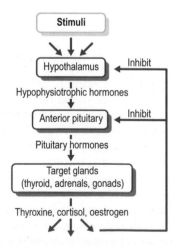

Figure 11.5 The principle of negative feedback in hormones of the hypothalamic–anterior pituitary axes.

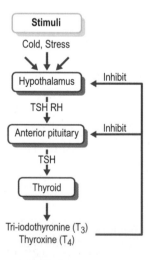

Figure 11.6 The hypothalamus–anterior pituitary–thyroid axis – the HPT axis.

Table 11.3 Effects of hormones secreted by the hypothalamus on the anterior pituitary gland

| Hypophysiotrophic hormones | | Effect on secretion of |
Name	Abbreviation	anterior pituitary hormones
Corticotrophin releasing hormone	CRH	↑ ACTH (corticotrophin)
Growth hormone releasing hormone	GHRH	↑ human growth hormone (somatotrophin)
Growth hormone release inhibiting hormone (somatostatin)	GHRIH	↓ human growth hormone (somatotrophin)
Luteinizing hormone releasing hormone	LHRH	{ ↑ FSH / ↑ LH
Prolactin inhibiting hormone	PIH	↓ prolactin (luteotrophin)
Prolactin releasing hormone	PRH	↑ prolactin (luteotrophin)
Thyrotrophin releasing hormone	TRH	↑ TSH (thyrotrophin)

thyroid axis (Table 11.3 shows hypothalamic and anterior pituitary hormones with their abbreviations):

- thyroid stimulating hormone releasing hormone (TSHRH) or thyrotrophin releasing hormone (TRH) – produced by the hypothalamus
- thyroid stimulating hormone (TSH) or thyrotrophin (also referred to as TSH) produced by the anterior pituitary
- thyroxine (T_4) and tri-iodothyronine (T_3) produced by the thyroid.

The thyroid hormones are regulated by the hypothalamo–anterior pituitary–thyroid axis (HPT axis) (Fig. 11.6). The hypothalamus releases thyroid stimulating hormone releasing hormone (TSHRH), which travels to the anterior pituitary via the small portal blood supply that runs down the stalk connecting the two tissues.

In response to TSHRH, the appropriate cells in the anterior pituitary release their hormone, thyroid stimulating hormone (TSH), which is taken up by the second capillary bed and transferred via the general circulation to the thyroid gland. Attachment of TSH to the membrane receptors of the thyroid cells will result in the production and release of the thyroid hormones tri-iodothyronine (T_3) and thyroxine (T_4). In the jargon of the axis system, these are the 'end organ' hormones. T_3 and T_4 act as a negative feedback on TSH and TSHRH production and to a lesser extent, TSH acts as negative feedback on TSHRH. At each stage there are also other inhibitors which fine tune the axis and increase the level of control.

The axis is stimulated at the hypothalamic level by stimuli from other centres in the hypothalamus itself, for example the heat regulating centre (see below), or from other brain areas. The balance between forward stimuli and negative feedback can be illustrated by considering the response to a change in blood temperature. One of the effects of thyroid hormones is to produce an increase in metabolic rate and hence heat production (thermogenesis); T_3 and T_4 are therefore important in the maintenance of body temperature (see Ch. 17).

When blood temperature is reduced, the hypothalamic heat regulating centre stimulates the centre, which produces TSHRH. The increased level of activity in the axis subsequently causes the production of increased T_3 and T_4, which in turn increase cellular heat production. A maintained rise in blood temperature removes the stimulus at hypothalamic level and the increased T_3 and T_4 act as negative feedback. As long as the ambient temperature remains low, however, the forward stimulus will outweigh the negative feedback, the T_3 and T_4 levels will remain high and extra heat continues to be produced. This is an adaptive mechanism which allows the body to respond to ambient temperature. It takes several weeks to become completely adapted and holidaymakers who go to a warm climate are usually just adapted when they come home, where they find that they feel uncomfortably cold until they (or their thyroid glands) re-adapt to a lower ambient temperature.

FUNCTIONS OF THE HORMONES OF THE HPT AXIS

TSHRH (thyroid stimulating hormone releasing hormone)/thyrotrophin releasing hormone can be considered as a release agent for TSH.

TSH (thyroid stimulating hormone) or thyrotrophin has a number of functions. It is sometimes referred to as a trophic hormone since the thyroid cell size and cell number is dependent on TSH. TSH also increases blood flow to the thyroid; it therefore increases the supply of oxygen, iodine and the other substrates required by the thyroid cells. Both the production and the release of T_3 and T_4 are stimulated by TSH.

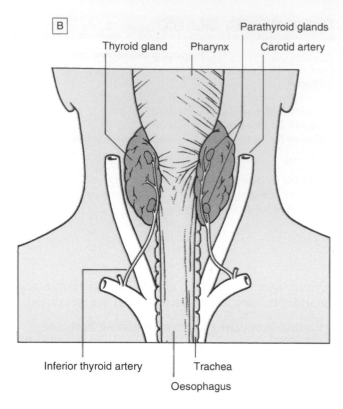

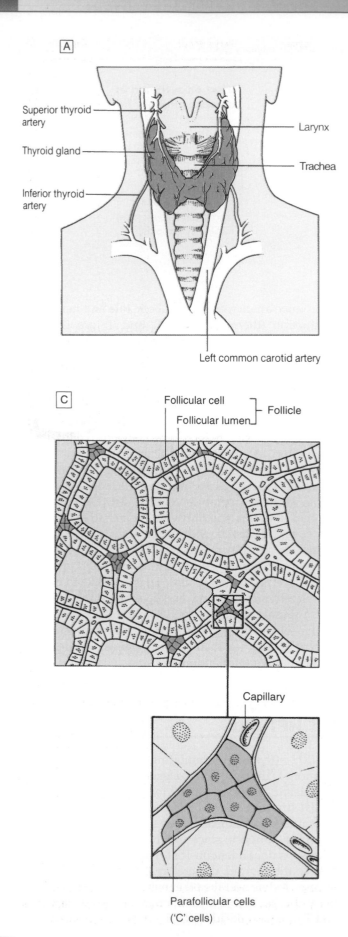

Figure 11.7 The thyroid gland. A, Position in the neck as viewed from the front. B, Position in the neck as viewed from behind, showing the parathyroid glands. C, Tissue structure. (From Rogers 1992, with permission of Elsevier.)

THE THYROID GLAND

The thyroid gland lies over the front of the trachea just below the larynx (Fig. 11.7A & B). Enlargement of the thyroid becomes visible as goitre.

On the back of the thyroid, four small parathyroid glands are visible (Fig. 11.7B). These are concerned with the regulation of plasma calcium balance (see Ch. 14).

Thyroid tissue is made up of groups of cells (follicles or acini) interspersed by blood and lymph capillaries (Fig. 11.7C). The follicles consist of a layer of cells – the follicular cells – enclosing a lumen filled with a colloid, the main constituent of which is thyroglobulin.

A microscopic section shows cells clearly visible outside the follicles; these are the parafollicular or 'C' cells. The 'C' cells produce the hormone calcitonin, hence the 'C', which is involved in the regulation of plasma calcium.

The hormones produced by the follicular cells are those usually known as 'the thyroid hormones', T_3 and T_4.

Thyroid hormones

- Tri-iodothyronine T_3
- Thyroxine T_4.

Synthesis

T_3 and T_4 are formed by the attachment of iodine to the amino acid tyrosine units on thyroglobulin. The first stage is the formation of mono-iodotyrosine (MIT or T_1) and di-iodotyrosine (DIT or T_2). These units are then coupled together to give T_3 and T_4 as in

$$T_1 + T_2 = T_3$$
$$T_2 + T_2 = T_4$$

Still attached to thyroglobulin, T_3 and T_4 are passed into the lumen to be stored within the colloid.

When stimulated by TSH, droplets of the colloid are taken back into the follicular cell. T_3 and T_4 are detached from thyroglobulin and passed into the general circulation (Fig. 11.8). Any MIT and DIT attached to the thyroglobulin is de-iodinated and the iodine is recycled or excreted.

Both hormones circulate bound to transport proteins, e.g. thyroxine binding globulin.

T_3/T_4 characteristics

T_4 has a longer half-life and lower biological activity than T_3 and is usually regarded as the reservoir form of T_3; it is converted to T_3 in the target tissues. A further refinement to the control of the thyroid hormones is at the stage of the conversion of T_4 to T_3. This conversion yields not only T_3 but an inactive version of the molecule, reverse T_3 (rT_3). The amounts of T_3 and rT_3

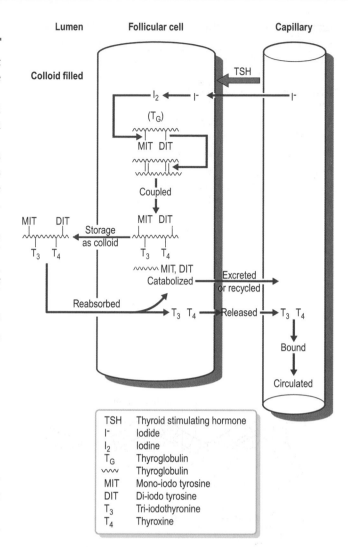

TSH	Thyroid stimulating hormone
I⁻	Iodide
I_2	Iodine
T_G	Thyroglobulin
∿∿∿	Thyroglobulin
MIT	Mono-iodo tyrosine
DIT	Di-iodo tyrosine
T_3	Tri-iodothyronine
T_4	Thyroxine

Figure 11.8 Synthesis of thyroid hormones.

can vary and some conditions such as starvation, some wasting diseases and even some stages of the response to trauma can produce an increase in the proportion of rT_3 with a resulting slowing of metabolic rate. This may be an adaptive mechanism which preserves energy stores in times of shortage. The lumen storage, the binding for transport and the degree of conversion of T_4 to the much more active T_3 all act as modifications which increase control. The thyroid hormones are referred to in the following sections as T_3/T_4 although the active substance is assumed to be T_3.

T_3/T_4 functions

The thyroid hormones have a wide range of effects.

- Most obvious is the effect on the rate of cellular activity. An 'overactive' thyroid can greatly increase basal metabolic rate (BMR) and, before sensitive tests of thyroid function were available, BMR was sometimes measured as part of the diagnosis of thyroid dysfunction. Heat is generated as a product of this activity and the thyroid hormones are an important part of body temperature regulation in the longer term.

- The hormones are required for the development and maintenance of the nervous system and even for body growth, where they act along with growth hormone and insulin.
- T_3/T_4 increase the number of adrenoceptors and therefore increase the effectiveness of adrenaline and noradrenaline. This becomes evident in thyroid disorder, and tachycardia even at rest is a characteristic of thyroid overactivity.
- Thyroid hormones have effects on nutrient metabolism mainly by increasing the consumption of stores such as body fat and protein by other hormones. T_3/T_4 also promote the uptake of carbohydrate from the gut and raise plasma glucose during feeding; the overall effect is to raise plasma glucose.

As always, some of these effects are most easily seen when thyroid function is abnormal. The use of the HPT axis simplifies prediction of the site of origin of the abnormality, i.e. whether it is thyroid, pituitary or hypothalamic in origin (Fig. 11.9). Measurements of indices such as TSH, T_3 and T_4 are used to confirm this in clinical practice.

Thyroid hormone excess and deficiency

T_3/T_4 excess

If T_3/T_4 are elevated, whatever the source of the dysfunction, they will give rise to the typical symptoms of hyperthyroidism. Most of the symptoms can be predicted as exaggerations of the normal effects of the hormones.

- The subject feels hot, looks flushed and feels uncomfortable in a warm environment. However, body temperature is likely to be normal due to vasodilation and sweating, provided hydration is adequate.
- Heart rate is elevated even at rest, systolic pressure is raised although diastolic may be significantly lowered by vasodilation. Pulse pressure is wide.
- The subject finds it difficult to rest although easily fatigued; muscle tremor is evident particularly in outstretched arms.
- Body weight is lost despite a good appetite and food intake.
- Tendon reflex time is shortened.
- There may be metabolic disturbance, e.g. raised plasma glucose.

The commonest form of overactivity is that seen in Graves' disease. In this condition an antibody is formed to TSH, referred to as thyroid stimulating immunoglobulin (TSI)

TSI stimulates the thyroid in the same way as TSH but is outwith normal negative feedback. If hormone levels in the axis are measured, T_3/T_4 are raised, TSH reduced and the presence of TSI is noted. Since TSI has similar properties to TSH, it not only stimulates the production of the thyroid hormones, it has a trophic action on the thyroid gland, increasing the size and number of the cells and producing the thyroid swelling known as goitre. This form of hyperthyroidism is often characterized by retraction of the eyelids and protrusion of the eye (exophthalmos), giving the subject a wide stare.

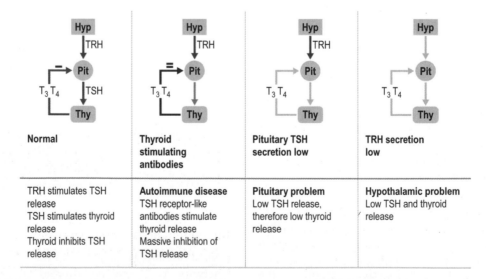

Figure 11.9 HPT axis abnormalities. (After Greenstein 1994 Endocrinology at a glance. With permission of Blackwell Science Ltd.)

This condition is treated by removal of part of the thyroid either by destruction of follicular cells by radioactive iodine or, less usually, by surgery. Drugs such as carbimazole limit the activity of follicular cells and can be used as conservative treatment, but they must be used over a long period of time and their success is somewhat limited. The adverse effects of excess T_3/T_4 on the heart can be blocked by an adrenoceptor blocker and this is useful as an adjunct to other treatment regimens.

Another example of axis abnormality is found in cases of pituitary excess, perhaps due to a functioning tumour of TSH producing cells. Analysis of the hormone levels in this case would show elevated T_3/T_4 due to elevated TSH, the presence of goitre (due to the TSH) and if the level of TSHRH were to be measured, one could predict that it would be low.

Treatment in this case requires identification and treatment of the pituitary site.

T_3/T_4 deficiency

Underactivity in the thyroid gland with low levels of T_3/T_4 shows symptoms many of which are clearly attributable to lack of the normal hormone activity. The condition in its severe form is called myxoedema.

- The subject is cold and often has a low body temperature. Thyroid function should be considered in patients admitted in a hypothermic state.
- Heart rate is slow and blood pressure, particularly systolic, is reduced.
- Tendon reflex time is prolonged.
- Neural signs such as apathy or forgetfulness may be present.
- Weight gain without excessive food intake is common.
- Lack of activity in skin, hair cells and sweat glands makes the dry and scaly skin a typical sign.
- Oedema, particularly facial oedema, is common due to the deposition of mucopolysaccharides in the tissue spaces.

If the site of dysfunction is the thyroid itself, e.g. if the cells have been destroyed by antibodies or radiotherapy or surgery (hypothyroidism is a common result of treatment for hyperthyroidism), the axis would show low levels of T_3/T_4 but elevated TSH. If the thyroid cells are unresponsive to TSH there may be no goitre.

This condition is treated by lifetime use of thyroxine. The term 'endogenous' is used for a substance which is produced by the body. If that same substance is administered, it would be described as 'exogenous', i.e. hypothyroidism is treated by exogenous thyroxine.

Congenital hypothyroidism

Congenital hypothyroidism occurs when the thyroid fails to function in the fetal stages. In the uterus, the infant usually develops normally using maternal thyroid hormones. However, after birth, if the condition were to go undetected, neural development and body growth would be impaired. This condition is sometimes known as cretinism. A blood test is carried out on babies soon after birth and if the condition is detected, thyroxine given from then on, and for life, avoids the retardation and damage that would otherwise occur.

Iodine deficiency hypothyroidism

Hypothyroidism such as myxoedema, which is pathological, can be contrasted with the condition known as endemic goitre, which is due to a nutritional deficiency of iodine. Endemic goitre is a worldwide problem with severe consequences. It occurs in areas of the world where soil is poor or leached out by very high rainfall and the food crops produced are deficient in iodine. The prolonged shortage of iodine results in low or barely adequate levels of T_3/T_4 with elevated TSH due to lack of negative feedback. The enlarged gland may make maximum use of the iodine available and may be able to just maintain normality but at the expense of a large goitre, hence the description endemic goitre. The goitres themselves may be disabling, causing respiratory or feeding difficulties, they are easily damaged and bleed copiously. The possible clinical deficiency of thyroid hormones may lead to an inability to work in a region where there is no public support or benefits system. An even more serious consequence may be damage to the offspring of the community who may be iodine deficient in the early stages of neural development, with consequent permanent impairment.

Treatment of nutritional hypothyroidism is by supplementation of iodine, which can be added to a staple food such as flour or salt.

THE HYPOTHALAMUS, ANTERIOR PITUITARY AND THE HORMONES OF THE ADRENAL CORTEX – HPA AXIS

This axis works to the same pattern as the thyroid axis, this time with the end organ the adrenal cortex. The hypothalamic adrenocorticotrophic hormone releasing hormone (ACTHRH) or corticotrophin releasing hormone (CRH) acts as the release hormone for the anterior pituitary hormone ACTH or corticotrophin,

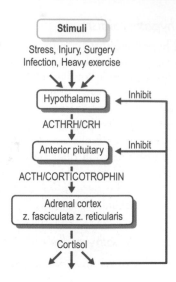

Figure 11.10 The hypothalamus–anterior pituitary–adrenal cortex axis – the HPA axis.

followed in turn by the adrenocortical hormone cortisol (Fig. 11.10).

THE FUNCTIONS OF THE AXIS HORMONES

ACTHRH (CRH)

ACTHRH (CRH) acts as the release hormone for the anterior pituitary hormone ACTH. Its output has a circadian rhythm, with levels highest in the early morning and lowest about 12 hours later. The normal output is pulsatile. The output is increased by stress, injury, surgery, infection, even heavy exercise. Disturbances in fluid balance or plasma glucose or even extremes of ambient temperature affect ACTHRH. Changes in ACTHRH are reflected in the levels of the other axis hormones. The forward stimuli at the hypothalamus are balanced by negative feedback from the axis hormones, particularly cortisol, but the greater the stimulus driving the axis, the higher the output of cortisol is likely to be.

ACTH (corticotrophin)

ACTH is produced in the anterior pituitary in response to ACTHRH. It is produced from a much larger precursor molecule, pro-opiomelanocortin (POMC), which also yields melanocyte stimulating hormone (MSH) and other neural peptides. As its name suggests, ACTH is a trophic hormone for the adrenal cortex and is required for the growth and maintenance particularly of the two inner zones of the cortex (see Fig. 11.12). If ACTH is withdrawn or suppressed, the cortex will

shrink. Conversely, if ACTH is present in excess, the cortex will hypertrophy in response. ACTH also promotes the release of cortisol from the adrenal cortex.

THE ADRENAL GLAND

The two adrenal glands are situated one at the top end of each kidney (Fig. 11.11).

The glands are composed of two parts:

- the adrenal medulla, derived from neural tissue in the embryo, produces the catecholamines adrenaline and noradrenaline (see p. 219)
- the adrenal cortex, which is endocrine tissue, produces the adrenal steroid hormones.

The adrenal cortex

The adrenal cortex consists of three zones, named according to their histological appearance and before there was any knowledge of their function (Fig. 11.12A & B):

- zona glomerulosa, the narrow outer zone (cells look as though grouped in small knots)
- zona fasciculata, the middle zone, the largest zone (cells look as though arranged in rods)

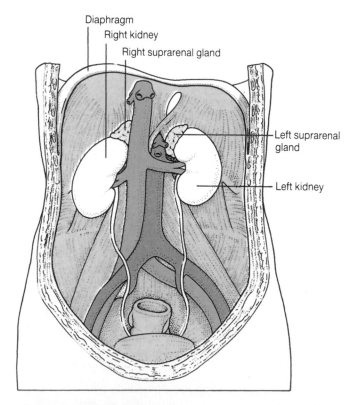

Figure 11.11 The adrenal glands. (From Rogers 1992, with permission of Elsevier.)

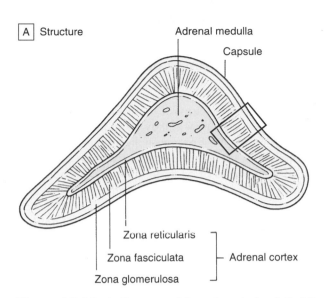

A Structure

Adrenal medulla

Capsule

Zona reticularis
Zona fasciculata ⎤
⎬ Adrenal cortex
Zona glomerulosa ⎦

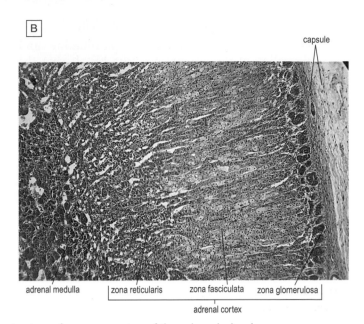

B

capsule

adrenal medulla | zona reticularis | zona fasciculata | zona glomerulosa
adrenal cortex

Figure 11.12 A, Structure of the adrenal gland. B, Microscopic view of a cross-section of the adrenal gland.

• zona reticularis, the inner zone (cells look as though arranged in a network).

Adrenocortical hormones

The cortical cells synthesize a variety of steroid hormones all of which are derived from cholesterol. These are:

• adrenal androgens (mainly zona fasciculata and reticularis)
• adrenal oestrogens (mainly zona fasciculata and reticularis)
• glucocorticoid – *cortisol* (zona fasciculata and zona reticularis)
• mineralocorticosteroid – *aldosterone* (zona glomerulosa).

(The adrenal androgens and oestrogens are not produced in sufficient amounts to have reproductive effects, but their pathological effects become important when there is overproduction.)

Steroid hormones enter target cells and bind with cytoplasmic, then nuclear, receptors.

CORTISOL

Cortisol is essential for survival. Without it, it would not be possible to withstand stress or injury. Cortisol is described as glucocorticoid, referring to its role in carbohydrate metabolism. While the term is accurate as far as it goes, it does not take account of the other metabolic actions or the anti-inflammatory properties of cortisol which make it essential for survival.

When released, cortisol is bound to a transport protein, e.g. cortisol binding globulin (transcortin) or to albumin. Over 90% of circulating cortisol is bound. The equilibrium maintained between the bound cortisol and the unbound active cortisol provides an additional layer of control over plasma levels.

Actions of cortisol

Most body tissues are sensitive to cortisol. Cortisol is a survival hormone, and its widespread actions promote the parameters important to the body's survival. The inflammatory response is necessary to combat injury and infection, but, if left unchecked, it might jeopardize blood pressure and therefore survival. Cortisol acts as an anti-inflammatory agent, moderating the response. It defends blood pressure so that tissue can be supplied and its metabolic effects ensure that plasma glucose is maintained in order to supply the brain.

Anti-inflammatory activity

Cortisol stabilizes blood vessel walls, making them less sensitive to the chemicals released as a result of injury. These inflammatory substances would otherwise cause vasodilation and increased permeability, both of which would reduce blood pressure. Cortisol also suppresses immune function, therefore reducing at source the amount of circulating vasodilator chemicals. In doing so, however, cortisol compromises immune defence, making the injured or already sick individual less resistant to infection.

Maintenance of blood pressure

Even in normal health, cortisol is required to maintain blood pressure. In addition to its stabilizing effects on blood vessels, it has a minor aldosterone-like effect on electrolytes, retaining sodium (therefore water) and excreting potassium.

Permissive effect on catecholamine activity

Cortisol affects the synthesis of adrenaline and noradrenaline in the adrenal medulla by altering the relative proportions of the two. It also cooperates in fat mobilization by the catecholamines and subsequent use of the derivatives for energy.

Metabolic actions of cortisol and maintenance of plasma glucose

Cortisol promotes the breakdown of both body protein and fat. Amino acids from the protein can be used as an energy source and some can be used as a source of glucose (gluconeogenesis); fat breakdown products can be used as an energy source and the small amount of glycerol released is used as a source of glucose. Cortisol therefore spares carbohydrate and promotes the use of protein and fat for fuel. Its overall effects are hyperglycaemic (see Chs 10 and 18).

Pharmacology

Cortisol, used pharmacologically as an anti-inflammatory substance under the name hydrocortisone, is only one of a large number of steroid anti-inflammatory drugs, many of them more potent than cortisol/hydrocortisone itself. The conditions in which they are used are wide-ranging: asthma, skin disorders, muscle and joint disorders, autoimmune conditions such as systemic lupus erythematosus where the disordered immune system has attacked host tissue and even some types of clinical shock where blood vessels have become lax and permeable. While steroid drugs can be life-saving, their use is not without problems; they do after all have the same properties as cortisol. They must be used with care since they are catabolic to protein and fat and may damage vulnerable tissue or may affect blood pressure or plasma glucose regulation. Their systemic use may, unless carefully managed, have adverse effects on the user's own HPA axis and put at risk their capacity to deal with stress.

An exogenous steroid will affect the HPA axis in the same way as the endogenous cortisol. Prolonged use at high enough levels will inhibit the production of ACTH, the trophic effect on the adrenal cortex will be withdrawn and the cortex will shrink. If the individual is then subjected to stress such as injury or surgery, the adrenal cortex will be unable to supply the cortisol required to withstand the stress. The exogenous steroid, likely to be at a relatively small fixed dose, is also insufficient and the unchecked inflammatory response may cause a profound drop in blood pressure, i.e. clinical shock. To protect the adrenal cortex and avoid this risk, steroids are usually given at the lowest dose possible and may be intermittent to allow the mass of the cortex to be maintained.

Excess and deficiency of cortisol

Cortisol excess

Excess production of cortisol is called Cushing's syndrome. The dysfunction may be at the adrenal cortex or the pituitary or, unusually, at the hypothalamus; the word 'syndrome' can be used to describe the effects of all three. If the dysfunction is pituitary, several hormones and hormonal axes may be involved and the condition would be complicated by excess of all the hormones affected. Cushingoid symptoms can also be due to exogenous steroids, described as iatrogenic Cushing's syndrome.

Many of the symptoms of excess cortisol can be predicted by exaggerating the effects of cortisol at normal concentrations:

- the individual loses skeletal muscle mass especially from the limbs, skin is thinned and loses stretch
- fat is redistributed from limbs to trunk, face and neck
- sodium and water are retained in excess, raising blood pressure and causing oedema, particularly evident in the face.

The combination of these effects produces the classic description of 'moon face oedema and large trunk with stick-like limbs'. About 20% of patients with Cushing's syndrome are hyperglycaemic to the point of diabetes.

Cortisol deficiency

Pathological deficiency of cortisol is rare and likely to be combined with deficiency of aldosterone in Addison's disease and is covered in the paragraphs on aldosterone (below). Deficiency of endogenous cortisol as a result of steroid therapy may occur when there is unexpected stress, and it is likely to show itself as inability to maintain blood pressure and possibly fasting plasma glucose.

ALDOSTERONE

Aldosterone is a corticosteroid hormone which provides useful areas of contrast with cortisol. It is produced by the adrenal cortex from zona glomerulosa, a zone which, once formed, is relatively independent of the requirement for ACTH for its maintenance. Like all steroids, aldosterone can penetrate target cell membranes and therefore occupies intracellular receptor sites.

Actions of aldosterone

Aldosterone is classed as a mineralocorticoid since its action is to retain sodium and excrete potassium at the distal renal tubules, gut and from sweat and tears. It has no metabolic or anti-inflammatory effects.

Regulation of release

It is not primarily regulated by the HPA axis, although in stress situations, the high levels of ACTH promote the output of aldosterone. It is instead parameter regulated, the parameters being:

- blood pressure (the renin dependent mechanism) (see Ch. 12)
- plasma potassium and, to a lesser extent, plasma sodium (the renin independent mechanism) (see Ch. 14).

Regulation by blood pressure

Regulation of aldosterone release in response to blood pressure is achieved using the renin, angiotensin, aldosterone mechanism (see Fig. 12.10, p. 236). A reduction in blood pressure at the kidney causes the release of renin from the juxtaglomerular apparatus. This acts on the circulating but inactive angiotensinogen to produce angiotensin I, which is converted to angiotensin II by a converting enzyme mainly in the pulmonary circulation. Angiotensin II in turn stimulates the adrenal cortex to produce aldosterone. The restoration of blood pressure at the kidney will inhibit the release of renin and act as a negative feedback on aldosterone release.

Regulation by electrolytes

Regulation of aldosterone in response to plasma potassium and sodium is the 'renin independent' mechanism. A rise in plasma potassium or a fall in plasma sodium will promote the release of aldosterone by acting directly on the cells of zona glomerulosa. The restoration of the electrolyte levels acts as a negative feedback on aldosterone and inhibits further release.

Excess and deficiency of aldosterone

Aldosterone excess

Excess aldosterone may be the result of a functioning tumour of the zona glomerulosa (primary aldosteronism) or a response to chronic low blood pressure or fluid shifts to a non-vascular compartment, for example in ascites (secondary aldosteronism). The results are a maintained elevation of blood pressure (BP) either to hypertensive levels or to approximately normal in the case of chronic losses of pressure.

Elevated BP may be attributable to many different causes but in the case of aldosteronism, the ratio of sodium to potassium is abnormal with hypernatraemia and hypokalaemia. The drug spironolactone competes for aldosterone receptors and may be useful in aldosterone excess.

Aldosterone deficiency

Deficiency of aldosterone occurs in Addison's disease where it is usually accompanied by cortisol deficiency. There is marked sodium loss resulting in water loss, with raised plasma potassium. The subject experiences muscle fatigue (electrolyte imbalance) and inability to maintain blood pressure, sometimes so severe that 'Addisonian crisis' is said to have occurred. If the subject is to survive, exogenous steroids including aldosterone are required.

THE HYPOTHALAMUS, ANTERIOR PITUITARY AND GROWTH HORMONE

This is a variation on the previous axes. It also features a number of confusingly similar hormone names. The hypothalamus produces a pair of hormones, growth hormone releasing hormone (GRH) and growth hormone inhibitory hormone (GIH or somatostatin). Both act on the anterior pituitary to stimulate or inhibit the production of growth hormone (or human growth hormone) (HGH) or somatotrophin. HGH has a number of direct and indirect effects. The indirect effects are mediated through a 'third organ', a tissue however not normally described as endocrine tissue – the liver (Fig. 11.13).

Indirect actions of HGH

The effect of HGH on the liver is to produce a number of somatomedins or growth factors now usually called insulin-like growth factors – IGFs. The actions of HGH are mediated mainly through IGF-1, the effects of which are to stimulate growth in bone, protein synthesis in muscle and lipolysis in fat. (The IGFs are often listed among the cytokine group along with other growth factors such as nerve growth factor (NGF), epidermal growth factor (EGF) and platelet derived growth factor (PDGF).)

Direct actions of HGH

HGH also has direct actions on fat cells and liver and muscle which are not growth promoting. In fact, they are sometimes referred to as anti-insulin or diabetogenic effects. It causes the breakdown of both fat and muscle, the resulting glucose produced by gluconeogenesis bringing about a rise in plasma glucose.

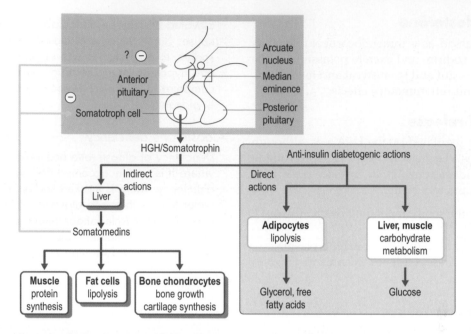

Figure 11.13 The actions of human growth hormone (HGH) or somatotrophin. (After Greenstein 1994 Endocrinology at a glance. With permission of Blackwell Science Ltd.)

Regulation of release of growth hormone

The regulation of the 'axis' is by IGF-1, which acts on the hypothalamus to inhibit GRH and stimulate somatostatin.

The levels of HGH rise early in sleep, in adults as well as children.

Excess and deficiency of HGH

Excess HGH

The most common cause of excess is a pituitary tumour. In children who are still growing, excess HGH causes gigantism. In adults whose long bones can no longer be extended, the condition is known as acromegaly.

In acromegaly, the lower jaw shows excessive growth and the small bones in hands and feet become enlarged. There is also increased coarsening of soft tissue in face, hands and feet. Glucose tolerance is impaired in many people with acromegaly, and diabetes (type 2) becomes overt in about one in ten. Some drugs, for example bromocriptine, reduce the secretion of HGH, or surgery (hypophysectomy) or irradiation may be appropriate.

Deficiency of HGH

This may be due to receptor insensitivity to the hormone, or may be due to pituitary insufficiency (primary pituitary dwarfism). Hypothalamic dwarfism, due to lack of release hormone, is much rarer. The condition can be treated with recombinant HGH.

Overgrowing

Growth hormone is of major importance in controlling growth from birth to adolescence. In certain circumstances, because of disorders due to tumour of the pituitary gland, there is an uncontrolled and excessive secretion of growth hormone. If this happens in childhood it leads to exaggerated growth known as gigantism.

In gigantism, growth is gradual but continuous and consistent; the affected person, with bones in normal proportion, may attain a height of 8 feet. Muscles may be well developed but later undergo some atrophy and weakening. The life span is shorter than normal because of a greater susceptibility to infection and metabolic disorders. The susceptibility arises because of compression of the pituitary gland from a (normally) benign tumour which originates from cells within the gland. One of the glands affected is the thyroid, leading to inadequate production of the hormones responsible for regulating metabolism and hence to metabolic disorders. Among such disorders is nutritional deficiency in which body-building and energy-yielding foods are not utilized. The consequence is progressive weight loss and weakness. Opportunistic organisms, which are normally harmless, take advantage and invade the body giving rise to gastrointestinal or parasitic disorders. It is thus the general deficiency of other pituitary hormones that usually causes death in early adulthood.

An excessive production of growth hormone in an adult results in enlargement of skeletal extremities, a condition known as acromegaly. For instance, the bones and soft tissues of the hands, feet, face and lower jaw become enlarged and the skin becomes coarse.

Growth hormone can also stimulate the growth of connective tissue such as ligaments, capsules and synovial membranes. A combination of connective tissue growth and hypertrophied bones compresses the local nerves causing pain, burning sensation in the joints, stiffness in the limbs, and tingling and numbness in the hands. These tumours may be surgically removed and the patient's symptoms of acromegaly may regress over time. Another condition commonly associated with acromegaly is diabetes mellitus (see Ch. 18). It affects, to some extent, up to 25% of people with acromegaly because growth hormone causes tissue resistance to insulin.

In both gigantism and acromegaly, apart from the physiological traumas that result from the excessive production of growth hormone, there are also problems in adapting to an altered body image that can cause great embarrassment.

THE ADRENAL MEDULLA

ADRENALINE AND NORADRENALINE

The adrenal glands are made up of two types of tissue. The inner neuroendocrine part, the medulla, is composed of chromaffin cells and is a modified sympathetic ganglion. It is supplied by sympathetic preganglionic nerves.

The medulla secretes two neurohormones, adrenaline (epinephrine) and noradrenaline (norepinephrine) in the proportions of about 4 to 1. They are known by their chemical group name as the catecholamines. They are both synthesized from phenylalanine, the last step being the conversion of noradrenaline to adrenaline by the enzyme PNMT (phenylethanolamine N-methyltransferase) They are stored in granules within the cells until release.

Effects of adrenaline and noradrenaline

The catecholamines have widespread effects on tissue cells. Their effects are determined by the receptor site type on the cells, but the response is affected by the numbers of receptors and the concentration of the catecholamine. Adrenoceptors are classified as alpha (α) and beta (β) and further divided into a number of subtypes. Table 5.3 (p. 94) shows the action of the catecholamines at the various site types (see Ch. 5).

Regulation of release

When the sympathetic nervous system is stimulated, the preganglionic fibres supplying the medulla release acetylcholine, bringing about the release of the catecholamines into the general circulation. As the level of sympathetic activity increases, for example in exercise or flight or fight, so does the medullary activity – this is the sympathomedullary or sympathoadrenal response.

In addition to blood received from the adrenal artery, the medulla receives blood drained from the adrenal cortex and carrying the steroid hormones. Cortisol has the effect of increasing the effect of PNMT, consequently increasing the proportion of adrenaline produced.

Metabolism of catecholamines

The catecholamines are broken down extracellularly by catecholamine-O-methyl transferase (COMT). Adrenaline and noradrenaline are also taken back into the cells producing them and broken down intracellularly by monoamine oxidase (MAO).

Excess catecholamine secretion

The chromaffin cells occasionally develop functioning tumours, i.e. a tumour which produces the secretion appropriate to the cell type but in excess amounts. The condition is called phaeochromocytoma. It causes paroxysmal production of the catecholamines, often brought on by bending or coughing or defecation, i.e. raising the intra-abdominal pressure. The attacks result in bursts of extreme hypertension and heat production. It is also characterized by hyperglycaemia. This usually benign tumour is treated surgically.

Pharmacology

Many drugs have been developed which make use of the receptor sites, either as agonists or antagonists. The greater the specificity for the site, the fewer unwanted effects the drug will have. Reducing the workload of the heart by the use of a β blocker has been part of clinical practice for many years, but the use of cardioselective β blockers has made it possible for people with asthma to use the drugs. The nonselective version affected β_1 in the heart so reducing its workload, but it also blocked the β_2 sites in the airways, an effect which caused bronchoconstriction. The cardioselective blocker has its effects on β_1 without significantly affecting β_2.

Agonists such as the β_2 agonist salbutamol have widespread use in the treatment of asthma. Salbutamol mimics the effects of adrenaline on β_2 receptors in airway smooth muscle, causing muscle relaxation and appreciable bronchodilation.

REFERENCES AND FURTHER READING

Berne R M, Levy M N 2000 Principles of physiology, 3rd edn. Mosby, St Louis

Brook C, Marshall N 1996 Essential endocrinology. Blackwell Science, Oxford

Campbell E J M, Dickinson C J, Slater J D H, Edwards C R W, Sikora E K 1984 Clinical physiology, 5th edn. Blackwell Science, Oxford

Ganong W F 2001 Review of medical physiology, 20th edn. McGraw-Hill Education, Philadelphia

Greenstein B 1994 Endocrinology at a glance. Blackwell Science, Oxford

Guyton A C, Hall J E 2000 Textbook of medical physiology, 10th edn. Saunders, Philadelphia

Guyton A C, Hall J E 2001 Guyton and Hall Pocket Companion to Textbook of medical physiology. Saunders, Philadelphia

Laycock J, Wise P 1996 Essential endocrinology. Oxford Medical Publications, Oxford

Porterfield S 2000 Endocrine physiology, 2nd edn. Mosby, St Louis

Rogers A W 1992 Textbook of anatomy. Churchill Livingstone, Edinburgh

12 Supplying the tissues

In practice you may be asked to consider the following:

1. A young man who has lost a significant amount of blood, but who is clearly still alive, appears to have an almost undetectable radial pulse?

2. This same patient is oliguric. What has caused this?

3. A patient with right heart failure has been prescribed a drug which 'will reduce preload'. Please explain.

4. A 50-year-old man who has pulmonary oedema is breathless. A change in posture eases his shortness of breath. Why is this?

5. The same patient's blood gases show a degree of hypoxia but normal carbon dioxide?

6. An elderly woman who has been prescribed a diuretic because of hypertension has refused to continue taking it because 'it gives me palpitations'. Can you explain to her why this is?

7. A woman with a history of hypertension has now had a diagnosis of phaeochromocytoma. She would like to know why her usual prescription has been temporarily changed to a β blocker.

8. A patient who has a history of hypertension, with a chronically elevated diastolic pressure, has developed a degree of cardiomegaly and reduced ejection fraction. Why? And what is the significance of this development?

9. A patient prescribed a diuretic has complained about its 'side effects'. It apparently causes his feet to be cold! Please explain.

10. An elderly man has complained of swollen ankles. He took the advice to sit with his feet raised, walk more etc., but this had no effect. He was prescribed a diuretic, which reduced the swelling. After some weeks he collapsed and was eventually found to be hypokalaemic. Explain all.

The circulatory system exists for one reason only, to meet the needs of the tissues. If the pump fails and perfusion stops, death is only four minutes away.

Reconciling the body's requirement for a steady internal environment with the rigours of the outside world and the very variable demands of the tissues has led to the evolution of a very sophisticated perfusion and exchange system which manages to meet the requirements. Even in circumstances where the tissue demands are extraordinary (e.g. at the limits of extreme exercise) or where the system itself is under threat (e.g. a large loss of blood), the coping mechanisms evolved (usually) manage to meet the need.

Although the cardiovascular system has refinements far outstripping modern engineering, it uses many of the same principles which apply to non-biological pumps and pipes. It is ironic to think how often we have had to invent things using the principles before we could recognize their biological forerunners.

VESSELS IN PARALLEL

Perfusion in the overall systemic circulation is arranged so that the main arteries supplying the organs are *in parallel*, not literally but functionally (Fig. 12.1). This is a familiar 'plumbing' design where several targets receive a fresh supply from a single line. Large arteries such as those supplying the liver, gut, kidneys, limbs etc. come directly from the aorta, so that the blood is at high pressure and fully oxygenated. The pressure in each of the supplies then has to be stepped down and the flow slowed down before exchange can take place in the capillary beds of that organ.

VESSELS IN SERIES – PORTAL CIRCULATIONS

The other 'plumbing' arrangement of 'pipes' is where the vessels are *in series*, i.e. one set of vessels following another.

In physiological terms this would be a *portal circulation*. Instead of the usual arrangement (Fig. 12.2) of

Artery → arteriole → capillary → venule → vein

the vessels in a portal system are arranged with two sets of capillaries linked by venules and veins. The layout is as follows (see Fig. 12.3):

first
artery → arteriole → capillary → venule → vein →
bed
second
venule → capillary → venule → vein
bed

This arrangement gives a way of using a series of vessels, anatomically close to one another, in a chain of processes, for example, where material taken up at the first capillary bed is to be deposited at the second. This description could, of course, be applied to the whole circulatory system. Blood enters the right heart, passes through the pulmonary vessels where gas exchange takes place, then through the left heart and on to the systemic vessels where the tissues are supplied, i.e. vessels in series. It would be unusual to include the whole system in a list of serial circuits, however, and more usually the following examples are given.

The first to be identified was the hepatic portal system, where blood takes up nutrients at the first set of capillaries as it passes through the intestine, then releases them to the liver at the second set of capillaries (see Chs 9 and 10). The hepatic portal system got its name from the fact that it enters the liver at the porta hepatis, the gate of the liver. Since that time, 'portal' has been used as a general term to describe this type of two-stage circulation.

The other portal venous link is that between the hypothalamus and the anterior pituitary gland (see Ch. 11). The first set of capillaries takes up hypothalamic releasing hormones which are delivered to the anterior pituitary by the second set. The anterior pituitary responds to the hypothalamic release hormones by releasing the appropriate anterior pituitary hormones.

A similar but arteriolar portal system is that at the nephron in the renal glomeruli (see Ch. 8).

Here the arrangement is:

first
artery → arteriole → capillary → arteriole →
bed
second
capillary → venule → vein
bed

Anatomically, the vessels are (Fig. 12.4):

afferent arteriole → glomerulus → efferent arteriole → peritubular capillaries → tubular venule

The purpose here is to use the first set of capillaries (the glomerulus) as a filter which will retain cells and plasma proteins in blood and filter off the fluid which will become tubular fluid. The second set of capillaries (the peritubular capillaries) is used to retrieve substances such as glucose and electrolytes reabsorbed by the nephron, or to secrete substances into the tubular fluid for excretion. The process of filtration diverts about 10% of the blood entering the kidney into the tubules (assuming glomerular filtration rate is approximately 120 ml per minute). This would normally cause a drop in pressure in the vessels following the glomerulus, but this has been avoided by having the

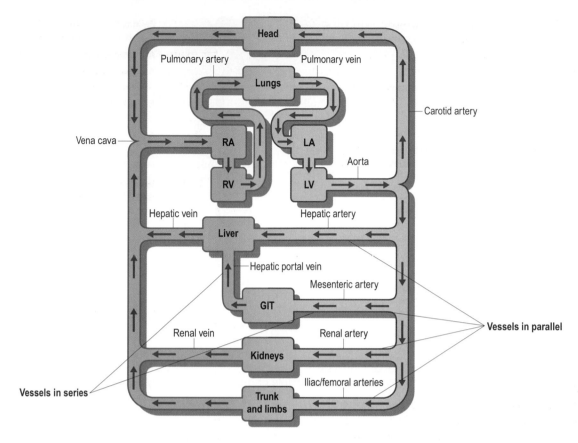

Figure 12.1 Blood vessels in parallel and in series. RA, right atrium; RV, right ventricle; LA, left atrium, LV, left ventricle; GIT, gastrointestinal tract. (After Watson 1999, with permission of Elsevier.)

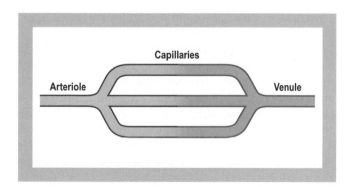

Figure 12.2 Conventional arrangement of vessels: arteriole – capillary – venule.

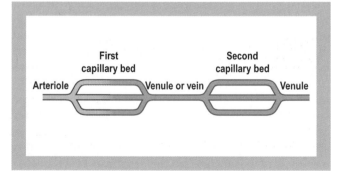

Figure 12.3 Diagrammatic representation of a portal venous system.

efferent arteriole narrower than the afferent – a strategy designed to maintain the pressure.

These are structural adaptations to suit a particular purpose. In the case of the series or portal circulations, the requirement is for an intermediate stage. This may be uptake from one site and delivery to another, or it may be a physical process such as filtering. There are benefits from these adaptations but there are also costs. Series circulations are always at risk. The second organ receives blood at a lower pressure and with a lower oxygen content; therefore, if there is a fall in systemic pressure, the downstream organ is at risk of damage. Renal tubular damage is a well-known complication of a catastrophic fall in blood pressure.

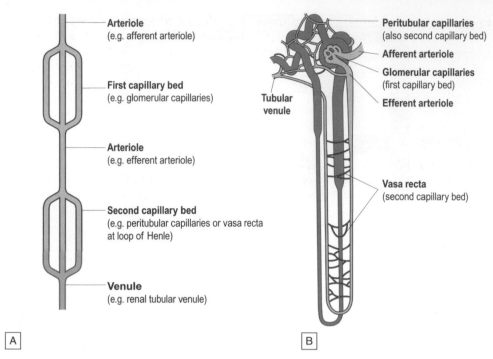

Figure 12.4 A, Portal arteriolar system. (Reproduced with permission from Watson 1999.) B, Renal microcirculation as an example of a portal arteriolar system.

SPECIALIZED CIRCULATIONS

Blood vessels are sometimes described as though they behave in the same ways wherever they are and whatever tissue they supply. Although vessels of any one type will have general characteristics, there are numerous adaptations to fit them to particular requirements. It could be argued that since all tissues have their own specialized functions, they would have their own specialized circulations. However, some circulations have very particular conditions to meet and are adapted accordingly. The adaptations may be structural or functional, e.g. the degree of permeability, the level of basal tone or the response to vasoactive substances.

CORONARY CIRCULATION

Since the heart muscle acts as the driving force for the whole system, it is essential that this muscle, above all, is well supplied. The supply must match the demand, and, even at rest this is considerable, about 20 times that of resting skeletal muscle. In exercise, the heart's requirement may increase by five times. One problem encountered by the coronary circuit is that during every systole, parts of it are obstructed as the myocardium contracts down on to the blood vessels. At rest, about 80% of flow occurs in diastole but it is less than that at active rates; therefore all the adaptations must maximize the supply (see Ch. 6).

The coronary circulation is the shortest in the body. Blood traverses the heart at rest in about 7 seconds, and, since the coronary arteries emerge from the aorta immediately after the aortic valve, systolic pressure is close to ejection pressure. The capillaries are very short and so numerous that almost every myocardial cell has its own capillary, keeping diffusion distance to a minimum and increasing the rate of transfer of oxygen and nutrients.

The coronary vessels are very sensitive to local blood gases and metabolites, and dilate promptly in response to local hypoxia and hypercapnia. In the normal heart perfusion is therefore matched to work done by the muscle. This increase in blood flow is referred to as metabolic hyperaemia. Sympathetic fibres supply vessel tone in the coronary circuit; the effect of metabolic hyperaemia is to overcome the tone and cause an increase in flow. The vessels also have β_2 adrenoceptors which cause dilation in response to adrenaline.

In addition to all the vessel adaptations, the myocardial cells are adapted to extract much more oxygen from blood than other tissues. At rest, about 75% of oxygen is extracted compared with 25% for the rest of the body at rest.

SKIN CIRCULATION

The skin circulation is adapted to allow the skin to act as part of the temperature regulatory system of the body (see Ch. 17). It has numerous arteriovenous (AV) shunts which are temperature regulated. When the body temperature is beginning to rise, the hypothalamic heat regulating centre inhibits the sympathetic output to the smooth muscle in the shunts, which consequently dilate; warm blood can then flow nearer to the body surface where it can be cooled. When blood temperature is low, sympathetic activity keeps the shunts constricted so that heat is conserved.

Similar local effects are produced by local mechanisms, e.g. using prostaglandins or changing the rate of the membrane pump activity.

By constricting and dilating, the skin circulation prevents the effects of changes in ambient temperature penetrating to the body core.

CEREBRAL CIRCULATION

The cerebral blood vessels have a highly engineered 'sprinkler system' type of arrangement called the circle of Willis by which pressure can be maintained equally around the many units which make up the brain. The carotid arteries have baroreceptors which monitor the main cerebral supply of blood but the brain vessels are independent of the baroreceptor reflex and, even when blood pressure is low in the rest of the system, cerebral vessels do not constrict. The brain has overall control over blood pressure and can maintain its own supply at the expense of all other tissues except the heart. The flow rate is very high and the high capillary density provides rapid and efficient transfer of materials (see Ch. 6 at 'Capillaries – the exchange vessels').

Blood–brain barrier

The exchange into brain tissue itself is controlled by the blood–brain barrier. The environment of the brain is very tightly controlled so that the brain is not exposed to the fluctuations in electrolytes and other solutes tolerated in the rest of the body. The capillaries supplying the brain cells allow the passage of water, carbon dioxide and oxygen, and there are special channels for glucose, amino acids and other organic acids. Lipid-soluble substances penetrate the barrier more easily than water-soluble substances.

Some areas of the brain are 'outside' the barrier. The posterior pituitary gland, for example, can release its hormones into the general circulation (see Ch. 11) and the osmoreceptor region of the hypothalamus is exposed to the osmolarity of the body fluids. The blood–brain barrier is not fully developed at birth. In a newborn baby, exposed to severe jaundice, the bile pigments will penetrate to brain tissue and can damage areas such as the basal ganglia. Bile pigments (and bile salts) will not penetrate the adult blood–brain barrier.

PULMONARY CIRCULATION

This is the circulation which takes up the oxygen upon which all the tissues depend. The pulmonary vascular system is the most atypical of all the 'specialized circulations'. It depends on being a low pressure system, in order that fluid can be reclaimed and removed efficiently from lung tissue. If the pressure is too high, pulmonary oedema forms. The distance between air in the alveoli and the blood which will carry the gases increases to the point where the diffusion distance is too great and oxygen uptake is jeopardized. Carbon dioxide is usually less affected because it is a more soluble gas and is less affected by diffusion distance.

Distribution of blood flow is uneven in the lung. When standing, the base of the lung is much better perfused than the apex; in fact, perfusion at the apex only happens during systole. The base of the lung is also better ventilated than the apex and the net result is that, overall, gas exchange is less good at the apex. When lying down, these differences disappear and gas exchange becomes more even throughout the lung.

Pulmonary vessels also behave quite differently when exposed to hypoxia and hypercapnia. Where other circulations dilate, pulmonary vessels constrict. This is not as contrary as it might seem when the function of the pulmonary circuit is considered. The aim is to take up oxygen and unload carbon dioxide for the benefit of the body as a whole. There is little to be gained from increasing perfusion in areas of lung which are poorly ventilated and therefore are poor sources of oxygen and already rich in carbon dioxide; better to direct the blood to more favourable areas of the lung. The giving of therapeutic oxygen to a hypoxic patient is important to maintain the patient's blood oxygen levels, but even more important is the fact that therapeutic oxygen reduces the pulmonary vessel constriction which would otherwise limit oxygen uptake.

THE PRINCIPLES OF EXCHANGE

The finely engineered circulatory route and all the modifications in the circuits serve only one purpose – to allow tissues to exchange material when required and at the rate required. The principles underlying the process of exchange are important. If a fault develops and is not corrected, it can lead to damage, or even death of the tissue.

The physical conditions at the capillary bed are central to the exchange process. All the mechanisms which control the activities of the cardiovascular system and many of those controlling other systems such as the kidneys, are aimed at providing the correct conditions in the capillary beds to meet the requirements of the tissue (see also Ch. 14).

THE MECHANISM OF EXCHANGE

The principle of exchange is fairly simple, the process itself is far from simple. The principle, first put forward by Starling in the 1890s, was that there was a balance between hydrostatic pressure pushing fluid out of vessels and osmotic pressure pulling it in. At the arteriolar end of the capillary bed, where hydrostatic pressure exceeds osmotic pressure, fluid leaves the vessels to become tissue fluid. Pressure and flow rate are reduced as the single stream (the arteriole) is divided into several smaller streams (the capillaries), and as the venular end of the capillaries approaches, hydrostatic pressure is now less than osmotic pressure. Fluid can now re-enter the vessels. Figure 12.5 shows this principle with the Starling figures which are still in use.

However, capillary exchange is not quite as straight-forward. When conditions were measured in capillary beds, it became apparent that neither permeability nor osmotic pressure was constant along the length and that pressure was still pulsatile in capillaries. It would appear that the effect of the pulsing pressure is to drive more fluid out at systole and pull more in at diastole. The increased permeability of the capillary near the venules may increase solute and fluid recovery in the diastolic phase. These mechanisms are described more fully in Chapter 14.

THE FACTORS WHICH AFFECT EXCHANGE

The volume and rate of exchange at capillary beds, although modified by pulsatile pressure, are primarily affected by:

1. Hydrostatic pressure – pressure pushing fluid out
   - pressure
   - resistance
   - flow.
2. Osmotic pressure – pressure pulling fluid in or retaining it.
3. Permeability – number and size of gaps.

HYDROSTATIC PRESSURE

Hydrostatic pressure literally means the pressure of a liquid against a surface and refers to the pressure of the blood against the vessel walls. 'Blood pressure' is hydrostatic pressure.

Pressure

Blood pressure measurements used clinically

- Systolic pressure – pressure at the peak of ventricular ejection, usually measured at the brachial artery.
- Diastolic pressure – pressure of blood in the vessels when the heart is not contracting, usually measured at the brachial artery.
- Pulse pressure – the numerical difference between systolic and diastolic pressures.
- Mean arterial pressure – arterial pressure oscillates between systolic and diastolic, but spends more time nearer the diastolic value. Mean arterial pressure (MAP) is a time weighted average which can be estimated using the following expression:

$$\text{MAP} = \text{diastolic pressure} + \frac{\text{pulse pressure}}{3}$$

- Capillary pressure – pressure is still pulsatile and varies along the length, higher at arteriolar end lower at the venular end.

The effect of hydrostatic or blood pressure is to push fluid along a vessel if the walls are impermeable, or out of the vessel where the wall is permeable. Fluid will only move from an area of higher pressure to an area of lower pressure, i.e. in response to a pressure gradient. The larger the difference between the two pressures, the steeper the gradient will be and the greater the movement. In the body, hydrostatic pressure is highest nearest the pump, i.e. the heart, which provides the head of pressure.

Hydrostatic pressure is measured in mmHg or in the SI unit kilopascal (kPa) (1 mm Hg ≈ 0.133 kPa). The former and more traditional unit reflects the method of measuring hydrostatic pressure using a column of mercury, i.e. in a sphygmomanometer. The greater the pressure pushing the lower end of the column, the more

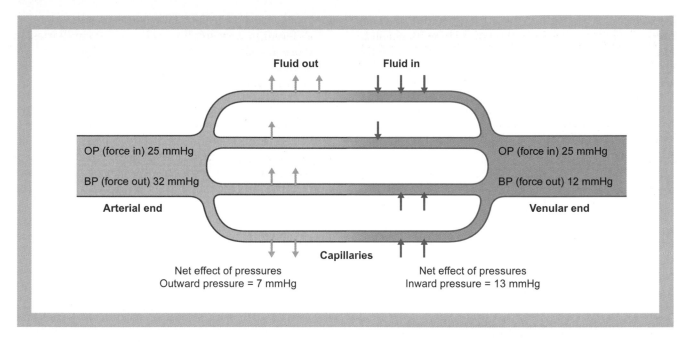

Figure 12.5 Fluid exchange at capillaries. OP, osmotic pressure; BP, blood pressure. (After Watson 1999, with permission of Elsevier.)

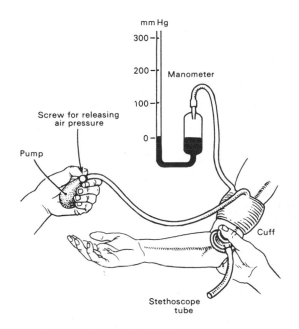

Figure 12.6 Column method of measuring pressure. (From Emslie-Smith et al 1988, with permission of Elsevier.)

mercury enters from the reservoir, and the higher the column rises (Fig. 12.6). The column method also illustrates the principle that the pressure in the column at the base is greater because of the gravitational effect of the column above it. Exactly the same principle applies to the leg veins when an individual stands. The venous pressure is higher in the feet and ankles because

of the column of blood above, less fluid is returned to the veins from the tissue and the result is the ankle swelling common when people have to stand still for long periods.

Atmospheric pressure

Hydrostatic pressure is pressure in addition to atmospheric pressure. This is variable, but the value under standard conditions is 760 mmHg. A systolic pressure of 120 mmHg is in fact a true pressure of 760 + 120 mmHg = 880 mmHg. A 'negative' pressure, which can occur in the right atrium at diastole, is a pressure below atmospheric pressure, for example 760 − 2 mmHg = 758 mmHg. In practice, however, atmospheric pressure values are ignored and physiological pressures are taken as the values above and below atmospheric pressure. In the case above, right atrial pressure at diastole would be expressed as −2 mmHg.

Resistance

Since blood in the circulatory system is travelling along a series of vessels which have the physical characteristics of pipes, the effect of resistance to flow becomes significant. Arterioles are sometimes called the resistance vessels. Their narrow bore and muscular walls allow them to change the pressure in the vessels and use the property of resistance to affect the degree and direction of flow:

$$\text{flow} = \text{pressure}/\text{resistance}$$

The effect of a hydrostatic pressure gradient is to cause fluid to move from A to B, the effect of resistance is to oppose or resist the flow. The greater the resistance the greater is the pressure required to overcome it and achieve flow.

Resistance is governed by three main factors:

- the radius of vessel
- the flow characteristics of blood itself
- viscosity.

Radius of vessel

The bore or calibre of a vessel greatly affects the resistance to flow. Poiseuille described this in 1840 and his work has been one of the cornerstones of the understanding of flow dynamics in the cardiovascular system ever since. Poiseuille's law states that flow is proportional to the radius to the power 4 (r^4) of the vessel and inversely proportional to the viscosity (i.e. the narrower the bore, the smaller the flow, and the thinner the liquid, the greater the flow). It is clear that an increase in resistance causes a reduction in flow. However, because of the fact that radius is to the power 4, a very small change in radius makes a very large difference to the resistance. Peripheral resistance is mainly due to arterioles. Their property of varying pressure and hence resistance gives them a very large influence on pressure and perfusion.

Flow characteristics of blood

Blood is not a perfect fluid, it is a fluid system made up of liquid plasma and cells which behave rather like droplets. This causes blood to flow differently in different sized vessels.

1. *Laminar streamlined flow.* In large vessels, blood behaves as a simple fluid, adopting a laminar streamlined flow (Fig. 12.7A). Blood flows along the vessel in concentric layers like cylinders, with the central cylinders moving slightly faster. Resistance is created more by the layers dragging on one another than by the drag of the outer layer on the vessel wall.
2. *Turbulent flow.* When laminar flow is disturbed, the flow becomes turbulent (Fig. 12.7B). Turbulence increases the resistance to flow and therefore the pressure required to maintain flow. It also produces sounds which can be heard if amplified, e.g. with a stethoscope (laminar flow is silent). Turbulence occurs if there is an obstruction to flow, e.g. the heart's valves cause turbulence which can be heard as one of the normal heart sounds. It can occur at high flow rates; sometimes flow in the aorta can be heard at peak ejection. Turbulence also occurs in less normal circumstances, for example if there is an irregularity such as atheroma in the vessel surface or where blood viscosity is low in anaemia.
3. *Axial or single line flow.* Flow patterns are very different in very small vessels such as capillaries. In these vessels, where the diameter is close to or smaller than the diameter of the red cell, laminar flow would not be possible.

It had been observed by Whittaker and Winton in the 1930s that the viscosity of blood in small vessels appeared to be about half that when blood was measured in a viscometer. As the vessel size decreases below that of small arterioles, the viscosity decreases until, at the radius of capillaries, it reaches a value close to that of plasma.

This effect is due to axial streaming (or single line flow). The forces (shear stress) exerted on the blood by the geometry of the vessel cause the flexible red cells to adopt a more elongated shape or folded 'jelly fish' shape and make their way to the axis of the stream. In small arterioles this leaves a thin layer of plasma along the vessel wall, which reduces friction. In capillaries, the elongated cells move along in a single line, an adaptation which maintains flow in a very narrow vessel (Fig. 12.7C).

Viscosity

Viscosity affects resistance and flow rate. As can be seen from the previous section, blood viscosity is not a simple matter. With a simple fluid, such as water or oil, viscosity is independent of the radius of the vessel in which it flows.

It is useful to compare the viscosity of biological fluids, such as plasma and whole blood, with that of water at the same temperature. This allows the term 'relative' viscosity to be used and avoids the necessity for the inclusion of the units (newtons per second per metre squared ($N\,s\,m^{-2}$)). When tested in a viscometer, i.e. in vitro, the relative viscosity of plasma at 37°C is about 1.8 times that of water; whole blood is about 4 times, the increase being related to the percentage of the volume occupied by the cells (haematocrit) (see Ch. 3). In vivo, however, due to axial or single line flow, the viscosity of peripheral blood is much less. In vessels which are approximately the radius of many arterioles, the relative viscosity is about 2.5 that of water and in capillaries it is reduced to about that of plasma, i.e. near the value for water.

Viscosity of blood depends mainly on haematocrit. In a viscometer, an increase in red cell number greatly increases viscosity. In vivo, however, while the increase in viscosity can affect flow in large vessels, the change in small vessels is much less. These smaller vessels, i.e. less than 30 μm radius, include arterioles, capillaries and venules, which make up the greater part of the circulatory system. Haematocrit changes therefore have little effect on peripheral flow except when they are very large.

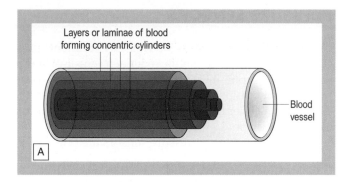

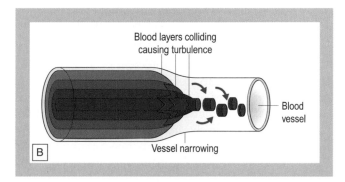

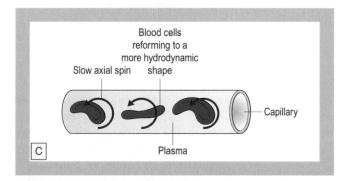

Figure 12.7 A, Laminar blood flow in large vessels. B, Turbulent flow. C, Axial or single line flow in small vessels. (After Watson 1999, with permission of Elsevier.)

In disease states, such as sickle cell anaemia, where the abnormal haemoglobin precipitates at low oxygen levels and stiffens the cell, or spherocytosis, where the cell cannot support folding, axial flow is not possible. The flow in the all-important capillary beds is impaired and the tissue becomes damaged and painful.

OSMOTIC PRESSURE

Osmotic pressure is the pressure which causes the movement of water through a permeable membrane in response to the presence of particles retained on the other side (see Ch. 14).

It is often taken that osmotic pressure (OP) is due largely to the plasma proteins. In fact only a small proportion is due to them, a much larger contribution coming from the electrolytes, glucose and urea. The significance of the proteins is that they are largely retained within the vessels, unlike sodium and other species which can move freely through the capillary membranes. The plasma proteins provide the effective osmotic pressure which is important to the operation and stability of the exchange system. Since osmotic pressure attracts water, its effect is to pull fluid into the vessel or to retain fluid within the vessel. A reduction in the concentration of plasma proteins (hypoprotinaemia), which can occur in liver disease (see Ch. 10), is characterized by oedema due to a reduction in osmotic pressure. To make matters worse, liver disease is often accompanied by an increased hydrostatic pressure at the capillary beds, a combination leading to an increased fluid shift to extravascular space, i.e. increased oedema and even ascites.

The difference between hydrostatic pressure pushing fluid out of the vessel and osmotic pressure pulling fluid in is also a gradient. The same rule applies – the larger the difference between the two pressure values, the steeper the gradient and the greater the fluid movement.

PERMEABILITY

Capillaries are permeable, although not all equally so (see Ch. 6). As with any sieve, the size of the holes has a large effect on the rate of flow through them. Small ions can pass through easily, larger particles cannot. Even within one type of capillary, permeability can vary, capillaries have been shown to be more permeable towards the venular end. Permeability can be altered by local conditions. In an inflammatory state, for example, mediators such as histamine and cytokines such as IL-1(interleukin 1) and TNF (tumour necrosis factor) (see Ch. 16) increase the gap size between the cells of the capillary membrane, allowing increased fluid to escape to the tissues. In more severe cases, plasma proteins can escape into the tissue space, greatly increasing the OP there and causing water to move into the space. The evidence of inflammation is clear from the swelling and, if close to the surface, the presence of blisters.

REGULATING EXCHANGE – THE IMPORTANCE OF HYDROSTATIC PRESSURE

The purpose of the circulatory system is to meet the very variable requirements of the cells. Different tissues have different needs. If brain and skeletal muscle are compared, the brain requires about 54 ml per minute per 100 g (a large part of which goes to supply the grey matter) and skeletal muscle at rest about 2.5. Tissues may have different requirements depending on the level of activity. In heavy exercise, the demand of skeletal muscle increases from the resting 2.5 to about 50 ml per minute per 100 g. At maximum exercise, the requirement may be about 30 times the resting requirement.

A major factor in the control of delivery to tissue cells is the pressure gradient at the capillary beds. Osmotic pressure is not normally altered rapidly and changes in permeability have the effect of facilitating flow rather than acting as a control. The regulating factor capable of rapid response is hydrostatic pressure. To this end, the mechanisms which control the activities of the cardiovascular system, and many of the other cooperating systems, are sensitive to changes in pressure and will respond by modifying the pressure to meet the need.

Although blood pressure is measured routinely in clinical practice, to be useful, it must be measured under standard conditions. In daily living, blood pressures are not constant but are constantly being adjusted to requirement.

THE REGULATION OF SYSTEMIC PRESSURE

Blood pressure, although variable, is maintained within a range of 'normal' values, 'normal' for sleep, 'normal' for exercise, and so on. The body has a complex array of mechanisms available to alter all the aspects of blood pressure. For example, systolic pressure and diastolic pressure can be adjusted independently. Blood can be moved from one circulation to another and adjustments can be made over a variety of time scales. Blood pressure must be able to respond to circumstances, to rise in activity and increase the supply to the capillary beds, and conversely to fall when the body is at rest. Even at rest, the pressures will move to the upper end of their normal resting range, then they will be brought down to the lower end of the range, to move up again, a phenomenon known as 'hunting'. Those small adjustments are not usually obvious to the subject; they can be measured but the changes are small. When a large and sudden adjustment to pressure is required, the activities of the systems producing the adjustment will show as symptoms.

The areas of control operate by a large number of pathways and over different time scales. It takes only a few seconds to change pressure by changing heart rate but much longer to change pressure by changing intravascular volume. The short-term regulation of blood pressure is mainly neural; longer-term regulation is mainly hormonal.

PRESSURE SENSORS

As with all aspects of the internal environment, pressures are continuously monitored. Each sensor provides the sensory input into a reflex arc; the central component is the hypothalamus and brain stem, and the effector arm either the autonomic nervous system or the endocrine system.

The major groups of pressure sensors are (Fig. 12.8):

- high pressure baroreceptors in the aortic arch and the carotid sinuses, so called because of their sites in high pressure vessels
- low pressure baroreceptors, also called volume receptors or cardiopulmonary receptors, in the low pressure atria and pulmonary circuit.

Baroreceptors are mechanoreceptors and fire when they are subjected to deformation. The endings are embedded in an area of stretchy tissue within the vessel wall so that any increase in pressure is amplified by stretch. Their effects are inhibitory, reducing sympathetic drive and increasing parasympathetic drive. When pressure rises, their firing rate increases; when pressure is reduced, their firing rate and therefore their inhibitory influence are reduced.

The baroreceptor reflexes have wide influence (Fig. 12.8).

The *high pressure receptor reflexes* affect heart rate, the bore of blood vessels, renal handling of fluid and the output of the catecholamines whose actions include the metabolic effects of adrenaline. Although the reflexes are continuously adjusting pressure, their effects are most clearly identified when pressure falls significantly, for example the familiar rise in heart rate and vasoconstricted cold skin of the patient who has become acutely hypotensive. In the same patient, less evident, but equally important, is the venous constriction which occurs in gut and liver, shifting blood into the central veins and helping to increase venous return. Sympathetic stimulation in the kidney will increase the retention of the volume.

The *low pressure receptor reflexes* also have inhibitory effects, again most easily seen when pressure is suddenly and significantly reduced. These include peripheral vasoconstriction, which decreases capacity and redirects blood flow, and an increase in the release of arginine vasopressin (AVP) (also called antidiuretic hormone (ADH)) which causes reclamation of water. At higher concentrations AVP is also a potent vasoconstrictor.

Other sensors which affect pressure are:

- hypothalamic and peripheral chemoreceptors which also regulate ventilation (see Ch. 7)
- hypothalamic osmoreceptors which regulate volume and osmolarity (see Ch. 14).

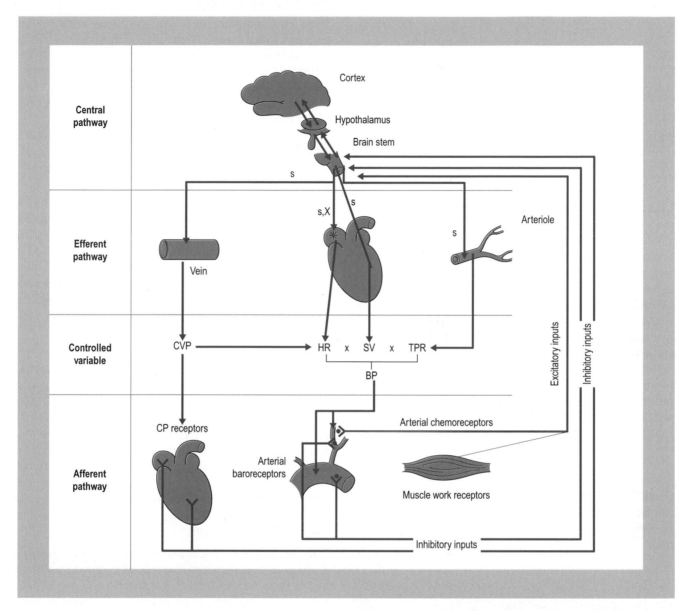

Figure 12.8 Baroreceptor effects – schematic overview of the reflex and central control of the circulation. CP, cardiopulmonary receptor group (heterogeneous); CVP, central venous pressure; SV, stroke volume; HR, heart rate; TPR, total peripheral resistance; BP, arterial blood pressure; s, sympathetic fibres (noradrenergic) (excitatory output); X, vagal cardiac fibres (cholinergic). Neuroendocrine reflexes and cerebellar relay are not shown. Terms 'inhibitory input' and 'excitatory output' refer to the net effect of receptor activation on cardiac output and blood pressure. (After Levick 1991 An introduction to cardiovascular physiology 3E (Arnold 2000). Reprinted by permission.)

THE MAJOR AREAS OF PRESSURE REGULATION

The major areas of adjustment of systemic pressure are shown below as separate entities. Although this is convenient as far as the text is concerned, it is an over-simplification of a complex integrated organization where signals indicating a need to alter pressure are likely to affect several of the control systems and effector tissues.

The main elements of pressure management are (Fig. 12.9):

• pump output – the heart
• vascular capacity – the vessels
• intravascular volume – blood volume.

Cardiac output is the volume of blood pumped out of the ventricles per minute and it provides the head of pressure which can then be altered to suit requirements.

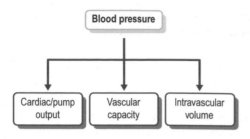

Figure 12.9 Major areas of blood pressure regulation.

Changes in cardiac output are related to systolic pressure.

Vascular capacity is the size or capacity of a vessel or of the overall system. Altering the radius of the vessels will alter pressure. Vasoconstriction reduces radius and capacity and will raise pressure within the vessel, vasodilation will enlarge the vessel and lower the pressure. Changes in arterial vessel capacity are likely to affect diastolic pressure (afterload). Changes in venous capacity will affect venous return (preload). (In addition to being used to alter the overall pressure, control of vessel radius can be used to alter resistance within a vessel and redirect flow of blood from one area to another or to alter the rate of flow to a particular tissue.)

Intravascular volume is the volume of blood within the vessels. When volume is reduced (if there is no compensation), pressure will decrease and vice versa. Since volume takes longer than cardiac output or vessel capacity to alter, control of volume provides a stabilizing influence over pressure regulation. Changes in volume will affect both systolic and diastolic pressures.

MECHANISMS ADJUSTING BLOOD PRESSURE

CARDIAC OUTPUT AND BLOOD PRESSURE

Cardiac output is the product of heart rate and stroke volume. It is directly related to arterial blood pressure; therefore a change in either heart rate or stroke volume will alter blood pressure (see Ch. 6). In practice, usually, both are affected, either directly or by one another.

Heart rate

Regulation of heart rate is carried out by a series of autonomic reflexes and it is affected by factors such as hormones and local chemicals.

Baroreceptor reflexes

Both high pressure and low pressure baroreceptors respond to increased stretching of the vessel wall, i.e. increased pressure, by increasing their firing rate. Their effect on the control centres in the brain stem is inhibitory and the result is a reduction in heart rate and force of contraction, so lowering cardiac output. A fall in blood pressure would have the opposite effect.

Baroreceptors are part of the short-term regulation of blood pressure.

Higher centre stimulation

Heart rate and stroke volume are also affected by the sympathetic nervous system in response to stimulation from higher brain centres by fear, anger and so on. The adrenal medulla is also stimulated, releasing adrenaline and noradrenaline and augmenting the sympathetic effects. This produces the familiar effect where the after-effects of fright, for example, go on longer than might be expected.

Hormones

In addition to the neurohormones adrenaline and noradrenaline, other hormones can change heart rate. The thyroid hormones, for example, increase heart rate by upregulating the adrenoceptors (see Ch. 11) and increasing the effectiveness of adrenaline and noradrenaline. One of the characteristic features of overactivity of the thyroid gland is rapid heart rate (tachycardia) even at rest, and a slow heart rate (bradycardia) typifies the underactive thyroid.

The Bainbridge effect

This is another mechanism allowing the heart to manage a change in input and is stimulated by stretching of the atrial muscle. It is a short-lived rise in heart rate, lasting for only 10 to 20 beats, produced by over-filling the atria, perhaps by a long filling period or infusion of fluid. It can sometimes be seen in practice at the beginning of an infusion. It is called the Bainbridge effect after the physiologist who first recorded it.

Stroke volume

Each change to stroke volume will, in turn, affect arterial blood pressure. Details can be found in Chapter 6. The following is a summary.

Stroke volume can be affected by the following:

1. Changing ventricular contractility
   - increased by sympathetic stimulation or by circulating catecholamines
   - increased by stretching the ventricular muscle during filling.

2. Changing the size of the ventricle (less usual). Altered ventricular volume is an effect of training and muscle enlargement. There is a limit to the benefit achieved by enlarging the heart because, when the walls of the chambers are over thickened, they become more difficult to contract.

3. Changing the volume returning to the heart as venous return. Venous return provides the volume some of which will become stroke volume. Venous return is very variable, affected, for example, by posture, movement and ventilation. Stroke volume must, therefore, also be variable to some extent, although the input (venous return) and the output (stroke volume) are kept in step with one another by the Frank–Starling mechanism. Even with changes in stroke volume, cardiac output is kept relatively steady, at least at rest, by compensating changes in heart rate.

VESSEL CAPACITY AND BLOOD PRESSURE

The overall or systemic pressure is the background pressure, which can be modified to suit particular local needs. Perfusion of tissues and the supply of materials depends on the ability of blood vessels to respond to the control mechanisms which alter systemic pressure, as well as to local mediators affecting pressure in the area. As an example, vasodilation to supply more blood to exercising muscle has more effect if systemic pressure rises enough to drive it there.

Overall or systemic changes to vessel capacity will affect mainly diastolic pressure. Local changes can produce pressure gradients to redirect blood from one area to another according to their relative needs.

Regulation of vessel capacity

Vessel size can be altered by numerous mechanisms either systemically or locally. Among the factors which produce dimensional changes in vessels are:

- autonomic effects
- neurohormones
- other hormones
- temperature
- local regulatory mechanisms.

Autonomic effects

These can be divided into the following:

- effects arising from the brain stem and hypothalamus, e.g. the baroreceptor reflex
- sympathetic effects stimulated by the higher brain
- sympathetic cholinergic effects

- parasympathetic effects on blood vessels in an important minority of tissues.

Reflex sympathetic effects (baroreceptor reflexes)

The baroreceptor reflexes, in addition to their effects on the heart, also affect blood vessels. The sympathetic pathways to the vessels are continuously (tonically) active and keep the vessels in a sustained state of partial contraction or tone. Some vessels show higher levels of basal tone than others, depending on their function. Vessels which are likely to have to dilate significantly, such as those in skeletal muscle, must have a high basal tone to start with. The reflex works by raising and lowering the level of activity in the mechanism rather than switching it on and off. A rise in blood pressure increases baroreceptor activity; this increases inhibition of the brain stem area which maintains the level of vasoconstriction and consequently, vasoconstriction is reduced. The opposite effect happens if blood pressure falls, baroreceptor activity is reduced, inhibition is reduced and the resulting vasoconstriction raises blood pressure. The sympathetic transmitter is noradrenaline and the receptor sites which bring about constriction are α_1.

Sympathetic effects stimulated by higher brain centres

The effect produced by the stimulation of the sympathetic system from the higher brain is not part of the reflex system. The cerebral cortex can directly affect the brain stem so that stimuli such as fear or excitement or embarrassment may affect blood vessels, i.e. 'pale with fear' (vasoconstriction) or 'red with embarrassment' (vasodilation).

Sympathetic cholinergic effects

These fibres are controlled by the forebrain and supply very few tissues, some skeletal muscle blood vessels and the sweat glands. They are unusual in being sympathetic and using acetylcholine as a transmitter and, more than that, some are examples of co-transmitter use, the other transmitter being non-adrenergic non-cholinergic (NANC), for example vasoactive inhibitory peptide (VIP) (see Ch. 5).

The effects are vasodilatory. The result produced in skeletal muscle is probably not a significant increase in perfusion, as there are not enough sites for it to be effective. It may be that the vasodilation is enough to reduce afterload at the beginning of muscular effort when cardiac output must rise rapidly.

Parasympathetic effect on blood vessels

The parasympathetic system supplies only a few vascular sites, for example the blood vessels in the salivary glands, the tongue and the external sex organs. The effect at all these blood vessels is to cause vasodilation.

The effect is not tonic (i.e. it can be switched on and off), separate sites can be selected and it is controlled from the forebrain. The vasodilation is produced partly by acetylcholine as would be expected, but these sites are also examples of the use of NANC co-transmitters. In the case of the gut, the NANC co-transmitter is VIP.

Parasympathetic activity at these sites has little effect on overall blood pressure, but the local effects are important. For example, the vasodilation in the salivary glands provides the extra fluid required for the increased flow of saliva when eating and the vaso-dilation at penis and clitoris allow engorgement and erection of the tissue.

Circulating noradrenaline/adrenaline

This is part of the much wider sympathomedullary response, i.e. the response of the adrenal medulla to stimulation by the sympathetic system and the release of adrenaline and noradrenaline. This mechanism, which can maintain blood pressure and at the same time redirect blood flow, depends on the ability of the catecholamines to use more than one type of adreno-ceptor site (α_1 constrictor, β_2 dilator). The combined effects, constriction in some vessels and dilation in others, cause blood to move from the high pressure, constricted area to the low pressure, dilated area.

This effect is very obvious when there is a large drop in blood pressure, due perhaps to haemorrhage, and blood is redirected from skin to vital organs. The resulting cold skin is clear evidence that the skin blood vessels can constrict almost to the point of closure.

Other hormones

A number of hormones released by the endocrine glands are vasoactive.

Atrial natriuretic peptide (ANP)

This hormone is released by the atria in response to stretch, by rapid filling or large preload. It causes arteriolar vasodilation. It also affects the kidney where it increases the excretion of sodium and water (see Ch. 8), thereby affecting both capacity and volume.

Cortisol

Cortisol has a very wide range of actions (see Ch. 11) which make it essential for survival. At blood vessel walls, it has the stabilizing effects of maintaining the tone and reducing permeability (see Ch. 19).

Arginine vasopressin (AVP) (or antidiuretic hormone (ADH))

As its alternative names suggest, this hypothalamic hormone is a potent vasoconstrictor when circulating at higher concentrations. It also acts on renal tubules, where it increases the retrieval of water, again affecting both capacity and volume (see Chs 8 and 11).

The effects of temperature on blood vessels

Temperature affects blood vessels overall by affecting heat regulation in the hypothalamus, and locally at the vessels themselves.

The central effect is achieved by altering the sympathetic tone of the vessels, particularly in skin. A reduction in (core) blood temperature causes vaso-constriction and, conversely, a rise in blood temperature causes vasodilation. The skin circulation is also parti-cularly sensitive to external changes in temperature and shields the core from environmental changes (Ch. 17).

The local effect of temperature is local dilation as temperature rises and local constriction as the tem-perature falls. The mechanism is not centrally mediated, however; it is a direct effect on vascular smooth muscle.

Autoregulation

It might appear that perfusion in any one area is mainly under the control of central mechanisms, either neural or hormonal. In fact, tissue circulations can refine their own perfusion by autoregulation. These processes may be either inherent in the smooth muscle itself, i.e. smooth muscle autoregulation (myogenic auto-regulation), or may be induced by local conditions such as pH or blood gas concentrations.

Smooth muscle (myogenic) autoregulation

This is likely to be due to the property of all muscle to contract following stretch. As the pressure rises in the blood vessel within a tissue, the vessel stretches, moderating the rise. When pressure drops, the vessel constricts and the pressure is raised. In this way, the flow rate is kept steady. Probably the best example of this is the autoregulation seen in the renal circulation.

Metabolic autoregulation

When an athlete is in training, the assessment of oxygen usage and carbon dioxide production can be used as a measure of effort. Blood vessels can use the same indicators but use them to regulate supply.

Metabolic autoregulation is the main regulator of flow in the coronary circuit, but the principles apply to other circulations with the exception of the pulmonary vessels. Here the principle of local regulation applies but the response from the vessels is atypical. In all other circulations, vasodilation is caused by increased levels of carbon dioxide, lactate and hydrogen and potassium ions and by decreased levels of oxygen. These conditions are characteristic of the working tissue and the phenomenon is described as metabolic hyperaemia.

In a resting skeletal muscle, perhaps 50% of capillary beds are not open. Metabolic hyperaemia does not simply increase blood flow to the open vessels; it relaxes arterioles supplying capillary beds, opening up those which were not active. This greatly increases exchange area and reduces the diffusion distance between the cells and their nearest capillary.

The system is precisely geared to requirement. As the tissue works, the metabolites accumulate, causing the vessels to dilate and the metabolites to be washed away. As the concentration is reduced, the dilator effect is reduced and constriction re-established.

Locally acting agents (vasoactive chemicals)

Many vasoactive chemicals produced locally act locally (see Table 6.1). These include the prostaglandins, serotonin, bradykinin, histamine and nitric oxide. Some, like nitric oxide, are produced by the endothelium, some by cells activated in the area, e.g. histamine released from mast cells. Some of the chemicals, for example the prostaglandins (PGs) and nitric oxide (NO), are the mediators through which other mechanisms work. PGs are a group of substances from a common origin, arachidonic acid, but with different effects; the PGF series is constrictor, the PGE series is dilator. Some of these local agents are involved in the response to injury sometimes called the triple response (see Ch. 19 at 'Wounds and wound healing').

INTRAVASCULAR VOLUME AND BLOOD PRESSURE

Regulation of intravascular volume (blood volume) is an important contributor to the regulation of blood pressure and a good example of multi-system co-operation since it involves, not only the nervous system and several endocrine systems, but heart, vessels and kidney, with contributions from gut and liver.

Although two of the hormones, AVP and ANP, provide a fairly rapid adjustment, changes in volume take longer to achieve than changes in either heart rate or vessel capacity. This slower rate of change, however, tends to have a stabilizing effect.

Hydrostatic pressure is regulated in parallel with osmotic pressure and some of the mechanisms are stimulated not only by changes in blood pressure but by changes in volume and osmotic pressure.

Fluid retention or excretion by the kidney (see Ch. 8) is the most closely controlled process of fluid regulation, although fluid exchange also takes place at the gut and skin.

The mechanisms of adjustment use:

- AVP (ADH)
- renin, angiotensin, aldosterone system
- atrial natriuretic peptide (ANP)
- fluid recovery from tissues.

Arginine vasopressin (AVP) (antidiuretic hormone (ADH))

AVP is a hormone produced in the hypothalamus and released from the posterior pituitary gland. It causes the reabsorption of water at the distal nephron. At higher concentrations, as its alternative name suggests, it is a potent vasoconstrictor. Details of AVP can be found in Chapter 11.

The release of AVP is stimulated by a drop in blood pressure, signalled by both high pressure and low pressure cardiopulmonary baroreceptors (or volume receptors). Their activity inhibits the production and release of AVP. When their firing rate is decreased as pressure falls, the inhibitory effect is reduced and AVP is released. The retention of water by AVP plus its vasoconstrictor effect raises pressure, acting as a negative feedback on the reflex. If blood pressure is raised, inhibition of AVP will cause less water to be reabsorbed at the kidney, fluid output is increased and blood pressure reduced. The action of AVP on the kidney is rapid, within a few minutes, and, with a half-life of about 15 minutes, it is relatively short-lived.

If pressure is adequate but body fluids are over-concentrated, AVP would again be released. This time the stimulus comes from osmoreceptors in the hypothalamus sensitive to changes in concentration. The retention of water at the kidney by AVP has the effect of diluting body fluids and restoring osmotic pressure to normal (see Ch. 14). In physiological terms, hydrostatic pressure takes precedence over osmotic pressure, and where blood pressure is severely reduced, water will be reclaimed even if body fluids are already dilute.

Renin angiotensin aldosterone mechanism

This system takes longer to adjust blood pressure than AVP but it can be maintained over a long period. It is initiated by a fall in blood pressure at the kidney and the release of the substance renin. This sets in train the series of reactions, the end result of which is the reabsorption of sodium ions at the nephron and the osmotic reabsorption of water with the sodium (Fig. 12.10).

The mechanism has the added advantage that angiotensin II acts as a vasoconstrictor of arteries and arterioles, reducing the overall capacity. It also promotes thirst and the intake of fluid. The whole mechanism, therefore, produces a rise in blood pressure by several regulatory routes.

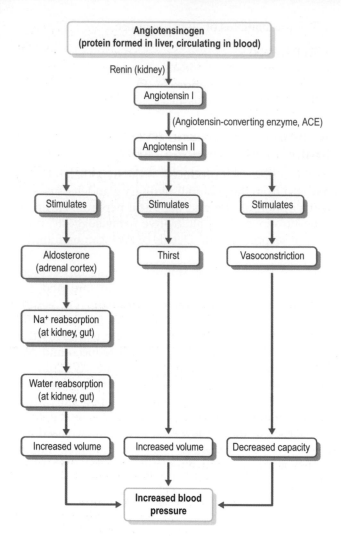

Figure 12.10 Renin, angiotensin, aldosterone mechanism. (After Watson 1999, with permission of Elsevier.)

The importance of this mechanism in the control of blood pressure can perhaps be appreciated when one realizes the large number of drugs developed to interfere with it. For example, a number of drugs which inhibit the activity of angiotensin-converting enzyme (ACE) have been developed. These are the ACE inhibitors such as captopril and enalapril which are used as antihypertensive agents. Spironolactone, a much older drug, is an antagonist to the receptors for aldosterone. It has a specialist use in some forms of liver disease and is not generally used as an anti-hypertensive agent.

Atrial natriuretic peptide (ANP)

ANP is a chemical mediator released by the cells of the atria in response to excess filling of the atria. Its presence would indicate venous return at either high volume or high pressure. It increases sodium (therefore water) output by the kidney, therefore reducing intravascular volume and systolic pressure. It also causes some vasodilation, particularly at small arteries and arterioles, thereby reducing peripheral resistance and diastolic pressure. ANP therefore reduces pressure by more than one regulatory route and reduces both systolic and diastolic pressures.

Fluid recovery from tissue

Tissues contain fluid surrounding the cells, mainly in the form of a gel. If blood pressure drops to a value below that in the tissue, fluid will migrate into the vessels. In an adult, in extreme hypotension, up to 500 ml can be retrieved. This is sometimes called internal fluid transfusion and evidence for its effectiveness can be seen in patients who have a low haematocrit following the loss of a large volume of blood.

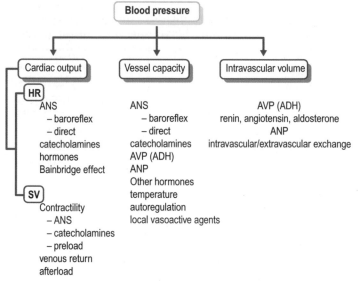

Figure 12.11 Summary of the mechanisms regulating blood pressure. ANS, autonomic nervous system; ANP, atrial natriuretic peptide; AVP, arginine vasopressin; ADH, antidiuretic hormone; HR, heart rate; SV, stroke volume.

SUMMARY OF MECHANISMS ADJUSTING BLOOD PRESSURE

Mechanisms adjusting blood pressure are summarized in Figure 12.11.

SYNCOPE – EVIDENCE OF COMPENSATORY ACTIVITY

In most normal circumstances, there will be no evidence of all the regulatory activity for either the subject or the observer. Even the individual who feels dizzy on standing up or getting out of bed is not conscious of 'postural hypotension'. They merely experience a brief tachycardia and the dizziness disappears.

Fainting or syncope can be an extension of the hypotensive effect of standing up. The individual loses consciousness due to lack of adequate cerebral perfusion. Inadequate venous return, due perhaps to pooling of the blood in the legs while standing in the heat, results in reduced cardiac output and a drop in arterial blood pressure. Falling to the ground (if done carefully) is probably the best remedy for fainting since venous return is greatly improved in a supine position. Some of the signs and symptoms of the compensatory mechanisms, pallor, tachycardia and so on, can be found among those listed in Table 12.1. A variant of syncope occurs when loss of consciousness is due to profound bradycardia and vasodilation, sometimes called a vaso-vagal attack. This may be a response to fear or emotional disturbance and results in a fall in sympathetic drive and an increase in vagal output. The initial symptoms are those of a simple faint, tachy-cardia, sweating etc., but the bradycardia which follows is profound and may last for several minutes. The response is thought to be analogous to the 'playing dead' response shown by some animals when attacked. Again, the action of bystanders should be to keep the individual in a supine or a recovery position. It is a mistake to try to prop this person up.

EVIDENCE OF RESPONSES TO A LARGE AND ACUTE DISTURBANCE IN BLOOD PRESSURE

The wide spread of responses to pressure disturbance can most easily be seen when the disturbance is large. Smaller disturbances will be compensated by all the mechanisms above, but the effects may not be visible and may not even be measurable. A large haemorrhage, however, produces such an acute loss in pressure that signs of the compensatory mechanisms in action become obvious.

The list of symptoms of acute haemorrhage shown in Table 12.1 can be found in many textbooks and will be familiar to many practitioners. The cardiovascular symptoms here are shown as either 'effect', i.e. which can be attributed to the low pressure itself, or 'response', where they are due to physiological compensation for the fall in pressure.

Table 12.1 Symptoms of acute haemorrhage

Hypotension	Effect
BP values	low systolic pressure, low volume venous return, low output – *effect*
	elevated diastolic pressure, reflex vasoconstriction – *response*
	narrow pulse pressure – result of the above
Tachycardia	baroreceptor reflex – *response*
	circulating catecholamines – *response*
Cold, pale skin	baroreceptor reflex vasoconstriction – *response*
	sympathomedullary response, redirection of flow – *response*
	angiotensin II – *response*
	AVP/ADH – *response*
Oliguria	AVP/ADH – *response*
	renin, angiotensin, aldosterone – *response*
	low glomerular filtration rate – *effect*

REFERENCES AND FURTHER READING

Aaronson P I, Ward J, Weiner C M, Schulman S P, Gill G S 1999 The cardiovascular system at a glance. Blackwell Science, London

Berne R M, Levy M N 2000 Cardiovascular physiology, 8th edn. Mosby, St Louis

Caro C G, Pedley T J, Schroter R C, Seed W A 1978 The mechanics of the circulation. Oxford University Press, Oxford

Clancy J, McVicar A J 1995 Physiology and anatomy – a homeostatic approach. Edward Arnold, London

Emslie-Smith D, Paterson C R, Scratcherd T, Read N W (eds) 1988 Textbook of physiology, 11th edn. Churchill Livingstone, Edinburgh

Ganong W F 2001 Review of medical physiology, 20th edn. McGraw-Hill Education, Philadelphia

Guyton A C, Hall J E 2000 Textbook of medical physiology, 10th edn. Saunders, Philadelphia

Guyton A C, Hall J E 2001 Guyton and Hall Pocket Companion to Textbook of medical physiology. Saunders, Philadelphia

Jordan D, Marshall J (eds) 1995 Cardiovascular regulation. Portland Press, London

Levick J R 1991 An introduction to cardiovascular physiology. Butterworth-Heinemann, London

Pocock G, Richards C D 1999 Human physiology: the basis of medicine. Oxford University Press, Oxford

Rogers A W 1992 Textbook of anatomy. Churchill Livingstone, Edinburgh

Simmons M L, Hicks G H 2000 Cardiopulmonary anatomy and physiology workbook. Saunders, London

Watson R 1999 Essential science for nursing students. Baillière Tindall, London

Just for interest

Chapman C B, Mitchell J H 1965 Starling on the heart. Dawsons, London

Te Koers H E D, Noble M M 1988 Starling's law of the heart revisited. Kluwer Academic, Dordrecht

13 Acid–base balance

In practice you may be asked to consider the following:

1. Acidity is due to the hydrogen ion (H+). As its concentration increases – what happens to pH?

2. Plasma pH is 7.35 to 7.45 – acidic? Or basic?

3. Buffers moderate changes in pH by taking up or giving up H+. Which is the 'renewable' buffer?

4. What is the role of haemoglobin in the maintenance of acid–base balance? What might be the effect on acid–base balance of a significant reduction in haemoglobin levels?

5. Chemoreceptors monitor CO_2 and H+. What is the effect on breathing of an increase in CO_2 production?

6. Voluntary hyperventilation or over-breathing can cause paraesthesia and cramp in the fingers and toes. Explain this. What simple therapeutic measure can help (apart from persuading the over-breather to try to breathe normally)?

7. What will be the renal compensation for voluntary hyperventilation?

8. Chronic hypercapnia will have the effect of dulling the response of the central chemoreceptors to CO_2. Breathing is then driven by peripheral hypoxic drive. What is this? What is the effect of giving oxygen to such a patient?

9. Chronic hypercapnia is likely to result in what type of acidosis? What confirming evidence would be available from plasma results?

10. What are the compensatory effects of metabolic acidosis, e.g. ketoacidosis? What confirming evidence would be available from plasma results?

This chapter is concerned with the regulation of one very important constituent of body fluids – the hydrogen ion (often written as H+). Homeostatic mechanisms exist within the body to ensure that conditions around body cells (including free, i.e. unbound, H+ levels) are maintained within acceptable limits. If this were not so, rapid fluctuations in the concentration of H+ would disrupt the delicate ion balance critical to the activity of excitable cells (muscle fibres and neurones). Furthermore, the forces which ensure the precise folding of the amino acid sequence of proteins, and therefore protein function as enzymes etc., would be disrupted. Severe changes in cell activity would result.

The various mechanisms which act to maintain free H^+ levels within a range compatible with life preserve what is collectively known as acid–base balance.

DEFINITIONS

An acid is a substance which dissociates when dissolved in water to yield free H^+ ions. Some physiological examples include:

- hydrochloric acid (HCl) produced by the stomach (see Ch. 9)
- carbonic acid (H_2CO_3) formed by all cells
- lactic acid ($CH_3.CHOH.COOH$) from anaerobic glycolysis (see Ch. 10).

These free H^+ released from acids have the potential to cause biological damage. A *strong* acid dissociates completely to yield a large number of free H^+ while a *weak* acid does not dissociate significantly. Many of the H^+ are not released but remain bound as a molecule; only free H^+ are acidic.

Using HCl as an example:

$$\underset{2}{\overset{1}{HCl \rightleftharpoons}} H^+ + Cl^-$$

$$\text{Acid} \qquad \text{Hydrogen ion}$$

If reaction 1 occurs to a large extent, the acid will be described as *strong*. If reaction 1 proceeds to a minor extent and reaction 2 occurs so that any free H^+ formed immediately recombine, then very little free H^+ will be produced and the acid is referred to as *weak*. HCl is a strong acid, reaction 1 dominates and a large number of free H^+ are released.

A base is a molecule within body fluids which has the ability to combine with free H^+. It is thus able to counteract large increases in body H^+ levels. Again the terms strong and weak may be used. A *strong* base rapidly binds (removes) free H^+ from solution. A *weak* base is not so powerful in this respect (Fig. 13.1).

MEASUREMENT OF [H⁺] LEVELS IN BODY FLUIDS

(The sign [ ] denotes the molar concentration of a substance per litre of solution, see below.)

Rapid changes in H^+ levels in body fluids represent a serious threat to health. It follows that it is important to monitor changes in body fluid H^+ levels and this can be done by monitoring fluid H^+ levels or pH.

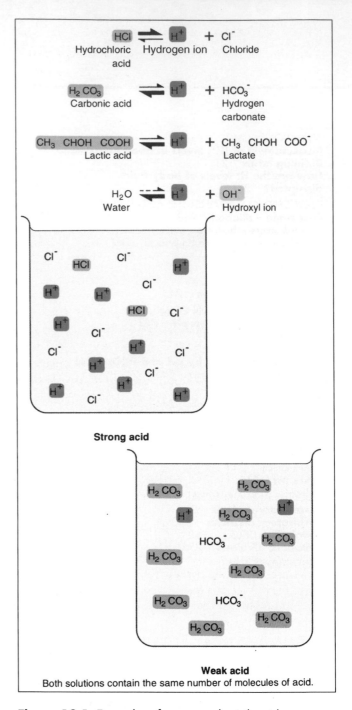

Figure 13.1 Examples of strong and weak acids.

The H^+ concentration levels can be quoted directly as moles per litre or, because there are actually very few free H^+ and the numbers become easier to manage, as nmoles/l (where nanomoles represent 10^{-9} moles).

An alternative method is to express each H^+ concentration as pH where pH = $-\log [H^+]$ (Table 13.1).

This calculation of pH can only be done if the $[H^+]$ is first expressed in mol/l. pH values and $[H^+]$ reported in terms of nmol/l are much easier to handle and

Table 13.1 Different units used to describe the concentration of hydrogen ions

[H⁺] mol/l		pH	nmol/l
1	10^0	0	
0.1	10^{-1}	1	
0.01	10^{-2}	2	
0.001	10^{-3}	3	
0.0001	10^{-4}	4	
0.00001	10^{-5}	5	
0.000001	10^{-6}	6	1000
0.0000001	10^{-7}	7	100
		7.4	40
0.00000001	10^{-8}	8	10
0.000000001	10^{-9}	9	1
0.0000000001	10^{-10}	10	0.1

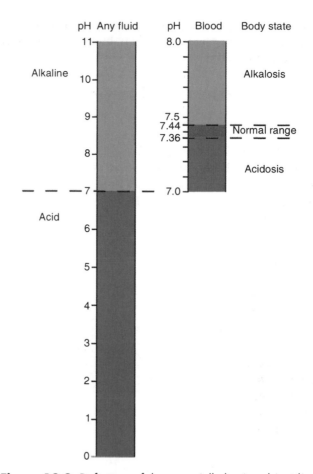

Figure 13.2 Definition of the terms 'alkaline' and 'acid', and 'alkalosis' and 'acidosis'.

laboratories within the UK may use either of these two methods. The important point is that if [H⁺] for example rises, then the value of pH will fall because the latter is a negative logarithmic scale, i.e. the more acidic, the lower the pH. The higher the pH value, the fewer the H⁺ there will be and the more basic or alkaline the solution.

DEFINING TERMS

A chemist would describe a neutral solution as one with a pH of 7.0. It is neither acidic nor basic. Solutions of pH less than 7.0 are referred to as *acidic* while those of pH greater than 7.0 are referred to as *basic* or *alkaline*. Although the latter two terms do not strictly mean the same thing, they are often used interchangeably.

It is important to remember that the normal ranges within arterial plasma for [H⁺] (36 to 44 nmol/l) and pH (7.44 to 7.36) are the reference points for describing the [H⁺] or pH of blood.

When H⁺ accumulate, the blood will become more acidic, [H⁺] exceeds 44 nmol/l and the blood is termed acidaemic (aemia – blood). Similarly, if H⁺ levels fall, the blood effectively becomes more alkaline and the term alkalaemic is applied when [H⁺] is less than 36 nmol/l or pH >7.44.

The change in body physiology that promoted the acidic conditions in body fluids is termed acidosis while alkalosis refers similarly to some disease or body conditions that promoted alkaline conditions (Fig. 13.2).

HOW ARE THE H⁺ LEVELS OF BODY FLUIDS DISRUPTED?

While the final sections of this chapter will consider disease states which can disrupt body H⁺ levels, it is important to appreciate that normal body metabolism generates a large number of H⁺ which represent a potentially serious threat to homeostasis (see Table 13.2). The low number of H⁺ actually found in body fluids is a tribute to the body's mechanisms for dealing with them.

In health these accumulating H⁺ are temporarily contained (by mechanisms to be described below) and then eliminated from the body.

H⁺ are generated in the following ways:

1. Carbon dioxide, which reacts with water to form carbonic acid, is produced by body cells. The equivalent of 13 moles of acid are formed in this way each day. Two points are important: (a) mechanisms must exist within the blood to ensure that the free H⁺ generated by the cells in the above reaction are transferred safely to the lungs (this is the job of blood buffers described in the following section); (b) in the lungs this reaction is reversed. Thus when respiration keeps pace with body metabolism, serious disruption of body H⁺ levels due to the accumulation of free H⁺ is avoided. The CO_2 is eliminated from the body. It

follows, however, that should the lungs become less efficient, serious changes in body H^+ levels will result (see equation below):

$$\text{tissue} \searrow \quad CO_2 + H_2O \rightleftarrows H_2CO_3 \rightleftarrows H^+ + HCO_3^- \rightleftarrows H_2O + CO_2 \quad \nearrow \text{lungs}$$

2. Breakdown of dietary protein and fat also yields acidic compounds. In addition, anaerobic muscle activity produces lactic acid.
3. Certain conditions may also yield acidic compounds, e.g. ketoacids are produced when fat is broken down in, e.g., diabetes (see Chs 10 and 18).

This production of acidic compounds by normal body activity is considerable and continuous (see Table 13.2) and although there are also sources of alkaline-promoting compounds in body metabolism, generally the acid threat to body homeostasis is of greater magnitude.

BODY DEFENCES AGAINST THE ACID THREAT

The defences of the body can be viewed in four stages:

- dilution
- buffering
- excretion at lungs
- excretion by kidneys.

FIRST STAGE – DILUTION

The first stage is very simple and relatively instantaneous in effect. H^+ produced are diluted in the large water content of the body. By dilution the strength of the acid threat is reduced.

SECOND STAGE – BUFFERS

The second line of defence is also quick to act and involves chemicals present in body fluids called buffers. Remember that only free hydrogen ions are acidic and therefore dangerous; bound or complexed H^+ are not acidic. Buffers chemically bind free H^+ so that they are locked to a molecule and no longer acidic.

In practice a buffer is composed of two compounds; one which will bind H^+ when they are in excess while the other yields H^+ when their numbers in the surrounding fluid start to fall. In this way $[H^+]$ are maintained within an acceptable range – neither too low nor too high.

Three important body buffer systems are hydrogen carbonate/carbonic acid, phosphate and proteins.

Ketoacidosis

During periods of prolonged starvation, the body's energy requirements are met by the breakdown of stored fats and proteins, rather than by a continuing intake of carbohydrates. Similarly, in untreated or poorly controlled type 1 diabetes, a deficiency of insulin prevents the effective use of glucose for energy production by insulin-sensitive cells. Consequently, fats and proteins are used instead. Even at rest, the body is still using energy, for example to keep warm, for new cell production, tissue repair, enzyme and hormone production, maintenance of muscle tone and respiration. Metabolism of fats under such conditions – starvation or uncontrolled diabetes mellitus – leads to the accumulation of ketone bodies in the bloodstream (see Chs 10, 15 and 18) and, consequently, in the urine, where they may be detected by the use of dipsticks. Ketone bodies consist of β-hydroxybutyric acid, acetoacetic acid and acetone, the first two being acids. Ketosis is the state where there is an accumulation of ketone bodies. Ketoacidosis exists where the acidity can no longer be compensated and plasma pH is actually reduced. Ketoacidosis is a form of metabolic acidosis (see p. 250).

Hydrogen carbonate/carbonic acid

$$CO_2 + H_2O \rightleftarrows H_2CO_3 \rightleftarrows H^+ + HCO_3^-$$

The hydrogen carbonate/carbonic acid buffer (or bicarbonate buffer) system is the most important buffer existing in the interstitial fluid around cells and in plasma. This importance stems from two facts: (i) a high concentration of buffer constituents exists in extracellular fluid (ECF) and (ii) two buffer constituents can be regulated – CO_2 by the lungs, and HCO_3^- by the kidneys. This system is sometimes referred to as the 'renewable' buffer.

Phosphate

Disodium hydrogen phosphate (Na_2HPO_4) and sodium dihydrogen phosphate (NaH_2PO_4) together form a buffer system because this pair of compounds can accept or donate a H^+ when it is necessary to maintain pH. This buffering system is very important inside body cells. It also plays an important role as a urinary buffer and enables large amounts of acid to be excreted safely in the urine (see Chs 8, 14).

Proteins

Proteins can act as buffers, binding and releasing hydrogen ions, because they contain some amino acids like aspartic acid that are acidic and some like lysine that are basic.

Table 13.2 Acids and bases formed in body metabolism

Acid	Source	Base
Carbonic acid	Carbon dioxide	Hydrogen carbonate
Lactic acid	Anaerobic glycolysis	Lactate
Aceto-acetic acid	Ketone bodies from fat metabolism	Aceto-acetate
Beta-hydroxybutyric acid		Beta-hydroxybutyrate
Sulphuric acid	Sulphur-containing amino acids	Sulphate
Phosphoric acid	Nucleic acids	Phosphate
Uric acid	Purines in nucleic acids	Urate
Acetic acid	Metabolism of dietary fibre by colonic bacteria	Acetate
Propionic acid		Propionate
Butyric acid		Butyrate
Ammonium	Protein metabolism	Ammonia

Proteins act as buffers both outside and inside cells. The plasma proteins (see Ch. 3) act as buffers in blood plasma. Of the huge variety of intracellular proteins, haemoglobin in the erythrocytes (see Chs 3 and 7) is of note. It buffers the H^+ derived from carbonic acid and thus facilitates the transport of carbon dioxide in blood to the lungs (see Ch. 7).

THIRD STAGE – LUNGS

The third line of defence against the acid threat is the body's respiratory system. The lungs, by changing the depth and frequency of respiration, can alter the amount of CO_2 lost from the body. The equation showing the generation and subsequent excretion of CO_2 (see p. 242) shows why a change in CO_2 levels will produce a change in levels of $[H^+]$ in blood or, conversely why a change in H^+ production changes CO_2 output.

FOURTH STAGE – KIDNEYS

The final and fourth line of defence is the kidneys. This response to an acid–base disturbance is slow. Responses one and two are virtually instantaneous, the respiratory response occurs within minutes, while the kidneys may take several hours or even days to correct, i.e. compensate for a change in body $[H^+]$. However, any shortcomings in terms of speed are counterbalanced by the power of the response. The kidneys can bring about the correction of altered $[H^+]$ by

- changing the amount of H^+ secreted in urine
- changing the amount of HCO_3^- secreted in urine
- by generating new HCO_3^- to raise plasma levels.

RESPIRATORY REGULATION OF pH

The large amount of carbon dioxide produced in metabolism is a continual threat to the maintenance of pH. However, carbon dioxide is safely transported to the lungs by the buffer systems as HCO_3^- and carbaminohaemoglobin (see Ch. 7). It is then efficiently excreted by the lungs and the amount excreted can be altered by changing the ventilation of the lungs.

EFFECTS OF VENTILATION ON pH

If ventilation increases, more fresh air is added to the gas mixture inside the lungs, and the concentration of carbon dioxide in alveolar air decreases. As a result, the gradient for the diffusion of carbon dioxide from the blood to the alveolar air gets steeper and more carbon dioxide is eliminated from the blood per minute. Thus, the concentration of carbon dioxide in body fluids decreases and the amount of carbonic acid (and thus H^+) in the body fluids decreases also. In other words, the pH increases.

Hyperventilation

Voluntary over-ventilation of the lungs, or over-breathing, can decrease the $[H^+]$ of blood from 40 to 32 nmol/l (pH 7.4 to 7.5) within a matter of seconds, causing dizziness. The dizziness is caused by the increase in pH and decrease in carbon dioxide concentration. These changes provoke a variety of effects including cerebral vasoconstriction and a decrease in the concentration of free calcium in body fluids. Both of these effects influence nerve cell function indirectly and directly. A period of hyperventilation is followed by apnoea (no breathing) during which the CO_2 levels can build up enough to trigger breathing. Many people

The ventilated patient

We automatically adjust the rate and depth of our respirations throughout the varying events of a normal day – walking to work, running up stairs, relaxing after a meal, and sleeping. Unless our breathing becomes very fast or laboured, we are probably quite unaware of the changes which occur. By contrast, a patient on a ventilator in an intensive care unit is usually unable to make such adjustments for himself. Often, such a patient is sedated, and his voluntary muscles (including those involved in respiration) are paralysed by means of drugs, so that he does not struggle to breathe against the machine but allows it to breathe for him. Consequently, once the ventilator is set to deliver a certain volume of air a number of times per minute, this 'minute volume' does not vary.

Regular analysis of arterial blood gases is carried out in order to ascertain that PO_2, PCO_2 and pH are within normal limits. If, for example, blood levels of CO_2 rise, and the pH falls, the ventilator may be adjusted to deliver a slightly greater volume of air at each stroke, or a higher number of strokes per minute, or both. (Note that increasing the oxygen intake would not bring down a raised PCO_2 level.) The danger is that prolonged inadequate ventilation of a patient, together with infrequent blood gas analysis, may lead to a rise in PCO_2 and a fall in pH (i.e. an acidotic state).

Patient restlessness may sometimes (but not always) be attributable to changes in CO_2 levels. For example, if the PCO_2 rises because of, say, inadequate ventilation, this will stimulate the patient's respiratory centre, causing him, if under-sedated, to breathe against the ventilator. (That is, he attempts to breathe for himself, his own respiration rate going against the rhythm of the ventilator.) Raising the ventilator's minute volume may help calm the patient by reducing his CO_2 level and, therefore, his respiratory drive. Patient restlessness is likeliest to occur when his sedation and paralysing drugs are wearing off.

Similarly, when a patient is being 'weaned off' a ventilator PCO_2 is allowed to rise by, for example, reducing the ventilator's stroke volume or decreasing its rate per minute. Consequently, when the effects of sedative and paralysing agents have worn off, the patient's respiratory drive is enhanced by the increased carbon dioxide level.

Hyperventilation and tetany

Hyperventilation raises the pH sufficiently to cause a reduction in the free calcium ion concentration in ECF. Muscle contracts and is unable to relax – tetany – and the parts most affected are fingers and toes which curl up giving the characteristic signs of carpo-pedal spasm. The remedy is to persuade the individual to rebreathe their own air from a bag or a cup. The higher concentration of CO_2 in the expired air raises plasma CO_2, lowers pH and allows the concentration of free calcium ions in ECF to increase.

Correcting severe acidosis

In the event of cardiac arrest, the victim's respirations will cease within a short time of the heart stopping. (Indeed, cessation of breathing may have been the cause of cardiac arrest.) As a consequence, the concentration of CO_2 in the patient's body fluids will rise, and the pH will fall. This is because carbon dioxide is no longer being blown off from the lungs at each expiration. Instead, it is accumulating in the body. At the same time, the lack of delivery of oxygen to the tissues results in the formation of lactic acid by anaerobic glycolysis. This makes the pH fall even further and depletes hydrogen carbonate in the body fluids.

First-aid measures consist of mouth-to-mouth resuscitation and cardiac massage until more effective artificial ventilation can be attempted using an endotracheal tube, through which high levels of oxygen can be delivered. Further resuscitation measures will include the administration of drugs and/or direct current electric shocks but, unless the patient's acidotic state is reversed, these will be to no avail. The longer the patient remains without adequate ventilation and circulation, the deeper will be his acidotic state.

High levels of oxygen delivered via an endotracheal tube, together with effective cardiac massage, should be successful in achieving circulation of well-oxygenated blood, an increase in the PO_2 of the body fluids and, because CO_2 is now being blown off, a fall in PCO_2. The pH should rise and the patient's acidotic state will be reversed. In the event of extended resuscitation measures, intravenous sodium bicarbonate (sodium hydrogen carbonate) 8.4% will be given to counteract the patient's low pH. However, this infusion should not be required if successful resuscitation is achieved quickly.

have seen an example of this when a screaming child suddenly stops breathing, much to the consternation of those around.

Hypoventilation

Conversely under-ventilation, or breath holding, leads to the retention of carbon dioxide, and therefore of acid, within the body. Consequently the [H⁺] increases (pH decreases). Most people can hold their breath for at least half a minute. In this time, blood pH decreases from 7.4 to 7.35. There is a limit to how long you can hold your breath. When CO_2 and H⁺ reach a critical level the brain stem centres will compel you to breathe.

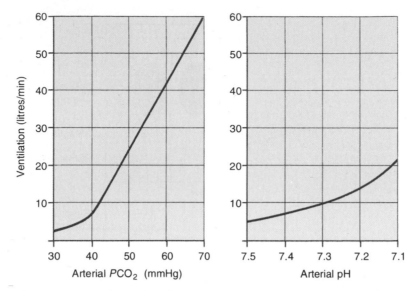

Figure 13.3 Relationships between blood PCO_2 and pH, and ventilation of the lungs. CO_2 is a more effective stimulant of breathing than is blood pH. (After Guyton 1986, with permission of Elsevier.)

CONTROL OF VENTILATION BY pH AND PCO_2

Normally, ventilation of the lungs is reflexly adjusted by the nervous system in such a way that arterial blood pH and arterial PCO_2 are stabilized at 7.4 and 40 mmHg (5.3 kPa) respectively. The effects of arterial pH and CO_2 on ventilation are illustrated in Figure 13.3. Even small changes in PCO_2, above and below the normal arterial value of 40 mmHg (5.3 kPa), cause significant changes in the rate and depth of breathing. This is strikingly different from the effects of oxygen (see Ch. 7), and makes clear how important CO_2 is as a regulator of breathing.

The respiratory centres (see Ch. 7) are influenced by impulses from chemoreceptors, some of which monitor the composition of the arterial blood (peripheral chemoreceptors), and some the extracellular fluid in the brain (central chemoreceptors) (Fig. 13.4).

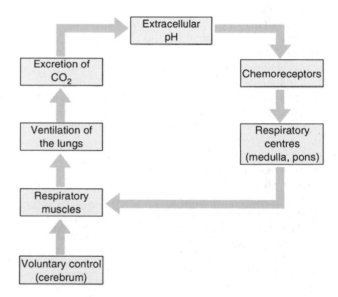

Figure 13.4 Control of extracellular pH by regulating the ventilation of the lungs.

Peripheral chemoreceptors

The peripheral chemoreceptors are the same as those that respond to the PO_2 of blood. They are located on the main arteries leaving the heart.

These receptors are only weakly responsive to changes in arterial CO_2 (unlike the central chemoreceptors in the brain – see below). However, changes in arterial [H$^+$] do induce changes in ventilation, e.g. a rise in [H$^+$] will stimulate respiration in ketoacidosis. The peripheral chemoreceptors play an important role in alerting the brain to changes in arterial [H$^+$] not caused by changes in CO_2 levels. If [H$^+$] increases (i.e. pH

decreases), the chemoreceptors are stimulated, and ventilation of the lungs reflexly increases. As a result, the elimination of carbon dioxide is enhanced, the concentration of carbonic acid in body fluids decreases and [H$^+$] is stabilized (Fig. 13.5).

Central chemoreceptors

The central chemoreceptors are situated close to the front (ventral) surface of the medulla oblongata, near to the respiratory control centres (Fig. 13.5 and Ch. 7).

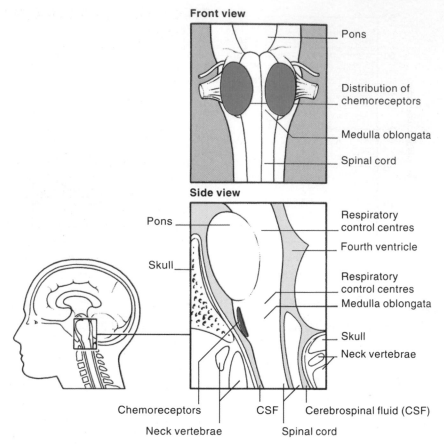

Figure 13.5 The situation of the central chemoreceptors in the brain in relation to the pons and medulla of the brain stem (top) and cerebrospinal fluid and base of the skull (bottom).

These receptors are responsive to changes in arterial CO_2 levels. The relationship is indirect, for the CO_2 is able to cross the blood–brain barrier, enter the brain ECF, and there react with water to release H^+. It is this ion that stimulates the respiration

$$CO_2 + H_2O \rightleftharpoons H_2CO_3 \rightleftharpoons H^+ + HCO_3^-$$

The lack of protein in the brain ECF means that there is less buffering of the H^+ and the H^+ is free to stimulate the central chemoreceptors. Only a small increase in arterial PCO_2 is needed to change the $[H^+]$ significantly to excite the central chemoreceptors.

The presence of the blood–brain barrier also explains why the central chemoreceptors are not directly affected by $[H^+]$ changes in blood (Fig. 13.6).

RENAL REGULATION OF pH

The excretion of acid and base by the kidneys inevitably occurs over a longer period of time than the minute to minute adjustments made by the respiratory system. The kidneys contribute in three main ways to acid–base balance. They:

- allow the excretion of bases such as HCO_3^-, SO_4^{2-}, HPO_4^{2-}
- recover and manufacture HCO_3^-
- excrete H^+.

EXCRETION OF BASES

The filtration of between 150 and 200 litres of fluid per day allows many compounds to be cleared from the blood, including bases gained in the diet or produced in metabolism. Provided that there are no specific uptake mechanisms which retrieve them from the tubular fluid, and provided they do not escape from the tubular fluid by passive diffusion (see Chs 8 and 14), bases will be automatically excreted in the urine. Drugs like salicylate and their metabolites are cleared from the body fluids in this way (Fig. 13.7).

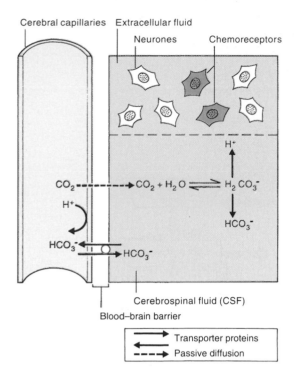

Cerebral capillaries   Extracellular fluid

Neurones   Chemoreceptors

Cerebrospinal fluid (CSF)

Blood–brain barrier

→ Transporter proteins
----> Passive diffusion

Figure 13.6 Relationships between cerebral capillaries, cerebrospinal fluid and neuronal extracellular fluid. The central chemoreceptors are excited by an increase in hydrogen ion concentration in the extracellular fluid, but not by an increase in H^+ in the blood. H^+ ions cannot easily cross the blood–brain barrier but CO_2 can. CSF H^+ concentration is regulated in the long term by the transport of hydrogen carbonate across the blood–brain barrier.

Testing urine pH can provide valuable information about a patient's physiological condition. For example, if the pH of a patient's urine was acidic and then rises, this may have been caused by changes in diet, medication or the effectiveness of respiration. Alkaline urine may, in some circumstances, prompt arterial blood sampling for blood gas analysis, and this may show a raised HCO_3^- level.

Bases that are vital constituents of the body such as hydrogen carbonate (see below), hydrogen phosphate and sulphate are normally recovered by specific transport mechanisms, but are excreted in the urine if they are present in excess. For example, if there is an excess of HCO_3^- in the plasma, the amount of HCO_3^- delivered to the tubules in the filtrate is greater than the absorptive capacity of the tubules for this ion, and the surplus is excreted in the urine in the form of sodium hydrogen carbonate. This makes the urine alkaline.

RECOVERY AND MANUFACTURE OF HCO_3^-

About 0.33 kg of $NaHCO_3$ are filtered by the renal glomeruli each day. This is 7 to 8 times the total amount present in the body as a whole. As HCO_3^- is part of one of the buffer systems that help to stabilize pH, its fate in the kidney tubules (whether it is recovered or eliminated) is crucial to the maintenance of homeostasis. HCO_3^- is recovered from the tubular fluid by the processes shown in Figure 13.8A. Hydrogen ions secreted by the tubular cells combine with HCO_3^- in the tubular fluid forming CO_2. CO_2 diffuses easily into the cells and is used to recreate HCO_3^- which is then secreted into the blood. In effect, H^+ recycle between the cells and the tubular fluid while HCO_3^- is reabsorbed. The process is catalysed by the enzyme carbonic anhydrase (see Chs 3 and 8).

The amount of HCO_3^- recovered by the kidneys depends upon several factors including the pH and PCO_2 of the plasma. When the body contains more acid than usual, all the filtered HCO_3^- is recovered but, in addition, new HCO_3^- is manufactured by the cells and secreted into the blood (Fig. 13.8A). This replenishes the lowered stocks of HCO_3^- in the extracellular fluid, which were used up in buffering the extra acid.

Likewise, if the PCO_2 is greater than normal (as for example when ventilation is impaired) more carbonic acid is formed by the convoluted tubules and more HCO_3^- is generated and secreted into the blood. Simultaneously, H^+ are excreted into the tubular fluid and voided in the urine (Fig. 13.8B).

EXCRETION OF H^+

H^+ are secreted into the tubular fluid by the tubular cells in exchange for sodium ions (Figs 13.8 and 13.9). Secreted H^+ that are not used to recover hydrogen carbonate are mopped up mainly by two urinary bases, hydrogen phosphate (HPO_4^{2-}) and ammonia (NH_3), and are excreted in the urine in the form of dihydrogen phosphate (H_2PO_4) and ammonium ion (NH_4^+) respectively (Fig. 13.9). This allows H^+ to be excreted in large amounts without causing a large change in urine pH.

Dihydrogen phosphate

Disodium hydrogen phosphate (Na_2HPO_4) and sodium dihydrogen phosphate (NaH_2PO_4) form a buffer system (see p. 242). As H^+ are added to the tubular fluid, disodium hydrogen phosphate is converted into sodium dihydrogen phosphate. The sodium released is absorbed and the H^+ are safely eliminated in the urine in the form of sodium dihydrogen phosphate (Fig. 13.9).

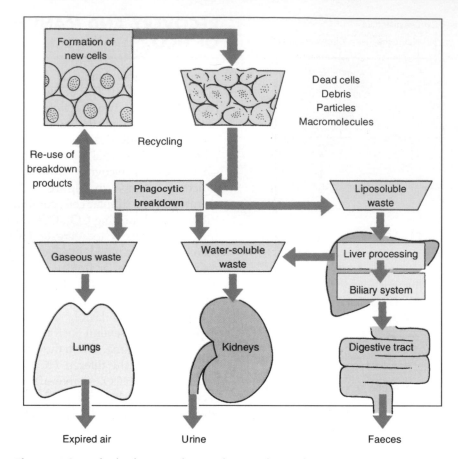

Figure 13.7 The body's recycling and waste-disposal systems.

Ammonium

The cells of the distal convoluted tubule manufacture ammonia from glutamine. The reaction is catalysed by the enzyme glutaminase, whose activity is affected by the pH of the intracellular fluid. Under acid conditions enzyme activity increases, and more ammonia is formed. Ammonia (NH_3) is soluble both in water and in lipids and diffuses quite freely from the cells into the tubular fluid. Here it combines reversibly with any secreted hydrogen ions to yield 'ammonium' (NH_4^+). The ammonium group does not diffuse easily across cell membranes. Consequently, H^+ secreted into the tubular fluid are trapped there and eliminated in the urine chiefly as ammonium chloride.

$$NH_4^+ \quad + \quad OH^- \quad + \quad H^+Cl^- \rightarrow NH_4Cl \quad + \quad H_2O$$

ammonium + hydroxyl ion + hydrochloric acid → ammonium chloride + water

This is another example of a buffer system. The reaction between ammonia and H^+ ions can be represented as:

$$NH_3 + H^+ \rightleftharpoons NH_4^+$$

Whenever there is net secretion of acid in the urine, some will always be excreted in the ammonium form.

When conditions require the conservation of acid and the excretion of an alkaline urine, ammonium disappears from the urine.

URINE pH

The pH of the urine can range between 4.5 and 8.4. Most often the pH is acid, simply because the consumption of diets containing meat inevitably generates acid for excretion. During fasting, the pH of urine will be acid also because of the catabolism of endogenous proteins. On a vegetarian diet, however, urinary pH may be alkaline because the metabolism of such diets may yield an excess of base.

ACIDOSIS AND ALKALOSIS

A disturbance of acid–base balance in the body, i.e. a deviation from the normal range of [H^+], can arise either from a change in the activity of the respiratory system or by the loss or accumulation of [H^+] as a result of some change in metabolism. Thus the cause

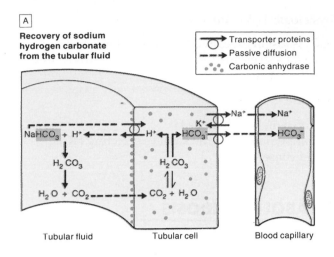

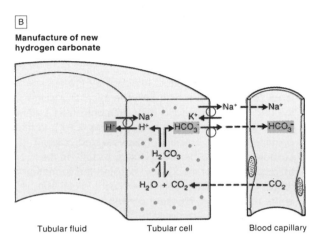

Figure 13.8 Processes involved in (A) the recovery and (B) the manufacture of hydrogen carbonate (HCO_3^-) by the kidneys.

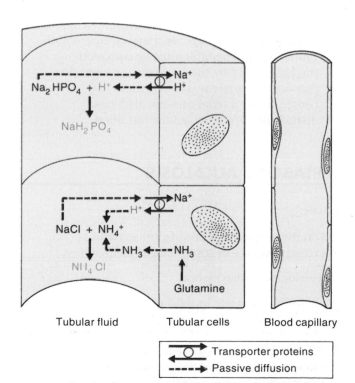

Figure 13.9 Renal excretion of H^+ in the form of dihydrogen phosphate ($H_2PO_4^-$) and of ammonium (NH_4^+).

of the change can be a respiratory or metabolic problem. If the change causes a rise in $[H^+]$, it is termed a respiratory or metabolic acidosis, while a fall in $[H^+]$ will result from a respiratory or metabolic alkalosis.

Two important points: A respiratory cause which alters $[H^+]$ will be evident as a change in plasma CO_2 levels – the lungs are either retaining or exhaling too much CO_2 and it is this change which is altering $[H^+]$. However, if the change is an accumulation of H^+ from acids produced by metabolism, the body responds first by attempting to buffer these ions with HCO_3^-. Thus a metabolic cause of acid–base disturbance will be evident as a change in plasma HCO_3^- levels.

RESPIRATORY ACIDOSIS

Cause:

- chronic obstructive pulmonary disease
- breath holding
- chemical or physical damage to the respiratory centres in brain stem.

Renal calculi: the pH of urine

Of the many causes of urinary tract calculi (stones), one is the tendency of certain substances (including the minerals calcium and phosphates) to be deposited in urine of a particular pH. Urate and uric acid stones, for example, can form in urine with a low pH. Following removal of such calculi, either surgically or, more frequently, by being passed spontaneously via the urethra, prevention of recurrences consists of a high fluid intake in order to dilute the urine, and drugs such as potassium citrate which, by generating hydrogen carbonate, increase the base content of the body and raise urinary pH.

Conversely, urinary tract infection by *Proteus* species leads to urine with a high pH. The microorganisms split the uric acid in urine and form ammonia (NH_3) which reacts with water to form hydroxyl ions (OH^-). In this alkaline medium, calcium phosphate and calcium carbonate tend to be precipitated, usually in the inflamed pelvis of the kidney, causing the formation of large, chalky calculi. Sometimes such calculi can fill the entire renal pelvis, blocking passage of urine and causing severe renal damage. The shape of such calculi gives rise to their somewhat imaginative name: staghorn calculi. A large calculus such as a staghorn used only to be removed by surgery, but newer methods have been developed which cause the stone to disintegrate. (Examination of specimens of calculi will demonstrate that phosphate and calcium carbonate stones are much more brittle and 'crumbly' than the smoother, harder uric acid and urate stones.)

Physiological consequence:

- CO_2 retained accumulates
- $[H^+]$ rises (pH falls), equation below moves to the right:

$$CO_2 + H_2O \rightleftarrows H_2CO_3 \rightleftarrows H^+ + HCO_3^-$$

Response to a rise in $[H^+]$:

1. Buffers absorb excess $[H^+]$.
2. Long-term compensation is via the kidneys, causing retention of HCO_3^- to counteract the accumulated $[H^+]$. NB, if the lungs are damaged, they cannot compensate for their own shortcomings.

RESPIRATORY ALKALOSIS

Cause:

- hyperventilation.

Physiological consequence

- CO_2 is lost in excessive amounts and as a result the $[H^+]$ falls (see equation above, equation driven to the left).

Response

1. Buffers in body release H^+.
2. Compensation via the kidneys excreting HCO_3^- and conserving H^+.

METABOLIC ACIDOSIS

Cause:

- production of lactic acid following excessive exercise
- production of ketoacids in diabetes mellitus
- severe diarrhoea leading to loss of HCO_3^-
- renal disease (H^+ not excreted).

Physiological consequence:

- accumulation of H^+ or loss of HCO_3^-.

Response:

1. Chemical buffers bind to excess H^+.
2. The lungs blow off CO_2 in an attempt to lower $[H^+]$ (see equation in col. 1 on p. 242).
3. The kidneys excrete H^+ and conserve HCO_3^-. However, if the cause of this disturbance was renal disease, this final response, renal compensation, cannot occur. The fault must be corrected predominantly by the respiratory system. In practice, this system is less efficient and consequently a renal cause of acid–base disturbance is a very serious condition.

METABOLIC ALKALOSIS

Cause:

- vomiting leading to loss of stomach acid
- excessive intake of some antacid medications.

Physiological consequence:

- fall in $[H^+]$ and rise in $[HCO_3^-]$.

Response:

1. Chemical buffers release $[H^+]$.
2. Respiration rate is reduced, thus CO_2 is retained. This in turn generates H^+, and is respiratory compensation.

CASE STUDIES

When interpreting a potential acid–base disturbance it is important to

- consider blood pH or H$^+$ and whether there is evidence of alkalaemia or acidaemia
- check out the blood CO_2 level
- check the blood bicarbonate level
- consider the case history – has the acidaemia/alkalaemia been present for some time (in which case compensation has had time to become effective) or has the condition occurred relatively recently?

Consider the following two case studies.

A young woman became very nervous and anxious as she waited for her appointment time in the dentist's surgery. The following blood analysis results might have been obtained: [H$^+$] = 30 nmol/l is low, CO_2 is low, and HCO_3^- is normal.

The [H+] result suggests an alkalaemia (see Fig. 13.2), while the change in CO_2 levels suggests a respiratory disturbance. The case details of rapid onset and the lack of change in levels of HCO_3^- suggest that there has been insufficient time for metabolic compensation by the kidneys to occur. Thus this case represents a primary respiratory alkalaemia.

The second case study is more complex and *all* the information in the case history is relevant.

An elderly man is admitted to hospital with chronic bronchitis. The [H$^+$] is normal. However, the CO_2 levels and HCO_3^- levels are raised.

The [H$^+$] is apparently normal but two important determinants of plasma H$^+$ levels are altered (HCO_3^- and CO_2). The chronic nature of the condition and the fact that the man suffers from bronchitis are relevant. There has been sufficient time for compensation to occur, and the apparently normal [H$^+$] suggests that the disorder is fully compensated.

The presence of bronchitis will cause retention of CO_2 (raising CO_2 levels and [H$^+$]) which in time will trigger renal compensation which will promote retention of HCO_3^- in an attempt to counter the raised [H$^+$]. The underlying condition (bronchitis) has not changed but the acid–base disturbance has been fully compensated by the action of the kidney.

This study illustrates the difference between *acidaemia* – a term used to describe the [H$^+$] within blood, and *acidosis* – a term used to describe the original cause of the disturbance.

The above case study describes a fully compensated respiratory acidosis.

'Air hunger' in diabetic ketoacidosis

Air hunger is a form of dyspnoea where the patient entering a ketoacidotic state takes rapid, deep sighing breaths. It can be distressing both for the patient (if conscious) and for the relatives. An alternative name for air hunger is Kussmaul respirations. In ketoacidosis, respirations increase in both rate and depth in response to [H$^+$]. This increase in carbon dioxide breathed out compensates for the metabolic acidosis.

REFERENCES AND FURTHER READING

Abelow B 1998 Understanding acid-base. Williams & Wilkins, Baltimore, MD

Anderson J R (ed) 1980 Muir's Textbook of pathology, 12th edn. Edward Arnold, London

Carroll H J, Oh M S 1989 Water, electrolyte and acid–base metabolism: diagnosis and management, 2nd edn. J B Lippincott, Philadelphia

Goldberger E 1986 A primer of water, electrolyte and acid–base syndromes, 8th edn. Lea & Febiger, Philadelphia
Advanced, clinically oriented text. Large well-referenced section on acid–base balance. Useful for following up original work

Guyton 1986 Textbook of medical physiology, 7th edn. W B Saunders, Philadelphia, p 508

Guyton A C, Hall J E 1996 Textbook of medical physiology, 9th edn. W B Saunders, Philadelphia

Hainsworth R (ed) 1986 Acid–base balance. Physiological Society Study Guide No. 1, Manchester University Press, Manchester
Detailed explanation of all aspects of acid–base balance for students and teachers

Higgins C 2000 Understanding laboratory investigations. Blackwell Science, Oxford

Sherwood L 2000 Human physiology from cells to systems, 4th edn. Brooks/Cole, Pacific Grove

Workman L M 1991 Introduction to fluids, electrolytes and acid–base balance. W B Saunders, Philadelphia
Clear basic text describing and explaining fundamental principles as well as examining causes and consequences of common disturbances

In practice you may be asked to consider the following:

1. On average, which are wetter, men or women? By how much? And why?

2. A severely hyperkalaemic patient is prescribed intravenous insulin and glucose. How does this lower the plasma potassium level?

3. A 50 kg elderly patient has been receiving 3 litres of normal saline daily since her operation three days ago. She has developed severe oedema. Why?

4. A patient admitted through Accident and Emergency has a plasma osmolality of 315 mosmol/kg (normal range 285–295). What could be causing this elevation?

5. Microalbuminaemia has been detected in a patient following surgery. The patient has developed postoperative oedema. Should he be given 10% albumin as a plasma expander?

6. Why does infusion of potassium chloride injection hurt?

7. Why must infusions of potassium chloride be mixed well and administered slowly?

8. Salt substitute contains potassium chloride. Why is this supposed to be less hypertensive than sodium chloride?

9. A patient recently admitted to the spinal ward has a plasma calcium of 2.7 mmol/l. What are the common causes of elevated calcium levels and how should this be treated?

10. An elderly woman who is showing signs of prolonged starvation is being started on intravenous nutrition. The pharmacist has suggested that the first day's regimen should contain only half the normal daily amount of phosphate. Why?

INTRODUCTION

One of the major functions of the circulatory system is to keep the total amount of water in the body constant, a process known as fluid balance. This it has to do in spite of the amount we drink. In addition, the circulation has to exchange fluid between the blood and the cells in order to deliver food and gases and remove waste products. This process is known as fluid exchange. This has to be achieved while keeping the levels of sodium, potassium, calcium, magnesium and phosphate within a narrow concentration band in both the plasma and the cells. This chapter describes fluid balance and exchange, the concepts of fluid compartments, and highlights the relevance of fluid and ion balance on health.

WATER

Water is the most abundant constituent in the body. However, measurement of the total amount is difficult as it is unevenly distributed between different body tissues. In order to estimate total body water (TBW), physiologists arbitrarily divide the body into two theoretical compartments: the body fat compartment, generally called the fat mass (FM), and the fat-free compartment or the lean body mass (LBM). The fat mass contains almost no water or potassium whereas the lean body mass contains almost all of the body's water. Various chemical techniques suggest that water accounts for 70–78% of lean body mass with a mean value of 73%. This varies by approximately 2% per day from morning to night and with food intake.

DISTRIBUTION OF TOTAL BODY WATER INTO BODY FLUID COMPARTMENTS

The 35–50 litres of total body water has to be given 'physical structure' or we would all be distinctly pear shaped. It is therefore wrapped up inside membranes. These fluid-containing membrane systems are arbitrarily considered to form three separate major fluid compartments; namely the plasma (the water in the circulatory system), the intracellular space (the water inside the cells) and the interstitial space (the water outside the cells but not in the plasma). In addition, about 3 litres of water is contained in the structure of bone. These fluid compartments are illustrated in Figure 14.1.

MOVEMENT OF FLUID BETWEEN THE MAJOR FLUID COMPARTMENTS

The amount of water in each compartment is governed by the balance of two pressures: the osmotic pressure which draws fluid into the compartment, and the hydrostatic pressure which forces water out of the compartment (Fig. 14.2).

The osmotic pressure of both plasma and cells is slightly greater than that of the interstitial compartment. As a result, there is a negative pressure of –1 to –2 mmHg in the interstitial space. Fluid balance between all fluid compartments is achieved when all the hydrostatic and osmotic pressures reach equilibrium (Fig. 14.3).

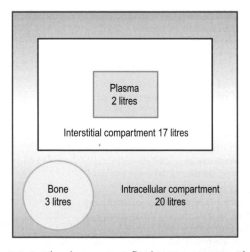

Figure 14.1 The three major fluid compartments. The cell membranes enclose about 23 litres of water in the intracellular space (including the 3 litres in bone). The plasma (excluding the red cells) contains about 2 litres of water. The interstitial compartment (lying outside the circulatory system and the cells) contains about 17 litres of water. Bone contains about 3 litres of water.

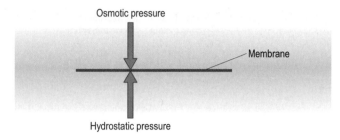

Figure 14.2 Forces involved in fluid exchange. In each compartment the hydrostatic pressure is a 'pushing out' pressure. The osmotic pressure is a 'pulling in' pressure.

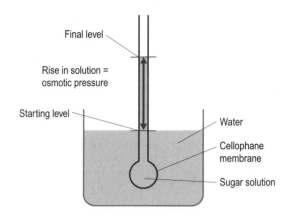

Figure 14.4 Visualizing osmosis. The sugar solution inside the membrane draws water through the pores. This rises up the tube until the weight of the column of liquid in the tube is equal to the osmotic pressure of the sugar solution.

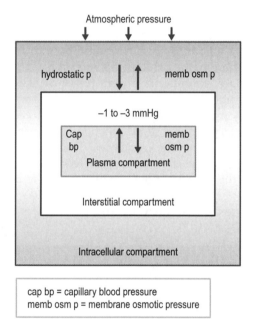

Figure 14.3 Hydrostatic and osmotic pressures operating in the body fluid compartments. Fluid balance is achieved when the hydrostatic and membrane osmotic pressures are in equilibrium in all the compartments.

OSMOLALITY AND OSMOLARITY

The gram molecular weight of any substance always contains the same number of molecules. For example, 360 g of sugar (the molecular weight of sucrose) contains 6.022×10^{23} molecules; 60 g of urea (the molecular weight of urea) contains the same number. The osmotic pressure can therefore be related to the molar concentration of the osmotically active material. The measurement of the number of particles is called either the osmolarity or the osmolality. If the measurement is the number of particles per volume it is called the osmolarity, if it is the number per weight it is called the osmolality. As human plasma contains large amounts of proteins and fats, 1 ml of plasma weighs less than 1 g. The osmolality is about 7% higher than the osmolarity. Osmolalities are used as the standard within medicine. The osmolality is a measure of the number of particles per weight of solution, which approximates to its molar concentration per weight.

Membrane osmotic pressure and colloid osmotic pressure (COP)

In the body, the pores in the capillary walls are much bigger than they are in cellophane. They allow free passage of ions and small molecules such as urea and glucose. However, large molecules such as albumin or globulin are retained within the plasma. The osmotic pressure, generated across the capillary wall between the plasma and the interstitial fluid, is caused by these large molecules. The membrane osmotic pressure, sometimes called the oncotic or colloid osmotic pressure (COP), is the measurement of the osmotic pressure generated across a membrane with pores of a

OSMOTIC PRESSURE, OSMOLALITY AND MEMBRANE OSMOTIC PRESSURE

Osmosis is the movement of water through tiny holes (pores) in a membrane from an area of high to an area of low concentration. You can visualize osmosis by putting a sugar solution into a cellophane bag and tying this onto the end of a hollow glass tube. If the bag is immersed in a cup of water the solution in the glass tube will slowly rise. The height of the rise of water is the osmotic pressure of the sugar solution (Fig. 14.4).

The osmotic pressure is dependent on the number of particles of sugar in the solution.

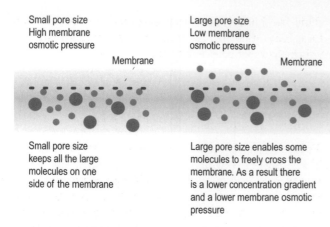

Small pore size
High membrane
osmotic pressure

Membrane

Large pore size
Low membrane
osmotic pressure

Membrane

Small pore size
keeps all the large
molecules on one
side of the membrane

Large pore size enables some
molecules to freely cross the
membrane. As a result there
is a lower concentration gradient
and a lower membrane osmotic
pressure

Figure 14.5 Relationship between membrane osmotic pressure and pore size.

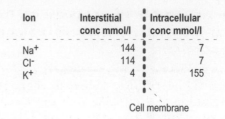

Ion	Interstitial conc mmol/l	Intracellular conc mmol/l
Na^+	144	7
Cl^-	114	7
K^+	4	155

Cell membrane

Figure 14.6 Sodium and potassium distribution across the interstitial fluid membrane. The intracellular pores prevent free movement of ions. Sodium is actively transported out of the cells and potassium is pumped in.

known size. The membrane osmotic pressure depends on the number of molecules on either side of the membrane that are unable to pass through the pores. This in turn is dependent on the pore size (and charge) of the membrane (Fig. 14.5).

Difference between osmolality and MOP

Membrane osmotic pressure or colloid osmotic pressure (COP) is a measure of the pressure caused by non-diffusible molecules at a membrane surface. Osmolality is a measure of the total number of particles in a solution.

Two types of membrane fluid exchange

The components which contribute towards the membrane osmotic pressure are very different at the interface between the cells and the interstitial fluid, and the plasma and the interstitial fluid.

Factors contributing to the cell/interstitial membrane osmotic pressure

The membrane dividing the interstitial fluid and the cell contents actively transports potassium into the cell and excludes sodium, a process driven by Na^+/K^+ ATPase, 'the sodium pump'. The membrane osmotic pressure across the cell membrane results mainly from the differences in ionic concentrations (Fig. 14.6).

The total concentration of ions inside the cells is very slightly greater than the total concentration of ions in the interstitial fluid, resulting in a membrane osmotic pressure gradient which draws water into the cells.

Factors contributing to the plasma/interstitial membrane osmotic pressure

The membrane osmotic pressure between the plasma and the interstitial fluid is very different. The pores are much larger and allow ions to freely diffuse across the membrane. However, human plasma is a mixture of small, medium and very large molecules. The large molecules (albumin and immunoglobulin) provide most of the osmotic drive at this interface.

There are various sizes and types of pore in the capillary membrane ranging from very small pores (probably molecular aquaporius or glycoprotein pores) to much larger pores (tight junctions between cells) at the venous end of the capillaries. The small pores are too small to be detectable by electron microscopy whereas the tight junctions are big enough to be visible by light microscopy. The relationship between membrane osmotic pressure and pore size is complex (Fig. 14.7).

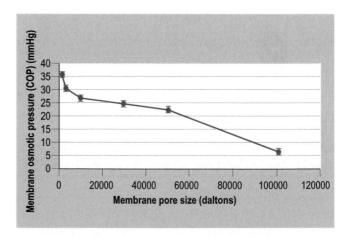

Figure 14.7 Change in membrane osmotic pressure with pore size for human plasma. At small pore sizes (1000–3000 Da) molecules, such as glucose, and ions are large enough to contribute to the membrane osmotic pressure. The smaller the pore size the greater their contribution. Between 10 000 and 30 000 Da the major contributor is albumin. At 100 000 Da immunoglobulins contribute most of the membrane osmotic pressure.

Differences in blood pressure on the two sides of the heart and their influence on fluid exchange

The blood pressure on the systemic side of the circulation (120/80 mmHg falling to about 50 mmHg at the beginning of the capillary) is much higher than that on the pulmonary side (30 mmHg falling to 5–10 mmHg in the capillary). Fluid exchange is therefore different on the two sides of the circulatory system.

SYSTEMIC CAPILLARY FLUID EXCHANGE

In 1896 Starling demonstrated that there was a fall in capillary pressure from about 30 mmHg at the arterial end of the capillary to about 10 mmHg at the venous end. His measurements suggested that the colloid osmotic pressure of plasma was about 20 mmHg. He assumed that the osmotic pressure was constant down the length of the capillary. As his measurements suggested that the arterial capillary blood pressure was greater than the osmotic pressure, he proposed that fluid would be forced out of the capillary in the first half of the capillary. As the venous capillary blood pressure was lower than the osmotic pressure, fluid would be drawn back into the plasma in the second half of the capillary. Thus fluid exchange consisted of movement of fluid out of the capillary at the arterial end and its return at the venous end (Fig. 14.8). Fluid balance would be achieved when the volume forced out was equal to the volume drawn back.

This mechanism has been accepted for the last 100 years. However, two fundamental problems with this hypothesis have been identified:

1. Capillary permeability doubles from the arterial to the venous end.
2. The capillary pressure is not constant but inherently pulsatile.

Pulse reverse osmosis (PRO) is a new hypothesis of fluid exchange that attempts to address these anomalies. It assumes that the change in permeability represents increasing pore size down the length of the capillary. The increasing pore size results in decreasing membrane osmotic pressure (MOP) down the length of the capillary. This decrease in MOP is equal and opposite down the length of the capillary. As the two pressures are equal there is no fluid movement and fluid balance is achieved. However, the blood pressure in the capillary is not constant but pulsatile. During the systolic phase of the pulse the blood pressure is higher than the MOP, resulting in fluid movement out of the capillary. During diastole the blood pressure is less, resulting in the return of fluid. The pulsing of the blood pressure therefore drives fluid exchange (Fig. 14.9).

PULMONARY CAPILLARY EXCHANGE

Capillary fluid exchange in the lungs differs from that in the systemic circulation as the blood pressure is lower in the pulmonary circulation (the pulmonary artery

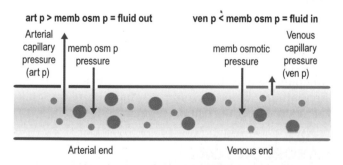

Figure 14.8 The Starling hypothesis of fluid exchange. Starling suggested that the arterial capillary pressure was greater than the arterial osmotic gradient, resulting in fluid movement out of the capillary. At the venous end the venous pressure was less than the osmotic pressure, resulting in fluid movement back into the capillary. Fluid balance is achieved when the volume filtered out at the arterial end is equal and opposite to the volume osmotically reabsorbed at the venous end of the capillary.

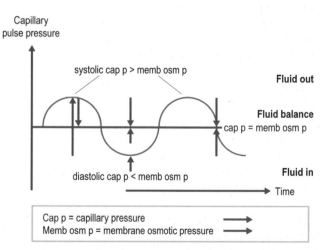

Figure 14.9 Pulse reverse osmosis. PRO suggests that fluid balance is achieved when the mean capillary pressure is equal and opposite to the membrane osmotic pressure. During the systolic phase of the pulse wave, the capillary pressure exceeds the membrane osmotic pressure, resulting in fluid movement out of the capillary. During diastole the membrane osmotic pressure exceeds the capillary pressure, resulting in fluid being drawn back into the capillary.

pressure ranges from 16–30 mmHg at systole to 4–13 mmHg at diastole). The difference in lung pressure between inspiration and expiration also adds to the pressures involved in fluid exchange. The major function of this part of the circulatory system is gas exchange. Fluid balance is still achieved when the mean capillary blood pressure is equal and opposite to the membrane osmotic pressure, but diffusion probably has a larger role in fluid exchange as there is a much shorter distance between the capillaries and the walls of the alveoli.

FLUID BALANCE

The major fluid compartments described above contain about 42 litres of water. This total volume needs to be maintained to prevent dehydration and death. The body continually loses water through the skin, the lungs, the urine and in the stools. We need to drink to replace these losses. There are three mechanisms which trigger thirst and encourage us to drink.

FINE TUNING OF FLUID BALANCE – ARGININE VASOPRESSIN (AVP)/ ANTIDIURETIC HORMONE (ADH) RELEASE

AVP or ADH (antidiuretic hormone), as the name implies, reduces water loss in the urine. Its release is triggered by specialist cells called osmoreceptors. These cells dangle in the circulation just below the hypothalamus. These cells are surrounded by semi-permeable membranes, which have a membrane osmotic pressure just like the capillary walls. If the concentration of plasma components unable to pass through the membrane is high, fluid is drawn out of the cell and the osmoreceptors shrink. This triggers the release of AVP into the bloodstream. Osmoreceptors are sensitive to concentrations of sodium, mannitol and glucose (without insulin) but are not affected by changes in urea concentration. If insulin is given at the same time as glucose the pores in the osmoreceptors are opened and no longer respond to plasma glucose concentrations.

If the osmolality (the total concentration of particles in the plasma) is above 280 mosmol/kg, AVP release is triggered, which slows down the rate of excretion of water and sodium by the kidney. If the osmolality of the plasma is below 280 mosmol/kg, AVP secretion is minimal. However, if the osmolality rises above a threshold value osmoreceptors are progressively stimulated, increasing AVP release. Once the osmolality has risen above 290–292 mosmol/kg, AVP reaches its maximum level of about 5 pg/ml. A change in

Table 14.1 Factors that affect AVP release

Agents known to cause increased AVP levels	Agents known to decrease AVP levels
Nausea	Noradrenaline
Emetics	Haloperidol
Hyperglycaemia	Fluphenazine
Pain	Promethazine
Stress	Morphine antagonists
Hypoxia	Alcohol
Angiotensin II	
Acetylcholine	
Adrenaline	
Histamine	
Bradykinin	
Prostaglandins	
Dopaminergic drugs	
Morphine	
Vincristine	
Cyclophosphamide	
Apomorphine	
Nicotine	

Most of the factors that increase AVP also increase capillary permeability.

osmolality of about 3% leads from minimal to maximal AVP release. AVP produces its effects by causing vasoconstriction. In the kidney AVP reduces glomerular filtration and reduces sodium transport in the collecting tubule. The half-life of AVP is 10–20 minutes so the effect of AVP is relatively short.

If the osmolality rises above 295 mosmol/kg, other osmoreceptor neurones are triggered which stimulate thirst. Water taken orally is absorbed rapidly and rapidly fills the fluid compartments, diluting the plasma and turning off AVP release. There are several other factors that can affect AVP release (Table 14.1).

Changes in AVP release represent the fine tuning of whole body fluid balance. The overall volume is maintained by controlling the rate of excretion, vascular tone and thirst. However, in serious fluid balance situations, where there is a 10% or greater change in circulating blood volume, baroreceptors take precedence over the osmoreceptors.

BARORECEPTORS

There are two types of baroreceptors, those located in low and those located in the high pressure areas in the circulatory system (see also Ch. 12).

Low pressure baroreceptors

Normal pressures are 1–5 mmHg in the right atrium of the heart, and slightly higher in the left atrium, 6–11 mmHg. Stretch baroreceptors located in the atria sense increased pressure. This triggers nerve impulses to cardiac centres in the brain stem and the medulla which block sympathetic vasoconstriction and reduce AVP release. Reduction of atrial pressure produces the opposite effects.

High pressure baroreceptor control

The pressure in the aorta pulses between 70 and 140 mmHg. High pressure baroreceptors are located both in the aortic arch and in the carotid sinus. Increase in circulating volume triggers these stretch receptors which reduce sympathetic nervous activity, AVP release and increase parasympathetic nerve activity. A decrease in circulating volume stimulates the opposite effects.

There is another high pressure baroreceptor system in the juxtaglomerular apparatus of the kidney. Increase in renal artery pressure triggers this baroreceptor to reduce the amount of renin released. This in turn reduces the levels of angiotensin II. This hormone powerfully constricts smooth muscle in the circulatory system, increases adrenaline and aldosterone levels, and stimulates AVP release and thirst.

The baroreceptors respond to acute and large changes in blood pressure and volume. The osmoreceptors and AVP perform the fine tuning. Both systems keep the volume of fluid in the body constant.

ATRIAL NATRIURETIC PEPTIDE (ANP)

ANP is a hormone manufactured in the atria of the heart. Increase in atrial pressure and pulse rate stimulates its release. ANP causes dilation of vascular smooth muscle, and inhibits the release of renin, and aldosterone, the sodium retaining hormone. Increased levels of ANP lower AVP secretion, reduce sodium loss by increasing glomerular filtration and reduce sodium transport in the renal collecting ducts. Reduction in atrial pressure and pulse has the opposite effect.

FLUID BALANCE IN THE WARD SITUATION

In the ward situation it is possible to administer fluids more rapidly than they can be eliminated by the body. Thirst can also be suppressed by drug therapy. The patient is frequently denied access to drink (nil by mouth etc.) as part of the protocol for a range of diagnostic tests. It is therefore essential to ensure that each patient gets sufficient fluid to maintain fluid balance. This is one of the most challenging tasks on the ward, particularly in the intensive care situation.

Table 14.2 Insensible losses

Route of water loss	Range of daily losses (ml/day)	Loss per kg body weight (ml/kg/day)
Skin	300–500	5.7
Lungs	140–470	4.4
Total insensible losses	700 ml/day	10 ml/kg

Calculated from Geigy Scientific Tables 1981; 1: 108–112.

Fluid balance is the process in which the patient's fluid intake is matched to the fluid output.

$$\text{Fluid balance} = \text{fluid in} - \text{fluid out}$$

Water is lost through the skin, through the lungs, in the urine and in the stools. The losses through the skin and lungs are called insensible losses as they are 'invisible'. Normal daily insensible losses are given in Table 14.2.

Total insensible losses amount to about 10 ml/kg per day or about 700 ml for a 70 kg person. This is often the only volume that can be given to patients with severe renal disease.

Losses in the urine

The losses from the urine are very variable and depend on the volumes taken either orally or intravenously (Table 14.3).

Ideally urine volumes should be measured, as they are so variable.

Losses from the gastrointestinal tract

Losses from the gastrointestinal (GI) tract are in the range of 30–160 ml per day during health. However, losses can be several litres during intestinal diseases. In such situations an estimate of gut losses should be attempted even if this is very unpleasant.

Table 14.3 Urine losses

Route of water loss	Range of daily losses (ml/day)	Loss per kg body weight (ml/kg/day)
Urine, male	690–2690, mean 1360	20 ml/kg/day
Urine, female	490–2260, mean 1130	16 ml/kg/day
Oliguric patients	100 ml	
Anuric patients	50 ml	

Calculated from Geigy Scientific Tables 1981; 1: 55.

The losses from the skin, urine and stools can be considered to be the daily baseline fluid losses.

Baseline water losses = insensible losses + urine losses + stool losses

This is the amount of fluid that needs to be given daily to prevent dehydration.

DESIGN OF FLUID THERAPY

Replacement fluid can be given orally (preferably) or intravenously if fluid cannot be given via the GI tract. The most common intravenous (IV) infusions are listed in Table 14.4.

Although these infusions are frequently considered to be inert, this is not the case. The first rule of fluid therapy is 'water flows where the ion goes'. Sodium is the major extracellular ion. Infusion of normal saline delivers this ion to the extracellular compartment (the plasma + the interstitium). Over 90% of the water administered with this sodium remains in the extracellular space. Very little diffuses into the cells. In order to get water into the cells, potassium, the major intracellular ion, has to be infused. To get the correct distribution of water into both the intracellular and extracellular compartments, a regimen is required that contains sufficient sodium and potassium to replace the body's daily losses of these ions.

The second rule of fluid therapy is 'any IV infusion administered should have an osmolality as close as possible to that of plasma', i.e. 287 mosmol/kg. Infusions that are half normal (i.e. have an osmolality of approx 150 mosmol/kg or less) dilute the plasma to such an extent that fluid is drawn into the red blood cells, which makes them swell. If solutions with a lower osmolality are infused, the red cells swell to such an extent that they burst, a process known as haemolysis. Infusion of concentrated solutions (above twice normal, i.e. 600 mosmol/kg) such as glucose 10% cause fluid to move out of the red blood cells causing them to shrivel, a process known as crenation. Low and high osmolality solutions cause pain and damage at the site of the infusion.

Concentrated IV feeding solutions, for example glucose or amino acids, must be infused via a central vein where the large volume and rapid flow reduce the damaging effects of the high osmolality.

Correction for additional patient fluid losses

In many situations additional fluid is removed from the patient via nasogastric suction, or tissue drainage. A volume equal to that removed should be added to the baseline amount to provide the correct volume. The replacement solution should be selected to have an ionic composition which is closest to the suction fluid being removed. Table 14.5 gives the ionic composition of a range of body fluids.

Table 14.4 Composition and osmolality of common IV infusions

Infusion	Composition	Osmolality (mosmol/kg)
Normal saline infusion	Sodium chloride 0.9% in water	285
Half normal saline	Sodium chloride 0.45%	144
Glucose infusion	Glucose 5% in water	278
	Glucose 10% in water	554
Compound sodium lactate infusion		260

Table 14.5 Ionic composition of body fluids

Fluid	Na (mmol/l)	K (mmol/l)	Ca (mmol/l)	Mg (mmol/l)	PO$_4$ (mmol/l)
Plasma	135–145	3.5–5.0	2.2–2.6	0.7–0.9	0.8–1.35
Normal stool	20–40	30–60	7.5–33 mmol/day	2.3–5.5 mmol/day	10–25 mmol/day
Diarrhoea	30–40	30–70			
Ileal fluid	140	11	4	3	
Urine	70–160	40–120	6 mmol/day	5 mmol/day	20 mmol/day
Sweat	15–25	3–4	0.73	0.13	trace

From Willatts (1982) and Lentner (1984).

Corrections for the initial state of hydration of the patient need to be incorporated into the fluid regimen. Patients who have been unable to eat for a prolonged period before admission have a higher proportion of water than those who have had a normal diet. The initial volume in malnourished patients may need to be decreased to avoid fluid overload.

The initial calculated baseline volume needs to be adjusted over long-term fluid therapy according to the changing needs of the patient. In hospitals, fluid therapy is usually monitored by using a fluid balance chart. These charts record the daily oral and intravenous fluid input and the daily urine and drain output. Insensible losses are rarely included. The standard practice of giving patients the same volume as they excrete is fraught with problems. Monitoring fluid therapy to fluid balance charts is far from ideal.

The most accurate way of monitoring fluid balance is measuring and recording the patient's daily weight.

Any rapid weight changes are most likely to be due to accumulation or excretion of water. The volume in the regimen should be adjusted to keep the patient's day-to-day weight at the prescribed level.

As stated above, the body performs the fine tuning of fluid balance through the effect of plasma osmolality on the release of the AVP (ADH). Plasma osmolality can therefore be used as a guide to the state of hydration of the patient. Normal plasma osmolality is in the range 282–295 mosmol/kg. A plasma osmolality above 300 mosmol/kg suggests dehydration, and an osmolality below 280 suggests overhydration. Good fluid balance will help to maintain the patient's blood pressure and reduce the chance of oedema and shock.

OEDEMA

Oedema is a clinical condition where there is an increase in interstitial fluid. As this fluid contains 140 mmol of sodium per litre of water, it is frequently described as sodium retention. It is better to consider it as salty water retention. There are several theories that suggest mechanisms for its formation. The forward theory suggests that a failing heart reduces the renal artery pressure so much that water is not filtered out properly in the kidney. The build-up of water results in the oedema. The backward theory suggests that a failing heart results in pooling of blood in the veins. This causes an increase in venous pressure and a decrease in the renal elimination of water. Another theory suggests that increased plasma renin, aldosterone and AVP levels

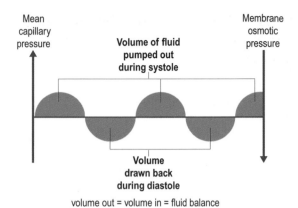

Figure 14.10 Fluid balance.

result in insufficient removal of fluid by the kidney with resultant increase of fluid in the interstitial space. All are more or less based on the Starling hypothesis of fluid exchange. PRO suggests that fluid balance is achieved when the volume of fluid forced out during the systolic phase of the pulse is equal and opposite to the volume drawn back during diastole (Fig. 14.10).

If the capillary pressure is greater than the membrane osmotic pressure, more fluid will be forced out into the interstitium during systole than is osmotically drawn back during diastole. This will result in fluid build-up in the interstitial compartment. This increase in fluid will present as oedema (Fig. 14.11).

Treatment of oedema

Oedema is treated with diuretics, usually loop diuretics. These drugs cause the excretion of salt and water from the loop of Henle in the kidney. Oedema therapy should be monitored against the daily weight of the patient. Weight loss of about 1 kg per day over the first few days is generally maintained until the mass of the oedema fluid is removed.

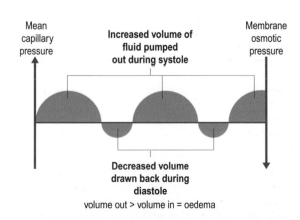

Figure 14.11 Oedema.

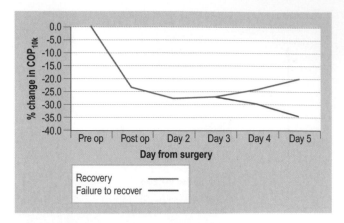

Figure 14.12 Daily change in COP following GI surgery. The COP falls to a minimum 2–3 days following GI surgery. The COP then slowly returns to normal over days 4–7 in patients who recover. Failure to recover may be associated with a falling COP. (COP_{10k} = COP measured on a membrane with a pore size of 10 000 Da.)

SHOCK FOLLOWING SURGERY

The hypoxia, increase in inflammatory mediators and increase in cytokine release following surgery increases capillary permeability to such an extent that albumin can leak out of the plasma. This results in a profound fall in COP, a marker for membrane osmotic pressure, and a fall in blood pressure. This condition is called the 'leaky capillary syndrome'. The drop in COP can be as much as 50–60% below the starting value. The typical standard pattern of change is demonstrated in Figure 14.12.

The degree of drop appears to mirror the 'stress of surgery'. The length of time to return to normal may be a useful prognostic index of recovery.

Fluid therapy following surgery

The fall in blood pressure is generally treated by infusing large volumes of normal IV fluids. However, although this maintains the blood pressure, the extra fluid further lowers the plasma albumin concentration, lowering the membrane osmotic pressure and increasing the risk of oedema formation. Leaky capillary syndrome is generally treated with plasma expanders.

Plasma expanders

Plasma expanders increase the number of large molecules in the plasma. These large molecules osmotically draw fluid into the circulation from the interstitial compartment and expand the plasma volume. Artificial expanders are derivatives of gelatin, dextrans or starches. Natural expanders such as albumin and plasma protein solution are made from human blood.

The molecular weight of albumin is 69 000 Da and immunoglobulins about 200 000 Da. Plasma expanders should therefore have a molecular weight of at least 70 000 Da. Table 14.6 lists some commonly available plasma expanders.

Gelatins are used, particularly in Europe, for non-complicated therapy, as a routine expander during and after surgery. Although their molecular weight is small (about half that of albumin), the molecules of gelatin are very sticky and form a gel which has the osmotic effect. Dextrans are now rarely used as they occasionally cause serious allergenic reactions. Starches are expensive and therefore often restricted to those procedures where there is the risk of capillary leak. In all cases infusion volumes should be limited to the manufacturer's maximum daily infusion dose.

Albumin infusion should increase the colloid osmotic pressure, decrease oedema and improve clinical

Table 14.6 Types of plasma expanders

Expander	Particle size (Da)	Comments
Gelatin	30 000	Commonly used as a cheap expander
Dextran 40	40 000	Rarely used now as risk of anaphylactic reaction
Dextran 70	70 000	
Dextran 110	110 000	
Hetastarch	200 000	Used in capillary leak
Hespan	500 000	
Albumin solution 5% and 20%	69 000	Used for replacement of the body's natural albumin
Plasma protein solution 4.5% containing 80% albumin and 20% globulin	69 000 / 200 000	Used for replacement following blood loss

outcome. In the treatment of shock, albumin infusion increases the plasma COP but has little positive effect on outcome, and may be harmful. During capillary leak, albumin is believed to leak out of the capillary, raising the interstitial concentration of albumin. As a result, there is an increase in albumin concentration on both sides of the capillary membrane, and the membrane osmotic pressure will be lower. As oedema occurs when the blood pressure exceeds the membrane osmotic pressure, this will make the oedema worse. In shock syndromes, trauma, sepsis and toxaemias, infusion of albumin may make the oedema worse.

SODIUM

Sodium is the major extracellular ion. There is about 80 g in the average male and 60 g in the average female. About half of this is in the extracellular fluid, 40% is in bone and about 10% inside the intracellular fluid. The different concentrations in the three fluid compartments are shown in Figure 14.13.

The intracellular membrane selectively controls the entry of ions and other small molecules. As a result, there is a large sodium concentration gradient across the cell membrane. The plasma membrane is much less restrictive to small molecules. Ions distribute unevenly across the plasma membrane depending on their charge, an effect known as the Donnan equilibrium. Monovalent cations (+ ions) have a lower concentration on the interstitial side of the membrane (96% of the plasma value). Monovalent anions (– ions) have a greater concentration on the interstitial side (104.2% of the plasma level). The sodium concentration gradient across the capillary membrane is therefore much smaller.

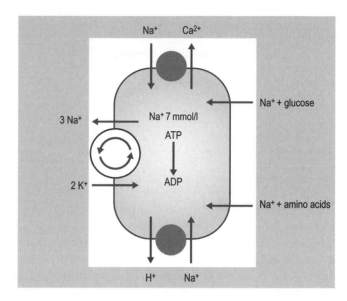

Figure 14.14 Control of intracellular sodium. Although there are several mechanisms in which sodium is transported into the cell, the sodium potassium pump ensures that intracellular sodium is kept down to about 7 mmol/l.

CONTROL OF INTRACELLULAR SODIUM

Sodium enters the cell though specific sodium channels. This can be as part of the transport of glucose and amino acids into the cells, or as part of the counter transport system where intracellular H^+ and Ca^{2+} ions are exchanged for sodium (Fig. 14.14). This influx of sodium is pumped out of the cell by the sodium potassium pump, under the action of sodium/potassium ATPase. Three sodium ions are pumped out for every two potassium ions absorbed. In this way the intracellular concentration of sodium is kept at about 7 mmol/l depending on the type of cell.

CONTROL OF EXTRACELLULAR SODIUM

Extracellular sodium levels are a balance between sodium intake and renal sodium excretion. They are also affected by 'water' balance, dehydration elevating and overhydration lowering the sodium levels.

Sodium intake

Daily sodium intake varies widely between countries. The average North American diet contains about 170–200 mmol, the Japanese 400 mmol and the British 160 mmol. This sodium is completely absorbed from the GI tract.

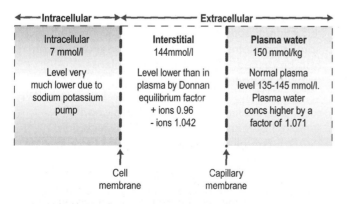

Figure 14.13 Sodium concentrations in the major fluid compartments.

Table 14.7 Daily ion losses (mmol)

	Normal daily amount	Na	K	Ca	Mg	PO$_4$
Sweat	300–500 ml	15–25	3–4	0.2–0.4	trace	trace
Faeces	100–200 g	7	11	17	5	10–25
Renal	500–2700 ml	150–220	70	6	5	25–65

Figures from Lentner (1984).
Sweat losses are much higher in hot climates. Faecal losses are greater during diarrhoea.

Sodium excretion

Excretion of sodium occurs in the sweat, faeces and in the kidney. The amounts (mmol) lost by each route are given in Table 14.7.

Sodium is mainly excreted in the kidney. The mechanisms are covered in detail in Chapter 8. The fine tuning of the levels is achieved through the balance of two hormones, aldosterone which retains sodium, and the atrial natriuretic factor which causes its elimination. In combination with the factors that control water balance these two hormones keep the sodium level in the plasma within the normal range 135–145 mmol/l.

DAILY SODIUM REQUIREMENTS

Taking too much salt may be harmful. The INTERSALT study showed that high salt consumers had elevated blood pressures and a higher stroke mortality than those taking more normal sodium levels. Dietary salt intake is one of the main factors that determines calcium excretion. A high sodium intake increases urinary excretion of both sodium and calcium. This may be related to subsequent reduction in hip bone density. Increased sodium intake also raises plasma concentrations of parathyroid hormone and increases hydroxyproline excretion. Both of these are indicators of decreased bone mineralization. High salt diets may therefore be related to decreased bone density in later life.

If the daily salt intake is reduced from 10 g (160 mmol) to 5 g (80 mmol) there is a decrease of 1–1.5 litres in extracellular volume and a corresponding weight loss of 1 to 1.5 kg. Several authors have therefore suggested that 70 mmol per day should be the baseline amount of sodium given as standard in fluid therapy and total parenteral nutrition (TPN) regimens. However, long-term biochemical monitoring of TPN suggests that this amount is too low. A three-year analysis of home TPN patients reported that the mean amount of sodium required to maintain normal plasma levels was 176 mmol daily. A similar study investigating hepatic TPN patients for 31–145 months gave a similar sodium requirement of 146 mmol/day.

Fluid regimens should provide about 2 mmol of sodium per day for uncomplicated fluid replacement.

SODIUM IMBALANCE

Hypernatraemia

Hypernatraemia is a biochemical diagnosis made when the plasma sodium is above 150 mmol/l. The symptoms are lethargy which can progress to coma and convulsions. There is muscular tremor with rigidity and hyperactive reflexes. Normal saline infusion contains 154 mmol of sodium per litre. Plasma contains about 140 mmol/l. Infusion of large volumes of sodium chloride infusion can cause the plasma sodium level to rise above 150 mmol/l. Most hospital-acquired hypernatraemia is iatrogenic and preventable. Hypernatraemia is generally treated by slowly infusing glucose 5% over 2–3 days. Other causes of hypernatraemia are excessive sodium administration or intake, inadequate water intake and excessive water loss.

Hyponatraemia

Hyponatraemia is a biochemical diagnosis made when the plasma sodium level falls below 130 mmol/l. Symptoms are mental confusion and disorientation progressing to convulsions and coma. The condition can be either true hyponatraemia; a deficiency in sodium or pseudohyponatraemia; or a reduction of sodium levels due to large amounts of lipids or proteins in the blood. Hyponatraemia can also be related to problems in the release of AVP following surgery or over-infusion of 5% glucose solutions. Conditions which cause an increase in AVP, such as some tumours, several drugs and the symptom of inappropriate AVP/ADH secretion (SIADH) can all cause hyponatraemia. Note that the convention now is to use the name AVP rather than ADH; however, the change has not made its way to SIADH, SIADH remains SIADH. Sodium should be replaced slowly to avoid the osmotic demyelination syndrome, and given intravenously rather than orally to avoid nausea and vomiting.

POTASSIUM

Potassium is the major intracellular ion. There is about 94–140 g in the average male and 70–90 g in the female. Potassium content is greatest in muscle (90 mmol/kg fat free tissue). The two major roles of potassium are nerve conduction and as the major intracellular osmotic component. The potassium concentration in the three main body compartments is given in Figure 14.15.

CONTROL OF INTRACELLULAR POTASSIUM

Insulin, alkalosis and acidosis, exercise, bicarbonate levels and β_2 adrenergic drugs all affect intracellular levels of potassium (Figure 14.16).

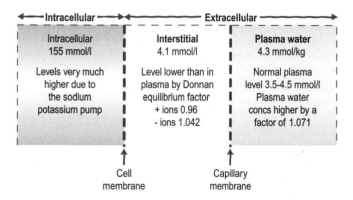

Figure 14.15 Potassium concentrations in the three major fluid compartments.

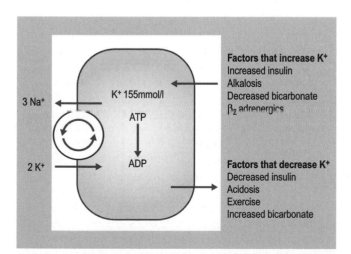

Figure 14.16 Control of intracellular potassium.

Increased insulin levels increase the levels of glycogen. One gram of glycogen raises the intracellular levels of potassium by 0.33 mmol/l. Alkalosis moves potassium into the cell, acidosis has the opposite effect. β_2 adrenergics such as isoprenaline increase adrenaline levels. β blockers inhibit this effect.

CONTROL OF EXTRACELLULAR POTASSIUM

The potassium levels in the extracellular fluid are a balance between the amount absorbed in the diet and the amount excreted in the kidney. These are illustrated in Figure 14.17.

Potassium intake

Both the North American and the British diet provide about 50–100 mmol of potassium per day. This is completely absorbed in the GI tract.

Potassium excretion

Excretion occurs in the sweat, stool and in the urine (Table 14.7). The major route of excretion is the kidneys. In general potassium excretion is 80 mmol/day.

DAILY POTASSIUM REQUIREMENTS

Daily potassium requirements are about 80 mmol.

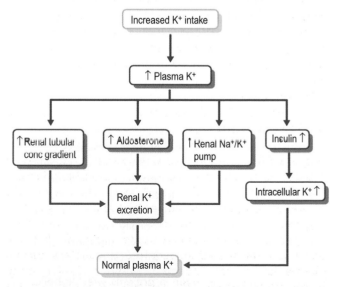

Figure 14.17 Control of extracellular potassium.

POTASSIUM IMBALANCE

Hyperkalaemia

Hyperkalaemia is a biochemical diagnosis made when the plasma potassium exceeds 5.5 mmol/l. It is life-threatening when the level exceeds 6.5–7.0 mmol/l.

Hyperkalaemia results in abnormalities in cardiac rhythm and conduction. Cardiac arrest may occur. High levels of potassium are used in cardioplegic solutions to stop the heart during heart surgery. If 15% potassium chloride injection is added to a drip it is possible to get layering. In this situation the potassium chloride forms a concentrated layer in the infusion which does not readily mix with the rest of the infusion fluid. Injection of this concentrated layer can cause cardiac arrest. It is very important to shake potassium chloride additives thoroughly after admixture to ensure that this concentrated layer is dispersed. Several deaths have resulted from 'layering' of potassium chloride injection.

Numerous factors affect extracellular potassium levels. Acidosis (following cardiac arrest or diabetic ketoacidosis) increases potassium levels (a fall in pH of 0.1 increases plasma potassium by 0.4–1.5 mmol/l). Haemolysis of a blood sample will cause falsely elevated values for plasma potassium. Conditions which result in haemolysis in the body, e.g. incompatible blood transfusion, disseminated intravascular coagulation or falciparum malaria, can cause very large increases in measured plasma potassium.

Acute treatment aims to reduce the cardiotoxicity with IV calcium chloride or gluconate. Injection of 50% glucose containing insulin should shift potassium into the cells and lower the plasma level. The acidosis may be counteracted with sodium bicarbonate infusion. If the acute treatment is successful, Resonium A or calcium resonium can be given rectally or orally to absorb potassium from the GI tract and bring down the levels.

Hypokalaemia

Hypokalaemia causes mild muscle weakness increasing to paralysis depending on the deficiency level. Severe hypokalaemia can cause life-threatening cardiac arrhythmias due to a greatly increased membrane potential on the surface of the nerve cells. Low potassium levels are generally caused by insufficient administration of potassium (particularly in long-term infusion therapy), large GI or renal losses.

Hypokalaemia can occur in patients with diabetic ketoacidosis treated with glucose and insulin infusion, in asthmatic patients on β adrenergics, or any condition that increases aldosterone levels such as renal artery stenosis or Bartter's syndrome.

Diarrhoea and vomiting cause decreased levels partly because of direct loss but also due to renal losses caused by the concurrent metabolic alkalosis. Epidemics of diarrhoea in disaster areas lead to malnutrition and hypokalaemia. In a recent outbreak in Rwanda, 1–3% of children treated with Ringer's lactate infusion died suddenly. Sudden deaths such as these were prevented by changing the infusion solution to potassium-containing saline and glucose infusions.

Most cases of hypokalaemia are caused by too little being included in fluid therapy, enteral or parenteral feeding regimens. Vomiting, nasogastric suction or fistulae are other less common causes of potassium deficiency. Drug-induced potassium deficiency is relatively common, particularly in the elderly, and is generally precipitated by diuretics or steroids.

Hypokalaemia is generally treated with saline containing potassium at a rate no faster than 10 mmol/hour and a concentration no higher than 40 mmol/l. Higher concentrations cause intense pain at the infusion site.

CALCIUM

The body contains 25 000–28 000 mmol (1000–1110 g) of calcium in the average male and 16 000–21 000 mmol (630–850 g) in the average female. Most of this is in the bone and teeth (99%). Calcium is involved in blood clotting, nerve conduction and muscle contraction. The concentrations of calcium in the three major fluid compartments are given in Figure 14.18.

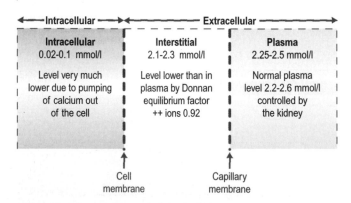

Figure 14.18 Calcium concentrations in the three major fluid compartments.

CONTROL OF INTRACELLULAR CALCIUM

Calcium enters the cells when specific protein calcium channels are opened. Influx of calcium into the cell results in muscle contraction, nerve conduction, exocytosis and glycogen metabolism depending on the type of cell. Calcium is actively pumped out of the cells by active transporter proteins which keep the level of intracellular calcium down to 0.02–0.1 mmol/l. In this process sodium is actively exchanged for calcium.

CONTROL OF EXTRACELLULAR CALCIUM

Only 1% of the body's total calcium is in the extracellular fluid. About half of this is bound to plasma protein. The remaining free calcium (approx 1.2 mmol/l) is physiologically active. The free calcium is kept constant by the interplay of intestinal absorption, bone metabolism and renal excretion mechanisms. Two main hormones are responsible for the control of these mechanisms, the parathyroid hormone (PTH) and 1,25-dihydroxyvitamin D_3 (1 alpha). The interactions between these mechanisms are shown in Figure 14.19.

Increase in PTH breaks down bone and releases calcium and phosphate, a process which requires vitamin D and magnesium. PTH also acts on the kidney to promote calcium absorption in the proximal convoluted tubule and increases urinary phosphate excretion. PTH stimulates the production of $1,25(OH)_2D_3$.

Vitamin D is also essential in calcium homeostasis. 7-dehydrocholesterol is converted under UV light in the skin to vitamin D_3. This is hydroxylated in the liver to 25(OH) vitamin D_3. In the kidney an extra hydroxy group is added to make $1,25(OH)_2$ vitamin D_3. This vitamin increases the incorporation of calcium into bone, decreases PTH secretion, increases calcium and phosphate absorption from the gut.

Calcitonin suppresses the osteoclasts, reducing bone breakdown. Hypocalcaemia reduces and hypercalcaemia increases the calcitonin levels.

Calcium intake

The normal adult diet in the UK and USA contains 20 mmol of calcium (800 mg). The UK daily reference nutrient intake (RNI) suggests 20 mmol (800 mg)/day at age 20 reducing to 5.75 mmol (230 mg) at age 70. The amount of calcium which can be absorbed from the gut (the bioavailability) is variable. It depends on the foodstuff in which it is contained and the individual's ability to absorb. However, 18–36% of ingested calcium is absorbed into the blood. Intravenous requirements are much lower at 5–8 mmol/day.

Calcium excretion

The routes and amounts of calcium excretion are given in Table 14.7.

CALCIUM IMBALANCE

Hypercalcaemia

Hypercalcaemia is a biochemical diagnosis made when the plasma level is greater than 2.6 mmol/l. Malignancy is the commonest cause, with bone calcium being released into the circulation. Hyperparathyroidism raises calcium levels. Prolonged immobility following surgery or change in muscle activity resulting from immobilization raises plasma calcium levels.

Severe hypercalcaemia is a medical emergency which needs urgent treatment. Patients are generally rehydrated with saline and given a loop diuretic such as furosemide (frusemide) to increase calcium excretion. Drugs such as thiazides or vitamin D which promote hypercalaemia should be discontinued. If the level remains high, bisphosphonates may be useful.

Hypocalcaemia

Hypocalcaemia is a biochemical diagnosis made when the plasma level is less than 2.2 mmol/l. Hypocalcaemia may develop following severe pancreatitis, acute renal failure, severe trauma and sepsis. TPN has been reported to induce metabolic

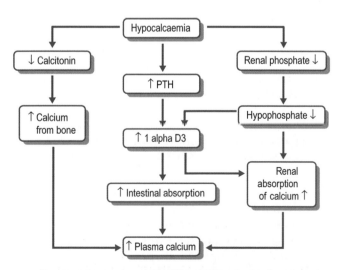

Figure 14.19 Factors involved in calcium homeostasis.

bone disease and hyperuricaemia. Some authors suggest that this may be due to either increased levels of plasma insulin or high levels of amino acids increasing calcium excretion. However, it may be due to increased losses such as that following small bowel resection.

Hypocalcaemia is treated by giving oral or IV calcium.

MAGNESIUM

Most of the magnesium in the body, about 60%, is in the bone with the remainder inside the cells. Magnesium is involved in the electrical potential of nerves and muscle fibres, as a co-factor for ATP-requiring enzymes, and in the synthesis of DNA and RNA. Magnesium and calcium metabolism are intimately related. Calcium homeostasis is partly controlled by a magnesium-requiring mechanism which releases parathyroid hormone. Chemical analysis suggests that there are 19 mmol/kg lean body mass. The concentrations of magnesium in the three major fluid compartments are shown in Figure 14.20.

CONTROL OF MAGNESIUM

Magnesium absorption from the gut is increased by increased levels of vitamin D. Magnesium release from bone is controlled by parathormone and calcitonin. Parathormone increases magnesium excretion. Calcitonin increases magnesium excretion. Potassium and magnesium metabolism is closely linked, with a deficiency in one usually being accompanied by a deficiency in the other.

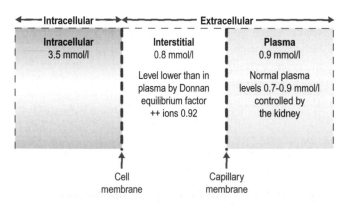

Figure 14.20 Magnesium concentrations in the three major fluid compartments.

Magnesium intake

The daily requirement to maintain normal plasma levels is 10–12 mmol per day. This is equivalent to 0.14–0.17 mmol/kg/day.

Magnesium excretion

Routes and amounts of magnesium excretion are given in Table 14.7. Normal daily losses are in the region of 10 mmol per day.

MAGNESIUM IMBALANCE

Hypermagnesaemia

Hypermagnesaemia is unusual in people taking a normal oral diet. However, over-infusion of magnesium or regular magnesium taken as a laxative can result in high plasma levels that can be toxic or even fatal, particularly if there is pre-existing renal disease. Hypermagnesaemia interferes with nerve transmission, which can cause paralysis and death. Treatment includes slow IV infusion of calcium together with large volumes of saline infusion. Loop diuretics also lower magnesium levels. Potassium and calcium supplements may be required to prevent hypokalaemia and hypocalcaemia developing during this treatment.

Hypomagnesaemia

Magnesium deficiency is common in patients with excessive GI losses such as those with Crohn's disease, and usually occurs with concomitant hypokalaemia and hypocalcaemia resistant to oral supplementation.

Starvation, malabsorption syndromes, acute pancreatitis, alcoholism, prolonged diarrhoea or vomiting are almost always accompanied by hypomagnesaemia and concurrent hypocalcaemia. The symptoms are very much the same including life-threatening cardiac arrhythmias. The treatment involves administering additional magnesium either intravenously or intramuscularly.

PHOSPHATE

There is 14–17 mmol (420–510 g) of phosphate in the average male and 11–13.0 mmol (330–400 g) in the average female body. About 85% of this is present in the bones and teeth, and 14% is inside the cells. The remaining 1% is in the extracellular compartment. Intracellular phosphate is present in the nucleic acids, membrane phospholipids, and as high energy

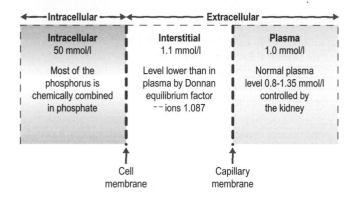

Figure 14.21 Phosphate concentrations in the three major fluid compartments.

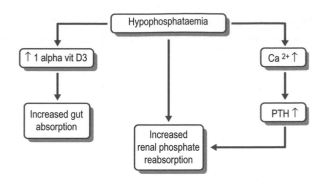

Figure 14.22 Renal and gut mechanisms which control extracellular phosphate.

compounds such as ATP, cAMP and NADP. Extracellular phosphate is present as phospholipids and inorganic phosphate. The inorganic form is present as either HPO_4^{2-} or $H_2PO_4^-$ in the ratio of 4:1. Fifteen per cent of this phosphate is plasma bound. Distribution is shown in Figure 14.21.

CONTROL OF INTRACELLULAR LEVELS

Any stimulus that causes intracellular phosphate deficiency increases phosphate uptake into the cell. Glucose and insulin stimulate intracellular movement of phosphate. Decreased PCO_2, increased pH, PTH and extracellular volume all increase intracellular phosphate.

CONTROL OF EXTRACELLULAR LEVELS

Extracellular phosphate is controlled by 1 alpha vitamin D_3. Hypophosphataemia stimulates the renal release of 1 alpha D_3 which in turn increases phosphate absorption from the gut. PTH has little direct effect but acts indirectly through its ability to increase 1 alpha D_3 production. In the kidney phosphate is freely filtered in the glomerulus. About 65% of this is reabsorbed in the proximal tubule. Increase in PTH reduces the amount of phosphate reabsorbed, thereby increasing its excretion (Fig. 14.22).

Phosphate intake

The normal daily phosphorus intake is 26–48 mmol (800–1500 mg). The Food and Nutrition Board in the USA and the Food Standards Agency in the UK recommend that the oral phosphate intake should be 12.9 mmol (400 mg)/day and that the phosphate: cal-cium ratio should be one, i.e. equal amounts of both should be included in the oral diet. The oral bio-availability is approximately 60% of the intake.

Long-term monitoring of TPN patients suggests that a minimum amount of 12 mmol (372 mg) to 13.1 mmol (406 mg) is required intravenously to maintain steady state plasma levels.

Phosphate losses

Routes and amounts of phosphate excretion are given in Table 14.7. Daily excretion is in the range 35–90 mmol/day.

PHOSPHATE IMBALANCE

Hyperphosphataemia

Hyperphosphataemia can result from under-elimination, e.g. renal failure, or overprovision of phosphate orally, rectally or intravenously. The biggest risk of hyperphosphataemia is precipitation of calcium phosphate in soft tissue of the kidney, heart, lungs, conjunctiva and skin.

Treatment options include phosphate-binding antacids, or in serious cases haemodialysis.

Hypophosphataemia

Symptoms of hypophosphataemia include irritability and confusion, which can develop into stupor, coma and seizures. Paraesthesias, muscle weakness and rhabdomyolysis can also occur. Muscle weakness resulting in both hypoventilation and impaired myocardial contractility can also occur.

There are three causes of hypophosphataemia: intracellular shift, reduced intestinal absorption, and increased urinary losses.

Intracellular shift

Acute respiratory alkalosis resulting from hypoxia, sepsis, cirrhosis, salicylate poisoning or burns can result in low PCO_2 levels and intracellular alkalosis. This activates phosphofructokinase, which causes increased phosphorylation of molecules within the cell using up the available phosphate. Extracellular phosphate is therefore drawn into the cell, resulting in a lowering of plasma phosphate levels. A fall in PCO_2 from 24 to 12 mmHg lowers the plasma phosphate level by up to a third within 1 hour. However, this is an intracellular shift of phosphate and is not a true hypophosphataemia.

Reduced intestinal absorption

Prolonged use of aluminium-, magnesium- or calcium-containing antacids can lower phosphate levels by increased phosphate excretion.

Administration of carbohydrate after long periods of starvation can precipitate hypophosphataemia. This 're-feeding syndrome' was studied in the Minnesota experiment reported by Keys et al in 1950. Six months of drastic food restriction in previously healthy subjects followed by subsequent re-feeding resulted in severe cardiopulmonary and neurological effects. This pathology was similar to that observed following administration of food to starving inmates of internment camps at the end of the Second World War. Following the introduction of TPN in the 1970s and 1980s the re-feeding syndrome was rediscovered.

In starved individuals the catabolism of fat and muscle leads to loss of lean muscle mass, water and minerals. The plasma concentrations of these depleted components including phosphorus generally remains normal due to adjustments in renal rates of excretion. When feeding is started, carbohydrate becomes the major energy source, insulin release is stimulated, and glucose, phosphorus and water and other components move into the cells. This results in a severe decrease in extracellular phosphate which in turn leads to depletion of ATP and other related compounds in red blood cells. In the circulatory system, cardiac decompensation, heart failure and depressed myocardial sarcomere contractility have been reported. In the nervous system, acute paralysis, diffuse sensory loss, cranial nerve palsies, paraesthesias, weakness seizures, rhabdomyolysis, Guillain–Barré-like syndrome have all been reported. In the respiratory system, acute respiratory failure is caused by a reduction in the amount of ATP available to enhance respiratory muscle contraction. In the blood, hypophosphataemia causes red cell dysfunction through alterations in shape, survival and physiologic capacity. Hypophosphataemia also causes granulocyte dysfunction through depressed chemotactic, phagocytic and bactericidal activity.

Increased renal losses

Hypoparathyroidism can cause hypophosphataemia because of increased phosphate excretion. Problems in vitamin D metabolism in vitamin D resistant rickets also result in low phosphate levels. Fanconi's syndrome results in a decrease in reabsorption of phosphate in the proximal tubules of the kidney. Oncogenic osteomalacia results in decreased phosphate due to prolonged loss of bone. The diuretic acetazolamide can also cause decreased phosphate levels.

Hypophosphataemia is treated by treating the underlying cause, replacing phosphate by increasing the oral intake or in severe cases by administration of intravenous phosphate.

REFERENCES AND FURTHER READING

Carroll H J, Oh M S 1989 Water, electrolyte and acid–base metabolism, 2nd edn. Diagnosis and management. Lippincott, Philadelphia

Cogan M G 1991 Fluid and electrolytes. Physiology and pathophysiology. Lange Medical Textbook, Prentice Hall International

Hill G 1992 Body composition research. Journal of Parenteral and Enteral Nutrition 16(3): 197–218

INTERSALT Co-operative research group 1986 INTERSALT study, an international co-operative study on the relation of blood pressure to electrolyte excretion in populations. 1. Designs and methods. Journal of Hypertension 4(6): 781–787
First of many references to INTERSALT study between 1986 and current date

Lentner C 1984 Geigy scientific tables. Ciba Geigy, Basel

Moore D F, Boyden C M 1963 Body cell mass and limits of hydration of the fat-free body: Their relation to estimated skeletal weight. In: Whipple H E, Silverzweig S, Brozwek J (eds) Body composition, pp 62–71. New York Academy of Sciences, New York

Prior F G R 1989 How to design intravenous fluid therapy. Pharmaceutical Journal (Hosp Pharm Suppl) (June) H5: 36–38

Prior F G R 1992 Designing basic TPN regimens, a practical guide. Geistlich Brothers

Prior F G R 1999 Plasma colloid osmotic pressure in the critically ill. Care of the Critically Ill 15: 167–172

Prior F G R, Gourlay T, Taylor K M 1995 Pulse reverse osmosis: a new theory in the maintenance of fluid balance. Perfusion 10: 159–170

Prior F G R, Morecroft V, Fergusson R, Gourlay T, Taylor K M 1999 Oedema, Starling and pulse reverse osmosis. International Journal of Artificial Organs 22: 138–144

Willatts S M 1982 Lecture notes on fluid and electrolyte balance. Blackwell Scientific Publications, Oxford

15 Nutrition

In practice you may be asked to consider the following:

1. Food provides energy, living and doing requires energy. What happens if intake exceeds output?

2. What approximate value might you give for your own BMR (basal metabolic rate)? Calculate your own BMI (body mass index).

3. Food may contain carbohydrate, fat or protein. Which of these has the most energy per unit weight (i.e. the highest energy density)?

4. Some dietary supplements contain essential amino acids? What does the term mean? Which are they?

5. The supplement's label identifies 'obligatory nitrogen loss'. Please explain.

6. A particular patient would benefit from an increase in dietary fibre. Why might an increase be beneficial? What sources can you suggest?

7. A patient has macrocytic anaemia. Which vitamin(s) might be needed? Please explain.

8. Microcytic anaemia is likely to require a mineral and possibly a vitamin. Which ones? Please explain.

9. A patient has undergone extensive surgery and has lost a considerable amount of weight. The loss is greater than can be attributed to reduction in intake. Why is this?

10. For the patient above, what changes will also have taken place in body composition?

In humans, food is an essential requirement for health and well-being. To survive it is essential that an adequate supply of energy and nutrients is available. The human body requires a continual supply of nutrients. This constant supply is maintained by control systems that regulate the intake of food and by hormones that regulate the storage and utilization of nutrients within the body between meals.

Food eaten consists of a complex mix of molecules, including macromolecules that, because of their size, are insoluble and cannot be utilized by the cells. These are broken down by the digestive system into smaller soluble units that can be taken up from the gut into the circulation and transported to the various parts of the body. The gut also has an immune system that plays an important role in protecting the body from harmful microbes present in food.

CELLULAR REQUIREMENTS

Cells require:

- energy
- raw materials
- supplementary materials and factors.

Energy powers cellular activity. Raw materials are used to build cellular components and manufacture products such as enzymes and hormones. Supplementary factors including minerals and vitamins participate in cellular activities and metabolism.

ENERGY

To supply energy to the cells, food is broken down (catabolized) to form high-energy phosphate compounds, e.g. ATP. The amount of energy provided by different nutrients is measured by burning food and measuring the amount of energy, measured as calories or joules, released as heat.

Calories and kilojoules

The combustion of a known quantity of a foodstuff is carried out in a sealed chamber (calorimeter). The heat generated raises the temperature in a water jacket which surrounds the combustion chamber. The change in the temperature of the water is recorded.

One calorie of energy is that needed to raise the temperature of 1 g of water by 1 degree Celsius.

1 kilocalorie (kcal) = 1000 calories

Currently the energy content of food is commonly expressed in SI units as joules (J) and kilojoules (kJ).

1 calorie = 4.184 joules
1 kilocalorie = 4.184 kilojoules

In food labelling the energy contents of food is usually stated in both calories and joules.

Table 15.1 Energy yielded by different foods and drinks

Food/drink	kcal/100 g	kJ/100 g
Tea (no milk/sugar)	<1	<1
Coffee (no milk/sugar)	2	8
Beer	33	139
Milk – whole	66	274
Wine (dry/sweet)	66/94	275/394
Vegetables:		
Potatoes boiled	72	306
Carrots/sprouts	24/35	100/153
Fruit:		
Apple/banana	47/95	199/403
Fish:		
Mackerel/cod	239/96	994/408
Lean meat:		
Beef/chicken	177/153	740/645
Egg, boiled	147	612
Bread:		
White/wholemeal	219/217	931/922
Peanuts	563	2337
Butter	744	3059
Corn oil	899	3696

Data from the Composition of Foods Sixth Summary Edition. Crown copyright. Reproduced with the permission of the Controller of HMSO and Queen's Printer for Scotland.

Energy content of foods

Different foods have different energy contents (Table 15.1) depending on the proportions of protein, fat and carbohydrate in the food. Protein and carbohydrate provide approximately 4 kcal/g and fat 9 kcal/g. Fatty foods such as cheese and butter are the most energy dense and weight for weight are the richest source of energy. Bread containing carbohydrate plus water is less energy dense. Carbohydrates and fats are fully broken down by the body to carbon dioxide and water, while protein is not completely broken down. The end products of protein metabolism are urea, uric acid and creatinine, all of which are eliminated in the urine.

Energy needs

The amount of energy that an individual needs depends on:

- age
- activity
- environment
- physical state
- emotional state.

Basal metabolic rate (BMR)

The minimum energy requirement of an individual who has not eaten for 12 hours and who is lying at rest

Table 15.2 Predicted basal metabolic rates of adult men and women of different ages, each weighing 65 kg*

Sex	Age range (years)	BMR		
		mJ/day	kcal/day	kcal/min
Male	18–30	7.07	1690	1.17
	30–60	6.82	1630	1.13
	>60	5.73	1370	0.95
Female	18–30	6.11	1460	1.01
	30–60	5.86	1400	0.97
	>60	5.32	1270	0.88

* Compiled from the report of a Joint FAO/WHO/UNU Expert Consultation 1985.

in a comfortable temperature is defined as the basal metabolic rate (BMR). In these circumstances energy is only required to maintain cell metabolism. (Table 15.2). The main influences on BMR are:

- cellular activity, controlled by hormones, e.g. produced by the thyroid gland
- body weight
- surface area of the body as this affects heat loss.

More energy is required to meet demands created by different activities and different environments. For example, any muscular activity increases energy requirements, as does shivering to generate heat in a cold climate. The energy needed in a variety of situations is illustrated in Figure 15.1.

Dietary requirements

A healthy diet has two aims:

- to provide adequate energy and nutrients to allow normal growth and replacement of tissue and also to allow normal physiological function to take place
- to provide protection against disease.

Recommended dietary targets for the UK population are:

- total fat intake <35% of energy (recommended intakes DH (1991)
- total carbohydrate 50% of energy (recommended intakes DH (1991)
- protein <15% of energy (recommended intakes DH (1991)
- fibre (non-starch polysaccharide) 18 g/day (figure expressed as NSP, from DH (1991))
- salt <6 g (DH (1994), COMA report, *Nutritional aspects of cardiovascular disease*).

To assist the public to understand what is meant by healthy eating 'The balance of good health' was launched in 1994 (HEA 1994).

A picture of a tilted plate is divided into five sections of differing sizes, each representing one of the five food groups. The plate model indicates the proportions of food in a well-balanced healthy diet. Information is provided about the appropriate number of servings from each group that should be aimed for on a daily basis. As different people need different amounts of food, a serving of a particular food is relative rather than specific.

The energy intakes currently recommended in several countries are listed in Table 15.3.

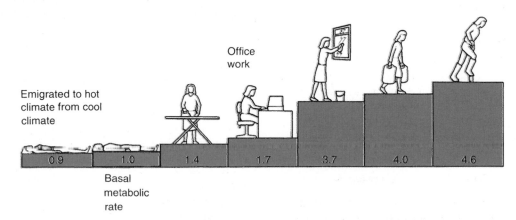

Figure 15.1 The relative energy costs of different activities undertaken by a woman as compared with her basal metabolic rate (BMR). General office work requires 1.7 times as much energy (1.7 × BMR) whereas walking with a heavy load requires four times as much (4 × BMR). The actual energy requirements in kilocalories or megajoules can be estimated from the data in Table 15.2. (After a report of a joint FAO/WHO/UNU Expert Consultation 1985, with permission.)

Table 15.3 Daily energy allowances recommended by different countries* for young adult (18–35 years) men and women of standard weight (by national standards†)

Country	Men kcal	Men kJ	Women kcal	Women kJ
Australia	2800	11 500	2000	8300
India	2400	10 000	1900	7900
Japan	2500	10 500	2000	8300
UK	2700	11 250	2200	9200
USA	2800	11 500	2000	8300

* Compiled from the Report of the Committee on International Dietary Allowances of the International Union of Nutritional Sciences 1975.

† The differences in energy requirement essentially reflect differences in body build.

RAW MATERIALS

In utero and through infancy, childhood and adolescence raw materials are needed for growth (see Ch. 31). In adults, the need for raw materials is normally limited to those required to replace items lost from the body. Losses include constituents of skin, hair and nails, secretions like sweat and mucus and the net losses occurring in faeces and urine. Other materials, derived from the breakdown of worn out cells and tissues, are recycled and re-used.

Cell debris is ingested and digested by phagocytic cells and the products are returned to the extracellular fluid (see Ch 14). For example, about 20 mg of iron are derived from the breakdown of old erythrocytes each day, and this is re-used in the formation of new haemoglobin. Consequently only 1 to 2 mg of iron are required per day to replace the net losses occurring from skin cells and body fluids.

Particular circumstances in adulthood which demand greater dietary intakes, because of the net gain of body tissues, include:

* pregnancy (growth of maternal and fetal tissues; Chs 30, 31)

Nutrition and surgery

Nutritional assessment and an appropriate nutritional intake pre- and postoperatively play a major role in recovery. Preoperative nutritional status has a significant impact on surgical outcome. There is an increased demand on the body's store of energy and protein postoperatively which will vary according to the degree of trauma and concurrent clinical factors.

The aims of adequate nutrition in surgical patients are to:

* facilitate wound healing
* reduce postoperative complications
* shorten the period of convalescence.

Table 15.4 Some of the products formed from amino acids in the human body

Name	Product Function/use	Chapter reference	Amino acid(s) used
Peptides	Hormones	11	All
Proteins	Enzymes		
	Receptors		
	Channels	1	All
	Cell structure		
	Antibodies	3,16	All
Purines and pyrimidines	Nucleic acids	1	Glycine Aspartic acid Glutamine
Creatine	Muscle metabolism	4B	Methionine Glycine Arginine
Melanin	Pigment	16	Tyrosine
Thyroxine	Hormone	11	Tyrosine
Adrenaline	Hormone	11	Tyrosine
Noradrenaline	Neurotransmitter	5	Tyrosine
Histamine	Inflammatory response	6,16	Histidine
Serotonin	Local vasoconstriction	3, 12, 16	Tryptophan

- physical activity that encourages muscle growth (Ch. 4B)
- restorative stages following illness or injury (Ch. 19).

Protein

Protein provides the same energy per gram as carbohydrate. However, protein is not used in the first instance as an energy source but in the growth, maintenance and repair of body tissue. Proteins are macromolecules made up of long chains of amino acids.

Table 15.5 The common amino acids found in proteins

Essential in the diet	Others
Valine*	Arginine
Leucine*	Glycine
Isoleucine*	Alanine
Threonine	Serine
Methionine	Cysteine
Phenylalanine	Tyrosine
Tryptophan	Aspartic acid
Lysine†	Glutamic acid‡
Histidine (in infancy)	Proline
	Histidine
	Hydroxyproline
	Ornithine

* Branched chain amino acids, e.g. valine

$$CH_3 \diagdown$$
$$CH_3 \diagup CH - CH_2 - COOH$$
$$\qquad\qquad | $$
$$\qquad\qquad NH_2$$

† Deficient in plant proteins other than those in peas and beans.
‡ Glutamate used in the food industry for giving meaty flavours to food.

Table 15.6 Daily intake of protein recommended for young adult men and women by different countries/ organizations*

	Protein intake (g/day)	
Country	Men	Women
Australia	70	58
India	55	45
Japan	70	60
UK	68	55
USA	65	55
WHO/FAO	37	29

* Compiled from the Report of the Committee on International Dietary Allowances of the International Union of Nutritional Sciences 1975.

Requirements

Amino acids are required for the synthesis of innumerable proteins and the manufacture of a variety of other products, examples of which are listed in Table 15.4 For the synthesis of any given protein to occur all the constituent amino acids must be available. If one of the amino acids is deficient, synthesis is interrupted and that protein cannot be formed. Twenty amino acids commonly exist in cells and tissues (see Ch. 1 and Table 15.5). Of these, in adulthood, eight must be present in the diet (essential amino acids) because they cannot be synthesized within the human body from other sources. Recommended intakes of protein are listed in Table 15.6.

Surplus amino acids

If there are plenty of amino acids in the bloodstream, surplus ones are deaminated, producing ammonia and a carbohydrate molecule. The carbohydrate can be used in mebabolism to form glucose and fat. Ammonia is incorporated into urea. The losses of urea and other products of amino acid metabolism in the urine represent a daily net loss of nitrogen from the body. Thus when dietary protein intake is high, urea excretion is greater than when it is not. Urinary losses of nitrogen

---

Health screening

Screening is now carried out to identify some of the possible errors in metabolism. One such error, which is genetic, is characterized by an inability to metabolize the amino acid phenylalanine normally.

Phenylalanine is an essential amino acid used in the synthesis of many proteins in the body and must be supplied by the diet. Within a normal diet there is an excess to requirements.

Surplus phenylalanine is converted into tyrosine, with the aid of the enzyme phenylalanine hydroxylase, and into phenylpyruvate (a phenylketone) with the aid of another enzyme, transaminase.

In people with phenylketonuria, phenylalanine hydroxylase is lacking and so phenylketones are formed in much larger amounts. They accumulate in body fluids and are excreted in the urine. This disorder, if undetected, is associated with nervous system abnormalities and mental retardation. Each child born has his or her urine analysed in order to detect the abnormality.

It is possible to implement a dietary control of phenylalanine until the child is 7 to 8 years old, when the brain becomes less susceptible to abnormal metabolites. Having a child on a special diet imposes many strains on a family and it is important that everyone involved in the child's care understands the diet and the reasons for the need for it.

Table 15.7 Plasma lipoproteins*

Relative size	Class	Source	% Composition				Functions
			Triglycerides	**Phospholipids**	**Cholesterol**	**Protein**	
◯	Chylomicrons	Intestine	90	3	5	2	Triglyceride transport
○	VLDL	Liver	55	20	15	10	
○	LDL	Plasma	8	22	45	25	Cholesterol transport
○	HDL	Various†	5	25	20	50	

* Compiled from Glickman & Sabesin 1988.
† Some HDL is secreted by intestinal and hepatic cells; some is formed in the plasma.
Key: VLDL, very low density lipoproteins; LDL, low density lipoproteins; HDL, high density lipoproteins.

provide useful information about the state of protein metabolism within the body when they are compared with dietary intake.

Nitrogen balance

If an individual's intake of nitrogen in protein is balanced by urinary losses of nitrogen in waste products the individual is in *nitrogen balance*. If growth is occurring, or there is considerable repair of tissues as in recovery from illness, then the loss of nitrogen may be less than that ingested and the individual is in *positive nitrogen balance*. Conversely, if net breakdown of tissues is occurring, then urinary losses may exceed intake and the result is a *negative nitrogen balance*.

Fats

Fats have a wide range of functions within the body. Fats are oxidized to provide energy for cells. This is the most concentrated form of dietary energy.
    Fat:

- provides essential fatty acids
- acts as a carrier for fat-soluble vitamins and antioxidants
- insulates the body against heat loss and provides protection for essential organs
- forms a structural component of brain tissue and the myelin sheath around nerves
- is essential in the formation of phospholipids and cholesterol which are vital constituents of cell membranes
- forms a substrate in hormone and prostaglandin synthesis.

Requirements

Like amino acids, fats are recycled and re-used. Often during this process they are broken down and reassembled in a slightly different form, as they are

during their digestion and absorption within the gastrointestinal tract (see Ch. 9). Fats are transported in the bloodstream largely in the form of lipoproteins (Table 15.7). Lipoproteins are molecular complexes consisting chiefly of:

- triglycerides
- phospholipids
- cholesterol
- specific proteins.

The complexes are dynamic structures that are being continually formed and degraded.
    Small losses of fat occur daily from shed cells, in secretions and in the faeces. These losses can be made good by the dietary intake of fat and by the synthesis of fats from glucose and from amino acids.

Essential fatty acids

Similar to amino acids, certain specific fats (essential fatty acids) need to be included in the diet, in adequate amounts. These fatty acids are:

- linoleic acid (found in plants)
- linolenic acid (rich source in marine life).

The essential fatty acids are required for the synthesis of prostaglandins which are regulators of cell function. The essential fatty acids are also constituents of some of the phospholipids in cell membranes and thereby influence membrane properties and functions.

Fat-soluble vitamins

An adequate intake of fat is required both to supply energy requirements and to provide the requisite amounts of essential fatty acids. In addition to this, an adequate intake of fats is needed to guarantee a tiny but vital intake of the compounds associated with them (fat-soluble vitamins) which are needed for cellular metabolism (Table 15.8).

Carbohydrates

Carbohydrates are needed to provide energy and form part of many cellular components, including DNA and RNA, and glycoproteins in cell membranes (see Ch. 1).

OTHER NUTRITIONAL REQUIREMENTS

Other required substances include:

- minerals
- vitamins.

Although many of these are recycled, there is always a dietary requirement to replace losses and meet additional demands imposed by growth and repair of tissue.

Minerals

These inorganic substances are either required in quantities measured in milligrams and tend to be called minerals or are required in quantities measured as micrograms and are called trace elements (Table 15.9).

Minerals include sodium, potassium, chloride, calcium, magnesium, iron and phosphorus. Trace elements include copper, chromium, manganese, iodine, molybdenum and selenium.

While elements such as iron and iodine are known to be important to health, the purpose of trace elements still needs some clarification. As a result, there can be variations in the recommended levels set by international advisory bodies.

Vitamins

Vitamins are organic compounds that are required in very small amounts to maintain normal metabolism and growth (Tables 15.7 and 15.10). Most vitamins cannot be manufactured by the body and so are similar to essential amino acids and fatty acids. They differ from them in that the amount required is very much smaller.

FOOD

The food we eat is either of animal, e.g. fish, meat, eggs, milk, or plant origin, e.g. cereal, fruit, vegetables, nuts, honey.

Food contains many different substances, not all of which are available to the body. Availability is improved by processing and cooking but these have their drawbacks as well as benefits.

Table 15.8 Fat-soluble vitamins

Vitamin	Alternative or equivalent name	Major sources	Reference nutrient intake*	Importance	Effects of deficiency
A	Retinol (β carotene)†	Butter, liver, fish liver oils, carrots	350–700 µg	Vision (see Ch. 24)	Night blindness Xerophthalmia
D	Calciferol	Action of sunlight on skin, fish, liver, oils, egg yolk	8.5–10 µg	Calcium metabolism (see Ch. 14)	Rickets Osteomalacia
E	Alpha tocopherol	Vegetable oils, eggs	‖	Antioxidant	‡
K	Menaquinone	Green leafy vegetables, bacterial metabolism (gut)	§1 µg/kg/day (adults) §10 µg/day (infants)	Synthesis of some blood coagulation factors (see Ch. 3)	Bleeding disorders caused by malabsorption (see Ch. 9)

* Dietary Reference Values for Food Energy and Nutrients for the United Kingdom. Report of the Panel on Dietary Reference Values of the Committee on Medical Aspects of Food Policy (1991) HMSO, London.

† Some foods such as carrots contain β carotene which is converted to vitamin A in the body. For this reason the vitamin A content of foods is quoted as 'retinol equivalents' in order to include this source of vitamin A.

‡ Vitamin E is so widespread in foods that specific deficiency hardly arises.

§ Production of vitamin K by intestinal bacteria makes estimation of dietary requirement difficult.

‖ The requirement for vitamin E is partly determined by the polyousaturated fatty acid content of the diet. Signs of clinical deficiency are unlikely to arise.

Table 15.9 Elements required in small amounts

Element	Symbol	Rich sources*	Reference nutrient intake for adults (mg/day)	(μg/day)	Effects of deficiency in humans
Iron	Fe	Treacle, liver, black pudding	8.7–14.8	–	Anaemia (see Ch. 3)
Zinc	Zn	Oysters†, meat, whole grains, legumes	7–9.5	–	Skin disorders Poor wound healing
Manganese	Mn	Plant foods (tea)	1.4	–	–
Copper	Cu	Green vegetables, liver	1.2	–	Anaemia (rare)
Molybdenum	Mo	Plant foods	§	–	–
Fluoride	F	Drinking water, tea	‖	–	Dental caries
Iodide	I	Seafood‡	–	14.0	Hypothyroid goitre (see Ch. 11)
Selenium	Se	Fish	–	60–70	Uncertain
Chromium	Cr	Widespread	–	¶	Insulin resistance

* Some foods that are less rich may contribute a large proportion of the dietary intake if they are eaten in large quantities. Cereals, for example, can be a significant dietary source of iron because of the amounts consumed each day.

† Oysters are exceptionally rich in zinc (10 to 20 times as much as in meat, legumes etc.).

‡ In some countries (USA, Switzerland, New Zealand but not the UK) iodine is also obtained from table salt which, in these countries, is iodized.

§ No RNI set, but safe intakes in adults between 50 and 400 μg per day.

‖ No RNI set, but the Panel suggest an upper limit on intakes of infants and young children of 0.05 mg/kg/day.

¶ No RNI set. A safe adequate level for children, 0.1–1.0 μg/kg/day and 25 μg/day for adults.

Table 15.10 Water-soluble vitamins

Vitamin		Other name	Rich* sources	Reference nutrient intakes† (mg/day)	(μg/day)	Role	Effects of deficiency
B group	B₁	Thiamin	Yeast	0.8–1	–	Involved in various aspects of cell metabolism especially enzyme activity	Polyneuritis Beriberi
	B₂	Riboflavin	Yeast, liver	1.1–1.3	–		Inflammation of the mouth
	B₃	Niacin	Yeast	12–18	–		Pellagra
	B₆	Pyridoxine	Liver	1.2–1.5	–		Rare
	B₁₂	Cobalamin	Liver, kidney, eggs	–	1.2–1.5		Macrocytic anaemia (see Ch. 3)
		Folic acid	Vegetables, yeast, liver	–	200		Macrocytic anaemia (see Ch. 3)
		Pantothenic acid	Liver	‡	–		Rare
		Biotin	Egg yolk	–	§		Rare
C		Ascorbic acid	Fruit, vegetables	40	–	Collagen formation Iron absorption Steroid synthesis	Scurvy

* Foods that are less rich may contribute a large proportion of the dietary intake because of the amounts consumed per day. Cereal based foods (such as breakfast cereals) and milk, for example, are good sources of the B vitamins.

† Range of recommended values from several countries (Australia, UK, USA) for adults.

‡ No biochemical method accepted for determining pantothenate status in humans. No signs of deficiency observed in UK on intakes between 3 and 7 mg/day.

§ No RNI set because of limited evidence; intakes of 10–20 μg/day considered safe and adequate.

Table 15.11 Differences in constituents between foods of animal and plant origin

Category	Exclusively animal	Richer in animal origin foods	Present in both	Richer in plant origin foods	Plant
Carbohydrates	Glycogen				Amylase (starch)
	Lactose				Cellulose
					Sucrose
Fats	Cholesterol	Saturated fats		Unsaturated fats	
Protein			Protein		
Vitamins	B$_{12}$*, D		A, B	C, E, K	
Minerals		Iron			
		Calcium			

* Produced also by microorganisms.

Table 15.12 Energy- and proteins-rich foods of vegetable origin*

Food		Energy (kcal/100 g)	Protein (g/100 g)
Class	**Example**		
Cereals	Soya flour		
	– full fat	447	36.8
	– low fat	352	45.3
	Wheat flour		
	– wholemeal	310	12.7
Cereal products	Meusli	363	9.8
	Oatcakes	412	10.0
	Bread		
	– naan	285	7.8
	– brown	207	7.9
	– white	219	7.9
Nuts	Peanuts	564	25.6
	Almonds	612	21.1
	Walnuts	688	14.7
Nut products	Peanut butter	606	22.6
Legumes	Lentils		
	– raw, dried	297	24.3
	– boiled	105	8.8
	Peas		
	– raw	83	6.9
	– boiled	79	6.7
	Red kidney beans		
	– raw, dried	266	22.1
	– boiled	103	8.4

Data from the Composition of Foods Sixth Summary Edition. Crown copyright. Reproduced with the permission of the Controller of HMSO and Queen's Printer for Scotland.

COMPOSITION

All food consists of the same constituents: carbohydrate, protein, fat, minerals, electrolytes, water and other organic molecules, including vitamins. Foods from different sources contain differing proportions of these constituents (Table 15.11). For example, protein is found in foods of both plant and animal origin while cellulose, a component of dietary fibre, is found only in food of plant origin. Some constituents of food such as dietary fibre are indigestible and some such as tannin and caffeine have no nutritive value. Other minor constituents are contaminants.

Vegetarian diets

More people today are choosing to follow a vegetarian diet. This choice is made for a variety of reasons including religious and cultural beliefs, moral and ethical reasons and health and environmental concerns. Vegetarianism is often more than an eating pattern. It is a philosophy that affects the individual's whole lifestyle.

Vegetarian diets can be nutritionally adequate if a sensible choice of foods is made. Vegan diets that do not include any animal products will be deficient in vitamin B_{12}, certain amino acids, iron and calcium. It is important to ensure that these requirements are met by supplementation. This requirement is particularly important in children and in women of childbearing age.

Another potential complication of a vegetarian diet is that it may consist largely of bulky, fibrous and watery foods. These easily make a person feel 'full up', but may not supply adequate amounts of energy and protein. This can be a particular nutritional risk for children. Foods of vegetable origin rich in energy and in protein, such as cereals, legumes and nuts, should be consumed in sufficient amounts to meet this need (Table 15.12).

Non-starch polysaccharide (dietary fibre)

Dietary fibre is the term used to describe the component of complex carbohydrate that is resistant to digestion (Table 15.13). The UK COMA panel in 1991 considered that the term dietary fibre should become obsolete and be replaced by the term non-starch polysaccharide (NSP). NSPs are a major component of plant cell walls and, as they can be clearly identified chemically, they can be precisely measured. Dietary fibre, however, remains the term familiar to the public.

In the UK, the average diet contains approximately 12 g of NSP per day (Bingham et al 1990). The COMA panel on Dietary Reference Values (DH 1991) proposed

Table 15.13 Dietary fibre

Examples	Source	Rich dietary sources
Cellulose	Constituent of plant cell wall	All vegetables
Hemicellulose		
Lignin	'Woody' plant tissues	Cereals
Pectin	Plant sap	Fruits
Gums		

that the adult UK intake should be 18 g fibre (NSP) daily from a variety of foods (Table 15.14). There is no specific recommendation for children other than that the intake should be proportionately lower. The fibre content of foods can be measured in different ways with the different methods resulting in different figures depending on the fibre fractions in the food. Currently in the UK data on the fibre content of food is measured both by the Englyst method, which measures the NSP content of the food, and by the Southgate method, which includes other carbohydrate that is not digestible, mainly resistant starch and lignin. As a result, analysis of dietary fibre using the Englyst method results in a lower figure than the Southgate method.

Diets low in fibre are known to be associated with an increased incidence of digestive and other disturbances. Dietary fibre:

- provides 'bulk' to a meal
- binds and adsorbs other substances
- is metabolized by colonic bacteria.

Bulking effect

The bulkiness of ingested food affects digestion and absorption in several ways. Firstly, in distending the stomach, a 'bulky' meal quickly evokes a sensation of 'fullness'. The desire to eat is thereby satisfied at a lower intake of available energy. Secondly, by 'diluting' the

Table 15.14 Some fibre-rich foods

Food	Dietary fibre (g/100 g)	Weight of average serving (g)
Wholemeal bread	5.0	50 (2 slices)
Muesli	6.4	50
Baked beans	3.7	60
Processed peas (canned)	5.1	60
Red kidney beans (boiled)	6.7	–

Data from the Composition of Foods Sixth Summary Edition. Crown copyright. Reproduced with the permission of the Controller of HMSO and Queen's Printer for Scotland.

available energy in the diet, the assimilation of nutrients in the small intestine will proceed at a more measured pace. Thirdly, distension of the digestive tract promotes motility and secretion, which in turn facilitate the digestive process.

Binding properties

Fibre clings to water and thus has a water-retaining effect which adds to its 'bulking' effect. This helps to make faecal residues softer and easier to evacuate. Some other substances are also preferentially adsorbed to dietary fibre. This reduces their concentration in the intestinal fluid and therefore limits their absorption. For example bile acids (see Chs 9 and 10) bind to dietary fibre. Consequently the loss of bile acids in the faeces is increased by a high fibre diet. Bile acids which are lost in the faeces are replaced by those newly synthesized from cholesterol (see Ch. 10). This contributes to the plasma cholesterol lowering effect that a high fibre diet is known to have. It has also been suggested that fibre may bind some potentially carcinogenic substances and therefore have a protective effect.

Bacterial metabolism

Although fibre is not broken down by gastrointestinal digestive enzymes, it is metabolized by the colonic bacteria, which use fibre as a source of nutrients and generate a variety of products from it including short chain fatty acids, and carbon dioxide, hydrogen and methane gases (see Ch. 9). Some of the fatty acids are absorbed. They also stimulate colonic motility and secretion.

Because fibre is food for colonic bacteria the numbers and the mass of bacteria increase when the dietary intake of fibre is high. This also increases the bulk of the residues in the colon. The well-known action of high fibre diets in promoting defecation is thus likely to be due to a combination of all these factors.

In Western society, affluence and other sociological factors have had an effect on fibre consumption. A preference for refined food and an increase in the use of prepackaged foods, which require a minimal amount of preparation and cooking, have contributed to a general reduction in fibre intake.

The increase of bowel cancer and diverticular disease in Western society has been linked to the decrease in fibre. Most people can rectify the deficiency by including more wholegrain bread and cereal and more fruit and vegetables in their diet.

Non-nutritive constituents

Any natural food may also contain tiny amounts of other substances (Table 15.15) including:

- substances peculiar to particular plant or animal species

Table 15.15 Some non-nutritive constituents of food

Type	Examples	Sources
Natural constituents	Alkaloids	
	– solanine	Green, sprouted potatoes
	– caffeine	Tea, coffee
	– pyrrmolizidine	Comfrey
	Cyanogenetic glycosides	Apricot kernels, cassava
	Flavenols	Tea
	Oxalic acid	Rhubarb
	Serotonin (5HT)	Bananas
Bacterial contaminants	Aflatoxins	Peanuts (mouldy)
	Amines	Mould on cheese
	Ergot alkaloids	Fungus on cereals
	Mycotoxins	Moulds
Contaminants arising from human activities	Antibiotics	Animal husbandry
	Cadmium	
	Mercury	Industrial pollution
	Lead	
	Pesticides	Agricultural practice
	Food additives (cyclamate, monosodium glutamate)	Food industry

- environmental contaminants
- bacterial contaminants.

Plants manufacture a variety of substances that are foreign to our cells. Some of these, such as caffeine, have a drug-like effect. Others such as the cyanogenetic glycosides are toxic.

Foods may also contain substances that have been taken up by the organism from the environment. Some of these may have been used by the farmer to maximize crop yield or to restrain pests and diseases. Animal foods may contain contaminants derived from the plants which the livestock have eaten, from the drinking water or, in the case of marine fish, from the sea in areas of pollution. Some substances, such as bacteria, which are passed on in this way may be made harmless by digestion, but others, such as mercury, are retained in the food chain and passed on to the human consumer. Food may also be contaminated by bacteria that generate harmful toxins.

Cassava, the principal food of many people in the tropics, contains a glyceride, linamarin, from which cyanide is released by enzymatic action. Before consumption, the roots are grated and sun dried to remove the cyanide. However, in West Africa an association has been found between cassava consumption and some neuropathies.

Food and drug interactions can occasionally occur. Tyramine, an amine formed from tyrosine by bacterial metabolism, is found in old or fermented food products where protein breakdown occurs. The older the food, the greater the bacterial contamination, the greater the amount of tyramine formed. Normally this is broken down by monoamine oxidase in the cells of the digestive tract and the liver so only small amounts enter the bloodstream. When monoamine oxidase inhibitors are prescribed for the treatment of depression, the breakdown does not occur and so larger amounts of tyramine circulate in the blood. One effect of tyramine is to promote the release of noradrenaline which produces a rise in blood pressure. For this reason foods high in tyramine such as cheese, yeast extracts and red wine are restricted if an individual is prescribed monoamine oxidase inhibitors (see Ch. 5).

Recently, genetic modification of food has caused concern among the public. Genetic modification (GM) is the technique of changing the genetic make-up of an organism by adding, removing or in some way altering individual genes to achieve a desired result. Genetic modification has been used for some years in food production. Crops have been modified to improve weed control or to make the plants more resistant to insects and therefore increase yield. However, many people have ethical concerns about GM foods and concerns about their long-term safety. In the UK the law ensures that if GM ingredients have been used in the production of a food product, it must be clearly indicated on the label.

AVAILABILITY OF NUTRIENTS

Nutrients present in a diet are not necessarily completely available to us. Some constituents, like dietary fibre, are indigestible whereas others, like iron, may be prevented from being absorbed by conditions in the digestive tract or by other substances in the diet.

Digestibility of food

Some polysaccharides and proteins cannot be digested easily by the enzymes present in the human digestive tract. This applies to some fibrous proteins, such as keratin in skin, and to the carbohydrate cellulose in plants. In some cases, particularly proteins, cooking begins the breakdown of such macromolecules, making them more vulnerable to enzymic attack and therefore to digestion.

Lactase deficiency

After early childhood, most of the world's population (85%) have a relative deficiency of the enzyme lactase, which breaks down the disaccharide lactose in milk to the monosaccharides glucose and galactose. Conse-

quently, lactose cannot be properly digested and, so, much of this carbohydrate in milk will be unavailable nutritionally (see Ch. 9).

Absorbability of nutrients

The absorbability of some substances, such as iron and calcium, depends on the form in which they are present in food and also on the blend of other substances in the diet, some of which may hinder their absorption.

Iron

Dietary iron, for example, is present in food in haem (from haemoglobin in meat) and exists in two inorganic forms ferrous (Fe^{2+}) and ferric (Fe^{3+}). Haem is readily absorbed whereas inorganic iron is not. However, Fe^{2+} is much better absorbed than Fe^{3+}. Conditions in the digestive tract that favour the formation of Fe^{2+}, and therefore the absorption of iron, include a low pH and the presence of reducing agents, like vitamin C, that convert Fe^{3+} to Fe^{2+}. If, however, the diet is rich in phytates (from unrefined cereals), insoluble salts of iron are formed and these cannot be absorbed. Consequently, iron deficiency can arise even though the total amount of iron in the diet appears to be adequate.

It is for these reasons that the dietary reference values of certain nutrients, such as iron (8.7–14.8 mg/day), far exceeds the amounts which need to be absorbed to maintain nutritional balance (iron: 1–2 mg/day).

FOOD PROCESSING AND PREPARATION

Food is usually processed before it is eaten, either during manufacture or in cooking.

Food processing

Processing enables natural products to be:

- preserved (frozen, canned, smoked, salted, irradiated)
- made palatable (attractive to eat)
- more digestible and of greater nutrient value
- safe to eat.

Sometimes different products are manufactured by processing, for example butter and cheese made from milk, and vegetable oils made from olives, peanuts, coconut etc.

Processing alters food. Its very real benefits, as listed above, have to be weighed against some drawbacks which may include:

- loss of fibre (in the refining of flour)
- losses of vitamins (in the heating required in canning and in thawing of frozen foods)

- undesirable effects of substances that are added (such as salt and sugar) or produced during processing (such as nitrosamines)
- changes in the chemical nature of some nutrients (such as fatty acids and amino acids) which make them less useful nutritionally.

Nutrient losses occur in fresh foods that have been in transit over time. In fruit and vegetables vitamins are particularly vulnerable. The only food that can be guaranteed as really fresh is that which is literally home-grown and eaten on the day it is picked.

Labelling

The Food Standards Agency (www.food.gov.uk) provides information about food labelling, health and safety.

Cooking

Cooking, whether in the course of manufacture or in the restaurant and home, makes food:

- safer to eat
- appetizing (usually!)
- digestible.

Food standards

Whilst food is essential for life, it may also cause illness if it contains:

- harmful bacteria
- viruses
- parasites – tapeworms or threadworms
- poisonous chemicals – pesticides etc.

National legislation within the Health and Safety Act (1974) sets compulsory standards for production, distribution and sale of foodstuffs. Hospitals, nursing and residential homes etc. all undergo regular inspections.
Important points in relation to food handling include:

- thorough defrosting of poultry and meat before cooking
- storage of cooked food and raw food separately
- avoidance of partial cooking of meat
- rapid cooking of food that is to be subsequently stored.

Food poisoning is a statutorily notifiable disease. Organisms cause food poisoning by direct invasion of the wall of the intestine, e.g. *Salmonella* spp., or by production of an enterotoxin, e.g. *Staphylococcus aureus*, and give rise to an acute illness, which usually includes one or more gastrointestinal symptoms.

Safety of food

Cooking can destroy harmful bacteria, toxins and viruses. Sometimes toxic chemicals, such as cyanogenetic glycosides (Table 15.15), present in the food are rendered harmless so that the food becomes edible.

Palatability of food

Cooking makes most foods more appetizing because new products are formed in the process. The blend of products depends on the form of cooking adopted, be it cooking in water or in fat, or by dry heat or radiation. Toast tastes different from bread because the charring produces dextrins from the carbohydrates. Sometimes the products generated, such as polycyclic hydrocarbons in barbecued foods, can be harmful if ingested in excess.

Digestibility of food

Cooking makes food more digestible because cells are ruptured, proteins are denatured, macromolecules are broken down and chemicals are released. Uncooked potato is not readily digestible, but cooking begins the breakdown and makes the nutrients present more available.

Minimizing losses of nutrients

Losses of nutrients in cooking can be minimized by:

- avoiding the use of too much water in boiling
- avoiding too high a temperature for too long
- keeping the time between cooking and serving food to a minimum.

NUTRIENT HOMEOSTASIS

The concentration of nutrients in the blood depends upon the balance between:

- intake
- metabolism
- losses.

For many nutrients, including glucose, amino acids and fats, dietary intake and metabolism are the key determinants of nutritional homeostasis. Both dietary intake and metabolism are regulated by neural and hormonal mechanisms in ways that maintain a supply of fuels for the production of energy and safeguard the plasma concentration of glucose.

Losses of nutrients in shed cells and tissues, faeces and body fluids are normally relatively small. Significant losses of water-soluble nutrients such as glucose and amino acids in the urine are normally prevented by their complete reabsorption from the glomerular filtrate in the renal tubules (see Ch. 8).

If more food is ingested than is needed the excess is stored chiefly as fat and weight is gained.

INTAKE

Diet is influenced by a number of factors including geographical factors, sociological factors, wealth, culture and religion. In humans, social factors play an important part in determining when food is eaten. The internal controls that register when the stomach is full and note the prevailing metabolic state may be overridden by voluntary or socially conditioned factors. As a result, humans find that they may eat more than is required in a way that animals do not.

Regulation of dietary intake

The major internal factors involved in the control of food intake are:

- gastrointestinal
  - distension of the stomach
  - cholecystokinin
- metabolic
  - plasma glucose
  - plasma free fatty acids.

Gastrointestinal factors

A bulky meal containing a lot of fibre will give rise to a sensation of fullness more quickly than one which is more readily digestible and may in fact contain more calories.

Cholecystokinin (see Ch. 9) is released from the small intestine by the presence of amino acids and fatty acids. In addition to its functions in stimulating the pancreas to secrete enzymes and the gall bladder to contract, cholecystokinin also acts on the hypothalamic cells which control feeding and contributes to the feeling of satiation. Because cholecystokinin is one of the factors that slows gastric emptying it also prolongs gastric distension which leads to a feeling of fullness. As a result, a meal with a high fat and protein content prolongs this feeling in a way that a meal high in carbohydrate does not.

Metabolic factors

Plasma concentrations of glucose and fatty acids are indicators of the metabolic state. In the fed state, high plasma glucose and low plasma fatty acid concentrations promote a feeling of satiety. Conversely in starvation a low blood glucose and a high circulating concentration of free fatty acids promote a feeling of hunger. One of the key controlling factors is the use of glucose by the cells of the hypothalamus. This is proportional to the plasma glucose concentration

---

Inflammatory bowel disease

Inflammatory bowel disease, predominantly Crohn's disease and ulcerative colitis, occurs as a result of a chronic non-specific inflammatory process which differs in terms of location and type of lesion. Malabsorption occurs in these disorders as the gastrointestinal tract has reduced enzyme secretion and lesions reduce the size of the absorptive area (see Ch. 9), which may lead to nutritional deficiency.

Dietary treatment of malabsorbtion requires an increased intake of the nutrients malabsorbed, or replacement with alternatives, concurrent with a reduction of bowel motility. A diet high in protein, calories and vitamins should be provided, with an increase in fluid intake if diarrhoea is present in order to prevent dehydration.

---

provided that the hormone insulin is also present in sufficient quantities. If it is not, as in diabetes mellitus, even though plasma glucose levels are high, all cells including the hypothalamic cells are starved of glucose. As a result, a person with diabetes mellitus can feel hungry when they are both hypo- and hyperglycaemic.

People who have diabetes mellitus are advised to include carbohydrate from complex fibre-rich foods that have a low glycaemic index. These include cereals such as oats, fruit and leguminous vegetables as this type of carbohydrate is slowly absorbed. Sugar can be included in modest quantities provided it contributes to a meal and is not taken in isolation. Large amounts of sugary food consumed alone cause a rapid increase in glycaemia because of its rapid absorption rate (See also Ch. 18).

Regulation of absorption

The rate of absorption of amino acids, monosaccharides and fats by the intestinal epithelium is determined by the:

- delivery of digested products to the epithelium
- absorptive capacity of the epithelium.

Delivery of nutrients

The factors which influence the delivery of digested products include the rate at which predigested chyme is emptied from the stomach into the small intestine and the rate at which proteins, carbohydrates and fats are broken down by digestive enzymes.

As described earlier, the rate at which the stomach empties depends on the nature of the meal. Meals containing a lot of fat are emptied more slowly than those which do not.

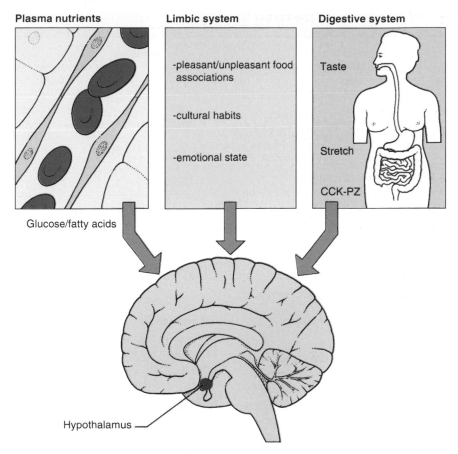

Figure 15.2 Information used by the hypothalamus in regulating the desire to eat and the consumption of food. CCK-PZ, cholecystokinin-pancreozymin.

Absorptive capacity

Virtually all the ingested carbohydrate and protein is digested and absorbed. Only small amounts escape into the colon to be metabolized by the colonic bacteria. Ninety-five per cent of the ingested fat is also absorbed. There are no digestive controls that stop us from absorbing too much other than those that regulate gastric emptying (see Ch. 9) and that control the desire to eat (Fig. 15.2).

In the case of nutrients such as iron and calcium, which are not completely absorbed, the amount absorbed can be regulated according to the requirements of the body. Iron absorption is increased in states of iron deficiency and decreased when the concentration of iron in the intestinal epithelial cells is high. The absorption of calcium is regulated by vitamin D (see Ch. 14).

METABOLISM

Once food has been ingested and absorbed the plasma concentrations of nutrients such as glucose, amino acids and fatty acids are adjusted by metabolic controls. In times of plenty, surpluses are stored; in deprivation, stores are used. The nutrient whose concentration is most closely regulated is glucose (see Ch. 18). A number of different mechanisms are involved in stabilizing its concentration in the face of the changing delivery of glucose to the body in feeding and fasting.

Feeding is normally an intermittent activity. In some societies food is consumed every few hours during the day so that fasting occurs only during the hours of sleep. In other societies, different cultural patterns and environmental constraints expose the body more frequently to periods of fasting, and even to starvation.

Stores

Absorbed items that are surplus to immediate requirements are stored in several ways (Table 15.16):

- glucose as glycogen in liver and muscle
- fats as triglyceride in adipose tissue
- amino acids are used to form proteins and surpluses are deaminated and then converted into carbohydrate or fat

Table 15.16 Nutrient storage in an average well-fed resting adult

| Nutrient | Form | Storage site | Amount | | | | Daily requirement |
			kg	g	mg	kcal	
Glucose	Glycogen	Liver	–	80*	–	320	
		Skeletal muscle	–	300*	–	1200	1500 kcal
Fats	Triglyceride	Adipose tissue	11†	–	–	100 000	
Iron	Ferritin	Liver mostly	–	–	500‡	–	1–2 mg
	Haemosiderin	All cells					
A, D, E, K	A, D, E, K	Liver					
B$_{12}$	B$_{12}$	Liver mostly	–	–	5	–	0.002 mg
Folic acid	Folic acid	Liver	–	–	8	–	0.3 mg

* From Astrand & Rohdahl 1986.

† From Garrow 1978.

‡ Amount varies considerably between men (1000 mg) and women (0–500 mg).

- some minerals and vitamins in the liver (iron, vitamins A, D, E and K, vitamin B$_{12}$).

Some of these substances, such as the fat-soluble vitamins, simply accumulate progressively if they are ingested in excess. Vitamins, though necessary for health, can be toxic if consumed in large amounts. There are few, if any, homeostatic control mechanisms limiting the plasma concentrations of fat-soluble vitamins and some other absorbed substances, such as cholesterol, to

an acceptable range. Consequently, plasma concentrations can exceed safe levels as well as fall below them. For example, hypervitaminosis can occur if the dietary intake of any of vitamins A, D or K is too large.

Glucose

Central to the control of metabolism is the absolute requirement of some cells for glucose. These cells include red cells, neurones and cells of the testes and

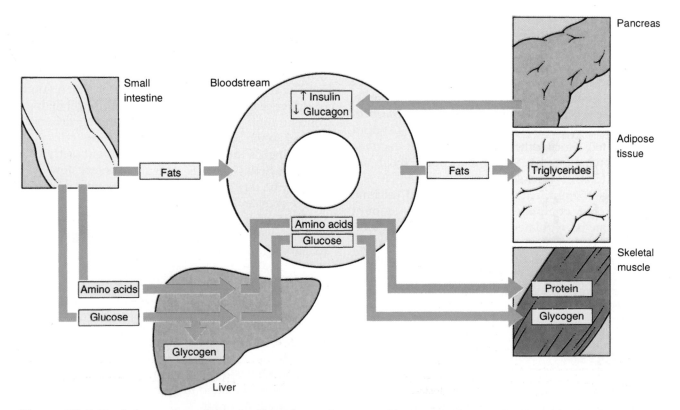

Figure 15.3 The fed state: fate of absorbed nutrients and patterns of hormone secretion after the ingestion of a meal.

renal medulla. The cells of the nervous system rely almost exclusively on glucose for the formation of ATP. Hypoglycaemia is therefore a threat to nerve cells and consequently to the body as a whole.

Normally, plasma glucose concentrations range between 4.5 mmol/l after an overnight fast to 10 mmol/l at the peak of absorption of a carbohydrate meal. Levels are normally kept within this range by metabolic adjustments which enable the surplus to be taken up after a meal and which maintain glucose supplies between meals.

After a meal – the fed state

When a meal is digested and absorbed most of the nutrients pass first to the liver before entering the general circulation (see Ch. 10). As soon as their concentration begins to increase in the arterial blood, the balance of hormones secreted by different endocrine tissues changes (see Ch. 11). The hormones enable glucose, amino acids and fatty acids to be taken up into cells and incorporated into macromolecules such as glycogen, proteins and triglycerides (Fig. 15.3).

Processing of nutrients by the liver

When food is available and digestion and absorption are proceeding, the concentration of absorbed nutrients in the venous blood from the gut increases. The liver is the first organ to be exposed to the nutrients, such as monosaccharides, amino acids, some vitamins and minerals, absorbed via this route (see Ch. 10).

Glucose is taken up by the liver (Fig. 15.4A) and converted into glycogen. Galactose, from the digestion of lactose in milk, is taken up and converted into glucose. The hepatic uptake of glucose is not insulin dependent.

Amino acids are taken up too (Fig. 15.4B). Some are used to form cellular and plasma proteins. Others are interconverted so that the proportion of different amino acids leaving the liver in the hepatic vein blood is not exactly the same as that entering it in the portal blood. Unbranched amino acids are preferentially used by the

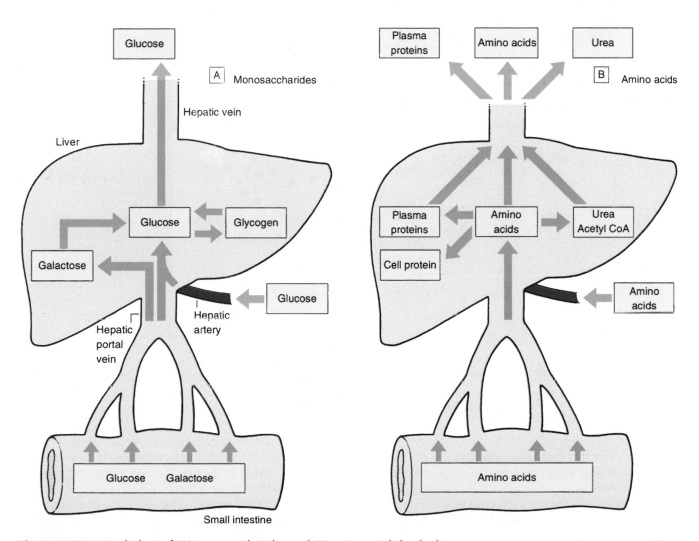

Figure 15.4 Metabolism of (A) monosaccharides and (B) amino acids by the liver.

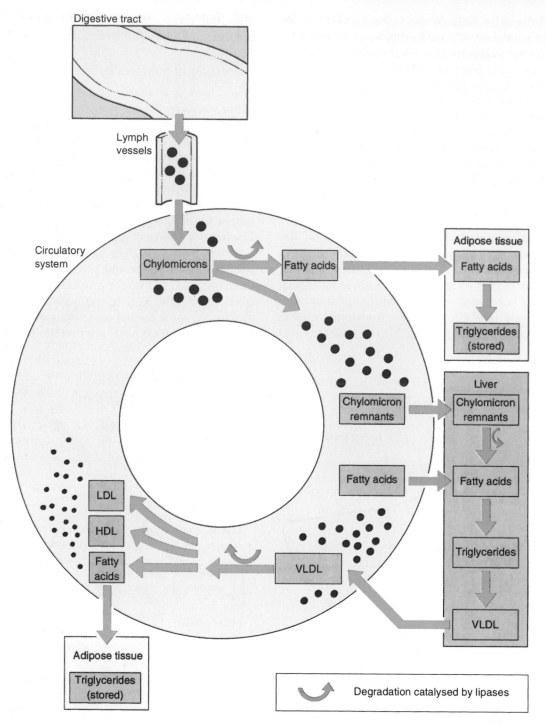

Figure 15.5 Metabolism of fats: roles of the circulatory system, adipose tissue and the liver.

liver with the result that the hepatic venous blood is relatively richer in branched amino acids (Table 15.5). Branched amino acids are used in large amounts by skeletal muscle.

Minerals such as iron, copper and lead are also taken up by the liver cells, as are several of the vitamins including vitamin B$_{12}$ and folic acid.

As a result of all this uptake and metabolism, the nutrient profile in the circulation as a whole is not the same as that in the venous blood draining from the gastrointestinal tract.

Absorbed fats largely bypass the liver, by entering the lymphatic vessels of the gut in the form of chylomicrons (Table 15.7 and Fig. 15.5). The lymph flows into the bloodstream via the thoracic duct. Triglycerides in the chylomicrons are then gradually degraded by enzymes (lipoprotein lipases) present in the capillaries of many tissues including adipose tissue and skeletal and cardiac muscle to yield fatty acids and glycerol. Fatty acids bind to plasma proteins, chiefly albumin, and circulate in the blood in this form.

Some fatty acids and what is left of the chylomicrons (chylomicron remnants) are taken up and processed by the liver and used to form new triglycerides. These triglycerides are packaged with other lipids to form very low density lipoproteins (VLDL) that are secreted by the liver into the blood. These lipoproteins are also attacked by lipoprotein lipase in the capillaries of the circulation yielding more free fatty acids and producing low density lipoproteins (LDL) and high density lipoproteins (HDL). LDL and HDL carry cholesterol in the bloodstream (see Table 15.7).

Hormonal control of metabolism

The rise in the concentrations of glucose and of amino acids in the circulation enhances the release of insulin

---

Nutrition and cardiovascular disease

Epidemiological studies highlight two important factors:

- cardiovascular disease (CVD) is environmentally determined (immigrant groups take on the incidence of their host country)
- there is a link between CVD and a high intake of saturated fat with a low intake of dietary fibre.

Low density lipoproteins (LDL) and high density lipoproteins (HDL) are good at carrying cholesterol in the blood, and a high intake of animal fats leads to raised serum lipids (see main text). Reducing the dietary intake of cholesterol specifically is only useful if the normal intake is high.

Polyunsaturated fats, mainly those rich in linoleic acid, tend to lower the serum LDL but their effect is only half as strong as the elevating effect of palmitic acid found in saturated fats.

Dietary fibre found in vegetables and fruit may have a positive effect of lowering blood lipids. Screening for hyperlipidaemia (high lipids in the blood) is now common. Concentrations of lipoproteins are decreased in obesity and increased by alcohol consumption.

Atherosclerosis occurs when fatty deposits rich in cholesterol develop within the inner lining of arteries, causing them to become narrow and reducing the blood flow.

When atherosclerosis occurs in the coronary arteries, ischaemic heart disease develops; when found within the cerebral arteries the individual is at risk of a cerebral vascular accident (stroke).

Much of this evidence is still under review.

---

and depresses the secretion of glucagon from the pancreas. These stimuli add to the stimulatory effects of the gastrointestinal hormones and the autonomic nervous system which occur during the digestion of the meal. The result is a substantial increase in the plasma concentration of insulin and a decrease in glucagon.

This change in the ratio of insulin and glucagon shifts the bias of metabolic activity towards the uptake of glucose, amino acids and fatty acids into cells and to their incorporation into glycogen, protein and triglycerides, respectively. This shift occurs chiefly in skeletal muscle and in adipose tissue. Some cells are not regulated by insulin in this way, including those which rely exclusively on glucose as the fuel for ATP production (neurones, red cells, kidney medulla) and the intestinal mucosa. In these cells uptake is permitted at all times.

Between meals – fasting

An average sized meal is digested and absorbed over a period of about 4 hours. Thereafter the concentration of nutrients in the blood falls gradually. As the concentration of glucose decreases, the balance of hormones secreted alters. The plasma concentration of glucagon increases and that of insulin decreases. This redirects body metabolism in such a way that the concentration of glucose in the plasma (and interstitial fluid) is protected and the supply of fuels for the production of energy is maintained (Fig. 15.6).

The concentration of glucose in the plasma is maintained in three ways:

- breakdown of liver glycogen (glycogenolysis)
- new synthesis of glucose (gluconeogenesis)
- sparing of glucose for selected tissues.

Glucogenolysis

It has been estimated that the amount of glycogen normally present in the liver of a well-fed adult could, on its own, maintain plasma glucose concentration in a resting adult for about 8 hours, say overnight. The glycogen stored in muscle cannot be drawn upon directly in the same way. Its primary function is to supply the energy needs of muscle cells. However, lactate released from muscle cells by anaerobic metabolism (see Ch. 10) can be converted back into glucose by the liver.

Gluconeogenesis

While glycogen stores are being depleted, the synthesis of new glucose (hence gluco-ineo-genesis) is stimulated by the increase in plasma glucagon and decrease in insulin. Amino acids, chiefly alanine derived from the breakdown of muscle proteins, and glycerol produced by the breakdown of triglycerides (lipolysis) in adipose

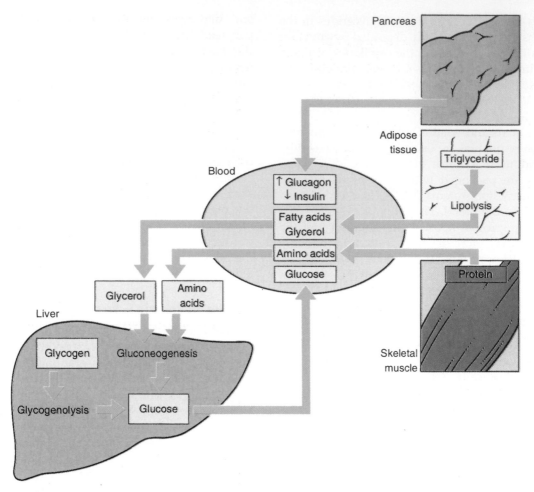

Figure 15.6 The fasting state: release and metabolism of stored nutrients, and pattern of hormone secretion.

tissue are converted by the liver (and also the kidneys) into glucose.

Glucose sparing

Fatty acids released by the breakdown of triglycerides in adipose tissue are used by some tissues, including muscles, as an energy source in place of glucose. During fasting the concentration of fatty acids in the blood increases (Fig. 15.7). In this way glucose is spared for those tissues which specifically rely on it (see Ch. 18).

Starvation

If food deprivation continues, fatty acids are metabolized in increasing amounts by the mitochondria and large quantities of acetyl CoA are formed. The surplus acetyl CoA formed within the liver overloads the liver's capacity to metabolize it via the citric acid cycle and increasing amounts spill over into the metabolic pathways leading to the formation of ketone bodies (Fig. 15.8).

Ketone bodies

Ketone bodies (or ketoacids) include aceto-acetic acid, acetone and beta-hydroxybutyric acid (also known as D-3 hydroxybutyric acid). Significant quantities of these products are detected in the blood after only a couple of days of fasting (Fig. 15.7). They can be used by various tissues, including brain, skeletal and cardiac muscle, as an alternative fuel to glucose. In the tissues they are converted back to acetyl CoA and metabolized via the citric acid cycle (see Ch. 10). Ketone bodies have an advantage over fatty acids in that they can gain access to cells much more readily because they diffuse more easily through cell membranes. Even brain cells can use ketone bodies because they can diffuse across the blood–brain barrier.

As starvation proceeds the body's requirement for glucose is progressively reduced. The increased concentration of ketone bodies in the blood inhibits the release of amino acids from skeletal muscle and slows the protein breakdown occurring there.

Protein energy malnutrition

Protein energy malnutrition (PEM) occurs in periods of starvation or as a result of stress associated with injury. Protein is catabolized to provide energy for the body.

Research demonstrates that no person should be without an intake of protein for longer than 5 days (Holmes 1986).

PEM is seen in the children in the developing world in two extreme forms:

- marasmus – more common where the diet is low in both protein and calories
- kwashiorkor – more common where the diet is low in protein but there is a relatively adequate energy (carbohydrate) intake.

PEM can also occur within hospitalized patients, especially following surgery and/or trauma, giving rise to a state of negative nitrogen balance. The extent of alteration in nutrient homeostasis is in direct proportion to the severity of the injury/stress and the individual's previous nutritional state. It is thus imperative that nutritional assessment is carried out prior to planned surgery and that nurses monitor, record and report on their patients' nutritional state and intake of nutrients.

The result is ketosis where high levels of ketone bodies are found in body fluids and the smell of acetone can be detected on the breath. Ketone bodies can also be detected in urine analysis. This test can be used to assist in the diagnosis of diabetes mellitus.

Digestive tract

In starvation, the gastrointestinal tract atrophies. This is partly due to the general breakdown of tissues that occurs with nutritional deficiency. However, it is also caused by the lack of activity in the digestive tract and by the lack of secretion of hormones, such as gastrin and CCK-PZ, which have a growth-promoting effect (trophic effect) on parts of the digestive system.

Patients who receive nutritional support via the intravenous route, as in total parenteral nutrition, for a prolonged length of time, will suffer from gastrointestinal atrophy. For this reason, when possible, the preferred route for nutritional support is nasogastric feeding via a tube or gastrostomy feeding.

Faeces continue to be formed even when no food is eaten. This is because the bulk of the faecal mass consists of bacteria. These continue to survive in the colon sustained by the nourishment they gain from shed cells and digestive secretions.

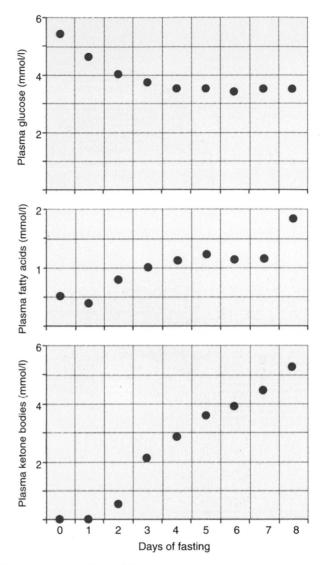

Figure 15.7 Effects of fasting on the composition of plasma: mean values from six subjects. (After Cahill et al 1966, with permission of American Society for Criminal Investigation.)

GAINING AND LOSING WEIGHT

Once adulthood has been attained, body weight changes very little. Tables of 'normal' weight for height have been compiled for many different populations worldwide. These tables are based on the normal statistics for the population as a whole. Guidelines for acceptable weights, such as those published by the BMA, represent the weights which are associated with the lowest mortality for that group (as researched for example by the Metropolitan Life Insurance Company).

Body weight

A change in body weight can be the result of one or more of several factors. It may represent changes in:

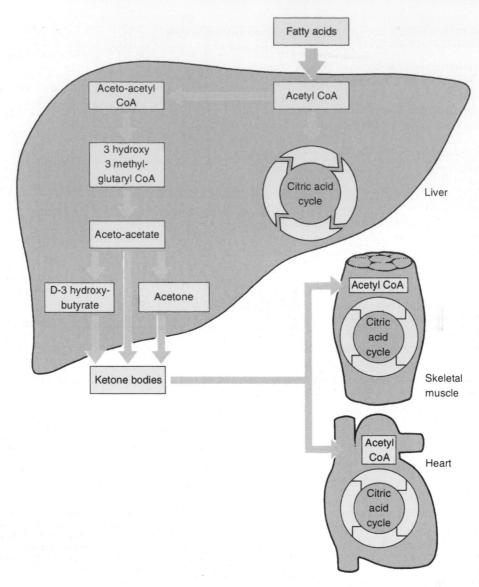

Figure 15.8 Formation and usage of ketone bodies. (Note: specific carbohydrates are needed to keep the citric acid cycle working. If these are deficient, as they are in diabetes mellitus, the concentration of ketone bodies in blood increases even more.)

- total body water
- muscle mass
- adipose tissue
- a combination of these.

Total body water

The factors which affect total body water are discussed in Chapter 14. Fluid retention and fluid loss are common causes of short-term changes in body weight. The dramatic effects of some slimming regimens probably have more to do with loss of water than with loss of fat.

Muscle mass

Gain and loss of muscle mass occur as a result of a change in physical activity. Losses also occur in star-

vation. However, large increases in muscle mass over and above 'normal' are not produced by overeating! As noted above, food surpluses are mainly converted into fat.

Adipose tissue

The factors that regulate the activity of adipose tissue and the storage of fat are not yet fully understood. What is clear is that, in the long term, if more energy is consumed than is required in metabolism the excess is largely converted into fat stores. It is not clear why some individuals seem more prone to obesity than others. Many factors are likely to contribute. These include:

- social and genetic factors
- emotional state

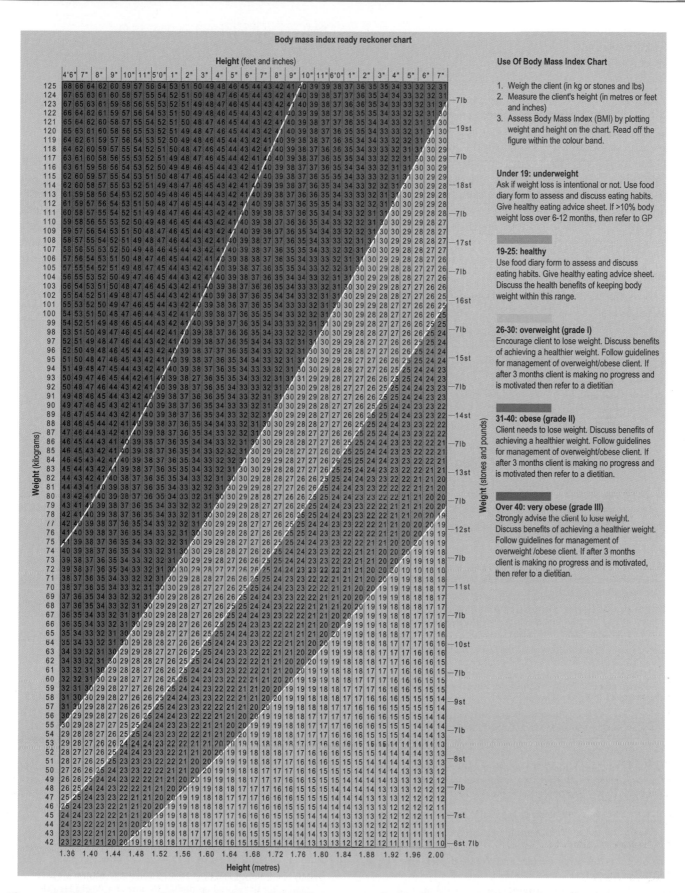

Figure 15.9 Body mass index ready reckoner chart. (After Garrow 1995, with permission of Lothian Health Board.)

- lack of physical activity
- dietary habits
- metabolic balance
- hormonal status.

The tendency to obesity prevalent in many technologically sophisticated societies is probably associated with a lack of physical activity (born of the growth in sedentary occupations, the development of the motor car etc.) coupled with an abundance of appetizing, easily assimilated, energy-rich, processed foods. Unless obesity is due to a metabolic disorder, the simplest strategy to adopt to lose weight is to limit the total amount of food/energy ingested and to increase the amount of exercise taken.

Body mass index (BMI)

Body mass index (BMI) reflects body fat stores and is calculated as:

$$\frac{\text{Weight (kg)}}{\text{height (m}^2)}$$

BMI can be interpreted as (Fig. 15.9):

<16 severely underweight
16–19 underweight
20–25 normal range
26–30 overweight
31–40 obese
>40 morbidly obese.

Difficulties arise in determining BMI accurately if it is not possible to measure weight and height. In some circumstances, for example the elderly, using height in the calculation does not take into account loss of height with increasing age. Recently waist circumference, which provides a guide to abdominal fat stores, has been used to provide a sensitive measure for long-term health risks (Lean et al 1995).

Waist circumference cut-off points (WHO 1989) suggest that men are at increased risk with a waist measurement ≥94 cm (37 inches) and women with a waist measurement ≥80 cm (32 inches).

REFERENCES AND FURTHER READING

Astrand P-O, Rohdahl K 1986 Textbook of work physiology – physiological basis of exercise, 3rd edn. McGraw-Hill, London

Bingham S, Pett S, Day K C 1990 NSP intake of a representative sample of British adults. Journal of Human Nutrition and Dietetics 3: 333–337

Cahill G F, Herrera M G, Morgan A P et al 1966 Hormone-fuel interrelationships during fasting. Journal of Clinical Investigation 45: 1751–1769

Cardiovascular Review Group Committee on Medical Aspects of Food 1994 Nutritional aspects of cardiovascular disease: report of food policy. HMSO, London

Department of Health Report of the Panel on Dietary Reference Values of the Committee on Medical Aspects of Food Policy (COMA) 1991 Dietary reference values for food energy and nutrients for the United Kingdom. Report on Health and Social Subjects 41. HMSO, London

Department of Health Report of the Cardiovascular Review Group of the Committee on Medical Aspects of Food Policy (COMA) 1994 Nutritional aspects of cardiovascular disease. Report on Health and Social Subjects 46. HMSO, London

Englyst H N, Cummings J H 1988 An improved method for the measurement of dietary fibre as the non-starch polysaccharides in plant foods. Journal of the Association of Official Analytical Chemists 71: 808–814

Food Standards Agency 2002 McCance and Widdowson's The composition of foods 6th summary edition. The Royal Society of Chemistry, Cambridge

Garrow J S 1978 Energy balance and obesity in man. Elsevier, North Holland

Garrow J S 1981 Treat obesity seriously. A clinical manual. Churchill Livingstone, Edinburgh

Glickman R M, Sabesin S M 1988 Lipoprotein metabolism. In: Arias I M, Jakoby W B, Popper H, Schacter D, Shafritz D A (eds) The liver: biology and pathobiology, Raven Press, New York

HEA 1994 The balance of good health. Health Education Authority in partnership with the Department of Health, MAFF and in cooperation with the Welsh Office, Scottish Office Home and Health Department and the Department of Health & Social Services, Northern Ireland

Holland B, Welch A A, Unwin I D, Buss D H, Paul A A, Southgate D A T 1991 McCance and Widdowson's The composition of foods, 5th revised and extended edn. The Royal Society of Chemistry & Ministry of Agriculture, Fisheries and Food, London

Holmes S 1986 Nutritional needs of surgical patients. Nursing Times 82(19): 30–32

Lean M E J, Han T S, Morrison C E 1995 Waist circumference as a measure for indicating need for weight management. British Medical Journal 311: 158–161

Royal College of Physicians 1983 Obesity. A report of the Royal College of Physicians. Journal of the Royal College of Physicians 17: 3–58

Thomas B (ed) in conjunction with the British Dietetic Association 2001 Manual of dietetic practice, 3rd edn. Blackwell Science, Oxford

Truswell A S 1986 ABC of nutrition. British Medical Association, London, p 37

World Health Organization 1989 Measuring obesity: classification and distribution of anthropometric data. WHO, Copenhagen (Nutr UD EUR/ICP/NUT 125)

World Health Organization 1998 Obesity. Preventing and managing the global epidemic. Report of a World Health Organization Consultation on Obesity. WHO, Geneva

16 Body defences

In practice you may be asked to consider the following:

1. The physiotherapist encourages coughing in a patient recovering from an abdominal surgery. Why?

2. A young man has his spleen removed and is advised to be vaccinated against *Streptococcus pneumoniae*. Why?

3. A podiatrist notices that a patient has an inflamed lesion on the anterior aspect of the foot. What signs and symptoms are indicative of inflammation?

4. Blood transfusions are a common type of transplant procedure. What distinguishes them from other types of transplantation?

5. A trainee hairdresser has to wear gloves when washing clients' hair because recently she has developed a rash (erythema with small blisters) on her hands. What type of 'allergy' does she have?

6. A middle-aged woman is stung by a bee. Moments later she collapses and loses consciousness. Why?

7. A 30-year-old woman has had one uneventful pregnancy. Her blood group is A Rh–. If she becomes pregnant again should she be concerned?

8. A 6-year-old schoolboy develops glomerulonephritis 10 days after complaining of a sore throat. Are the two events connected?

9. Patients with DiGeorge's syndrome have a developmental disorder that results in hypoplasia or aplasia of the thymus. Can they still make antibodies?

10. How are viruses and other obligate intracellular parasites eliminated from the body?

OVERVIEW

The immune system is a highly developed complex network of organs, cells and soluble factors whose function is to defend the body from injurious microbes, undesirable substances and foreign cells. The ability of these agents to harm the body is dependent upon their pathogenic potential (e.g. available virulence factors) and the integrity of the body's defensive system.

To successfully defend itself, the body must, in the first instance, possess the ability to prevent or limit access to it. Barriers, for example the skin, and the epithelia of the respiratory, gastrointestinal and genito-urinary tracts, restrict the entry of potentially injurious agents into the body. Despite this, some penetration inevitably occurs. Therefore, the body must also have an effective destructive facility and operate efficient waste removal systems.

The body's defensive system can be divided into two parts – innate immunity and adaptive immunity. The innate immune response is the first line of defence and is characterized by its speed. In contrast, the adaptive response is slower and is characterized by its specificity and memory. Although these two responses are usually considered separately, in practice there is a great deal of interaction between them. Both systems utilize many of the same cells, chemical mediators and cytokines. This cooperation results in a highly effective response.

BARRIERS TO ENTRY

The organs and tissues of the body are enclosed by a layer of tissue (epithelium) which acts as the first line of defence against the entry of unwanted substances. This defensive barrier includes (Fig. 16.1):

• the outer surface (the skin)
• several inner surfaces (those of the respiratory, digestive, urinary and genital tracts).

Each epithelium is specialized in ways that are appropriate to its particular function. Each is continually renewed by the growth and development of new cells.

SKIN

The skin (Fig. 16.2) consists of two layers:

• epidermis
• dermis.

It contains glands, blood vessels, and a variety of sensory receptors and defence cells. These all contribute to ensuring that the skin provides a hostile environment for microbes. Skin differs between different parts of the body. Skin that has hair follicles (hairy skin) has a thin epidermis and many sebaceous glands. Non-hairy (glabrous) skin, such as that on the surface of the palms, has a thicker epidermis and many more sensory receptors. There are variations between individuals, related to age, environment and ethnic origin.

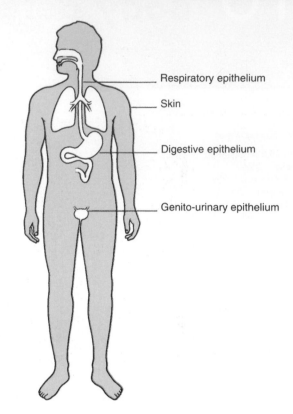

Figure 16.1 The epithelial barriers across which substances must pass to reach other cells, tissues and organs.

Labels: Respiratory epithelium; Skin; Digestive epithelium; Genito-urinary epithelium

Epidermis

The cells of the basal cell layer (also known as the germinal layer) (Fig. 16.2A) act as stem cells (see Chs 1, 3) from which the rest of the epidermis (Fig. 16.3) is formed. From the basal layer, cells are pushed towards the surface by the formation of new cells by the stem cells. It takes about 2 weeks for the cells to reach the surface. As these cells migrate they change in structure and activity so that they eventually form the impenetrable keratin layer of the stratum corneum (Fig. 16.3).

Dermis

The dermis (Fig. 16.2A & B) consists largely of a fibrous network of two kinds of protein, collage and elastin. These proteins are formed and secreted by cells, fibroblasts, scattered amongst the fibres. Collagen fibres give strength to the skin, whereas elastin provides flexibility.

Situated in the dermis are secretory glands, a variety of sensory receptors, and many defence cells.

Glands

The secretory glands originate embryologically from cells of the epidermis and all secrete their products on

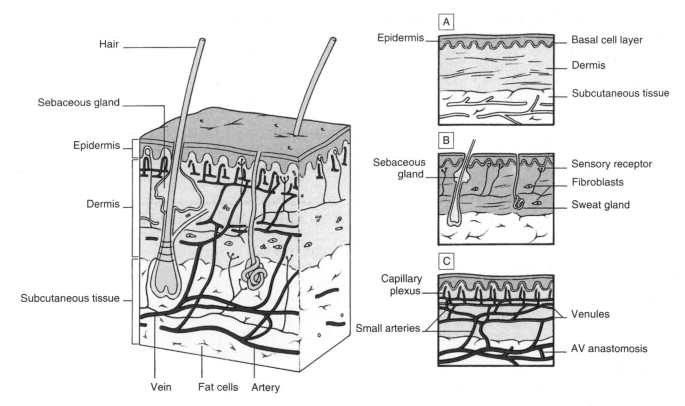

Figure 16.2 The structure of the skin. A, Layers. B, Component cells and structures. C, Blood supply.

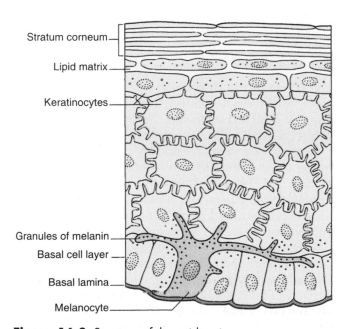

Figure 16.3 Structure of the epidermis.

to the skin surface. Sweat glands, which are widely distributed over the body, secrete a dilute solution of salts. Sebaceous glands are found everywhere except in areas lacking hairs (palms, soles). These glands secrete sebum which contains a mixture of unsaturated fatty acids, proteins and salt.

Other cells

The skin contains sensory receptors of various kinds. Most of these are situated in the dermis, but some such as free nerve endings are present in the epidermis. Some receptors are involved in activating protective reflexes, for example the withdrawal reflex (pulling your hand away from a painful stimulus) (see Ch. 20).

Other cells present in the skin include Langerhans' cells and mast cells, both of which are cells of the defence system.

Blood vessels

There are three interconnected networks of blood vessels associated with the skin (Fig. 16.2C):

- a capillary network (plexus) beneath the epidermis
- small arteries and venules in the dermis
- larger arteries and veins in the subcutaneous tissue.

There are variations in the precise arrangement and control of the cutaneous blood vessels in different parts of the body. This regulation of blood flow and capillary permeability plays a central role in the inflammatory process. Parts of the skin which play a large role in temperature regulation contain a large number of arteriovenous anastomoses, which link arteries and veins directly. These anastomoses are controlled by the nervous system, and enable blood to flow either in large quantities through superficial tissues, or to be diverted to deeper subcutaneous tissues (see Ch. 12).

Barrier function

The skin and mucous membranes provide both anatomical and physiological barriers to infection. Associated with these barriers are the microbes that constitute the body's normal flora. These microbes can assist in protecting the body by providing a hostile environment for potentially pathogenic species.

Intact skin provides a very effective barrier to microbial infection. The tightly packed layers of keratin-containing cells of the epidermis make a practically impenetrable barrier. Additionally, sebaceous glands produce the antimicrobial substance sebum. The pH (between 3 and 5), the relative lack of water and high osmotic pressure of the skin provide an environment that is inhibitory to most bacteria and fungi.

Mucous membranes are less effective in preventing microbial invasion than the skin. The production of mucus, tears, saliva and vaginal secretions protect the mucous membranes by entrapping, diluting and removing invading microbes. The action of ciliated epithelium and the protective reflexes of sneezing, coughing and vomiting also play an important role in the removal of unwanted microbes.

Harmless bacteria and fungi colonize the skin and mucous membranes. These microbes prevent potential pathogens from invading by competing for nutrients, producing harmful substances (such as bacteriocins) and by providing a hostile microenvironment, such as maintaining a low local pH.

MUCOUS MEMBRANES

The mucous membranes that constitute the body's inner surfaces act as the first line of defence against the entry of unwanted substances into the body and include the epithelia of:

- the respiratory tract (see Ch. 7)
- the digestive tract (see Ch. 9)
- the urinary tract (see Ch. 8)
- the genital tract (see Ch. 31).

These epithelia are more permeable than the skin as they are not keratinized and do not have a stratum corneum. Like the skin, they are continually renewed. This is essential for their barrier function.

The body is also defended at these sites by physiological and chemical factors including:

- protective reflexes (such as sneezing, coughing and vomiting) that forcibly expel noxious materials
- secretions (such as nasal secretions, tears and saliva) that trap, dilute and inactivate harmful substances before they are washed away.

The respiratory and digestive tracts are particularly vulnerable – the respiratory tract, due the large surface area of the alveolar epithelium, and the digestive tract due to its surface area and the huge variety of substances to which it is exposed.

Respiratory tract

The huge surface area of the alveolar epithelium (see Ch. 7) potentially offers unrestricted entry to any substance which is inhaled and can diffuse across it. Protective reflexes, secretions and macrophages all play their part in shielding this vulnerable epithelium. A key role is played by the nose.

Protective reflexes

Inhalation of noxious materials is resisted by several protective reflexes, such as sneezing and coughing, which inhibit breathing and force the inhaled materials out of the respiratory tract. These reflexes are evoked by sensory receptors in the respiratory epithelium (see Ch. 7). Sneezing is evoked by stimulation of receptors in the nose whereas coughing is a vagal reflex triggered by receptors in the larynx and tracheobronchial tree.

Secretions

The whole of the upper part of the respiratory tract (nose, nasopharynx, larynx, trachea and bronchi) is lined by a ciliated epithelium, embedded in which are goblet cells and seromucous glands (see Ch. 7).

Secretions are swept continually towards the pharynx by the action of the cilia: upwards from the trachea and bronchi and downwards from the nose. Thus, particles trapped in the mucus and substances dissolving in the secretions are carried away from the highly permeable and extensive alveolar epithelium.

Secretion by the seromucous glands is reflexly stimulated through cholinergic nerves resulting in a copious flow of a watery secretion.

Digestive tract

As the chief purpose of the digestive tract is the absorption of nutrients from the diet, this epithelium has to contend with all substances which we deliberately swallow in food and drink, some of which are potentially harmful. As in the respiratory tract, the most vulnerable epithelium (intestinal) is protected by reflexes, which control access to that epithelium and evict unwanted intruders.

In the digestive tract the reflex activity which expels unwanted material, as in vomiting and diarrhoea, is almost invariably accompanied by increased secretory activity too.

Protective reflexes

Upper digestive tract

Once material has been swallowed it may be rejected by activation of the vomiting reflex. Vomiting is controlled by a group of cells in the medulla of the brain (associated with the nucleus tractus solitarius) that are excited by signals arising from receptors in:

- the upper gastrointestinal tract (see Ch. 9)
- the chemoreceptor trigger zone (area postrema) in the medulla oblongata of the brain stem (see Ch. 20).

The vomiting reflex triggers:

- relaxation of the body of the stomach
- retroperistalsis in the upper small intestine.

These events hold substances in the stomach, preventing them from passing on into the small intestine. At the same time the glottis closes, thus sealing off the respiratory tract. Additionally, there is an increase in salivation and a generalized activation of the sympathetic nervous system, resulting in sweating, cutaneous vasoconstriction and tachycardia.

Lower digestive tract

Irritation of the lower digestive tract also provokes secretion and contractile activity that promotes the expulsion of irritants via the rectum, as in diarrhoea. The responses are mediated by the enteric nervous system (see Ch. 9) and are influenced by the autonomic nervous system. Effective stimuli include bacterial toxins (including cholera toxin) and plant products used as laxatives, such as cascara and senna.

Secretions

Both saliva and gastric juice contain antimicrobial agents that limit the numbers and activities of microbes entering the small intestine. The pH of gastric juice is effective in preventing growth of all but the specifically evolved bacterium *Helicobacter pylori* (Table 16.1).

PHAGOCYTOSIS

The integrity of the skin and mucous membranes can be breached through injury, injection, and disruption of the normal microflora populations or, on occasion, the action of specifically adapted pathogens. When this occurs, the body's innate immune system acts to remove the microorganism. This is accomplished by the destructive activity of specific leucocytes. Primarily this takes the form of phagocytosis. Phagocytosis is the

Table 16.1 Protective secretions of epithelial surfaces

Source	Antimicrobial component
Tears	Lysozyme, IgA, IgG
Wax	Cerumen
Mucus	Mucin
Saliva	Lysozyme, IgA, IgG, digestive enzymes
Sweat	Lysozyme
Sebum	Fatty acid, lactic acid
Gastric juice	HCl, digestive enzymes
Semen	Spermine

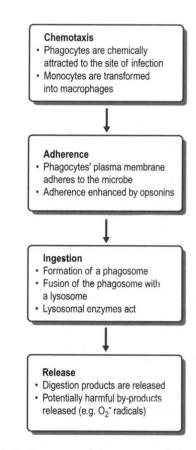

Chemotaxis
- Phagocytes are chemically attracted to the site of infection
- Monocytes are transformed into macrophages

Adherence
- Phagocytes' plasma membrane adheres to the microbe
- Adherence enhanced by opsonins

Ingestion
- Formation of a phagosome
- Fusion of the phagosome with a lysosome
- Lysosomal enzymes act

Release
- Digestion products are released
- Potentially harmful by-products released (e.g. O_2^- radicals)

Figure 16.4 Overview of the process of phagocytosis.

process by which microorganisms are engulfed and destroyed by granulocytes (specifically neutrophils and eosinophils) and activated macrophages (Fig. 16.4). The speed at which neutrophils are recruited and activated to destroy pathogens at the site of infection is central to the effectiveness of the innate immune response.

In addition to phagocytosis, other cells of the innate immune system possess the ability to directly or indirectly destroy pathogens. Natural killer cells (NK cells) are large granular lymphocytes that can be induced to secrete cytotoxic molecules called perforins which lyse virally infected cells and tumour cells. Basophils (circulating basic-staining granulocytes) and mast cells (located in connective tissue and mucosa) contain granules containing pharmacologically active substances which play a major role in inflammatory and allergic reactions.

Macrophages, which are much bigger cells (see Ch. 3), follow a little later. Both groups of cells are attracted to the site of action by chemicals produced locally. This process is termed chemotaxis.

The numbers of phagocytic and attacking cells found at different sites within the body reflect the degree of cellular breakdown occurring there and the degree of exposure of those sites to invading cells and toxins. Thus, large numbers of phagocytic cells are normally found within the respiratory tract (alveolar macrophages) and lodged in the liver (Kupffer cells).

ACTIVATION

The phagocytic activity of the macrophages depends upon several factors including:

- some that influence them directly
- some (opsonins) that make the target of their attack more attractive.

The factors that influence the macrophages directly come from several sources. Many of these substances attract mobile macrophages to cell debris and foreign cells, such as bacteria, by chemotaxis. They also transform and activate cells. Monocytes, for example, are transformed into macrophages as they migrate from the blood into the tissues. Within the tissues, macrophages are aroused to intense phagocytic activity by the action of cytokines, for example (see Ch. 11).

Opsonins are any factors that make substances more susceptible to phagocytosis. Antibodies secreted by lymphocytes act in this way, as does one of the products of the complement cascade, known as C3b. Opsonins bind to the foreign cell or protein and act as 'markers' singling out that cell or protein as a target for disposal and facilitating phagocytosis.

DIGESTION

Phagocytic cells contain vesicles (lysosomes) (see Ch. 1) containing a variety of enzymes (acid hydrolases). When bacteria or macromolecules have been engulfed, the vacuole formed fuses with a lysosome, and the acid hydrolases and other bactericidal agents, like hydrogen peroxide produced by the phagocyte, begin the process of degradation.

Some of the products generated in digestion, such as glucose and amino acids, are used by the macrophages in their metabolism. Others are excreted by the macrophages into the body fluids and may then be taken up and used by other tissues. Iron, for example, derived from aged red cells, is re-used by haemopoietic cells of the bone marrow in the manufacture of new red cells. In this way, macrophages participate in the economy of the body by enabling useful waste products to be recycled.

Some products generated by the macrophages become incorporated into the cell membrane of the macrophage and act as antigens which activate lymphocytes (antigen presenting function). This is important in the development of immunity (see p. 304).

Sometimes the material which has been engulfed by the macrophages cannot be digested. This applies to dust particles, asbestos and silica, for example. These remain within the cell for its life span. When the cell dies and is itself degraded and disposed of by the same system, these particles will become lodged in another macrophage. These materials are thus not readily eliminated from the body and, over a lifetime there can be a substantial build-up of such materials (Fig. 16.4).

SOLUBLE FACTORS

In addition to the function and structure of the anatomical barriers of the skin and mucous membranes, a variety of soluble factors contribute to the body's defence. These factors are primarily proteins or glycoproteins (Table 16.2).

INFLAMMATORY RESPONSE

When the body is injured by physical, chemical or infecting agents, a complex series of events takes place to ensure that the damage does not spread or worsen, and that the damage is repaired. These events are known collectively as the inflammatory response and involve vascular, cellular and chemical components.

MECHANISM

When a tissue is injured or infected many different chemicals are produced (Table 16.3). They originate from:

- damaged cells
- defending cells (such as macrophages and lymphocytes)
- invading cells (such as bacteria)
- plasma and interstitial fluid.

Table 16.2 Major soluble factors

Soluble factor	Source	Activity
Interferon (alpha, beta and gamma)	Leucocytes, fibroblasts	Induces an antiviral state in uninfected cells
Complement (over 20 glycoproteins)	Hepatocytes	Lyses cells, enhances the acute inflammatory response, enhances phagocytosis
Tumour necrosis factor (alpha and beta)	Macrophages, neutrophils	Enhances phagocytosis, involved in chronic inflammation
C-reactive protein	Hepatocytes	Enhances phagocytosis, activates the complement cascade

Table 16.3 Chemicals produced in response to injury or injection

Category	Examples	Source
Acute phase proteins	Fibrinogen	Liver
	C-reactive protein	
Amines	Histamine	Mast cells
	Serotonin	Platelets
Complement	C_1–C_9	Produced from plasma proteins secreted by the liver and macrophages
Cytokines	Interleukins	Activated lymphocytes and macrophages
	Tumour necrosis factor	
Eicosanoids	Prostaglandins	Many cells
	Thromboxane	
	Leukotrienes	
Kinins	Bradykinin	Produced from plasma proteins secreted by the liver
Lysosomal enzymes	Hydrolases	Macrophages

As well as influencing the activity of the defending cells they may locally:

- affect the circulation
- irritate sensory receptors
- promote tissue repair.

Following a brief period of vasoconstriction, many of the released chemicals cause local vasodilation and increased capillary permeability. This improves access to the site of injury for defending cells and increases the delivery of soluble factors and vital nutrients.

The increased blood supply raises the temperature of the tissue, so that the site feels warm (calor) and makes it appear red (rubor). The increased capillary permeability allows for the influx of cells, fluids and chemical mediators to the site of injury. The accumulation of fluid causes tissue swelling (tumour) and combined with the action of mediators on nerve endings, pain (dolor). These signs of inflammation combined with the transitory loss of normal function of the affected tissue (functio laesa) are known historically as the 'cardinal signs of inflammation'.

SENSATION

Sensory receptors that respond to noxious stimuli (nociceptors) (see Chs 20 and 21) are stimulated by chemicals such as histamine, prostaglandins and bradykinin. This results in discomfort ranging from an irritating itch, such as that produced by an insect bite, to pain (see Ch. 29).

TISSUE REPAIR

Tissue repair involves:

- formation of a connective tissue scaffold
- growth of new blood vessels
- replacement of specific tissue cells.

Soon after an injury a temporary scaffold of interlacing strands of fibrin is formed which seals off blood vessels and forms a crust over the wound. This is gradually replaced by a connective tissue scaffold formed by fibroblasts (see Ch. 19). The connective tissue knits the wound together forming strong scar tissue, walling off the injury from uninjured areas and providing a framework to guide the growth of the specialized tissue cells. Later on, macrophages clear away some of this scaffolding. This is why scar tissue formed after surgery becomes less prominent after months or even years.

If the connective tissue completely envelops a region of inflammation, so that bacteria and defending cells are completely walled off, the result is an abscess.

Delivery of vital supplies to the tissue under repair is guaranteed by the growth of new capillaries (angiogenesis). These develop from existing vessels. Capillary endothelial cells, stimulated by factors released locally, grow out from the capillary wall and penetrate the connective tissue.

New cells replace the lost specialized cells if the tissue is capable of regeneration. When this is not possible, connective tissue acts as infill (fibrosis). As the repair is completed and scaffolding is removed many of the new capillaries regress and the redness of the scar fades.

RECOGNITION OF FOREIGN MATERIAL

The main attribute of the body's defence system is its ability to recognize foreign material. Following recognition, the cells respond individually or with other cells of the defensive system. The functions of recognition and interaction are facilitated through the presence of a variety of surface molecules and receptors. Receptor activation usually results in intracellular signals being sent to the nucleus of the cell.

All nucleated cells of an individual have on their surfaces unique glycoproteins called MHC class I molecules. A restricted population of cells (macrophages, dendritic cells and B cells) also express MHC class II molecules. MHC stands for major histocompatibility complex. These molecules are the products of a tightly linked gene cluster found on chromosome 6 and are responsible for defining an individual's unique tissue type. There are many different forms of genes for each subregion of the MHC and this results in the large diversity of tissue types found in the population. It is through the recognition of identical MHC molecules that the body's defence system recognizes 'self'. Differences in these molecules signify the presence of a foreign cell, or 'non-self'.

Additionally, the cells of the immune system are able to identify other individual molecules and particular patterns of molecules on pathogens. For example, CD14, a molecule found on macrophages, specifically binds to the lipopolysaccharide (LPS) on Gram-negative bacteria. Once bound, the bacterium can be destroyed.

Other molecules found on the surfaces of cells are required for facilitating the various functions of the cells of the defensive system. These functions include directing cell migration, targeting specific tissue responses and activating inflammatory responses. The molecules responsible for this are part of a large group called adhesion molecules and belong to subgroups such as the selectin family, integrin family, or immunoglobulin superfamily. Specific cell types or restricted populations of cells express different adhesion molecules. Alteration in the pattern or number of these molecules results in activation of specific defensive mechanisms.

ADAPTIVE IMMUNE RESPONSE

The innate immune response exhibits a degree of specificity, in that a distinction between foreign material and self is made. However, this specificity is limited to extracellular pathogens, can be damaging to normal tissue and does not provide for improved future protection.

For a fully functioning defensive system, there is a requirement for the recognition and successful elimination of specific pathogens and foreign molecules (antigens). This recognition must be sufficiently accurate so as to be tolerant (non-reactive) of self-molecules and innocuous substances. Additionally, there is a need for a heightened response upon subsequent exposure. These roles are fulfilled by the adaptive immune response.

The adaptive, or specific immune response involves the interaction of two groups of cells: antigen-presenting cells and lymphocytes. Antigen-presenting cells, such as macrophages, are also central to the innate immune response. Lymphocytes can be found in the blood and lymphatic systems, and in lymphoid tissues. They are the cells that through their actions confer the attributes of specificity, tolerance and memory on the adaptive arm of the immune system.

LYMPHOCYTES

There are two main classes of lymphocyte:

- T lymphocytes (T cells)
- B lymphocytes (B cells).

T and B lymphocytes differ in their life histories and they specialize in different activities.

T cells are not mature when they leave the bone marrow. They mature in the thymus gland. Mature T cells express a receptor on their surfaces (TCR or

T cell receptor). This receptor associates with other membrane glycoproteins to form specific recognition complexes. When presented with foreign material (antigen) they are then primed for their terminal differentiation events. B cells mature fully in the bone marrow and remain 'naive' and only respond when they encounter a specific antigen. Again receptor molecules facilitate this response. The lymphoid tissues provide the microenvironment required for effective antigen presentation.

Both T and B cells respond to a wide variety of materials, including proteins, bacteria, viruses and aberrant cells. T cells, however, tend to be most effective against abnormal cells and those infected by pathogens (viruses, bacteria, fungi) whereas B cells tend to recognize pathogens encountered outside cells. Individual lymphocytes differ from one another in the different proteins they manufacture to use in defence. Some of the proteins are inserted into the cell membrane as receptors. Others are secreted as antibodies which latch onto foreign or abnormal cells or macromolecules.

When a T or B lymphocyte encounters a cell or macromolecule which is able to interact with the specific protein receptors in its cell membrane, the interaction stimulates the lymphocyte to:

- proliferate
- differentiate.

The events that follow differ for B and T cells. Activated B cells produce antibodies that disable the antigen (humoral immunity) whereas T cells respond in a variety of ways collectively referred to as cellular immunity.

HUMORAL IMMUNITY

Once a B cell encounters an antigen, it becomes activated to proliferate and differentiate into a plasma cell (Fig. 16.5). The antigen can be encountered in association with a T cell (initiating a T cell dependent response) or without a T cell (initiating a T cell independent response).

Plasma cells manufacture and secrete large amounts of protein which 'recognize' the cell or molecule encountered by the B cell. These secreted proteins – antibodies – bind to the antigen and this has several consequences each of which renders the antigen harmless (Fig. 16.6):

- preventing pathogen adhesion to mucosal surfaces
- neutralizing toxins
- coating of antibody opsonizes the antigen
- activating the complement system

- clumping of antigen–antibody complexes (agglutination).

Opsonization enhances the process of phagocytosis. Antibodies prime antigens for phagocytosis by actually linking them to the phagocyte. This triggers phagocytosis.

The complement system is a sequence of enzymatic reactions which generates a number of different products with wide-ranging effects including:

- inflammation (see p. 300)
- chemotaxis of phagocytic cells
- opsonization of antigen
- cell lysis (rupture of cell membranes).

Agglutination creates large particles from small ones. This limits the movement of the antigen and provides more binding sites for linkage to the phagocyte.

All antibodies have the same basic molecular structure (Fig. 16.7). Each molecule is a protein (immunoglobulin) consisting of four polypeptide chains linked together to form a 'stem' and two 'arms'. There are five different stems giving rise to five different families of immunoglobulins, IgA, IgD, IgE, IgG and IgM, but there are an infinite number of different 'arms' creating an infinite variety of antigen-binding sites.

Each class of antibody has a slightly different role to play in the immune response (Table 16.4). Within different parts of the body, different antibody classes predominate. Activated lymphocytes produce IgM first before switching to the production of one of the other classes, such as IgG, the main class of antibody in plasma. Both IgM and IgG are involved in opsonizing antigens. The IgA class has a different function. It tackles recognized antigens *before* they get into the body through the epithelial barriers of, for example, the respiratory and digestive tracts, or the ducts of exocrine glands. By binding to antigens, IgA class antibodies prevent their uptake into the body. IgE attaches itself to mast cells (see Ch. 3) and triggers their secretion of histamine and other chemicals of the inflammatory response.

CELL MEDIATED IMMUNITY

T cells have been subdivided into two well-defined groups according to their function:

- T helper cells (T_H)
- T cytotoxic cells (T_C).

Additionally these populations can be identified by the type of glycoproteins that they express on their surfaces. Generally, T_H cells express the CD4 molecule, whilst T_C cells have the CD8 molecule on their surfaces.

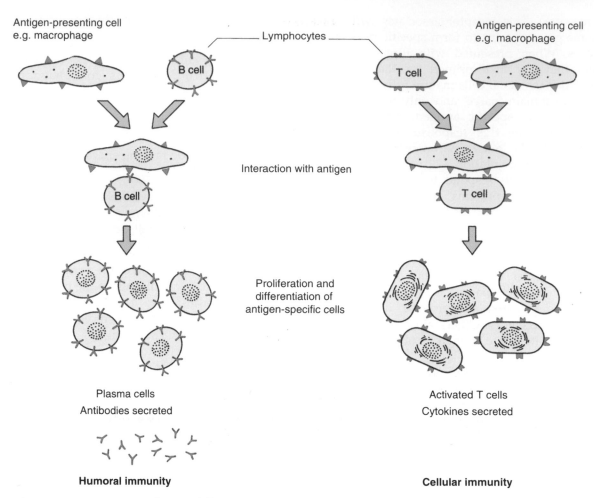

Figure 16.5 Sequence of events following an encounter between a B or a T lymphocyte and an antigen. (The antigen here is shown embedded in the membrane of the macrophage.)

A third group of T cells is thought to exist which has a suppressing function. However, no discrete surface molecule profile has been found for them.

When an antigen is encountered helper T cells secrete substances, referred to as cytokines (Table 16.5), that stimulate the activity of other defence cells, including B cells, cytotoxic T cells and macrophages (Fig. 16.8).

Activated cytotoxic T cells directly attack abnormal cells of the body. These abnormal cells may be ones that have become disordered, as in cancer, or cells that have been invaded by viruses. The T cells latch on to the target cell and release a protein (pore forming protein). The protein inserts itself into the membrane of the target cell making it more permeable so that the cell swells and dies.

Suppressor T cells appear to inhibit the immune response and may be important in preventing the response from getting out of control.

CYTOKINES

The complex interactions of the components of the innate and adaptive immune systems rely upon the mediating activity of a group of molecules called cytokines. Cytokines are short-lived, low molecular weight proteins or glycoproteins that are capable of being produced by most cells and have a wide variety of activities, such as inducing differentiation, proliferation or apoptosis. Cytokines can be grouped according to their biological activity (Table 16.5). They function over a small area as intercellular messengers and transmit their signals through binding with specific cell receptors (see also Ch. 11). Differential regulation of the immune system is modulated by the specific stimulation of cytokine production and the specific expression of cytokine receptors on target cells. Thus,

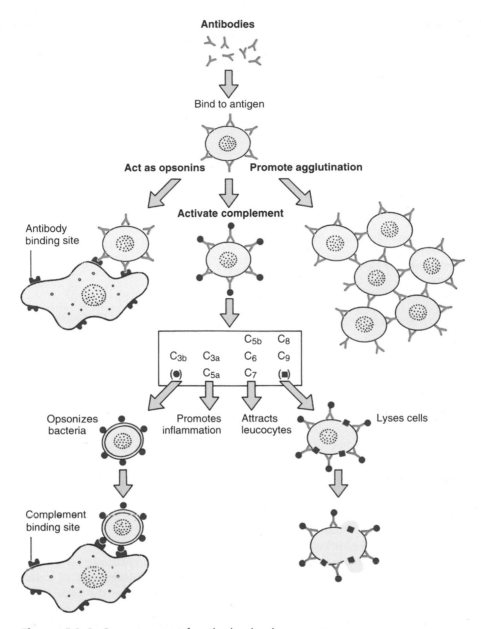

Figure 16.6 Consequences of antibodies binding to antigen.

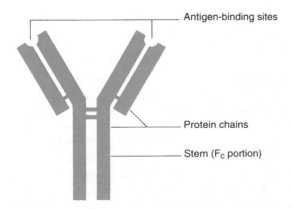

Figure 16.7 Structure of antibodies.

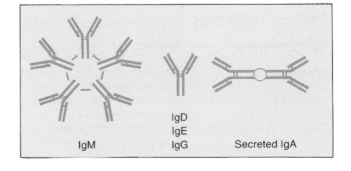

Table 16.4 Characteristic features of the five classes of immunoglobulins

Class	Features
IgM	Early antibodies formed by all plasma cells Effective as opsonins and in promoting agglutination; activate complement
IgG	Major class of immunoglobulin present in plasma Effective as opsonins; activate complement, disable bacterial toxins Able to cross the placenta
IgA	Secretory form secreted by epithelia (tracts and exocrine glands) Disable antigens before they penetrate the epithelial barriers
IgE	Attach to mast cells and trigger the release of histamine Role in allergic response and parasitic infections
IgD	Distinctive characteristics uncertain; possibly involved in differentiation

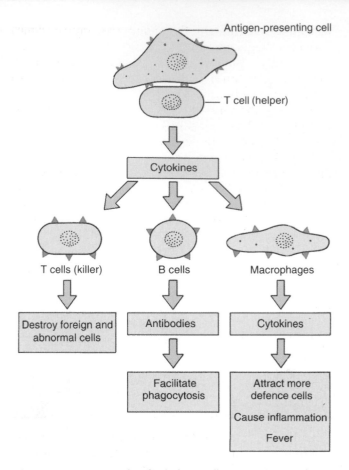

Figure 16.8 Key role of T helper cells in activating other defence cells by secreting cytokines.

the innate and adaptive immune responses are able to act together in order to provide a comprehensive defensive system.

DEVELOPMENT OF IMMUNITY

The initial encounter between lymphoctyes and an antigen usually only provokes a small response (primary immune response) which takes several days to develop. The sluggishness of the response is due to the time it takes for the challenged lymphocytes to multiply and differentiate into active cells producing antibodies and cytokines.

Some of the cells formed at this initial encounter continue to circulate within the blood and tissues for years after the original challenge has subsided. If the same antigen is encountered a second time, some time later, this circulating pool of cells (memory cells) is primed. Consequently, the response (secondary immune response) is quicker and more powerful than before. On repeated exposure the number of cells which can specifically react against a particular antigen

Table 16.5 Cytokines

Cytokine group	Notes	Activity	Example
Chemokines	Chemoattractant role, important in inflammatory response	Regulate leucocyte traffic	Macrophage inflammatory protein-1alpha (MIP-1α)
Interleukins	Produced by some leucocytes and act on others	Modulate lymphocyte function	IL-2
Colony-stimulating factors	Cause differentiation and proliferation of stem cells	Promote growth	Granulocyte-macrophage colony stimulating factor (GM-CSF)
Interferons	Type 1 have antiviral activity Type 2 act directly on effector cells of the immune system	Modulate intracellular killing	Interferon-alpha (INF-α)

increases. Consequently, the immune response becomes correspondingly greater.

Immunity develops in a specific way in each individual depending on his or her exposure to antigens throughout life, and on the development of tolerance to the cells and proteins that are 'natural' to that person. Development of immunity begins *in utero* (see Ch. 31) and continues throughout life.

If people are exposed to bacteria or viruses which are uncommon in their natural environment, their initial defence may be inadequate to prevent illness. Thus, travellers may succumb to bacteria which are tolerated by the indigenous populations. Similarly, travellers may import diseases which pose little or no threat at home but which are lethal in the country visited. Some protection can be conferred by vaccination in which a small or inactive quantity of the appropriate antigen is injected. Vaccination triggers the development of lymphocytes that can mount an attack against that antigen in the future.

INAPPROPRIATE IMMUNE RESPONSES

Usually the immune system efficiently recognizes, destroys and disposes of foreign material with little or no damage to the host. In some circumstances, the immune system over-responds or responds to material that is not foreign. Over-responsiveness of the immune system is called hypersensitivity or, more commonly, allergy. Immune response against self-components is known as autoimmunity.

HYPERSENSITIVITIES

Hypersensitivity responses occur as a result of either humoral or cell-mediated responses. They are classified into four groups:

- type I, IgE-mediated
- type II, antibody-mediated cytotoxic
- type III, immune complex-mediated
- type IV, cell-mediated.

As a rule, the hypersensitivities involving antibody occur quickly, from a few minutes to a few hours after exposure. Type IV hypersensitivity is also known as delayed type hypersensitivity and can take many hours to days to develop.

Type I hypersensitivity

Type I responses are more commonly known as allergic reactions. Some individuals have a predisposition to produce abnormal levels of IgE. This condition is known as atopy. For these individuals an initial exposure to an antigen is usually uneventful. However, subsequent exposures cause membrane bound IgE on mast cells and basophils to cross-link. This cross-linking causes these cells to degranulate. The granules contain pharmacologically active mediators that act on smooth muscle cells, small blood vessels, mucous glands and platelets. This leads to smooth muscle contraction, vasodilation, increased vascular permeability, platelet aggregation and increased mucous secretion. Most type I responses occur on mucous membrane surfaces and are the result of the inhalation or ingestion of the initiating antigen. Examples of this type of reaction are:

- hay fever
- asthma
- eczema
- food allergies
- systemic anaphylaxis.

Type II hypersensitivity

Type II hypersensitivity is also known as antibody hypes-mediated cytotoxic hypersensitivity. It is the result of IgG or IgM binding to cells, via cell surface antigens, and causing them to be destroyed by the actions of complement or cytotoxic T cells. Examples of this type of reaction are:

- transfusion reactions
- drugs
- Rhesus incompatibility (see Ch. 3).

Transfusion reactions are only seen when there has been a mismatch of blood groups. Drugs such as aspirin and penicillin are known to precipitate this type of reaction. Aspirin can bind to platelets, causing them to become targets for destruction and resulting in clotting disorders, and penicillin can bind to erythrocytes, resulting in their subsequent damage. Following a normal delivery of a rhesus D positive (Rh+) baby or a previous Rh+ blood transfusion, an Rh− mother can produce IgG antibodies against the erythrocytes of any subsequent Rh+ fetus she may carry. This results in the condition known as haemolytic disease of the newborn.

Type III hypersensitivity

When antigen–antibody complexes are deposited in various tissues the complement cascade is activated. This results in enhanced inflammation and neutrophil recruitment. The usual inflammatory response occurs and a large amount of lytic enzymes are released from the neutrophils. Complexes causing this type of reaction are either of great number, or of a size that cannot pass through the basement membranes of tissues. If the complexes are deposited at one site then localized damage occurs. However, systemic effects can be seen. Examples of this type of reaction are:

- post-streptococcal glomerulonephritis
- vasculitis
- farmer's lung.

Type IV hypersensitivity

This type of hypersensitivity is the only one that is cell mediated. Usually it occurs at least 24 hours following exposure to the initiating antigen. When an antigen cannot be phagocytosed, due either to the nature of the antigen (e.g. *Mycobacterium tuberculosis*) or to a defect in normal macrophage function, various cytokines are produced with the effect of accumulating a large number of activated macrophages at the site. These macrophages can then either wall off the antigen by forming a granuloma, or release lytic enzymes which cause localized damage. Examples of this type of reaction are:

- contact dermatitis
- tubercular lesions.

The mechanism of this hypersensitivity reaction has been exploited to form the basis of the TB test.

AUTOIMMUNITY

Autoimmune reactions occur when the immune system recognizes a self-molecule to be foreign. They arise due to the breakdown of self-molecule. The immune reactions to these antigens can cause serious damage to cells and organs. Autoimmune disorders can be characterized as either:

- organ specific
- systemic.

Organ-specific autoimmunity involves an immune response directed against a specific target organ resulting in direct damage to that organ or to its function. The immune response can involve the humoral response or the cell-mediated response. Self-antibodies (autoantibodies) can be directed against a specific component of an organ or they can bring about the over-stimulation or blocking of normal organ function. Direct cell damage occurs as a result of inflammation of or cell killing. Eventually, damaged cells get replaced by connective tissue. When the autoantibodies are directed against products or receptors of organs or glands, their function can be impaired. Examples of organ-specific autoimmune diseases include:

- insulin-dependent diabetes mellitus
- autoimmune anaemia
- Graves' disease
- myasthenia gravis.

Systemic autoimmune diseases involve widespread damage as the autoantibodies involved are directed at a large range of target antigens. Typically the damage is the result of a general fault in the regulation of the various mechanisms of the immune system. These diseases are the result of the activity of cytotoxic T cells, action of autoantibodies and/or the accumulation of immune complexes. Examples of systemic autoimmune diseases are:

- systemic lupus erythematosus (SLE)
- ankylosing spondylitis
- rheumatoid arthritis.

REFERENCES AND FURTHER READING

Cooke E M 1991 Hare's Bacteriology and immunity for nurses, 7th edn. Churchill Livingstone, Edinburgh
Clear basic text

Davies R, Ollier S 1989 Allergy, inflammation and the immune response. In: Davies R, Ollier S (eds) Allergy the facts. Oxford University Press, Oxford

Emslie-Smith D, Paterson C, Scratcherd T, Read N W (eds) 1988 Textbook of physiology, 11th edn. Churchill Livingstone, Edinburgh

Goldsby R J, Kindt T J, Osborne B A (eds) 2000 Kuby Immunology, 4th edn. W H Freeman, New York

Johnson A 1988 Natural healing processes. The Professional Nurse 3(5): 149–152

Lydyard P M, Whelan A, Fanger M W 2000 Instant notes in immunology. BIOS Scientific Publishers, Oxford

Mathew O P, Sant'Ambrogio G 1988 Respiratory function of the upper airway. Marcel Dekker, Basel
Collection of authoritative reviews of all aspects of the upper airways written for and by specialists

Millington P F, Wilkinson R 1983 Skin. Cambridge University Press, Cambridge
Review of the fundamental biology and mechanics of the skin. Useful for reference

Nilsson L, Lindberg J, Lindqvist K, Nordfelt S 1987 The body victorious – the illustrative story of our immune system and other defences of the human body. Faber & Faber, London
Superb pictures bringing this aspect of human biology to life

Parkin J, Cohen B 2001 An overview of the immune system. Lancet 357(9270): 1777–1789

Rang H P, Dale M M 1991 Pharmacology, 2nd edn. Churchill Livingstone, Edinburgh
Advanced textbook of pharmacology. Useful for further information

Roitt I M 2001 Essential immunology, 10th edn. Blackwell Scientific Publications, Oxford
Beautifully presented, advanced textbook. Useful for further information

Thody A J, Freidman P S 1986 Scientific basis of dermatology. A physiological approach. Churchill Livingstone, Edinburgh
Specialist text for reference

17 Thermoregulation – maintaining body temperature

In practice you may be asked to consider the following:

1. In the limbs, arterial vessels and venous vessels run close together but with the flow in opposite directions. How does this simple arrangement help thermoregulation?

2. The vascular basal tone in the skin circulation is important to maintaining core temperature. Please explain.

3. The very young have deposits of brown adipose tissue. How does this help maintain their core temperature?

4. A pyrexic patient is to be cooled. Use of a fan and sponging with tepid water are familiar remedies. Why use a fan and why tepid, not cold water?

5. The fever above was brought about by a microorganism, but how was the temperature disruption achieved?

6. The early effects of fever include shivering and vasoconstriction. What causes these effects?

7. A canoeist has been admitted to Accident and Emergency suffering from accidental hypothermia. He had overturned the canoe and had been coping with the situation well until his dry-suit had been torn. Very soon after that he was overcome by cold. Please explain.

8. A young man is brought into Accident and Emergency suffering from hypothermia. He had attempted to walk home from the pub, had fallen in the snow and was found by police during the night. He has no injuries. Please explain.

9. The young man above was found to have a very narrow pulse pressure. Why?

10. A holidaymaker ate lunch, enjoyed the wine and lay down in the sun. The temperature climbed to the high 30s and he slept on. He eventually woke, feeling very unwell. During the night his temperature continued to rise until he suffered a convulsion. What has happened to him?

Animals which do not closely regulate their body temperature, like lizards for example, have to wait around till the sun comes up. They are poikilotherms. Animals which do regulate their temperature (homeotherms) are independent of the outside temperature but must pay in energy terms for the freedom. Heat must be generated when the temperature threatens to fall and lost when the temperature rises; there is a constant need to balance losses against gains. If heat is lost by sweating and vasodilation, adjustments also have to be made to fluid balance and blood pressure.

The chemical reactions on which the cell depends are all affected by changes in temperature; for example, there may be a 10% increase in reaction rate for an increase of 1° Celsius (°C). In addition, the enzymes which drive the reactions work best at their optimum temperature and only work at all over a narrow temperature range. Temperature must therefore be maintained within that small range. One of the effects of fever is the malfunction of body systems, resulting in muscle rigor or central nervous seizures as the cell reactions become de-synchronized.

Body temperature is routinely measured in the outer ear or in the mouth, either site giving a result close to the temperature within the body, i.e. core temperature, although measurement in the mouth is open to error from the effects of recent food or drinks. Normal core temperature is approximately 36.3 to 37.3°C. The parts which make up the core are head, thorax and abdomen, but, in a warm environment, most of the body will have a temperature close to that of the core. The surface or shell temperature is lower, with the extremities lowest of all. The temperature of the core is tightly controlled; the shell temperature may vary over a wide range.

Within the body, different areas will have different temperatures. Rectal temperature during and after exercise may be significantly above 'normal' not because of heat generated there but because of the difficulty in dissipating the heat. The scrotum is maintained at a temperature significantly lower, about 32°C, to maintain the health of the sperm. Some of the variation between one area and another is evened out by the constant stirring action of the blood acting as a distributor of heat.

Core temperature is not a constant value. It varies from person to person; some healthy individuals have normal temperature of 36°C, normal for others may be a temperature of 38°C. Within one individual, temperature can vary over a number of days; females have a lower temperature after menstruating, rising about 0.5°C at ovulation. Over one day, the temperature varies, lowest during sleep at night and highest in the early evening. Superimposed on all of this are the constant small variations as temperature is adjusted to the set point or, more accurately, within its set range (see below). The temperature will rise as heat is produced and fall as heat is lost. When the low end of the range is reached, heat conservation begins and the temperature rises to the upper limit only to be reduced again. This constant adjustment up and down a range is referred to as 'hunting' and it is typical of systems where a range is maintained around a set value, for example, 36.8 to 37.2 with a set value of 37°C.

The body obeys the same laws of physics as any other solid object as far as temperature is concerned: it gains heat from warmer surroundings and loses heat to cooler surroundings. Unlike most other solid objects, however, it produces heat and it can regulate how much heat to retain or lose.

Metabolism is made up of many cell reactions, the end product of which is heat. The more active the tissue, the more heat is produced. In a cold environment, the heat is continually lost and, to maintain core temperature, the mechanisms of heat conservation must be used. In a warm environment, retaining heat is not a problem, and the mechanisms for losing heat may have to be employed. In extremely hot conditions, heat may even be transferred to the body, making it difficult to maintain core temperature by physiological means only and requiring some behavioural response, like getting out of the heat.

- The ambient temperature at which it is easiest to maintain body temperature is about 27 to 31°C without clothes and lower than this depending on what is worn.
- The temperature range at which heat gain is most easily balanced by heat loss is the thermoneutral zone and is equivalent to a skin temperature of about 33°C.

HEAT TRANSFER

Heat is transferred to the surroundings by:

- radiation
- conduction
- convection.

Radiation

Radiation is the transfer of thermal energy as infrared rays. Over half of the loss of heat occurs by this means. In a room, heat is transferred to walls, floor, ceiling and the contents of the space without direct transfer by touching. In a cold room, the room will gradually warm up as you get colder and colder. The sun will transfer radiant energy to the body, even if the air temperature is low. The effect is magnified by reflection of the rays from a surface such as snow, as skiers in shirtsleeves can testify.

Conduction

Heat is transferred from one object to another when they are in contact. Heat is transferred to or from clothes or the chair you are sitting on or whatever you may be leaning on. Much more significant, however, is the transfer made to the air even though it is a poor conductor of heat. Here it becomes more convenient to think of conduction and convection together.

Conduction and convection

Transfer of heat to or from the surrounding air is first by conduction to the very thin layer immediately in contact with the body surface. If the air is cooler, heat is lost to this nearest layer. The molecules which make up air are in constant movement and the temperature difference between the now warm air layer and the cooler layers outside will cause small currents of air, i.e. convection currents. The warmed air next to the body surface is immediately moved away, to be replaced by another layer of cool air to which more heat can be transferred. If the air movement were to stop and the air temperature were to match skin temperature, transfer of heat would come to a halt. The loss by conduction therefore requires convection to keep it going. This is the basis of 'wind chill'; a cold windy day can feel much colder than a still cold day even if the air temperatures are the same.

About 20% of heat loss occurs because of conduction and convection, although this is reduced by wearing clothes which trap an air layer next to the skin.

Air is a fairly poor conductor of heat compared with water and heat loss to water is much greater. Temperatures which can be tolerated in air, even without clothes, require a survival suit in water.

SWEATING

An important cooling mechanism uses the conducting property of water and adds another property – evaporation. This is the heat regulating mechanism of sweating.

Insensible loss

When water is converted from a liquid to a vapour, the process of evaporation requires heat, referred to as latent heat. (Latent heat is given out again as the water vapour (as steam) condenses, which explains why a steam burn is so much more damaging than a burn caused by the same volume of hot or boiling water.) As far as sweating is concerned, the extra latent heat needed to evaporate the water is taken from the body's heat, with the effect of reducing body temperature.

About 600 ml of water passes through the skin and mucous membranes in a day (insensible water loss) and is evaporated using about 450 kcal (1.9 MJ) insensible or evaporative heat loss. Even without the loss of heat to evaporate the moisture on the skin, the moist layer

has a cooling effect as body heat moves into it by conduction.

Sensible loss

When core temperature rises, sweating is increased in response to the sensory signals (hence the term 'sensible' sweating) about the degree of deviation from the core temperature set point. The process of cooling by evaporation is the same as above, but the rate of water loss can be many times greater than that of insensible loss and can be matched to the extra heat load.

Effective sweating depends on there being sufficient body water and the surrounding air being at a lower temperature. Convection currents are also needed to move the warm saturated air away. These principles are applied to the treatment of a pyrexic patient, who is sponged with tepid water (cold water would cause vasoconstriction and heat retention) and fanned gently.

TEMPERATURE REGULATION

Control over body temperature is organized along the same lines as other parameters in the body environment. Information about the state of the parameter is relayed from receptors to a central regulating area; this in turn causes activity in effector tissues to adjust temperature (Fig. 17.1).

THERMORECEPTORS

Thermoreceptors are sensory endings in skin (peripheral or shell receptors) and in the hypothalamus (central or core receptors). Other areas with receptors supplying temperature information include the spinal cord, lungs and the gut. The receptors respond to a rise in temperature from their base point, so for example,

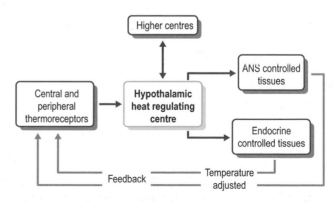

Figure 17.1 The principles of centrally controlled thermoregulation. (ANS, autonomic nervous system.)

there are receptors which are affected by a rise in temperature from a low temperature typical of some areas of skin, while others would respond to a rise from a much higher temperature. The receptor pathways have an 'order of precedence' with the highest priority signals relating to core temperature.

CENTRAL REGULATION

The hypothalamus regulates many other aspects of the internal environment in addition to core temperature; therefore information about temperature must be integrated with all the other sensory information. As well as the input from thermoreceptors giving information about temperature itself, the hypothalamus receives information about other parameters which are likely to impinge on temperature, for example blood pressure, fluid balance and gas balance. It also receives information about other activities going on, e.g. exercise, eating, sleeping, and about emotional states.

It has numerous routes of somatic, autonomic and endocrine output allowing the temperature to be adjusted by a variety of mechanisms (Fig. 17.2). The mechanisms can be divided into two groups, those which retain and/or increase heat (heat gain) and those which cause heat loss. The balance between the two groups of mechanisms is regulated by the thermoregulatory or thermogenetic centre in the hypothalamus.

The small adjustments, which are constantly being made, are usually unnoticed. As always, the evidence for the existence of the mechanisms is best seen where significant changes have to be made (see below).

Whatever adjustments have to be made, they must be integrated with the regulation of other parameters. A well-known clinical example is the pattern of blood pressure and temperature changes characteristic of situations where both are under threat (see below).

SKIN

Skin has a critical role in thermoregulation. It is the tissue which 'keeps the inside in and the outside out', a description which neatly fits its role in thermoregulation.

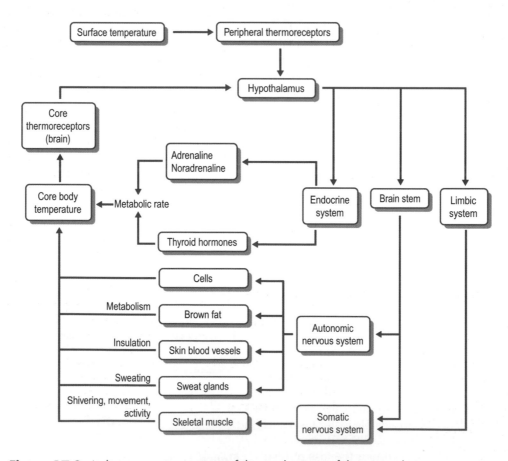

Figure 17.2 A diagrammatic summary of the mechanisms of thermoregulation.

Skin is the barrier between environments which may be at widely differing temperatures. The outside temperature may be many degrees below zero, or 45°C above, but the body core temperature must stay around 37°C. Skin allows water to permeate through (insensible loss) and has many sweat glands which have a controllable water output (sensible loss). The skin circulation has anastomoses which allow capillary beds to be closed to retain heat, or open and perfused to lose heat (see Ch. 12 at 'Specialized circulations'). Blood flow in a thermoneutral state is about 10 to 20 ml per minute per 100 g. Vasodilation to cool down can increase the flow to about ten times that and vasoconstriction may reduce the flow to only about 1 ml per minute per 100 g (see p. 318 – 'Cold-induced vasoconstriction–vasodilation). Blood vessels in skin have thermoreceptors which, in addition to relaying information to the hypothalamus, operate reflexly to change the degree of sympathetic stimulation of the blood vessels. A fall in temperature increases sympathetic discharge and the degree of vasoconstriction; a rise in temperature has the opposite effect.

TEMPERATURE ADJUSTMENT MECHANISMS

A rise in temperature can be achieved either by increasing the production of heat or by reducing its loss (in practice both would happen). A fall in temperature would be achieved by increasing loss and reducing heat production (Table 17.1 and Fig. 17.3); increasing loss is an immediate response, reducing production takes longer.

HEAT GAIN

Heat is generated by:

- Processing of food and subsequent cell activities (*dietary thermogenesis*).

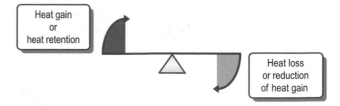

Figure 17.3 The principle of body temperature regulation – balancing heat gain against heat loss.

- Muscular work, including degree of muscle tone and shivering. When muscle contracts, ATP is metabolized and heat is produced. When one is cold, the behavioural response is to stamp feet, clap one's hands together and so on. Cold also increases the tone of muscles, so increasing heat production. If the temperature continues to fall, shivering begins. It is an involuntary effect although arising from somatic motor neurones. The muscles do not move the body or perform any task and the synchronized contractions serve only to produce heat. *Shivering thermogenesis* is not enough to maintain temperature if the ambient temperature is very low and, because it is very expensive of energy, it cannot be sustained over a long period.
- Increased catecholamine output. Cold stress rapidly stimulates the sympathetic nervous system and the adrenal medulla. Noradrenaline and adrenaline increase heart rate and vasoconstriction (noradrenaline) and increase the tone in skeletal muscle. Metabolic rate is raised by the catecholamines so increasing *non-shivering thermogenesis*.
- Increased thyroid hormone output (longer-term adaptation to cold). Cold stress increases activity in the hypothalamo–anterior pituitary–thyroid axis (see Ch. 11). The resulting rise in metabolic rate increases heat production. This is an adaptive response which may take several weeks to achieve, not a short-term response to sudden cold.

Table 17.1 Summary of temperature regulation mechanisms

Heat gain	Heat retention	Heat loss
Dietary thermogenesis	Vasoconstriction	Sweating
Muscular work	Countercurrent blood flow	Vasodilation
Muscle tone	Fat insulation	↑ Ventilation
Shivering	Clothing	Removing clothing
↑ Catecholamines	Behavioural responses	Behavioural responses
↑ Thyroid hormones		
Brown adipose tissue		
Behavioural responses		

• Brown adipose tissue. This is richly supplied by blood vessels (hence its name). When stimulated by noradrenaline, rather than being metabolized to lipid by-products, it yields a large proportion of reaction energy directly as heat. Babies and young animals of other species have significant deposits which are likely to be an important contributor to maintaining their body temperature (see p. 317 at 'Thermoregulation in the newborn').
• Behavioural responses such as increased food intake, hot drinks.
• Behavioural responses such as exercise.

Reduction in activity in the mechanisms above will reduce heat generation.

HEAT RETENTION

Heat loss is reduced by:

• Skin vasoconstriction.
• Insulation, e.g. superficial fat.
• Blood vessels in a countercurrent arrangement. In the limbs, arterial and venous vessels run alongside one another but with the flow in opposite directions, i.e. countercurrent. As warm blood from the core flows down a limb, it gives up heat to the cooler blood in the venous vessel returning to the core. Although the extremities might be cooler, vital heat is conserved at the core. Constriction of the skin blood vessels ensures that, in the cold, blood flow is kept deep in the limb (Fig. 17.4).
• Behavioural responses such as moving to somewhere warmer, putting on more clothes, curling up.

HEAT LOSS

Heat loss is increased by:

• skin vasodilation
• sweating
• increased ventilation (although panting is more effective in species such as the dog)
• behavioural responses such as
  – moving to somewhere cooler
  – being less active
  – removing clothes
  – applying cool water to skin
  – eating less; cold drinks.

In summary, thermoregulation is achieved by balancing heat gain against heat loss (Fig. 17.3):

• a rise in core temperature will prompt less stimulation of heat gain mechanisms and more stimulation of heat loss mechanisms

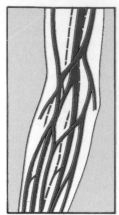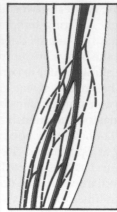

Figure 17.4 Two cooperative thermoregulatory adaptations – countercurrent flow and vasoconstriction/vasodilation. *Left*: Countercurrent flow. Warm arterial blood loses heat as it flows towards the periphery. However, the heat moves into the cooler venous blood returning from the periphery, minimizing heat loss. *Right*: As superficial blood vessels constrict or dilate in response to temperature, blood can be brought to superficial layers if heat is to be lost or can be diverted to deeper vessels if heat is to be retained. (After Emslie-Smith et al 1988, with permission of Elsevier.)

• a fall in core temperature will prompt more stimulation of heat gain mechanisms and less stimulation of heat loss mechanisms.

ABNORMAL TEMPERATURE STATES

As core temperature deviates from normal, characteristic effects begin to appear; the larger the deviation the more damaging the consequences (Fig. 17.5).

Reduction in temperature is better tolerated than a rise in temperature, although either is better tolerated if developed slowly and the exposure to the most extreme temperatures is not prolonged. The extremes compatible with life are about 23 and 45°C. The range of temperatures which can be corrected without outside help is much narrower, about 28 to 43°C.

HYPERTHERMIA

Fever – pyrexia

Fever is the best known of the temperature disturbances. Descriptions of fever are known from early history and some of the earliest remedies were attempts to treat it; for example, the use of willow bark which is a source of aspirin.

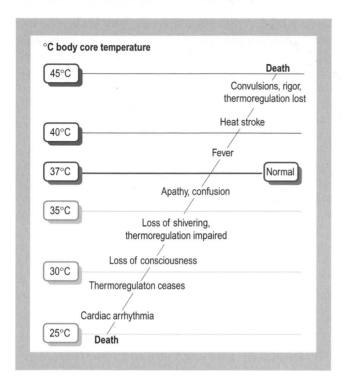

Figure 17.5 The effects of deviation from normal core temperature.

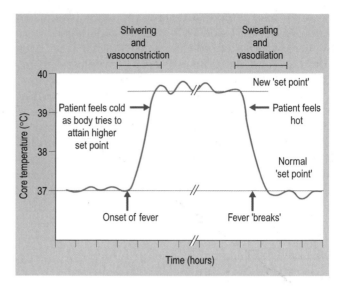

Figure 17.6 A diagrammatic representation of the time-course of a typical febrile episode. (After Pocock & Richards 1999 Human physiology: the basis of medicine. Reprinted by permission of Oxford University Press.)

Fever is not a response to heat; it is caused by an elevation of the set point by pyrogens. These are either endotoxins produced by bacteria or cytokines produced by the immune system cells in response to infection (see Ch. 16).

The altered set point stimulates the heat gain mechanisms and inhibits heat loss and, predictably, core temperature rises. The sufferer feels cold, the skin is cold and vasoconstricted, and shivering may be intense. Measurement will show that, in spite of the patient's own impression, temperature is high.

Fever has evolved as part of the response to infection and is considered part of the body defence system. However, prolonged fever can be damaging and is normally treated with an anti-pyretic such as aspirin. Thermoregulation is less efficient in small children, they may develop a high temperature quite rapidly and convulsions may occur in pyrexic children. Cooling a fevered child may avoid this.

After the effect of the pyrogen has passed, the set point re-sets. Core temperature is now above the healthy norm and the heat-losing mechanisms begin to act. The individual feels and looks hot (now vasodilated), sweats and feels thirsty. An inclination to sleep at this point often acts to reduce physical effort and muscle tone and, as the mechanisms take effect, temperature returns to normal (Fig. 17.6).

Heat stroke

Exposure to high ambient temperatures will produce hyperthermia when the thermoregulatory mechanisms are unable to compensate the heat gain. All the systems which cause heat loss and inhibit heat gain are employed, but the internal temperature continues to rise. When fluid reserves are no longer sufficient to produce enough cooling, the skin feels dry and core temperature rises rapidly. This is heat stroke. Abnormal osmotic pressure and electrolyte levels may cause muscle rigor and neural damage and dysfunction. The elevated temperature increases reaction rates in the cells so that more heat is produced. The rates are not equally affected and the normally integrated reactions become de-synchronized, adding to the dysfunction. If core temperature exceeds about 42°C death is likely unless the subject can be cooled.

Competing priorities – body temperature versus blood pressure

Heat stroke may produce measurable evidence of the defence of more than one homeostatic parameter at the same time. When body temperature is rising, fluid is lost in sweat and by ventilation, thereby potentially reducing blood pressure. Vasodilation, in an attempt to lose heat, increases the capacity of the vascular system. The combination of reduced volume and increased capacity will significantly reduce pressure (see Ch. 12).

The body's responses to pressure loss are to increase cardiac output, to vasoconstrict and to retain volume. There are, however, the underlying problems of an elevated core temperature and probably insufficient fluid. Vasoconstriction will increase core temperature by constructing an insulating layer over the core. Volume retention decreases sweat formation and, in any case, has limited effect if there is insufficient fluid.

A stage is reached where two homeostatic priorities, blood pressure and body core temperature, are in competition with one another. With no intervention, the body will lose fluid and vasodilate, so losing heat, until blood pressure reaches a critical low value. Then vaso-constriction and fluid retention are stimulated, raising pressure, until a critical high temperature is reached. At this point, the priority again becomes body temperature and the cycle begins again.

A series of temperature and blood pressure readings will show oscillation of both temperature and pressure as first one priority then the other is defended – at least as far as possible. Intervention in the form of cooling and the administration of fluids is essential to help the individual out of this situation.

Since osmolality and individual electrolyte levels will also have been affected by the mechanisms involved in maintaining temperature and pressure, the composition of the fluids is important and rehydration must be done with care.

Malignant hyperthermia

This is a relatively rare phenomenon but none the less clinically important. It is a response to an anaesthetic such as halothane or muscle relaxant such as suxamethonium (succinylcholine), where sustained breakdown of ATP and the muscle spasm produced causes rapidly developing hyperthermia. It is due to an inherited genetic disorder of calcium release channels. Contraction in muscle requires calcium to be released from intracellular stores via calcium release channels. Muscle relaxation requires that the calcium be taken back into store, a process fuelled by ATP. In an individual with this faulty gene, when halothane is present, the channels remain open, the process of ATP breakdown is continuous and the muscle spasm is maintained. The heat generated causes a catastrophic rise in temperature. If the subject is to survive, the agent must be removed and ice used to reduce the temperature. The condition is now treated with the drug dantrolene sodium, which closes the calcium channels even in the presence of halothane or suxamethonium.

HYPOTHERMIA

Despite the efficiency of all the complex mechanisms which maintain temperature, there can be circum-stances where they prove to be inadequate and the core begins to cool. Hypothermia may be accidental, developing rapidly if someone falls into very cold water, much more slowly in cold air. It may be induced clinically in some kinds of surgery, e.g. some open-heart surgery and neurosurgery. Since the cell rates of reaction are slowed as the temperature falls, cooling extends the time in which work can be carried out on tissues where normal perfusion is not available.

Hypothermia is usually taken to be a core temper-ature of 35°C and below. The systems of heat gain and preventing the loss of heat are likely to be operating, with shivering, vasoconstriction and the many behav-ioural responses. The effect of temperature reduction is to reduce reaction rates; therefore all the thermo-regulatory systems themselves begin to slow. The most obvious effects are slow heart rate and respiration rate. At about 34°C shivering is lessened and will cease as the temperature drops further. Voluntary movement

A familiar sight at the end of the London Marathon is of massed runners, all wearing shiny space blankets. They will have exercised hard and will be radiating increased amounts of heat from the surface of their bodies. The highly reflective nature of the space blanket limits loss of heat to the surrounding air (which may be comparatively cool, the Marathon being run in April). Despite their light weight, these blankets are an extremely good protection against heat loss, they can be used in mountaineering, in ambulances and in nursing the hypothermia victim in hospital.

Raising the core temperature in mountain rescue

Rewarming victims of hypothermia in mountaineering accidents, just like rewarming people rescued from the sea, is not simply a question of applying as much heat as possible as quickly as possible. *Gradual* warming is the key – along with prevention of further heat loss – so that blood from the body core is not transferred to the skin surface too quickly.

A relatively new method of rewarming the body core is the use of heated, humidified oxygen (or air) supplied through a face mask. With this equipment, which is portable, the deep tissues of the lungs, and thus the major vessels of the chest and neck, are warmed. (To appreciate the effectiveness of this method, consider which vessels return blood to the heart from the lungs, and how that blood is then pumped to the thorax, neck and head.) This method is of use only in conjunction with effective methods of preventing further heat loss from the victim's body.

becomes impossible and with it the behavioural response such as putting on clothes. Apathy and confusion add to the problems. It is not unknown for mountaineers who have become hypothermic to have unused extra clothing with them or in extreme cases to have taken off clothing before collapsing.

At about 32 to 30°C, the ability to regain normal temperature without external help is lost. Below this, about 28 to 26°C, cardiovascular function may become disordered and fibrillation may well be the cause of death. The lowest survivable core temperature for an adult is about 22 to 25°C; the lower the temperature the more difficult it is to re-warm.

Warming the hypothermic subject requires great care. If warmed rapidly and from the outside, skin vasodilation will allow very cold blood to move to the core, causing a further drop in temperature which may well be fatal. An insulating blanket and breathing warm air are safer.

Vulnerability to hypothermia

- As people get older, the sensitivity to temperature changes decreases. A young adult can detect ambient air changes of less than 1°C, while some elderly people cannot discriminate between temperatures different by 2.5°C. Elderly people may be less mobile for all sorts of reasons and may choose not to heat their living space. Metabolic rate is likely to be lower and adaptive changes to raise metabolic rate are less than in the young.
- There may be some degree of neural or endocrine dysfunction which would make it difficult to adapt to or respond to cold; for example, thyroid function should always be considered when an elderly person is found to be suffering from hypothermia.
- People who are immobile are at risk from hostile temperature conditions. In addition to their inability to move out of the cold area, they may have lost some of the involuntary responses such as shivering.
- Alcohol consumption can increase vulnerability to cold. Alcohol has vasodilator effects and reduces the effectiveness of the vasoconstrictor response. It may also blunt the sensitivity to cold and inhibit the behavioural responses which might be made to avoid hypothermia. Some aspects of hypothermic 'behaviour' may be mistaken for drunkenness and, when evidence of alcohol can actually be detected, the effect may be to mask the hypothermia and possibly reduce the chances of help being offered.
- Some drugs increase the risk of developing hypothermia. The drug chlorpromazine has the capacity to inhibit shivering and it can be used as an adjunct in surgery which involves the use of therapeutic hypothermia. Chlorpromazine, however, is also used in the treatment of psychoses and it follows that anyone taking chlorpromazine needs to be aware of the potential risk of accidental hypothermia.

Thermoregulation in the newborn

Babies have the problem of a very small volume with a large surface area, so losing heat is easy. They have (usually) only a thin layer of fat so heat conservation is difficult. The shivering mechanism is not well developed, making this form of heat generation inefficient. Premature babies are even more vulnerable.

On the other hand, their capacity per kg body weight to generate metabolic heat is about four times greater than that of an adult. Babies also have, in neck, shoulders, thorax and abdomen, disproportionately large deposits of brown adipose tissue which responds to noradrenaline and adrenaline by releasing large amounts of heat.

In spite of their heat generating capacity, newborn babies need to be kept reasonably warm. Thermogenesis either by overall body tissue or by brown fat is expensive in energy terms. An ambient temperature of about 33°C will usually maintain core temperature without the baby having to resort to extra heat generation.

LOCAL EFFECTS OF TEMPERATURE

LOCAL EFFECTS OF COLD

The immediate effects of cold are vasoconstriction and decreased cell metabolism. Skin colour can, with some experience, be an indication of the conditions within the skin. If vasoconstriction is intense the skin will be white in a fair-skinned person, and in a dark or black skin, it may acquire a greyish hue due to lack of blood in the capillaries. In a pale skin, a blueish tinge indicates stasis of the blood flow and the presence of deoxygenated haemoglobin. In extremely cold conditions, a cold red skin indicates that blood is present in the capillaries but oxygen has not been withdrawn from the haemoglobin either because the requirement of the cells is very low at that temperature, or the enzymes involved in the dissociation are below the temperature at which they can function.

Cold-induced vasoconstriction–vasodilation

If the skin temperature remains close to freezing, the phenomenon of cold-induced vasoconstriction–vasodilation is seen. A period of intense vasoconstriction allows metabolites to accumulate and the beginnings of tissue injury cause the release of the vasodilator nitric oxide. The cold itself may reduce the effectiveness of the vasoconstrictor control.

The response of the vascular smooth muscle is to relax. Blood flows into the area, warms it and limits the damage to the tissue served by the circulation. As soon as the dilated vessels begin to lose significant amounts of heat and the local dilator effect of the metabolites is reduced, vasoconstriction begins again. Although painful, this adaptive response has long allowed work to be done in extreme conditions.

Frostbite

Cold can cause injury, however – frostbite.

Frostbite is the localized freezing of peripheral parts of the body, usually fingers, toes, ears and nose. Frostbite can occur even if the core temperature is being maintained. It can happen in British winter mountaineering, but is much more likely where temperatures are lower. The early signs of superficial frostbite are white waxy tips to the fingers or toes affected and there may be superimposed blisters. If the area is painful, the nerves are still intact and treatment at this point is likely to be successful, if uncomfortable. Deeper frostbite, especially if sustained for some time, may result in gangrene, with the subsequent loss of the part affected. The full effects of frostbite cannot be cured, only amputated. Prevention is essential and a great deal of work has gone into the development of excellent mountaineering gear. Unfortunately, accidents and injuries still carry the risk of frostbite.

Unlike the gradual warming of the hypothermic body, where frostbite has occurred, rapid and prompt warming of the tissue is required. The longer the cells remain frozen, the greater the risk of permanent damage, but both the rescuer and the rescued should be aware that warming of extremely cold limbs causes severe pain.

LOCAL EFFECTS OF HEAT

Heat increases the rate of cell metabolism including the reactions concerned with replication and differentiation. Warm skin heals more rapidly than cold skin (see Ch. 19). The heat-induced vasodilation improves perfusion and the delivery of the cell's requirements. On the other side of the coin, however, too much heat damages cells. Even relatively modest temperatures (below 50°C) will cause denaturation of the proteins; higher temperatures will simply cook the tissue.

Damage can be caused by radiant heat or contact with a heat source. A particularly nasty burn can be caused by steam, which, as it condenses on the cool skin, releases latent heat. The burn is caused, not just by water at 100°C but by the large amount of extra heat given off in its conversion from a vapour (steam). The chemicals released at the wound site cause vasodilation and increased capillary permeability resulting in the familiar red blistered area (see Ch. 19).

The amount of damage can be limited by cooling the area rapidly in cold water (and continuing long enough for the tissue to cool down). This rapidly removes the damaging heat and minimizes injury.

REFERENCES AND FURTHER READING

Astrand P-O, Rodahl K 1986 Textbook of work physiology, 3rd edn. McGraw-Hill, New York

Case R M, Waterhouse J M (eds) 1994 Human physiology: age, stress and the environment. Oxford Science Publications, Oxford

Clancy J, McVicar A J 1995 Physiology and anatomy – a homeostatic approach. Edward Arnold, London

Emslie-Smith D et al 1988 Thermoregulation. In: Emslie-Smith D, Paterson C R, Scratcherd T, Read N W (eds) Textbook of physiology, 11th edn. Churchill Livingstone, Edinburgh

Ganong W F 2001 Review of medical physiology, 20th edn. McGraw-Hill Education, Philadelphia

Guyton A C, Hall J E 2000 Textbook of medical physiology, 10th edn. Saunders, Philadelphia

Krog J 1974 Peripheral circulatory adjustments to cold. In: Borg A, Veghte J H (eds) The physiology of cold weather survival. NATO: Agard Report No. 620

Pocock G, Richards C D 1999 Human physiology: the basis of medicine. Oxford University Press, Oxford

In practice you may be asked to consider the following:

1. Plasma glucose is maintained by several hyperglycaemic hormones and one hypoglycaemic hormone. Which are these?

2. Why is the maintenance of normal glucose levels so important?

3. In the event of lack of glucose, can the brain use any other fuel?

4. How is plasma glucose maintained by someone who does not eat carbohydrate?

5. Insulin facilitates glucose entry into the cells of insulin sensitive tissues. Which are these?

6. A patient has been found to have adequate levels of insulin in plasma, but still has low glucose tolerance. What might this be due to? He has been advised to lose weight. How might that help?

7. Is the patient above likely to develop ketosis?

8. A middle-aged man has suffered a myocardial infarct. A few hours later his plasma glucose is significantly elevated. He is in some pain, worried and frightened. He has no history of diabetes. Please explain.

9. A young woman who has had diabetes since childhood has developed an overactive thyroid. Her glycosylated haemoglobin levels have risen and she needs more insulin to get back to her normal level of control. Please explain.

10. The woman above has had a hypoglycaemic attack. On the following morning, she finds that her blood tests show plasma glucose to be elevated. She has the choice to increase her insulin dose or leave it at the usual number of units. If asked, what would be your advice?

DEFINING THE TERMS

Although glucose levels are often referred to as 'blood' glucose, the preferred term *'plasma glucose'* is more correct since most laboratories measure the concentration of glucose in plasma rather than whole blood.

The term 'plasma (or blood) *glucose*' is used where glucose itself is measured by enzymic methods, for example using an enzyme-impregnated 'stick' or by a laboratory method. Measurements of 'plasma (or blood) *sugar*' may use other non-enzymic methods and may include other sugar-related compounds.

This chapter uses the term 'plasma glucose'.

THE STABILITY OF PLASMA GLUCOSE LEVELS

Although the brain can use other fuels such as lactate and ketone bodies, glucose is the main source of energy for the central nervous system. The brain uses about 100 g of glucose per day and an adequate concentration gradient is required to maintain the supply. The central effects of hypoglycaemia can be loss of cognitive function extending to loss of consciousness and, if extreme and prolonged, loss of life.

Other tissues, although they also use glucose as fuel, have a wider choice and are unlikely to malfunction as dramatically as the hypoglycaemic brain.

The stability of glucose balance is therefore critical to normal function. It must be maintained not only when food intake is plentiful and regular, but also when there are long periods with no intake. The systems controlling glucose concentrations must be capable of causing storage in times of plenty and release on demand, i.e. managing an efficient banking system. In most individuals, possibly over 95%, glucose regulation is so efficient and robust that in spite of the present Western trend towards too much intake and not enough output of energy, plasma glucose remains normal.

Plasma glucose is maintained at between 3 and 8 mmol/litre. These are the outer limits of the normal range and the concentration is more likely to be within the tighter limits of 3.5 to 5.5 or 6 mmol/litre regardless of feeding or fasting. Plasma glucose concentration outside normal range is damaging. Low values (hypoglycaemia) are damaging in the short term since glucose is the major fuel substrate of brain and nervous tissue. Hyperglycaemia over a long period of time is damaging to all tissues and can lead to the complications associated with diabetes mellitus. Glucose regulation must be capable of withstanding large variation of input and expenditure of glucose and constantly maintaining a narrow range of concentration. The hormones involved must be capable of reducing plasma glucose during and after feeding, then raising plasma glucose from a variety of body stores (endogenous stores) over fasting periods which might extend not just for hours but for days or weeks.

There are many levels of control over glucose concentration.

- It is regulated by a group of hormones, each with its own set of modifying controls. Regulation of release

may be affected by the autonomic nervous system, by the levels of individual substrates such as amino acids and fatty acids, or by activities in the brain itself.
- The A and B cells of the pancreas, which release glucagon and insulin respectively, are themselves subject to a number of factors which alter the amount of hormone produced in response to the main stimulus. The particular chemical messengers present in circumstances such as feeding, exercise and stress will affect hormone release.
- Glucose regulation is also affected by the number and affinity of the hormone receptor sites, which in turn modify the effectiveness of the hormone (see pp. 323, 328).
- The metabolic pathways which store and release glucose are subject to the relative amounts of substrate present, the influence of the autonomic nervous system and the profile of other hormones present.

It must come as no surprise that, when the physiological regulation of glucose fails as, for example, in diabetes, and exogenous insulin must be used instead, the level of regulation, no matter how good, cannot match the body's own.

THE HORMONES OF GLUCOSE REGULATION

The hormones involved are insulin, glucagon, adrenaline, growth hormone, cortisol and the thyroid hormones. Of these, only insulin reduces plasma glucose; all the others, the counter-regulatory hormones, raise plasma glucose.

The terminology used to describe the counter-regulatory hormones is open to question. Insulin reduces plasma glucose concentrations and is indisputably a hypoglycaemic hormone, but the counter-regulatory hormones are sometimes referred to as 'glucogenic' or 'hyperglycaemic'. Some of the hormonal actions do cause glucose formation (glucogenesis) but others promote the use of alternative fuels or limit glucose uptake and are therefore glucose sparing. All the counter-regulatory hormones raise or maintain plasma glucose but their release is usually inhibited by hyperglycaemia. Neither 'glucogenic' nor 'hyperglycaemic' seems an accurate description in this context. This chapter uses the descriptor 'counter-regulatory'.

In the processes of glucose regulation, the individual hormones use a variety of substrates and operate over different time scales (Fig. 18.1).

The liver plays a central role in maintaining glucose balance. Its cells contain the enzymes for the metabolic

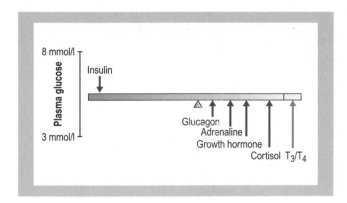

Figure 18.1 Glucose balance. (After Watson 1999, with permission of Elsevier.)

pathways which manipulate the nutrient substrates and it is sensitive to the hormones which can selectively stimulate or inhibit the pathways (see Ch. 10).

Nutrients enter the gut as protein, fat and carbohydrate and are successively degraded to amino acids, fatty acids and glycerol, and a variety of monosaccharides (see Ch. 9). At absorption, fatty acids and glycerol are reassembled to triglycerides and bound to transport proteins. The products of digestion are taken by the hepatic portal vein to the liver for processing, and it is at this stage that plasma glucose levels can determine how they are processed. These nutrients are termed exogenous since they are from an outside source.

Substrates can also be endogenous. These come from the body's own protein, fat and carbohydrate which are continually being broken down and replaced. A large proportion of the products of breakdown can be used as fuel.

ADJUSTMENTS TO PLASMA GLUCOSE

Plasma glucose is constantly being adjusted so that it stays within its reference range.

To raise plasma glucose:

- it can be released to plasma as it is absorbed from the gut
- it can be released from its storage form of hepatic glycogen (glycogenolysis)
- it can be formed from a non-carbohydrate source (gluconeogenesis).

To lower plasma glucose:

- it can be used to produce energy (glycolysis)
- it can be stored as glycogen (glycogenesis). Glycogen can be stored within liver, muscle and other tissues, but only hepatic glycogen can be broken down and exported to blood to raise plasma glucose levels

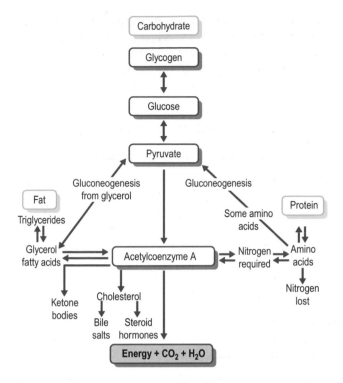

Figure 18.2 Interconversion of endogenous or exogenous nutrients.

- it can be converted to triglycerides for storage as fat (lipogenesis). About 90% of glucose is stored as lipid
- it also becomes attached to proteins such as haemoglobin (glycation or glycosylation) (see p. 328 at 'Type 1 diabetes').

The interconversion of the nutrients is the same whether from an exogenous or endogenous source. The biochemical pathways are covered in more detail in Chapter 10. An outline of the interrelationships is shown in Figure 18.2.

This chapter considers the main characteristics of insulin and glucagon including their role in glucose regulation. The other hormones in the group, the catecholamines, human growth hormone, cortisol and the thyroid hormones, are considered only from the point of glucose regulation. Other information about the latter hormones can be found in Chapter 11.

THE ENDOCRINE PANCREAS

The pancreas consists of two types of tissue, exocrine and endocrine. By far the larger part is exocrine tissue made up of the cells and ducts which produce pancreatic juice (see Ch. 9). The endocrine tissue, the islets of Langerhans, occupies only about 2% of the volume of the pancreas. The islets, each with a capillary

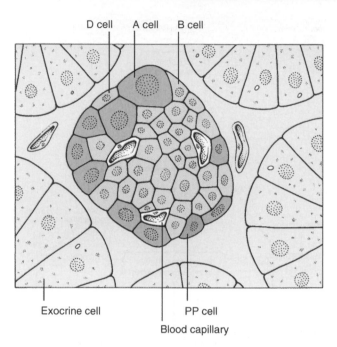

Figure 18.3 Islets of Langerhans.

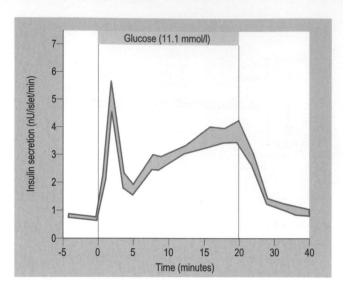

Figure 18.4 Biphasic secretion of insulin by isolated perfused rat islets in response to stimulation with 11.1 mmol/l glucose. (After Edwards 1986, with permission of Elsevier.)

system into which the hormones are passed, are clearly distinguishable, at microscopic level, from the surrounding tissue (Fig. 18.3). They are supplied by parasympathetic and sympathetic fibres.

The islets are made up of four different cell types A, B, D and PP (sometimes shown as α, β, δ and PP):

- A cells – glucagon, raises plasma glucose
- B cells – insulin, reduces plasma glucose
- D cells – somatostatin, inhibits the release of both insulin and glucagon
- PP – pancreatic polypeptide, affects the secretion of pancreatic juice.

INSULIN

Insulin is a large polypeptide hormone produced by the B cells of the pancreas. It is produced from a larger precursor molecule, proinsulin, which is cleaved at release to give insulin and C-peptide. C- peptide has no biological action and is excreted unchanged, but it can be used as a measure of the release of insulin (insulin has a short half-life and is degraded by a number of tissues, notably the liver).

In an adult, the islets contain about 150 to 200 units of insulin, and about 40 units are used daily. At release, insulin travels in the unbound state.

Insulin is released continuously at a basal rate supplemented by release at a higher or stimulated rate in response to a stimulus. When there is a long fasting period, insulin is released at a suppressed rate. Release in response to a stimulus has a characteristic biphasic pattern (Fig. 18.4). The early first phase takes place within a few minutes of stimulus, lasts for 5 to 10 minutes and insulin is released from a small storage pool. This is followed by phase 2, which lasts for about an hour and is mounted from a larger pool topped up by synthesis. At this point, maintaining the stimulus will cause continued release.

The liver removes about half of the insulin entering by the hepatic portal vessel. Insulin is filtered at the glomeruli and degraded by the kidney.

STIMULI TO INSULIN RELEASE

The primary stimulus to insulin release is rising plasma glucose; insulin is therefore parameter regulated (see Ch. 11). The amount of insulin released, however, is modified by many other factors, some of which stimulate secretion, some which inhibit. The B cell is therefore capable of producing a variable response to its primary glucose stimulus.

The groups of factors which modify insulin response to glucose are substrate, neural (autonomic) and endocrine.

Figure 18.5 shows some of the factors which increase or decrease the response to glucose. The modifying

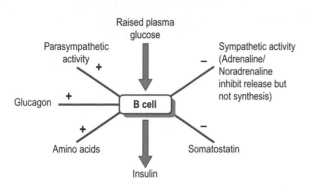

Figure 18.5 Factors influencing the B cell response to glucose.

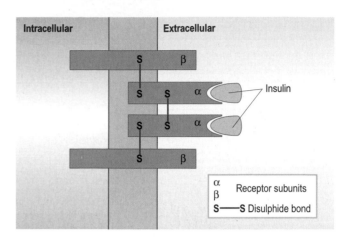

Figure 18.6 Diagrammatic representation of an insulin receptor site.

factors shown in Figure 18.5 give only an indication of how elegant the mechanisms are which keep plasma glucose within normal limits while taking other circumstances into account.

In a series of paracrine actions, insulin and glucagon inhibit the release of one another, and, since they have opposing actions, this may achieve a more positive response from each. On the other hand, both insulin and glucagon are inhibited by somatostatin from the D cells. This has a damping effect and reduces the tendency to abrupt changes in plasma glucose values caused by two opposing hormones.

An extension to the mechanism above is an example of control systems at their best. When adrenaline is released in an emergency, it inhibits insulin release so that plasma glucose can rise, but, better than that, it inhibits somatostatin so that glucagon can be released rapidly and add to the rise in glucose levels.

At a neural level, when, for example, there is a response to feeding, the parasympathetic division, which has a large role in gut function, also increases the response of the B cell, providing a rapid and early response to the incoming food. The opposite happens when in an emergency requiring a sympathetic response from heart, blood vessels and so on, the same sympathetic response also inhibits the release of insulin and allows plasma glucose to remain high enough to cope with the emergency.

Substrates such as amino acids, particularly leucine and arginine, stimulate the B cell and may contribute to the finding of an enhanced insulin response to a mixed meal. Fatty acids and ketone bodies also stimulate the B cell but much less strongly. Fatty acids and ketone bodies circulate at higher levels during fasting and this may be a mechanism to protect the fasting subject from ketosis (a low level of insulin is enough to inhibit the production of ketone bodies, see p. 327).

INSULIN RECEPTORS

Insulin's protein structure would suggest that its target cell receptors should be on the membrane surface and that a second messenger would be used. Instead of this, however, insulin uses a system in which the receptors link the outside and inside of the cell and, after binding, the receptor site and its hormone become internalized.

Insulin receptors consist of four subunits bound together. Two of the subunits are on the cell surface and the other two bridge the membrane; therefore the whole receptor is located both on the surface and in contact with the cell interior. When insulin binds to the two surface units, the change in the molecular shape is communicated by the two bridging units to the inside of the cell (Fig. 18.6). This sets in train the enzyme cascade which results in insulin's effects. After the insulin is bound, the whole assembly is taken into the cell by the process of endocytosis, the receptor part is returned to the membrane and the insulin is degraded. This internalization of the receptor may be part of the mechanism for regulating the number of receptor sites (see Ch. 11 at 'Target cell receptors').

THE EFFECTS OF INSULIN

The functions of insulin are to promote anabolism and inhibit catabolism and its actions can be divided into anabolic effects and anti-catabolic effects (Table 18.1). Insulin affects all tissues to some extent but its main target tissues are liver, skeletal muscle and adipose tissue. These are referred to as 'insulin-dependent tissues'. In muscle and adipose tissue, glucose entry to the cells is not rapid enough without insulin which activates glucose transporters and increases the uptake

Table 18.1 Anabolic and anti-catabolic effects of insulin

	Anabolic	Anti-catabolic
Carbohydrate	↑ glucose transport in skeletal muscle and adipose tissue ↑ glycolysis ↑ glycogenesis	↓ glycogenolysis ↓ gluconeogenesis
Lipids	↑ (liver) synthesis of fatty acids ↑ triglycerides synthesis	↓ lipolysis ↓ (liver) fatty acid oxidation ↓ ketogenesis
Protein	↑ amino acid transport ↑ protein synthesis	↓ protein catabolism

rate. Liver cells do not require insulin for glucose entry, but the intracellular metabolic pathways are influenced by insulin.

The anabolic effects are important after a meal when storage and the laying down of new tissue can take place. The anti-catabolic effects are equally important in the periods between food when they limit the amount of breakdown which might otherwise happen. In a fed state, the anti-catabolic effects limit the breakdown of stores already formed and avoid adding to the existing glucose. An important point is that insulin release at basal level is enough to limit catabolism, while many of the anabolic actions require higher levels. If insulin is absent, for example in untreated diabetes, the uninhibited catabolism causes the sufferer to lose very large amounts of body protein and fat.

Insulin is a potent hormone and the risks of hypoglycaemia have led to the evolution of a large number of counter-regulatory mechanisms, mounted not by one hormone but a group of hormones, each of which has its own individual controls.

THE COUNTER-REGULATORY HORMONES

GLUCAGON

Glucagon is a polypeptide hormone produced by the A cells of the pancreas. It binds to membrane receptors at the target cells and activates the cAMP second messenger system (see Ch. 11). Like insulin, it circulates in the unbound form.

Stimuli to glucagon release

Glucagon is secreted in response to falling plasma glucose concentrations and inhibited by rising concentrations. As with insulin, the amount of glucagon released is affected by a number of substrate, neural and hormonal factors (Fig. 18.7).

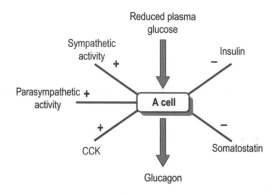

Figure 18.7 Factors influencing the A cell response to glucose.

In some examples of modifying influences, a factor will affect insulin and glucagon at the same time. This is not as contradictory as it sounds; in fact, as was the case with insulin, it adds to the refinement of the glucose-regulating systems.

For example, glucagon output is increased by sympathetic activity and causes a rise in plasma glucose, as would be expected. However, it is also stimulated by parasympathetic activity and is produced along with insulin during the early stages of digestion. The combination of the two hormones has the effect of limiting the reduction in glucose caused by early insulin at the beginning of a meal and before a significant amount of carbohydrate has been absorbed.

Both insulin and glucagon are stimulated by amino acids, particularly arginine. The combined effect may be to allow insulin to promote protein synthesis using the amino acids while glucagon maintains plasma glucose levels.

Effects of glucagon

Glucagon acts early and rapidly when glucose levels begin to fall and has the opposite effects to that of insulin. Its effects are:

- to raise plasma glucose by breaking down liver glycogen from which glucose can be released to the bloodstream
- to limit the uptake and storage of glucose by other tissues
- to cause the breakdown of lipid (lipolysis) to give fatty acids and glycerol and promoting their use as alternative fuel
- to increase the liver uptake of amino acids some of which can be used to provide more glucose by gluconeogenesis.

OTHER COUNTER-REGULATORY HORMONES

Information on the other counter-regulatory hormones can be found in Chapter 11. However, it is useful to recall here those activities which relate particularly to plasma glucose regulation.

Adrenaline

Adrenaline is one of the neurohormones secreted by the adrenal medulla. Its effect on α adrenoceptors on the B cell is to inhibit the release of insulin and allow plasma glucose to rise. It also has metabolic effects, working with glucagon, to cause the breakdown of liver glycogen. A further effect is to stimulate lipolysis. While this contributes little to plasma glucose levels apart from the small amount of gluconeogenesis from glycerol, it does provide an alternative fuel substrate which can be used to spare glucose. The overall effect of adrenaline is glucogenic and, if in excess, hyperglycaemic.

Human growth hormone (HGH)

HGH is produced by the anterior pituitary gland and its release is controlled by a complex interplay of hypothalamic releasing hormones and inhibitory hormones. It is also regulated by factors which are produced in response to it, for example insulin-like growth factors (IGF). It is affected not only by plasma glucose levels but also by the concentration in plasma of specific amino acids. Its effect is to inhibit glucose usage in skeletal muscle and increase plasma glucose. However, since HGH also increases insulin output, its net effect is glucose sparing, i.e. it diverts glucose from use as a fuel into pathways by which HGH and insulin can promote growth. At normal levels of HGH, and where adequate insulin can be produced, the hyperglycaemic effect of HGH is limited. In circumstances where insulin is suppressed, for example, by the catecholamines in an emergency, HGH can become a significant contributor to elevating plasma glucose levels.

Cortisol

Cortisol also raises and maintains glucose levels; it is both gluconeogenetic and glucose sparing. The time scale is longer than that of the previous hormones. Cortisol levels are highest in the early hours of the morning, causing a rise in plasma glucose coinciding with the end of the overnight fast, a phenomenon (*the dawn phenomenon*) seen in both non-diabetic and diabetic individuals.

Its actions provide glucose from large storage compartments unlike the limited glycogen store. It has a catabolic effect on protein and promotes liver conversion of some of the released amino acids to glucose (gluconeogenesis). It also causes the breakdown of adipose tissue providing some glucose from glycerol, but, probably more importantly, a large store of fatty acids as alternative fuel (glucose sparing). In normal circumstances, the breakdown of skeletal muscle and adipose tissue is a necessary part of overall tissue turnover. In a long period of fasting or stress, however, since both compartments are very large, they can be used to provide both energy and glucose over a period perhaps of many weeks.

Physiological stress such as injury or surgery is characterized by the elevated levels of cortisol necessary to withstand the stress (see Chs 11 and 19). The metabolic effects are to cause catabolism of body fat and protein so that weight loss becomes very evident. The elevation of plasma glucose in such stress states may be enough to produce clinical hyperglycaemia.

Thyroid hormones T_3/T_4

The thyroid hormones have metabolic effects which include sparing glucose as a fuel. While they do not normally play a large part in short-term regulation of plasma glucose, they do affect the rate at which fuel is consumed and become significant where conditions are in some way abnormal, for example in trauma or in starvation. Although in extreme states thyroid function would be reduced by the formation of more inactive rT_3 (reverse T_3; see Ch. 11), the overall effect is to raise plasma glucose.

FAILURE OF PLASMA GLUCOSE REGULATION

HYPOGLYCAEMIA

The symptoms of hypoglycaemia begin to appear at about 2.7 mmol/l but this is variable and affected by the rate at which plasma glucose is being reduced. The biochemical definition of hypoglycaemia is a glucose concentration of less than 2.2 mmol/l in venous plasma.

Hypoglycaemia may be due to a number of causes, for example some forms of liver disease or insufficiency of a counter-regulatory hormone, or it may occur in starvation or prolonged exercise when glycogen stores become exhausted. The commonest cause, however, is an imbalance between available glucose and exogenous insulin used in the management of insulin-dependent diabetes mellitus. The imbalance may be due either to insufficient food intake or unaccustomed level of activity or to an excess of insulin compared with requirement at that time.

The physiological responses to hypoglycaemia are typical of those produced in any emergency, plus those counter-regulatory responses to plasma glucose below the normal range. In addition, some symptoms are due to the effects of low glucose itself.

Symptoms

To some extent, symptoms vary with the individual and the rate at which hypoglycaemia has developed. However, many of the characteristic symptoms can be divided into two groups:

- adrenergic (sometimes referred to as 'autonomic')
- neuroglycopenic.

'Adrenergic' symptoms

The neural/neuroendocrine response includes an increase in sympathetic stimulation and the release of circulating adrenaline and noradrenaline, stimulating the production of glucose from hepatic glycogen and raising plasma glucose. This also causes the effects usually associated with the catecholamines, pallor, tachycardia, tremor and so on. These are often mistakenly described as the effects of hypoglycaemia, since they are the effects of the body's response to hypoglycaemia. However, they are recognized by the diabetic person as warning signs. Glucagon, HGH and cortisol are also released. They have their own less obvious but none the less important counter-regulatory effects.

(One difficulty experienced by people who have been diabetic for a number of years is that first the glucagon, and then the adrenaline/noradrenaline response becomes blunted. The sympathetic response may also be damaged by autonomic neuropathy, removing some of the warning signals. Those individuals must then monitor plasma glucose even more frequently and carefully to avoid unheralded hypoglycaemic attacks.)

Neuroglycopenic symptoms

If plasma glucose continues to fall, symptoms of shortage of glucose in the nervous system, neuroglycopenic symptoms, begin to appear. These may include aggression, apathy and poor coordination. These symptoms make it difficult for the sufferer to do anything to help himself, or for a helper to assist. Worse still, this state may be mistaken for drunkenness and the wrong action taken. Further reduction in glucose concentrations results in unconsciousness.

Left untreated, the individual's counter-regulatory mechanisms will usually raise plasma glucose and restore consciousness after a time.

Some circumstances make this unaided recovery difficult. Long-acting (depot) insulins and the sulphonylurea chlorpropamide, which has a long half-life, oppose the countermeasures and prolong the hypoglycaemic episode. Alcohol, which inhibits gluconeogenesis, impedes recovery.

Hypoglycaemic episodes may occur during sleep – *nocturnal hypoglycaemia*. The symptoms of sweating, tremor and tachycardia may not rouse the sleeper, who wakes in the morning cold, damp and with a headache. Timing the overnight insulin so that its peak of activity coincides with the early morning hyperglycaemia due to cortisol may avoid the problem of nocturnal hypoglycaemia, at the same time reducing the level of morning hyperglycaemia.

Hypoglycaemic episodes are followed several hours later by rebound (or response) hyperglycaemia due to the effects of the counter-regulatory hormones. This is called the Somogyi effect after the physician who described it. People who have type 1 diabetes should be aware of this and know not to increase the following doses of insulin solely in response to it.

Treatment of hypoglycaemia

Avoidance is the best treatment. However, this is not always possible. Most people aim at maintaining plasma glucose as close to normal as possible, but close to normoglycaemia is also close to hypoglycaemia. Sweets or some other readily available fast-acting carbohydrate taken at the first signs will usually halt the progress to hypoglycaemia. This should be followed immediately with a snack or meal containing complex carbohydrate. In the event of having to provide assistance, carbohydrate equivalent to about 75 g of glucose is required. If the patient has become unconscious, glucagon by injection will restore consciousness, but oral carbohydrate will still be required to restore plasma glucose levels.

HYPERGLYCAEMIA

Transient hyperglycaemia

Raised plasma glucose concentrations are characteristic of the body's response to stress such as illness, injury and trauma, all situations marked by increased levels of the catecholamines and cortisol (see Ch. 19). The physiological effects of the response may be to produce glucose levels above those which would be expected in a biochemically normal subject. In most cases, the concentrations found will be at the upper end of the normal range, but, in severe stress or in an individual whose glucose tolerance is fragile, clinically significant hyperglycaemia may be found. These are not normal circumstances, however, and when the effects of the stress disappear, plasma glucose regulation should return to normal.

Persistent hyperglycaemia

Failure of glucose regulation, characterized by repeated or persistent hyperglycaemia, is recognized clinically as diabetes mellitus (see below). Diabetes may be:

- primary where the fault in the regulatory system is lack of insulin or tissue resistance to it
- secondary to underlying pancreatic pathology or where there is excess production or administration of hyperglycaemic agents.

Ketosis/ketoacidosis

Ketone bodies consist of one ketone (acetone) and two acids, acetoacetate and β hydroxybutyrate. They are synthesized in the liver from acetyl CoA, much of which is derived from fatty acids (Fig. 18.2). Many tissues, including the brain, can use ketone bodies as an energy source when there is a lack of glucose, i.e. ketone bodies are glucose sparing. Insulin, even at low levels, inhibits the formation of ketone bodies (ketogenesis) and provided their rate of synthesis does not exceed their rate of use, ketone bodies do not accumulate.

Elevated levels of ketone bodies are sometimes found in starvation, where they have a glucose-sparing effect, but they are more often associated with uncontrolled or untreated insulin-dependent diabetes.

Insulin entry to cells is reduced by lack of insulin and the use of fats as alternative substrates increases the production of ketone bodies far beyond the levels at which they can be used. As they accumulate, the effects of the two acids on pH are compensated by hyper-ventilation and urinary excretion of the hydrogen ion (see Ch. 13). As long as the pH remains within the normal range, there is a state of *ketosis*. Ketone bodies will be found in excess in blood (ketonaemia) and in urine (ketonuria).

When pH compensation is overwhelmed, hydrogen ion concentration is increased, producing *acidosis*. The combined state is *ketoacidosis*.

This is a medical emergency requiring correction of hyperglycaemia, acid/base imbalance, intracellular and extracellular electrolyte imbalance, varying degrees of dehydration – amongst others!

DIABETES MELLITUS

Diabetes has been classified by type – types 1, 2, 3 and 4 (ADA 1997; WHO 1999).

Primary diabetes has been described as type 1 or type 2. People with type 1 diabetes are dependent on exogenous insulin; those described as type 2 are less likely to require insulin initially, but will require nutritional advice and may subsequently require the addition of oral hypoglycaemic agents and eventually insulin. Types 1 and 2 are not differences in severity of the same disorder, they have different patterns of inheritance, different factors which precipitate the condition and different aetiology.

Diabetes secondary to other pathological conditions is classified as type 3.

Gestational diabetes, classified as type 4, is described and classified separately in the criteria since the diagnosis is made retrospectively on completion of the pregnancy. If the diabetes remains after completion of the pregnancy, the diagnosis of type 1 or 2 would be made at that point.

PRIMARY DIABETES MELLITUS

To paraphrase the statement of SIGN (Scottish Intercollegiate Guidelines Network) 2001, 'Diabetes mellitus is a major and increasing health problem in all age groups. Accurate national prevalence data is unknown, but data from the Tayside Diabetes Registry suggest that prevalence is 2.6% and rising. Type 2 diabetes, in particular, is a growing problem with an ever-increasing prevalence due to the aging population and the increasing incidence of obesity.'

Diagnosis of diabetes mellitus is made according to the criteria set out in the recommendations of the World Health Organization (WHO 1985) and the WHO consultation document (1998). The American Diabetes Association (ADA) has published diagnostic criteria (1997) which differ in the use of some of the intermediate criteria and the use of the oral glucose tolerance test (OGTT), but do not differ materially in the overall diagnostic criteria. (From 1 June 2000 Diabetes UK recommended that health-care professionals adopted the new criteria set out by WHO (1999). This includes the categories IGT (impaired glucose tolerance) and IFG (impaired fasting glucose), not clinical entities in their own right, but considered to be risk factors for cardiovascular disease (IGT) and/or future diabetes (IFG).)

WHO criteria are as follows:

- the presence of diabetic symptoms (polyuria, polydypsia, unexplained weight loss)
  plus
- fasting plasma glucose >7.0 mmol/l
  or
- random plasma glucose >11.1 mmol/l.

In the absence of symptoms:

- 2 fasting plasma glucose samples >7 mmol/l
  or
- 2 random plasma glucose samples >11.1 mmol/l
  or
- one of each
  or
- >11.1 mmol/l 2 hours post 75 g glucose load (OGTT).

Type 1 (insulin-dependent) diabetes

In patients with type 1 diabetes, there is lack of insulin secretion. They are usually younger, children and juveniles; adults who develop type 1 diabetes are usually (but not always) below 40 years of age.

Antibodies to islet cells can be found, supporting the view that this is an autoimmune condition, or that an infection has altered B cell surface characteristics, rendering it open to attack by the immune system.

Type 1 diabetes can only be treated by the lifetime use of exogenous insulin or insulins. These were originally of animal origin, pork or beef (these are still in use). More commonly, however, the product is bacterially produced recombinant insulin matched to human insulin and known as 'human insulin'.

Continuing physical activity, healthy eating and weight control form the basis of general self-care.

Management of the condition requires extensive monitoring.

- Frequent measurement of plasma glucose concentrations by the person with diabetes will give indications of current glucose status.
- The level of glycated haemoglobin gives an indication of glucose regulation over a longer term. Glucose attaches to proteins, including haemoglobin, the amount attached being related to the glucose concentrations to which the protein is exposed. An assessment of a subfraction of the total glycated haemoglobin, $HbA1_c$, will give a measure of the plasma glucose levels over the half-life of the red cell, i.e. 60 days. The best long-term health outcome is related to $HbA1_c$ levels at or near normal non-diabetic levels.

Type 2 diabetes

Type 2 is by far the commoner of the two types; about 85% of the diabetic population is type 2. Its onset is insidious and reduced glucose tolerance may be present for some years before diagnosis and treatment.

It is characterized by insulin deficiency rather than absence of secretion, or normal or even higher output with a variable degree of insulin resistance. The population is usually older, although type 2 diabetes is increasingly being identified in obese young people.

Some people who are of normal weight and have type 2 diabetes may be found to have antibodies to insulin, or receptor defects or post-receptor defects.

Many people with type 2 diabetes, however, are overweight. A number of factors, including obesity, have the effect of downregulating insulin receptors and decreasing target cell response. Where the individual is overweight, weight reduction is strongly advised, since weight loss should improve glucose tolerance.

A number of oral hypoglycaemic agents are available, for example the sulphonylurea group, which increase insulin release from the pancreas, sometimes prescribed along with metformin which increases peripheral uptake of glucose (it also has the effect of reducing appetite). The prandial glucose regulators repaglinide and nateglinide also act by stimulating insulin release. Acarbose inhibits glucose uptake from the gut and the thiazolidinediones (glitazones) increase insulin sensitivity. Many type 2 patients use exogenous insulin, and it is important that this is introduced as soon as required rather than delayed until complications have become damaging.

PATHOPHYSIOLOGY OF THE UNTREATED DIABETIC STATE

The symptoms of diabetes in its developing stages are well known to patients and practitioners alike. A list of symptoms such as polyuria, polydypsia, thirst and so on is common material in textbooks. However, many lists are just that and give little help in understanding the progression of pathology as the condition worsens. The developing stages of diabetes are excellent examples of physiological cause and effect, when the normal homeostatic state is repeatedly threatened by abnormality and repeatedly compensated until, if there is no intervention, the pathology becomes overwhelming.

The symptoms of diabetes are due to:

- effects of insulin lack
- effects of the compensatory mechanisms
- effects which occur as compensation is overwhelmed.

There is a fundamental difference in the progression of type 1 and type 2. A factor which is central to the difference is the preservation of some output of insulin in type 2, albeit limited or fairly ineffective. This small amount is enough to limit the catabolism to some extent and certainly to avoid the rampant ketogenesis which takes place in untreated type 1. Type 2 is therefore much slower to develop and without the dramatic effects of large losses of weight and disturbances in acid–base balance. It is, none the less, a damaging condition.

The steps in the progress towards fully developed type 1 and type 2 are shown in Figure 18.8. The symptoms usually associated with untreated diabetes are indicated in bold italics. It should be noted that well-managed diabetes is not characterized by these symptoms.

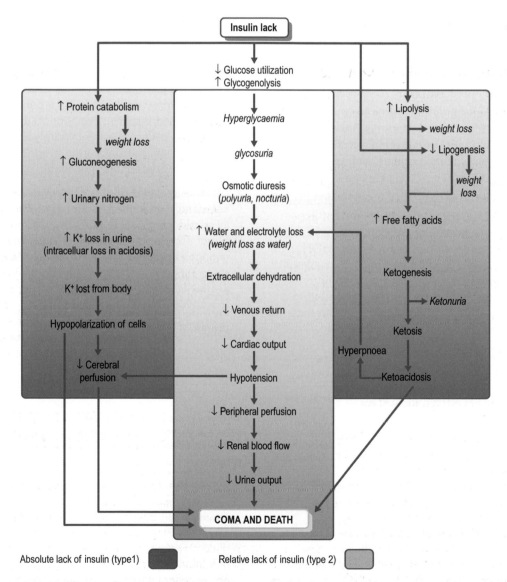

Figure 18.8 The pathophysiological effects of absolute and relative lack of insulin in uncontrolled diabetes mellitus. Type 1 – absolute lack of insulin – entire figure, shortened time scale in central panel. Type 2 – relative lack of insulin – central panel, extended time scale related to the retention of some insulin activity which prevents the rampant catabolism and ketogenesis characteristic of type 1. (After Hawker 1978, with permission of Elsevier.)

At one time, before the discovery in 1922 of insulin by Banting and Best, the progress of type 1 individuals towards death by the route in Figure 18.8 was relentless. Now it is unusual to see even the moderate symptoms, access to medical services is easy, diagnosis is swift and treatment well established. In some cases, however, even in well-managed diabetes of any type, some other illness may cause glucose regulation to become unstable, allowing some of the symptoms to surface.

TYPES 3 AND 4 DIABETES

Type 3 (secondary) diabetes

This may be caused by lack of insulin due to pancreatic disease such as pancreatitis, neoplastic disease or haemochromotosis. It may result from treatment of pancreatic disease, for example, pancreatectomy.

Secondary diabetes may also result from the production of excess endogenous counter-regulatory hormone (or hormones) or the administration of exogenous hyperglycaemic agents such as the steroid group.

There are several examples of secondary diabetes due to the overproduction of one or more of the counter-regulatory hormones. About 20 to 25% of people who have developed acromegaly (HGH excess) or Cushing's syndrome (cortisol excess) will develop diabetes. Even thyrotoxicosis can tip someone with less robust glucose tolerance into a diabetic state, or increase the dose of insulin required by an individual with pre-existing diabetes.

Steroid therapy may reduce glucose tolerance to a significant degree in some individuals and this must be taken into account when steroids are prescribed.

The effect of trauma, which is to produce increased levels of all counter-regulatory hormones, may be enough to produce glucose intolerance in some people (see Ch. 19). The effect may be mild and temporary, lasting only as long as the early response to the trauma and due mainly to insulin suppression by the catecholamines. Where the injury is large and the response prolonged, for example where there are extensive burns, the suppression of insulin in the early stages, followed by its antagonism by cortisol and the other counter-regulatory hormones, may be enough to produce a diabetic state which requires treatment.

Type 4 (gestational) diabetes

In pregnancy, insulin levels are increased in response to (mainly) placental hormones and a less than robust pancreas may not be able to respond to the demands for increased insulin. 'Gestational' diabetes is the term used to describe the hyperglycaemic state which can occur temporarily during pregnancy in a genetically susceptible individual.

Glycosuria found during pregnancy does not necessarily indicate gestational diabetes. The renal threshold for glucose, normally plasma glucose of about 10 mmol/l, is reduced (and variable) due to changes in glomerular filtration rate.

Since hyperglycaemia is associated with risk to the baby, if gestational diabetes is confirmed, that individual is treated as diabetic for the duration of the pregnancy.

REFERENCES AND FURTHER READING

ADA (Expert committee on the diagnosis and classification of diabetes mellitus) 1997 Report of the expert committee on the diagnosis and classification of diabetes mellitus. Diabetes Care 20: 1183–1197

Edwards C R W 1986 Endocrinology. Heinemann, London

Guyton A C, Hall J E 2000 Textbook of medical physiology, 10th edn. Saunders, Philadelphia

Hawker R W 1978 Notebook of medical physiology – endocrinology. Churchill Livingstone, Edinburgh

Porth C M, Hurwitz L S 1994 Diabetes mellitus. In: Porth CM. Pathophysiology, concepts of altered states. Lippincott, Philadelphia

Rogers A W 1992 Textbook of anatomy. Churchill Livingstone, Edinburgh

SIGN 2001 Diabetes 2001. Scottish Intercollegiate Guidelines Network (SIGN). On line. Available: http://www.sign.ac.uk

Watson R 1999 Essential science for nursing students. Baillière Tindall, London

WHO study group 1985 Diabetes mellitus. Technical Report Service 727: 10–20. WHO, Geneva

WHO (Expert committee on the diagnosis and classification of diabetes mellitus) 1998 Report of WHO Consultation. Part 1: Diagnosis and classification of diabetes mellitus. Diabetes Care 20: 1183–1197

WHO 1999 Definition, diagnosis and classification of diabetes and its complications. Department of noncommunicable disease surveillance. WHO, Geneva

Wilding J, Williams G 1997 Diabetes and disorders of intermediary metabolism. In: Souhami R L, Moxham J (eds) Textbook of medicine, 3rd edn. Churchill Livingstone, Edinburgh

Williams G, Pickup J 1999 Handbook of diabetes, 2nd edn. Blackwell Science, London

In practice you may be asked to consider the following:

Wounds and wound healing

1. Ms X has experienced a small cut wound caused by the edge of a sheet of paper. It was painful when it happened, the local area became reddened and slightly raised along and near the incision line. Explain the effects of the injury.

2. A climber has suffered a nasty friction wound caused by a climbing rope running through his closed hand. The wound has mainly affected the palm of his hand. He is young and healthy and physiologically the wound is likely to heal well. What circumstances might hinder the healing process?

3. Mrs Y is 80 years old and has always been fit and well. She broke her hip in a fall and unfortunately was not found for several hours, during which she lay on the floor. The surgery was prolonged and now she has developed a pressure wound. What factors in the case of Mrs Y would increase the risk of formation of pressure wounds ? Why do those factors cause an increased risk? Which dressing type would you recommend?

4. What are the physiological and biochemical factors which cause acute wounds to become chronic wounds?

5. What are the physiological factors which differentiate venous and arterial leg ulcers?

Systemic response

1. The victim of a road traffic accident has extensive trauma including head injuries. Shortly after the preliminary assessment, she is found to have plasma sodium of 133 mmol/l. The reduction in

sodium concentration is not due to administered fluids; what could be causing this?

2. A patient admitted through Accident and Emergency has a plasma osmolality of 315 mosmol/kg (normal range 285–295). What could be causing this elevation?

3. Narrow pulse pressure is a common finding following significant blood loss. Explain both the term and the narrowness.

4. Where there has been extensive trauma, it may be difficult to find a peripheral pulse. It may also be difficult to find a vessel where an infusion line may be entered. What is the cause of this?

5. A middle-aged man has suffered a myocardial infarct. Within a few hours, his plasma glucose has become significantly elevated. He has no history of diabetes. Explain the hyperglycaemia.

Illness

1. Oedema is a characteristic finding in many forms of liver disorder. Identify the factors in liver disorder which cause the beginning of oedema.

2. Where there is hepatic cirrhosis, the factors which allow oedema to persist and then develop into ascites can act as indicators of the progress of disorder. What are these factors and what evidence could be used to confirm their presence?

3. A patient has complained of angina and been prescribed GTN. What is this, how does it work and how will the patient know that it is having an effect?

4. The patient above has now suffered a myocardial infarct. What is the likely relationship between the angina and the MI?

5. What are the physiological responses to stress/trauma in the form of MI? Why in the case of MI are the responses not particularly helpful? Using that information, explain the rationale for the measures normally taken to treat MI.

INTRODUCTION

Injury and illness threaten and challenge the body's environment. Living creatures have always been at risk and over time have evolved elegant and complex ways of surviving, healing their wounds and recovering. Even now, the processes are still being unravelled, but with better understanding comes better treatment and care.

There is a characteristic pattern of response to threat to the internal environment which is almost independ-

ent of the cause. The body systems set about defending the major homeostatic parameters such as blood pressure and energy supply to the tissues particularly the brain, with the object of staying alive. There may well be no threat to life, but the response as it has evolved must have the capacity to cope with the worst eventuality. The predictability of the response has resulted in the use of more general terms such as 'the physiological response to stress' rather than 'response to injury' or 'response to trauma'. The term 'stress' can then be extended to include not only injury or trauma but other physiological stress such as that encountered in illness.

The response is mounted by the nervous system and all the systems it commands. The autonomic and endocrine effects are relatively well understood, and we are all familiar with the effects of fright or a minor accident, the racing heart, sweating palms and so on. However, the full effects of the response still have aspects which are unexplained; for example, the brain's manipulation of the immune system in injury and illness is far from clear. Where there is injury, the inflammatory and immune systems must be inhibited if the subject is to survive but not so inhibited that the subject has no resistance to even the smallest infection. The balance of effects and the identity of the agents which determine the balance are difficult to clarify. Among other problems, the potentially damaging process of inflammation appears to trigger many of the systemic responses which can ensure survival, and the wound mechanisms which bring about healing. On the other hand, over-activity in the same responses can delay recovery.

Wounds and trauma are essentially threats to the internal environment from the outside world. 'Illness' is usually brought about by a fault in the structure or the function or the control of function of the body's own components. Infection might be seen as coming somewhere between the two, a situation where an external agent enters the body and brings about dysfunction or adverse reaction in its systems.

This chapter is concerned with injuries and illness rather than infection. Details of responses to infection can be found in Chapter 16.

WOUNDS AND WOUND HEALING

Creatures have been wounding themselves and each other as long as there have been creatures. Wound healing has evolved to a complex series of actions and reactions which, in most cases, can produce regeneration of the tissue or, at the least, a very good repair. The very success of the process has allowed most of us to take it for granted.

Wounds and wound care, however, are expensive. Chronic wounds such as leg ulcers, pressure wounds and foot ulcers in diabetes are estimated to cost the UK National Health Service about £1 billion per year (Harding 1998). As the processes have become better understood, better wound care practices and products have been developed. However, a sound knowledge of the mechanisms, as they are currently understood, and an interest in wounds, can help in further progress and allow healthcare practitioners to make the best use of the body's own excellent systems.

Wounds have been part of experience for so long that some of the terminology predates the understanding of the events and may simply describe the outward signs. The phrases 'healing by primary intention' or by 'secondary intention' are not particularly helpful but are well understood by the practitioners who deal with such wounds. The term 'granulation' as in 'granulation tissue' remains in use, not because it accurately represents what the tissue is, but because the description is familiar, well known and good enough for people to identify tissue at this particular stage. Even the names of the phases of healing at a wound site remain descriptive terms.

THE PROCESSES OF WOUND HEALING

The same group of cellular and molecular processes is involved in the healing of all soft-tissue injuries, whether they are traumatic wounds, such as lacerations, abrasions and burns, surgically made wounds or chronic ulcerative wounds such as pressure wounds or leg ulcers.

The physiological processes involved in wound healing are conventionally divided into phases, which overlap and are in any case artificial and based on appearance. However, the 'phase' terminology is useful and widely used.

The phases typically described are inflammation, proliferation and remodelling, but it is useful to precede these with a haemostatic phase. Firstly, bleeding must be stopped when there has been an injury and, secondly, the cells involved in clotting, principally the platelets, release factors which begin the inflammatory phase of healing. Wound healing therefore begins almost as the wound is made.

This account describes four phases:

- haemostasis
- inflammation
- proliferation
- remodelling.

The phases are coordinated by a series of cytokines which include chemoattractants, growth factors and

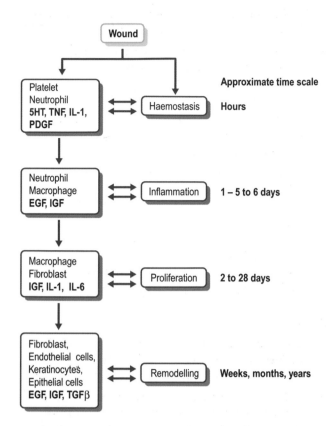

Figure 19.1 Stages in the process of wound healing. 5HT, 5-hydroxytryptamine, EGF, epidermal growth factor; IGF, insulin-like growth factor; IL-1, interleukin 1; IL-6, interleukin 6; PDGF, platelet-derived growth factor; TGFβ, transforming growth factor β; TNF, tumour necrosis factor.

growth inhibitors (see Chs 11 and 16). There are also cellular adhesives and enzymes which break down cellular adhesives. Yet more cytokines, along with neurotransmitters and hormones, act as links with the whole body response to injury. There is a complex interaction between the blood vessels, blood, dermal and epidermal cells and the extracellular matrix which changes from phase to phase (Fig. 19.1). The whole organization is under the control of an army of cytokines.

One characteristic of wound healing is that, at particular stages in the process, a cell type will play a predominant role, e.g. platelets in the haemostatic phase followed by neutrophils early in the inflammatory phase followed in turn by macrophages, then fibroblasts. In some cases the first type produces an attractant which recruits the second; in others, local conditions might have been changed to favour the second cell type.

The following is a summary account of wound healing; further details of individual reactions can be found in the chapters identified.

HAEMOSTASIS

When blood vessels are damaged, collagen is exposed and platelet adhesion is increased by agents such as tumour necrosis factor (TNF) and nitric oxide (NO) which are released by the damaged cells.

Platelets

Platelets have several functions in the healing process including the all important contribution to arresting bleeding. The platelets stick to one another and to the surface of the vessel, forming a plug. This platelet plug may be enough to stop blood loss in a minor injury.

The smooth muscle in blood vessels which have been cut constricts in response to signals from the autonomic nervous system and constrictors such as 5-hydroxytryptamine (5HT) (serotonin) released by platelets. The narrowing of the vessel temporarily reduces blood loss and increases the likelihood of the platelet plug remaining in place.

Contact of the platelets with exposed collagen triggers the release of a number of platelet factors, including adenosine diphosphate (ADP), 5HT and platelet factor 3. These stimulate further platelet aggregation, further local vasoconstriction (although this is temporary) and a cascade of enzymatic reactions which results in the formation of a clot (see Ch. 3). The fibrin matrix of the clot supports and reinforces the platelet plug.

Platelets perform a major role at this stage. Not only are they central to the successful arrest of bleeding, but the cells trapped within the clot, particularly the platelets, contribute to initiating the inflammatory response and activating the complement mechanism (see Ch. 16), i.e. the next stage in healing.

Platelets also release PDGF (platelet-derived growth factor), which stimulates growth in a number of tissues, notably blood vessels; therefore they contribute to the generation of the replacement tissue.

Fibrinolysis

The clot must be removed when it is no longer useful. The fibrin matrix is broken down by the enzyme plasmin, normally present in plasma in the inactive plasminogen form. When plasminogen is trapped along with blood cells, plasma and serum within the blood clot, it becomes activated by a number of factors, including tissue plasminogen activator (tPA) released by the injured tissue. The process of fibrinolysis yields fibrinogen degradation products and fibrin degradation products (FDP) (see Ch. 3).

Fibrinogen and fibrin degradation products can be found in any sample of blood but the level is substantially increased after injury.

Plasminogen has been found, in close association with macrophages and fibroblasts, throughout the entire period of wound healing. In addition to its role in the dissolution of fibrin associated with the clot, it has a role in the later removal of existing extracellular matrix (ECM) as new ECM is formed in the proliferative phase. There are other endogenous fibrinolytic agents of clinical importance. The kidney and urinary tract area, for example, has higher levels of the fibrinolytic enzyme urokinase and consequently has an increased tendency to bleed following injury or surgery.

INFLAMMATION (1 TO 5–6 DAYS)

'Calor, rubor, tumor, dolor' is the classical description of inflammation, that is, the affected area is hot, red, swollen and painful (see Ch. 16).

Vascular effects

On injury, damaged cells immediately release mediators such as histamine, TNF and substance P which, as its name suggests, causes pain. The cells of the vascular endothelium release nitric oxide (NO). NO, histamine and TNF are potent vasodilators and have the effect of increasing blood vessel permeability. The earlier vasoconstriction is overcome. The chemical vasodilation, plus the effects of local axon reflexes, reduces the pressure inside the vessel and further limits blood loss. The local dilation makes the area warm and red, with the beginnings of swelling.

Increased blood vessel permeability allows the easy passage of both fluid and phagocytes into the surrounding tissue space. The fluid lost to the tissue space may raise extravascular pressure enough to stop further blood loss into the tissues. The migration of phagocytes is important in limiting the activity of infective particles in the surrounding tissue.

The local area is now clearly swollen and there may be blistering or dysfunction if the oedema occurs in the area of a joint. The vascular effects of inflammation occur along with the cellular effects below.

Cellular effects

Neutrophils

In the early stages of inflammation, neutrophils migrate to the site of the wound in large numbers in response to several chemoattractant factors released by damaged cells and by factors produced by platelets. Neutrophils can be regarded as the first line of defence against infection entering at the site of the wound. They release a number of cytokine factors important in attracting other leucocytes such as lymphocytes, and proteolytic enzymes which contribute to clearing damaged tissue.

They also contain many intracellular proteolytic systems and serve an important role as very active phagocytes which can move easily between blood and tissue removing dead and damaged tissue, foreign material and infective organisms. They are the cell type dominating at this point.

Macrophages

Monocytes and tissue macrophages at the site of the wound are stimulated by a number of platelet and leucocyte factors to release mediators which are chemotaxic (i.e. attractant) and stimulatory to macrophages. Their numbers increase as neutrophil numbers decrease and they take over as prime mover in the sequence of healing.

1. Macrophages release a number of factors including TNFα, TGFβ (transforming growth factor β), interleukins, IGF1 (insulin-like growth factor 1) and PDGF (PDGF is produced from cells other than platelets) which are thought to coordinate the progress of healing from one stage to another (Cooper et al 1994).

2. They are large and very active phagocytes and play an important part in clearing the site.

   Some descriptions of wound healing include a separate 'destructive phase'. Tissue destruction must take place as new tissue is formed, but the process of removing tissue debris goes on continuously in the inflammatory and proliferative phases rather than in a separate phase. As the inflammatory phase proceeds, clearance of dead and damaged tissue, foreign particulate material and bacteria by phagocytosis and enzymic breakdown continues.

   Several enzyme systems are involved in the breakdown of structural tissue at a wound site. Some are the matrix proteinases, others are released by neutrophils and macrophages, and others are plasminogen activators such as the tissue plasminogen activator tPA. These enzymes break down not only cell structures but the adhesives like fibronectin which bind together the now damaged and denatured tissue. Without this breakdown, the solid mass of debris at the wound site remains longer and hinders the growth of new tissue. These adhesives, however, also bind together healthy new matrix, and excess of the enzymes, or lack of inhibition of their breakdown, leads to wound sites that are slow to heal.

3. Macrophages are not only able to destroy bacteria and remove tissue debris but they also produce growth factors that stimulate the formation of fibroblasts, the synthesis of the structural protein collagen and the process of angiogenesis. They also, in common with many other cell types, produce interleukins, for example, interleukin 1 (IL-1). This cytokine has many functions which include local effects, such as an increase in tissue adhesion and the attraction of lymphocytes to the injury site, and systemic effects, such as the induction of acute-phase proteins by the liver (see Ch. 16). Interleukin 1 also has a role (shared with IL-6) in stimulating activity in the hypothalamic–anterior pituitary–adrenocortical axis (HPA axis) (see Ch. 11), i.e. it is one of the agents bringing together the local and systemic responses to injury (see Fig. 19.5 and under 'Systemic response to stress').

PROLIFERATION (2 TO 28 DAYS)

Platelet activity during and following haemostasis and macrophage activity in the inflammatory phase have been found to recruit fibroblasts and other cells into the wound site and to stimulate their activity.

Fibroblasts

Fibroblasts are key cells in the formation of the extracellular matrix (ECM) by producing fibronectin and proteoglycans, e.g. hyaluronic acid (see Ch. 1). They also lay down collagen fibres of several types at the site of the wound.

Angiogenesis is stimulated by several factors including PDGF and new blood vessels start to infiltrate the wound. The new capillary loops are rapidly growing structures but fragile and easily damaged. Great care must be taken with dressings at this stage. The hormone leptin has been found to affect angiogenesis, acting as a growth signal in the pathways and promoting vascularization. Since it is also involved as a trigger for the inflammatory system, it may have an important role in wound healing (Frubeck & Salvador 2000).

The ECM plus the new capillaries is described as 'granulation tissue'. As well as being a physical structure, ECM provides a means of regulating cell-to-cell communication. It contains small soluble proteins provided by both fibroblasts and keratinocytes which become attached to the ECM. The integrins are cell adhesion molecules located on the cell surface. They provide mechanical connection between the components of the matrix and act as a 'pathway' for the chemical signals between cells. The signalling system and the integrins may be parts of a system that match the size, shape and direction of orientation of the parts which make up the area being repaired. We take it for granted that, when a wound heals, the new tissue will be running in the right direction, but it does not happen by magic!

There is a delicate balance between the formation of the right amount of new tissue and the concurrent degradation of the previous tissue. The role of the proteolytic enzymes such as the proteinases and their inhibitors is the subject of much research. The breakdown enzymes not only remove old tissue but restrict the amount of new tissue allowed to remain. Too much breakdown produces slow healing, too little produces excess ECM and hinders normal healing. Proliferation must not become hypertrophy.

As proliferation continues, inflammation begins to subside, the wound site and its surroundings become less red and angry, and organized tissue begins to fill the site.

Substrates and growth factors

Substrates, such as glucose, amino acids and the vitamins and minerals that contribute to tissue formation, are required for healing and one of the functions of the systemic response is to ensure that they are provided. These are only effective in the presence of growth promoters which regulate their incorporation and retention. Chronic wounds have been shown to have lower levels of a number of growth factors when compared with acute wounds which have healed well (Higley et al 1995).

There are several families of growth factor. Insulin-like growth factors (IGF) have been extensively studied. They are produced by a wide range of cells including macrophages and fibroblasts and promote many anabolic processes. Growth factors such as IGF attract endothelial cells and they are therefore involved in angiogenesis. They are also mitogenic to fibroblasts and therefore required for tissue construction (see Ch. 16).

Epidermal growth factor (EGF) is found in many tissues and is secreted by many cells. It is secreted by platelets, for example, in large enough quantities to stimulate mitosis and migration of cells, indicating that its local effects are important in the early stages of wound healing. EGF is also found in saliva, being produced by the submandibular cells – justifying the ancient practice of licking one's wounds perhaps.

Epithelialization

Epithelialization takes place from the margins of the wound towards the centre of the wound. Some keratinocytes proliferate at the wound margins. However, some are modified so that they gain phagocytic activity and can move across the bed of the wound. This keratinocyte migration along with contraction at the site causes epithelialization and closure of the wound.

REMODELLING (WEEKS, MONTHS OR YEARS)

In any injury involving skin loss, epithelial cells at the wound margins divide and begin to move over the newly granulating tissue. As this process is dependent on regulation by factors within the ECM, the cells can only move over living tissue and move best in a moist environment (see below at 'Moist wound healing'). They pass under any scab. When such cells meet other migrating keratinocytes, mitosis is reduced because of the increased concentrations of inhibitory factors as the advancing cells come together.

Wound contraction resulting from the activity of myofibroblasts helps to bring the wound edges together. Angiogenesis is also inhibited, leading to a progressive reduction in the number of blood vessels in the area. This gradually changes the appearance of the tissue from dusky red to white (blanching). The collagen fibres are reorganized, the degree of cross-linking increases and the wound tensile strength increases. After injury and repair, the scar tissue differs somewhat from that of the original healthy tissue and is not as strong or as flexible. The wound edges particularly are vulnerable, in some sites only about 50% of the normal skin tensile strength being regained within the first 3 months after injury.

> Contraction of the wound is important for closure, but in some areas, such as the face, it may distort the features. Expert remodelling using external pressure, for example from a partial mask, may be required. Fibrous tissue in the scarred skin may sometimes become greatly hypertrophied leading to keloid scar.

Healing of an incised wound ('healing by primary intention')

This is typical of a surgical wound or an accidental wound made by glass or a knife. The edges are close together and, although a number of blood vessels might be transected, little tissue is lost. There is little ECM (granulation tissue) formed and epithelialization is rapid. The wound edges produce a narrow scar which blanches rapidly. However, the recovery of full tensile strength may take some time (Fig. 19.2).

Healing of a large, open or ulcerated wound ('healing by secondary intention')

This type of injury requires considerable tissue refilling. A large amount of matrix and vasculature must be restored and epithelialization, by definition, must be over a much greater area. Infection risk is greater and healing, particularly remodelling, extends over a much longer period (Fig. 19.3).

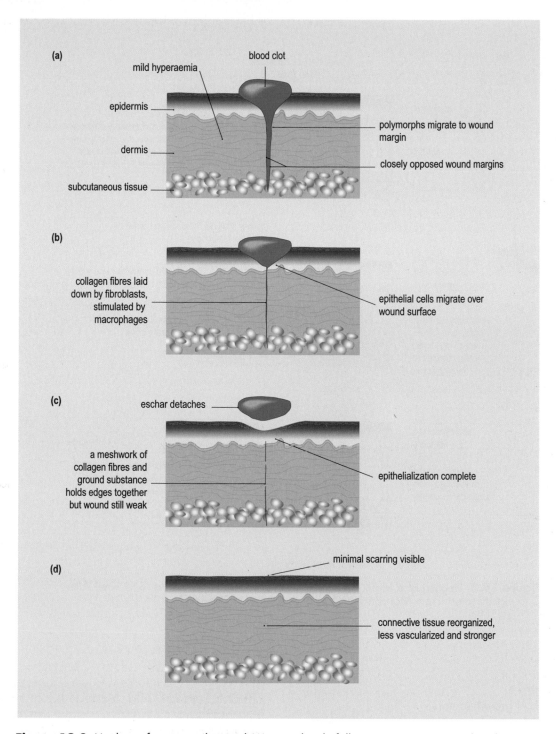

Figure 19.2 Healing of an incised wound (A) immediately following injury, (B) 2–3 days later, (C) 10–14 days later, and (D) 1 year later. (From Morison 1992, with permission of Elsevier.)

FACTORS WHICH AFFECT WOUND HEALING

The presence of the following factors may cause a wound to become a chronic wound.

Local factors include:

- poor perfusion
- infection
- foreign bodies such as metal or glass or fragments of road surface

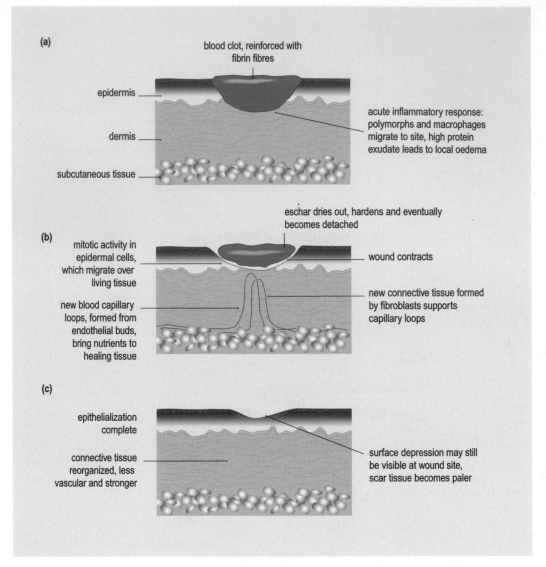

Figure 19.3 Healing of a large, open or ulcerated wound. A, 0–3 days; B, 1 week later; C, 6 months later. (From Morison 1992, with permission of Elsevier.)

- crushed tissue
- local lack of growth factors
- local imbalance of growth factors and inhibitors
- senescent cells (Stanley et al 1996).

Systemic factors include:

- poor nutrition, either general such as lack of total energy or nitrogen, or specific, such as deficiency of vitamin C, iron etc.
- metabolic disorder, e.g. diabetes
- system disorder, such as cardiovascular, renal or liver
- immobility
- steroid therapy, chemotherapy, radiotherapy.

MOIST WOUND HEALING

In the early 1960s a study by George Winter was published in the journal *Nature*, the results of which have gone on to influence the development of wound dressings over the last 40 years. The study demonstrated that, in experimentally created, acute, superficial wounds, which were kept occluded and thus moist, epithelialization occurred twice as quickly as in those wounds left exposed to air. This initial study was carried out in pigs. However, subsequent human studies demonstrated a similar effect on healing. Since these original studies, subsequent work by others has demonstrated that moist wound healing offers many advantages over dry wound healing, and that the effects of occlusion are not just limited to the epidermis. Some of the advantages attributed to moist wound healing include:

- increased rates of epithelial migration
- the facilitation of tissue rehydration and debridement
- increased cell contact with wound fluid
- improved granulation tissue
- pain relief
- infection control.

WOUND DRESSINGS

Dressings, if chosen to address specific wound requirements, can help provide an optimum healing environment. For example, wound dressings can be used to aid debridement, remove excess exudate, control bleeding and protect a wound. However, it is important to note that the application of any wound dressing is of little value unless a full assessment of all factors that may delay wound healing has been undertaken and any problems addressed.

Nowadays, choosing an appropriate dressing for a wound can be an extremely difficult and complex task due to the numerous products available. Having an understanding of the mechanism of action of the various types of wound dressings available, and a clear definition of the desired treatment outcome for a particular wound, may make this choice less arduous.

ALGINATES

Alginate dressings are derived from sodium and calcium salts of alginic acid, a polymer obtained from various types of seaweed. Alginic acid contains guluronic and mannuronic acid residues, and the differences in the amounts of these compounds affect how the dressing gels. When a dry alginate dressing comes into contact with wound exudate or other body fluids containing sodium ions, the calcium ions from the calcium alginate are replaced by sodium ions present in the fluid and calcium ions are liberated into the wound. This ion exchange causes the dressing to become a hydrophilic gel, which provides a moist wound environment that facilitates wound healing as well as allowing atraumatic removal of the dressing. Alginates also have haemostatic properties, as when the calcium ions are released into the wound, this activates the platelets and assists in haemostasis. Alginates are not suitable

for wounds that are dry or covered in hard, black necrotic tissue.

HYDROGELS

Hydrogels consist mainly of water and also contain a small amount of either starch or carboxymethyl-cellulose polymer which acts as a gel-forming medium. Hydrogels are able to donate or absorb fluid depending on the hydration of the wound and the formulation of the dressing product. It is, however, their high water content that makes them invaluable in the debridement of wounds. In contact with the wound bed, these dressings increase the moisture content of necrotic and sloughy tissue, facilitating enzymatic activity and thus enhancing autolytic debridement. Hydrogels can also be used on granulating and epithelializing wounds, although maceration may occur if the environment is too moist.

FOAM DRESSINGS

Foam dressings vary in their individual structure and performance characteristics. In general, however, most of these dressings consist of a highly absorbent foam between a low adherent facing and a semipermeable film backing. When applied to an exuding wound, the dressing will absorb excess fluid but maintain the wound surface in a warm, moist condition, providing an environment conducive to healing. Foam dressings can be used on a variety of exuding wounds, including leg ulcers, pressure sores, minor burns and donor sites. The dressing will, however, be of limited value on dry, necrotic tissue; before application this should be removed, either surgically, or by some other means.

HYDROCOLLOIDS

Hydrocolloid dressings consist of a micro-granular suspension of polymers, including carboxymethyl-cellulose and gelatin or pectin, in an adhesive matrix coated onto a sheet of foam or film, depending on the particular dressing. When the dressing comes into contact with exudates, the polysaccharides and other polymers absorb water and swell, forming a gel. The moist conditions produced under the dressing promote fibrinolysis, angiogenesis and wound healing. If applied to wounds containing dry slough or necrosis, the dressing prevents the loss of water vapour from the surface of the skin; this effectively rehydrates the dead tissue which is then removed by autolysis. Hydrocolloid dressings can be used on a variety of wound types, including leg ulcers, pressure sores, superficial burns, donor sites and minor abrasions.

HYDROFIBRE

The hydrofibre dressing is a soft, non-woven dressing composed of sodium carboxymethylcellulose (or hydrocolloid) fibres. This dressing acts by way of a hydrophilic action which absorbs fluid by vertical wicking and results in the rapid uptake of fluid directly into its fibres. Other fibrous dressings tend to trap exudates around the fibres. This mechanism allows the dressing to become a soft coherent gel that retains its integrity during handling and allows an increased amount of exudates to be absorbed into the dressing. As exudate is locked away, there is little release of fluid back onto the skin or wound surface and therefore less risk of skin maceration.

VAPOUR PERMEABLE FILMS

These dressings are thin sheets of polyurethane coated with a layer of acrylic adhesive. They are permeable to water vapour and gases, but not to liquids and microorganisms. The degree of vapour permeability varies between products. These dressings have no absorptive capacity and are mainly used to secure primary dressings and to encourage rehydration of wounds. They may be used in the treatment of scalds, first or second degree burns, minor injuries (including abrasions and lacerations) and for the prevention of superficial pressure areas. The various products have slightly different methods of application and the practitioner should be familiar with the method of dressing removal in order to minimize discomfort and trauma, especially in those patients with fragile skin.

ODOUR ABSORBENT DRESSINGS

These contain charcoal which, when used as a dressing, has the ability to adsorb toxins and wound degradation products as well as volatile fatty acids responsible for the production of wound odour. Some dressings also contain silver, which has an antibacterial action. Odour absorbent dressings are indicated for the management of malodorous wounds including fungating lesions, faecal fistulae, infected pressure sores and heavily exuding leg ulcers.

THE SYSTEMIC RESPONSE TO STRESS

Trauma might be described as an assault on the body environment from external sources. This may be surgery where the injury is clean and controlled, or accidental injury with all the contamination and complications typical of accidents. It may be the destructive effects of flames and excessive heat, or the equally destructive but less dramatic effects of pressure on an area of poor perfusion and fragile skin, i.e. a pressure wound. While the causes are many and varied, the response follows a similar and predictable course. In general, the magnitude of the overall response is related to the size or severity of the injury, the greater the degree of injury, the greater the whole-body response. The effectiveness, however, is dependent on factors such as the health and age of the individual.

Evolution favoured those who could survive unaided and therefore the response had to be funded from body stores. It is expensive in metabolic terms since the demand for energy and nitrogen are high in times of injury or illness at a time when intake is likely to be limited.

The response involves the defence of certain biological priorities, for example blood pressure, plasma glucose and the supply of energy to vital organs. Vital organs cannot function without at least a minimal blood pressure and an adequate energy supply, and brain function is jeopardized by lack of glucose. The aim is to keep brain and body alive.

MECHANISMS IN THE RESPONSE

The physiological response to the stress of trauma emanates from the brain and involves all the body systems and their controls in a complicated, beautifully orchestrated response. When there is danger, the brain is alerted by signals from the pathways which process sight, sound, smell and other external stimuli. The high alert state will in turn affect the brain areas which prepare the body to fight or run. This is the beginning of the response to stress.

Ascending signals from the body, for example pain and the circulating chemical messengers the cytokines, reinforce the central response to existing or impending trauma.

A change in blood pressure or blood gas concentrations will stimulate the hypothalamus; therefore the stress response, although moderated, occurs even in the deeply unconscious state.

The major central areas that operate the response are, in addition to the hypothalamus which has the prime role, the posterior and anterior pituitary glands, the brain stem and the spinal cord.

The hypothalamus is central to the normal regulation of the internal environment and to its protection when under threat. In addition to its countless incoming and outgoing pathways within the brain, it controls the activities of the autonomic nervous system (ANS), it has neural connections with the posterior pituitary gland, brain stem and cord, and endocrine links with the anterior pituitary. The anterior pituitary in turn regulates the end organ hormones of a number of hypothalamic–pituitary axes (see Ch. 11) and also produces other hormones which act independently of the axes. Therefore the hypothalamus and anterior pituitary gland taken as a combined unit can give rise to an immense range of effects. The hypothalamus is able to mount a fast neural response via the ANS and the neurohormones, and a slower but sustained response via the endocrine system.

In a state of stress, one of the major axes is the hypothalamic–anterior pituitary–adrenocortical axis – the HPA axis (see Ch. 11), leading to one of the main agents of control, the adrenal gland. Both component parts, the medulla and the cortex, are important contributors to survival under stress.

Figure 19.4 shows the wide spread of activities provoked in response to trauma.

The main points are summarized below.

1. The hypothalamus has control over the autonomic output and therefore the activities of the sympathetic and parasympathetic divisions.
2. It controls the activities of the adrenal medulla and the output of the catecholamines (the sympathomedullary response).
3. The hypothalamus produces the hormone arginine vasopressin or antidiuretic hormone (AVP/ADH) which is released from the posterior pituitary gland.
4. A number of hormonal axes (see Ch. 11) also originate within the hypothalamus. One of these is the HPA axis which regulates the production of the hormone cortisol. Cortisol is an essential component of the survival systems; without

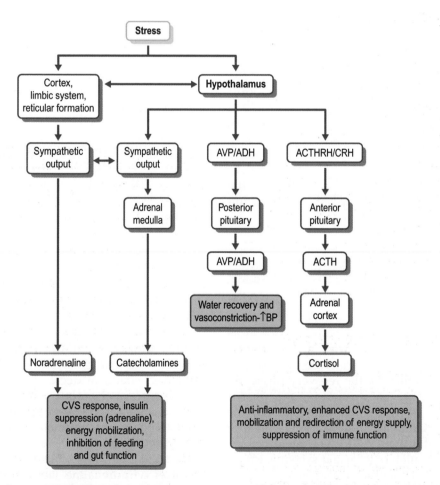

Figure 19.4 Physiological responses to stress. (After Berne & Levy 1993, with permission of Elsevier.)

it, survival of even moderate trauma is not possible.

The systems operating from the hypothalamus work on different time scales. The neural effect of the ANS output is rapid and is the first line of defence. The release of the neuroendocrine catecholamines and AVP/ADH is only slightly slower and augments the ANS effects. The endocrine axis effects are next in line and although slower to become effective, the effects can be maintained for a prolonged period of time. This arrangement allows the body to respond with a wide array of mechanisms, so increasing the range and scope of its defensive strategies.

Although the neurohormone adrenaline, from the adrenal medulla, is important to the management of stress in the early stage of the response, the presence of the hormone cortisol from the adrenal cortex is essential to survival. The body's defence against pathogens is its immune system (see Ch. 16). However, the inflammatory part of the immune system can overwhelm the injured subject. Cortisol moderates the effects of the immune system so that it defends but does not kill the host. In damping the inflammatory response, however, cortisol also suppresses the immune response; the injured subject is therefore more likely to survive but at the price of increased vulnerability to infections.

Although the response to stress works to defend as much of the internal environment as possible, when the stress is severe, some major parameters become priorities. For example, food intake is less important than maintaining blood pressure (BP) and, if necessary, gut function may all but cease as blood is diverted to maintain pressure at vital organs. Similarly the maintenance of osmotic pressure is a lower priority than hydrostatic pressure and BP will be maintained by the retention of water even to the point of significant dilution of the major electrolytes (see Ch. 14).

STRUCTURE OF THE RESPONSE

The effects of this array of mechanisms may be divided artificially but conveniently into phases, based on their different time scales. The phases are named variously as the acute or shock phase, followed by the hypermetabolic phase (sometimes referred to as the hypercatabolic phase), then by the recovery phase. As with the local response to wounding, the phases overlap and the divisions are not clear cut, but the system is clinically useful. They follow a similar pattern to the local effects at a wound site. The agents which bring about the integration of local and systemic effects (Fig. 19.5) are the subject of much research.

The acute phase is short and can last for 24 to 36 hours, the hypermetabolic or hypercatabolic phase

for several days, and the recovery phase may extend into weeks and months. The length of time depends on many factors. The severity of injury, the subject's state of health, intervening infection or surgery, the presence of pain, and many others, all affect the length of the phases and progress from one to the next. Clearly, a factor such as a further injury during a later phase may cause a return to the acute phase.

The course of the systemic response to stress can be followed from one phase to the next using the following examples:

- the maintenance of blood pressure
- the maintenance of plasma glucose and the supply of fuel.

MAINTENANCE OF MAJOR PARAMETERS

THE MAINTENANCE OF BLOOD PRESSURE

The brain and other vital organs cannot function without an adequate supply of blood carrying oxygen, water, nutrients and the many other factors which are required to keep cells alive. An adequate supply requires that an adequate blood (hydrostatic) pressure be maintained.

The normal regulation of blood pressure is achieved by making adjustments to cardiac output, vascular capacity and intravascular volume (blood volume). Cardiac output and vascular capacity can be altered rapidly, giving rapid changes in BP. Intravascular volume takes longer to change and consequently BP changes using these mechanisms happen more slowly (see Ch. 12).

Acute phase

In this first phase, during and immediately after the event, there is powerful stimulation of the sympathetic nervous system. Noradrenaline released from the nerve endings increases vasoconstriction in the arterioles and, to a lesser extent, increases heart rate and stroke volume. This has the result of increasing BP by the combined effects of decreasing vascular capacity and increasing cardiac output.

Sympathetic stimulation also increases the output of the catecholamines, adrenaline and noradrenaline, from the adrenal medulla (the sympathomedullary effect). Adrenaline's cardiovascular actions are different from those of noradrenaline (see Chs 5 and 6), its major effects being a significant increase in cardiac output and redirection of blood flow to vital organs. This

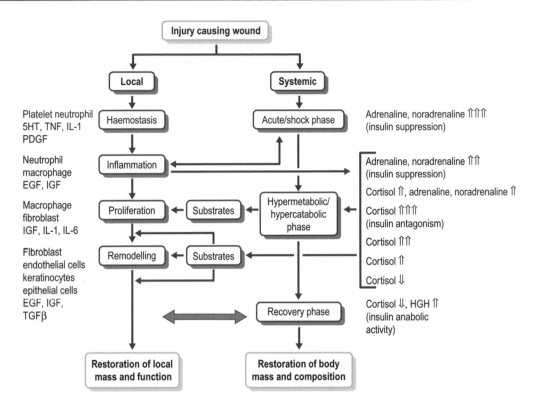

Figure 19.5 Integration of local and systemic effects. 5HT, 5-hydroxytryptamine; HGH, human growth hormone; EGF, epidermal growth factor; IL-1, interleukin 1; IL-6, interleukin 6; IGF, insulin-like growth factor; PDGF, platelet-derived growth factor; TGFβ, transforming growth factor β; TNF, tumour necrosis factor.

redirection of flow is achieved without a reduction in pressure by the combination of constriction mainly by noradrenaline and selective dilation by adrenaline. Constriction of blood vessels in less essential areas, such as skin and gut, allows blood to be diverted to vital organs and the lower pressure in the dilated vessels in these vital areas ensures that blood will flow there.

Arginine vasopressin or antidiuretic hormone (AVP/ADH) is also important in the early support of BP. It is promptly released from the posterior pituitary, following rapid synthesis by neurones in the hypothalamus. The effects of AVP/ADH are vasoconstriction, reducing vascular capacity, and retention of water, increasing intravascular volume. This addition of volume is an important step in the long-term preservation of BP.

In the acute phase, BP has been supported mainly by altering cardiac output and vascular capacity. However, the workload on the heart and the effects of vasoconstriction on peripheral circuits can be damaging if prolonged. The next phase is marked by more emphasis on retaining and increasing volume.

Hypermetabolic phase

The adrenocorticosteroid hormone aldosterone makes an important contribution to the maintenance of BP by regulating the electrolytes sodium and potassium, which in turn affects volume. Aldosterone effects overlap the first and second phase, an early response but capable of being sustained.

Aldosterone is stimulated (see Ch. 12) by the renin–angiotensin pathway in response to a fall in BP. It is also stimulated by a renin-independent mechanism when there is a rise in plasma potassium. This is a very effective stimulus and a useful one since raised plasma potassium is characteristic of tissue injury and its effects are damaging (see Ch. 14). The actions of aldosterone are to cause an increase in sodium retention and potassium excretion at the renal tubules, in the gut and at sweat glands. The effects are to achieve water retention as an osmotic response to sodium retrieval and at the same time, reduce the level of potassium if it is elevated.

As pressure begins to increase due to volume increase, the levels of AVP/ADH are reduced. While this reduces the water retrieval due to AVP/ADH, it also moderates the hormone's potent vasoconstrictor effect. Vasoconstriction can be useful, prolonged ischaemia is not.

Cortisol is necessary for survival in trauma or extreme stress. Without it the body's inflammatory mechanisms (see Ch. 16), which cause vasodilation and increased permeability of blood vessels, would make it very difficult if not impossible to maintain BP. Cortisol has the effect by stabilizing blood vessel membranes, reducing the dilation and making them less permeable. Pressure can be maintained and fluid loss to the tissues reduced. It also has a mild aldosterone-like effect which augments aldosterone itself, and, since cortisol levels are greatly increased in stress states, this contribution is important.

The increased volume increases the perfusion of tissues, in turn, increasing the chance of tissue survival and speeding healing.

Where fluid intake is plentiful, this retention of fluid may increase body weight, disguising the true loss of weight due to loss of body fat and protein.

Recovery phase

In the recovery phase, the stimuli to the neuro-hormones and hormones are reduced. As BP and the electrolyte levels return to normal, aldosterone levels are reduced. The drive from the hypothalamus is reduced and the plasma level of cortisol falls as the negative feedback regains its effect (see Ch. 11). Retention of fluid is reduced and normal fluid balance is recovered.

THE MAINTENANCE OF PLASMA GLUCOSE AND THE SUPPLY OF FUEL – THE METABOLIC RESPONSE TO TRAUMA

The effects of the overall response to trauma are extensive and cannot be covered adequately in this text. However, the selected aspects of the metabolic effects of stress and recovery outlined here are of major importance. Their effects will be very familiar to anyone who has cared for an injured person.

Most of us are familiar with the loss of weight, loss of muscle mass and effectiveness, and perhaps elevation of plasma glucose brought about by trauma. The metabolic sector of the response is concerned with the breakdown of body stores, glycogen, fat and skeletal muscle, to provide substrates for fuel and later for repair and growth. The demand for fuel is high following injury, particularly after the first few days. A severe extensive burn injury may double basal metabolic rate, and, although the energy requirement for activity may have been reduced to little or nothing, the high basal rate may be similar to that individual's normal active requirement prior to injury. An individual so severely injured is unlikely to be able to eat and even more unlikely to be able to meet this large requirement orally. Where intake is

less than requirement, the deficit will be met out of stores and that individual will lose weight. In trauma, or stress due to other causes, the neurohormones and hormones released favour the loss of tissue and weight loss becomes an almost obligatory state (see Chs 10 and 11).

Acute phase

In the acute phase, fuel, in the form of glucose, is supplied from the most rapidly accessed store, liver glycogen, initially made available by the effects of (mainly) glucagon. As glucose is released from the glycogen, plasma glucose begins to rise. This would normally be a stimulus to the release of insulin, which would immediately lower glucose levels. However, the release of insulin is suppressed by the catecholamines and a real increase is achieved. In some cases, for example sometimes immediately following surgery, the insulin suppression may be enough to cause hyperglycaemia and transient ketonuria. This is a manifestation of the normal response to stress and not an indication of any metabolic disorder. The ketone bodies produced can be used by the brain as a supplementary source of energy.

Liver glycogen is limited in quantity and the response moves on to other hormones and other fuel stores.

Hypermetabolic phase

Cortisol is again essential for survival, this time because of its metabolic effects. These are central to the release and conversion of body stores to make them available as substrates for energy, glucose and new construction material.

In this hypermetabolic phase, cortisol provides increased fuel and glucose availability by the breakdown of body fat and skeletal muscle (see Fig. 18.2). Together these make up a large percentage of the body's weight and can provide for a prolonged need, unlike hepatic glycogen which is of limited mass.

Body fat

Body fat is broken down and used as an alternative energy source, its normally large mass and high energy value making it an important contributor to survival. Very little is converted to glucose, only that portion which comes from the glycerol part of the triglyceride. However, it does have a small contributory effect in sparing glucose from other sources.

Body protein

Body protein or lean body mass (mainly skeletal muscle) is also broken down. Importantly, this also has a large mass and, in the context of trauma, has a more diverse range of uses than does fat.

Supply of energy as glucose

Some of the protein provides the continued glucose supply necessary for brain and nerve metabolism. This provision of glucose from amino acids (gluconeogenesis) is expensive, since the nitrogen part of the amino acids used in this way is detached and lost by excretion. Evidence for this can be found in the increased urinary nitrogen values of patients with injuries.

Plasma glucose is often elevated in this phase and the hyperglycaemia may be prolonged where the injury is severe or ongoing. Unlike the acute phase hyperglycaemia, however, this is due to the effects of insulin antagonism (mainly by cortisol) and tissue resistance rather than insulin suppression.

Hyperglycaemia following trauma has been known for many years. One of the very early reports was that by Claude Bernard in 1877 where hyperglycaemia was associated with haemorrhage (Bernard 1877). However, much of the investigative work now is on the insulin resistance causing hyperglycaemia rather than the hyperglycaemia itself.

Although insulin resistance is an integral part of the survival response, the effects are not all helpful. Insulin has important anabolic and anti-catabolic effects (see Ch. 18) and resistance to it increases the breakdown of body fat and protein. In practical terms, the greater the resistance is the longer is the time taken to recover.

The degree of resistance is related to the magnitude of the trauma or surgery (Thorell et al 1996a), other factors being loss of blood and the type of surgery. Biochemically, the degree of insulin resistance was found to be best related to the levels of IL-6 (Thorell et al 1996b). One factor that increases insulin resistance even in the healthy and uninjured is starvation. Investigations into the common practice of fasting patients prior to surgery have shown that fasting is associated with unnecessary discomfort for the patient, an increased degree of insulin resistance and impaired fluid homeostasis. Clinical studies have shown that the degree of insulin resistance can be reduced if the subject is given carbohydrate-rich fluids within 2–3 hours of surgery, so that he enters the trauma response in a fed rather than fasted state (Nygren et al 1998; Soop et al 2001). In studies of patients who have undergone elective surgery, the practical results of reducing insulin resistance are that a shorter stay in hospital can be achieved (Ljungqvist et al 2001).

The physiological outcome of reducing insulin resistance and thereby increasing its anti-catabolic effect is that less body nitrogen, i.e. lean body mass, is lost by gluconeogenesis.

Nitrogen for replacement

Some of the protein is used as a source of nitrogen for amino acids for repair at wound sites and replacement of proteins such as the clotting factors and plasma albumin lost at injury.

Nitrogen for bioactive components

Yet more nitrogen is used to produce the 'acute phase proteins'. These proteins are part of the inflammatory and immune response, e.g. inflammatory mediators, complement components and scavenger proteins such as the haptoglobins (see Ch. 16). They are produced by the liver and the cells of the immune system in response to cytokine stimuli.

Weight loss resulting from trauma

The weight loss induced by these catabolic activities cannot be reversed by simply increasing energy and protein intake. The hormonal balance must favour energy and nitrogen retention. As long as the effect of catabolic hormones, such as the catecholamines and cortisol, outweighs the anabolic effects of insulin, growth hormone and other growth-promoting hormones, little headway can be made in the accretion of new body mass, although losses can at least be minimized by adequate nutrition. Where there is physical injury, a similar situation exists at the wound site. Substrates provided by the systemic response may be present, but the balance between local growth-promoting cytokines and inhibitors of various kinds must be favourable before normal healing can take place.

Pre-existing poor nutritional status, hence reduced body stores, diminishes both the effectiveness of the systemic response and the healing of any wound present.

Evidence of these activities is clear, especially where there is a large wound, when there is very marked weight loss in the subject, although the true extent of the loss may be hidden by fluid retention. Small wounds show little evidence of this systemic activity, but even a moderate wound which persists, such as a leg ulcer or a pressure wound, becomes a drain on the nutritional economy.

Pain

Pain is a powerful stimulus to mechanisms of systemic catabolism; therefore inadequate or ineffective analgesia will inhibit wound repair and prolong particularly the hypermetabolic phase, leaving the subject nutritionally diminished and more vulnerable to infection.

Recovery phase

This phase may be difficult to differentiate from the previous phase until it has become well established.

It is the time when the metabolic balance due to hormones, cytokines and other chemical agents begins to shift from being predominately catabolic to predominately anabolic. In other words, recovery begins to gain ground.

The stress drive from hypothalamus is reduced and negative feedback from hormones such as cortisol becomes more effective. There is less antagonism to insulin and plasma glucose regulation becomes effective. Insulin's growth-promoting activity is increased and in turn this increases the anabolic effect of insulin-like growth factors (IGFs) and human growth hormone itself. The pattern of tissue restoration has been shown to favour first the accumulation of fat, then protein (Jeejeebhoy et al 1982). Later this fat mass is reduced and lean body mass increased; therefore although body weight is regained in this phase of the response, body composition is not restored for some time. This part of recovery may be prolonged. The number of weeks or months will depend on the severity of the trauma, the nutritional support available and the level of activity which is necessary to restore muscle mass and function.

ILLNESS

DISTURBANCE OF THE NORM

'Illness' can be regarded as the results of breakdown of a system or normal control of function. It is a threat to normality coming from within. How people feel is greatly affected by circumstances; what they are doing, who they are with, what the weather is like, all affect how one feels. Feeling well is a very subjective state, so also is feeling ill. Sometimes feelings of illness can be due to circumstances which are not purely physiological or biochemical; those feelings of illness are no less real but are beyond the scope of this chapter.

Feeling ill or being ill, however, is usually, but not always, due to changes in the internal environment which can be measured. Physical illness usually begins with a fault in a system or its regulation, sometimes called the 'primary defect'. Where there is an acute event such as myocardial infarct or haemorrhage, the onset is so rapid that it has many of the characteristics of injury. There will be an acute stress response, often tissue injury and, if the event is followed by surgery, there will also be surface and internal wound sites. Where there is a slowly developing illness, however, unlike injury or other traumatic happenings which are obvious and cannot be ignored, the original fault may well escape detection for some time with the individual being unaware of it or deciding to ignore it.

COMPENSATED DISTURBANCE

Someone out of breath climbing stairs may put this down to 'lack of exercise' or 'getting old' or 'too many cigarettes', but they do not usually imagine that they might have a degree of cardiac failure or obstructive airway disease. They decide instead to climb fewer stairs.

During this period of ignoring the situation, the body's compensatory mechanisms are working to readjust whichever parameter is threatened. The person who is chronically slightly out of breath, for example, could be hyperventilating for a number of reasons. The cause may be metabolic disorder, cardiac or respiratory disorder or a failure of adequate gas exchange. The parameter which is being adjusted is the same in each case, either carbon dioxide or hydrogen ion excess acting to stimulate ventilation which in turn reduces the level (see Ch. 13).

An individual who has cardiac or respiratory dysfunction may also be slightly hypoxic. The body compensates by releasing erythropoietin (see Ch. 9) in response to hypoxia. More red cells are produced and the oxygen-carrying capacity increases, so returning oxygen levels to normal. The evidence for compensation could be found in a higher red cell count and an increase in the percentage of reticulocytes (see Ch. 3). The underlying cause of the hypoxia is not relevant to the compensatory mechanism, it is simply a response driven by the stimulus of hypoxia.

The compensations may be enough to maintain a normal internal environment or at the least one which can be tolerated. It may become the accepted state for that individual and they fit their level of activity to their ability to carry it out. This may go on for some time, perhaps years. Some people who develop type 2 diabetes may have had the condition for many years before it is detected, by which time it may have done considerable damage (see Ch. 18).

EVIDENT DISTURBANCE

As the environment begins to be significantly disturbed, the level of stimulus to the mechanisms is greater and more obvious evidence of compensation begins to appear. In the example above, breathlessness might now be present even at rest. Even at this point, the parameter may still be within normal limits although the physiological effort to keep it normal is large and more and more mechanisms have to be recruited. Then, as the disturbance becomes still greater, symptoms emerge which reflect both the primary fault and the physiological efforts to correct it. Yet more symptoms begin to show some of the aspects of the response to stress.

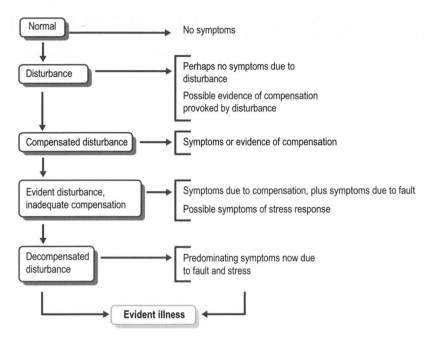

Figure 19.6 A general pattern of a developing state of illness.

Stress affects many physiological and biochemical parameters. Normal blood pressure may be altered; for example diastolic pressure may increase. Fluid may be retained and electrolyte levels altered. Cortisol output may be increased in response to stress in the shape of abnormalities in the internal environment, or perhaps in response to the individual's feeling of unwellness and anxiety.

DECOMPENSATED DISTURBANCE

When compensation is inadequate, the illness and the stress become evident. The primary fault, which has no doubt worsened, is now producing effects that have exceeded compensation. The characteristic symptoms of the fault have become apparent. The compensatory systems are still operating and producing their own effects, added to by the effects of the ancient response to ongoing stress. If there is pain, infection, surgery or pressure injury, the stress response is reinforced.

A PATTERN OF DEVELOPING ILLNESS

With knowledge of the workings of a particular system and its control agents, it is possible to anticipate the characteristics of illness related to that system. The ability to anticipate allows one to explain possible events or, sometimes more importantly, to spot the unpredicted event. Many specific conditions will have

been covered in the foregoing chapters as illustrations of physiology becoming pathophysiology, but it is worth considering some examples of 'illness' which show clear evidence of the pattern shown in Figure 19.6.

The pattern shown in Figure 19.6 is considered in the examples summarized below. A more detailed example of a pattern of development of illness in untreated types 1 and 2 diabetes mellitus is discussed in Chapter 18 and shown in Figure 18.8.

CARDIOVASCULAR SYSTEM DISORDER

The cardiovascular system provides examples of illness where progress is likely to be at predictably different rates.

MYOCARDIAL INFARCTION

Myocardial infarction (MI) is an example of an acute event more akin to injury rather than a progression towards developed illness, although there may have been earlier clues to an underlying problem. There is a severe fall in cardiac output, resulting in a large and rapid stress response where many of the effects are unhelpful to a damaged heart. As part of treatment of MI, many of these stress effects must be countered if the heart (and the victim) is to survive.

Physiological principles of treatment

The principles are aimed at safeguarding heart function. They include among others:

- provision of oxygen
- pain relief for patient comfort and reduction of sympathetic drive
- diuretic to reduce preload
- vaso- or venodilator to reduce afterload.

CHRONIC HEART FAILURE

More typical of disorders which are compensated in the early stages, but then become more and more difficult to compensate and tolerate, are left heart failure and right heart failure. Left and right ventricles have different properties, and, although both are pumps, they work in different conditions supplying and being supplied by different anatomical systems (see Chs 6 and 12). Chronic cardiac failure is the inability of the heart to maintain adequate tissue perfusion at normal cardiac filling pressure.

Left ventricular failure (LVF)

LVF is a reduced efficiency of the pump supplying the aorta, i.e. the main supply to body, brain and heart itself. There are many causes of LVF, such as coronary artery disease or other cardiac muscle dysfunction which reduces contractility. Another well-known cause is prolonged hypertension, particularly where there is elevated peripheral resistance causing an excessive afterload. The effect is an inability to clear the volume in the ventricle at the end of diastole, i.e. to achieve a good stroke volume. Heart rate is also affected as the heart becomes less sensitive to noradrenaline. As a result, cardiac output is reduced. At the same time, the pressure inside the ventricle is increased leading to back pressure on the left atrium and consequently on the pulmonary circuit. The compensatory responses to a fall in cardiac output all increase pressure, as does the stress response, so putting a further load on the failing heart.

The disorder becomes evident with symptoms such as breathlessness (due to pulmonary oedema), particularly lying down at night when lungs are less well drained. Fatigue and lack of cardiac capacity to cope with activity are distressing symptoms which unfortunately gradually worsen.

Physiological principles of treatment

Dysfunction which originates in the left heart is likely to affect the right heart. The general principles of treatment of the whole heart are shown below at 'right ventricular failure'. The early involvement of the pulmonary system, however, requires monitoring and possible treatment. Gas exchange becomes less efficient as fluid accumulates in the lungs and breathlessness is a common symptom. The individual will already have found that sleeping with the head and chest raised by several pillows is necessary, but in a severe attack, oxygen will have to be administered. Hypoxia in the pulmonary circuit causes pulmonary vessel constriction which exacerbates the poor gas exchange and early relief of hypoxia is advisable.

Right ventricular failure

Right heart failure (RVF) is also chronic heart failure, but the fluid mechanics differ from those in LVF and the symptoms and course of the condition are consequently different. RVF may be due to pulmonary hypertension in lung disease or dysfunction of the myocardial tissue. The great veins at the entrance to the right atrium are normally at a low pressure, only 2 to 3 mmHg; therefore even a moderate increase in the pressure in the right heart may be enough to cause back pressure in the veins, causing venous engorgement in the neck, oedema in the ankles when standing and in the sacral area when lying down.

Fluid shift to the tissue space causes a fall in intravascular volume, resulting in compensatory responses which retain fluid and compound the problem. A stress response added to this recruits all the mechanisms which would normally restore, but in this case increase, pressure. Increased pressure in the venous circuits causes more fluid shift and so on.

An aid to memory says of heart failure: 'left failure – oedema in the lung, right failure – oedema in the rest'. However, as heart failure progresses, both ventricles may fail and oedema will be found in the lungs and the periphery.

Physiological principles of treatment

The principles of treatment are based on correcting, if possible, the disordered physiology. If one considers the design of the heart, two pumps each of two chambers, working in synchrony, it is clear that whichever side is first affected, the second will be affected because of it. Treatment of chronic heart failure must consider the involvement of both sides of the heart.

Treatment may be one or other, or a combination of, the following:

- rest
- reducing workload on the heart by reducing preload and afterload (see Chs 6 and 12), reducing intravascular volume and increasing contractility

- reducing intravascular volume by diuretics or angiotensin-converting enzyme (ACE) inhibitors or the aldosterone site antagonist spironolactone
- increasing contractility using cardiac glycosides.

LIVER DYSFUNCTION

There are as many dysfunctions of the liver as there are functions. However, disruption of the liver's architecture in hepatic cirrhosis serves to illustrate the pattern of developing illness.

The liver has a very large flow of blood passing through it via the hepatic artery and the hepatic portal vessel. It is drained by the hepatic venous system (see Ch. 10). When passage of blood through the liver becomes obstructed by fibrotic or cirrhotic tissue, profound physical and chemical changes begin to take place. The changes are caused by circumstances such as hypoxia due to poor cardiac output, infection or inflammation in the liver or consumption of excess amounts of alcohol. The changes take place slowly. Fatty deposits appear which can be resolved if the primary cause is removed. However, if the cause persists, the deposits become more permanent and structurally more obstructive. The individual may still be unaware of any dysfunction at this stage.

As the obstruction increases, pressure changes begin in the vessels perfusing the liver. Pressure in the lower pressure hepatic portal vessel begins to rise due to back pressure from the obstruction and initially this is enough to maintain the flow as normal. Although the portal vessel has a lower oxygen tension than the arterial blood, because the flow rate is high, it makes a significant contribution to the oxygenation of the liver cells. The rise in pressure, however, has other effects and fluid begins to shift from the venous system to the tissue spaces and the early symptom of oedema begins to appear. As liver function declines, hepatic synthesis of plasma proteins is reduced and the resulting lower osmotic pressure combined with higher hydrostatic pressure increases fluid loss to the tissues (see Chs 12 and 14). In addition to the predictable symptom of oedema, there may be other signs of the liver's synthetic failing ability, for example bruising indicating a reduction in the production of clotting factors.

As cirrhosis advances, inflammatory activity in the liver causes increased permeability in the membranes surrounding it. These include the peritoneal membrane, so allowing fluid (and protein) to escape in abnormal quantities into the peritoneal cavity, i.e. allowing ascites to develop. Wherever there is oedema and movement of fluid to the extravascular space, the compensatory mechanisms of fluid recovery, such as the renin–angiotensin–aldosterone mechanism, are stimulated. These will have been active for some time, but the development of ascites now adds an extra stimulus since water and sodium move very easily into the space. The scene has now become one where an error signal, i.e. loss of fluid, continuously reinforces the mechanisms, which makes the situation worse.

Liver function by this stage has become such that the individual is ill, uncomfortable and unable to eat normally. The stress response, which has been in force for some time, adds to the physiological and biochemical disarray.

Physiological principles of treatment

Correction of the original fault would be a primary aim, especially if the condition is in the early stages, since the liver has considerable powers of regeneration.

The physiological principles of treatment in the later stages would include reduction in fluid load and management of nutrition and electrolytes.

The aldosterone response which brings about sodium retention with subsequent water retention can be inhibited by the aldosterone receptor site inhibitor spironolactone.

REFERENCES AND FURTHER READING

Wounds and wound healing

Bryant R 2000 Acute and chronic wounds, 2nd edn. Churchill Livingstone, Edinburgh

Carrougher C J 1998 Burn care and therapy. Mosby, St Louis

Clark R A F (ed) 1996 The molecular and cellular biology of wound repair, 2nd edn. Plenum Press, London

Cooper D M, Yu E Z, Hennessey P et al 1994 Determination of endogenous cytokines in chronic wounds. Annals of Surgery 219: 688–692

Frubeck G, Salvador J 2000 Is leptin involved in the signalling cascade after myocardial infarction and reperfusion? Circulation 101: e194

Harding K 1998 The future of wound healing. In: Leaper D J, Harding K G, Wound: biology and management. Oxford University Press, Oxford

Higley H R, Ksander G A, Gerhardt C O et al 1995 Extravasation of macromolecules and possible trapping of transforming growth factor-beta in venous ulceration. British Journal of Dermatology 132: 79–85

Hinman C D, Maibach H 1963 Effects of air exposure and occlusion on experimental human skin wounds. Nature 200: 377–378

Hunt T K 1990 Basic principles of wound healing. Journal of Trauma 30: 122–138

Leaper D J, Harding K G 1998 Wound: biology and management. Oxford University Press, Oxford

Morison M, Moffatt C, Bridel-Nixon J, Bale S 1997 Nursing management of chronic wounds, 2nd edn. Mosby, London

Phillips J 1997 Pressure sores. Churchill Livingstone, Edinburgh

Stanley A C, Park H Y, Phillips T J et al 1997 Reduced growth of dermal fibroblasts from chronic venous ulcers can be eliminated with growth factors. Journal of Vascular Surgery 16: 59–66

Winter G 1962 Formulation of the scab and the rate of epithelialisation in the skin of the domestic pig. Nature 193: 293–294

The systemic response to stress

Bernard C 1877 Lessons on diabetic and glycogenetic animals (Fr – trans). Baillière, Paris

Berne R M, Levy M N 2000 Principles of physiology, 3rd edn. Mosby, St Louis

Ellis K J, Eastman J 1993 Human body composition: in vivo methods, models and assessment. Plenum, New York

Ganong W F 2001 Review of medical physiology, 20th edn. McGraw-Hill Education, Philadelphia

Guyton A C, Hall J E 2000 Textbook of medical physiology, 10th edn. Saunders, Philadelphia

Jeejeebhoy K N, Baker J F, Wolman S I et al 1982 Critical evaluation of the role of clinical assessment and body composition studies in patients with malnutrition and after total parenteral nutrition. American Journal of Clinical Nutrition 35: 1117–1127

Ljungqvist O, Nygren J, Thorell A et al 2001 Preoperative nutrition – elective surgery in the fed or overnight fasted state. Clinical Nutrition 20(suppl 1): 167–171

Moulton C, Yates D 1999 Lecture notes on emergency medicine. Blackwell Science, Oxford

Nygren J, Thorell A, Soop M et al 1998 Preoperative insulin and glucose infusion maintains normal insulin sensitivity after surgery. American Journal of Physiology 275: E140–E148

Soop M, Nygren J, Myrenfors P et al 2001 Preoperative oral carbohydrate treatment attenuates immediate postoperative insulin resistance. American Journal of Physiology 280: E576–E583

Thorell A, Nygren J, Ljungqvist O 1996a Insulin resistance – a marker of surgical stress. Current Opinion in Clinical Nutrition and Metabolic Care 2: 69–79

Thorell A, Essen P, Andersson B et al 1996b Postoperative insulin resistance and circulating concentrations of stress hormones and cytokines. Clinical Nutrition 15: 75–79

Illness

Berne R M, Levy M N 2000 Principles of physiology, 3rd edn. Mosby, St Louis

Berne R M, Levy M N 2000 Cardiovascular physiology, 8th edn. Mosby, St Louis

Campbell E J M, Dickinson C J, Slater J D H, Edwards C R W, Sikora E K 1984 Clinical physiology, 5th edn. Blackwell Science, Oxford

Ganong W F 2001 Review of medical physiology, 20th edn. McGraw-Hill Education, Philadelphia

Guyton A C, Hall J E 1997 Human physiology and the mechanisms of disease, 6th edn. Saunders, Philadelphia

Guyton A C, Hall J E 2000 Textbook of medical physiology, 10th edn. Saunders, Philadelphia

SECTION 2
Interaction with the external environment

Section 2 is made up of two parts:

Part 2A – Sensing and responding to the external environment

Section 2 is concerned with the central nervous system. Part 2A gives an overview of the somatic nervous system, of its cell types, component structures and major pathways. The main characteristics of the sensory and motor systems are described with key aspects of each developed in subsequent chapters. Hearing, vision, taste, smell and proprioception are examined in this section as examples of sensory activity.

An examination of the motor system includes, in addition to body movement, a chapter on the important topic of communication.

Part 2A is supported by chapters on neurones and muscle (Excitable cells) in Part 1A.

Part 2B – Aspects of experience

This part includes chapters on complex topics such as emotion and behaviour, and learning and memory. A chapter on pain includes the mechanisms of different types of pain and information on anaesthesia and analgaesia.

20

The somatic nervous system: an introduction

The somatic nervous system controls all skeletal muscles within our bodies, and, as a result, controls our movements and actions. It also creates our personal consciousness of the world about us and of our place in it. It is a complex system about which a great deal is yet to be unravelled, but it is also fascinating in that its workings determine our personality, intelligence and skills. By knowing more about how the nervous system functions we may increase our understanding of our own experience and behaviour.

During in utero development, the nervous system develops from a cluster of primitive ectodermic cells to form the brain, spinal cord, and cranial and spinal nerves. Within the brain and spinal cord, neurones and their axons are grouped together to form many different structures, through the processes of differentiation and migration.

Interwoven amongst the neurones are supporting cells (glia) that do not conduct impulses but help to maintain the function of the nervous system. Preservation of nerve cell function is also the role of the blood supply, the blood–brain barrier and the cerebrospinal fluid, all of which will be discussed later.

The brain and the spinal cord are both enveloped by membranes (meninges) and housed within the bony chambers of the skull and vertebral canal.

UNDERSTANDING THE NERVOUS SYSTEM

The standard approach to studying the structure and function of the nervous system is to break it down into its component parts, e.g. nerves, muscles, electrical transmission. However, in doing this it is all too easy to lose sight of the overall working of the system. While there is a real advantage, in terms of simplicity, in investigating each part of the system separately, it should also be borne in mind that any results or findings should be viewed in the context of the whole nervous system. The study of the nervous system is often approached from two diverse areas, namely, physiology and psychology. Both subjects are concerned with understanding how our minds work and how we behave, but they usually approach the subject from different angles and use different methods of investigation. Often the physiologist looks narrowly at specific neural mechanisms and from this, attempts to build up a model of how the brain works and how this

Human functions, whether physiological or psychological, are so interrelated that professional care cannot be given if disease processes are considered without taking into account their effect on the individual and his family. This is the basis of the holistic approach to health care and nursing.

determines behaviour. Conversely the psychologist may first observe a person's behaviour and then attempts to infer how that behaviour is brought about. For a full understanding of our minds and behaviour, both approaches are necessary and insights from each subject need to be combined.

PHYSIOLOGICAL FRAMEWORK

Like the autonomic nervous system, the components of the somatic nervous system may be divided into three elements:

- sensory (input functions)
- motor (output functions)
- integrative.

Sensory systems are responsible for detecting changes in our external environment, for analysing this information, and for selecting what is transmitted to those parts of the brain that 'make sense' of the information and power our actions.

Motor systems control the contraction of skeletal muscle at an unconscious (reflex) and at a conscious (voluntary) level. These systems enable us to walk, run, stand, sit, make sounds, frown etc.

Integrative components blend information from our senses with commands issued to the muscles to produce sophisticated activities, such as thinking, writing and speaking, and other features of our personalities such as mood, emotion and motivation.

PSYCHOLOGICAL DIMENSIONS

Experience

What we experience depends in part on what our sensory receptors tell us about stimuli originating from outside and inside our bodies. Excitation of the brain provoked by activation of sensory receptors gives rise to the experience of sensation. For example, the absorption of light by receptors in the eye gives rise to the sensation of vision, whereas the excitation of nerve endings in the skin and elsewhere by injurious stimuli (e.g. tissue damage) gives rise to the sensation of pain. Receptors do not respond to vision or pain. Receptors

stimulate the brain areas that create these sensations in our minds. These sensations in turn alert us to changes both outside and inside the body.

Intelligence

Understanding what has been sensed depends upon the links or associations we make between different forms of sensory experience and also between present and past experiences. There is a difference between hearing the sounds of a teacher speaking and actually understanding what is being said, or between looking at a drawing in a book and knowing what it means. Sensation and perception are not the same thing. In sensing something, we register a change in some aspect of our internal or external environment; in perceiving it, we know what it is. We think about it.

Expression

We give expression to our understanding of our experiences in various ways, by what we do and say, by our laughter, tears, smiles and frowns. We convert our thoughts into activity. We react consciously and unconsciously to the stimuli acting on us. Sometimes we react instinctively (reflexly). At other times we make more considered choices, weighing up different strategies and choosing what, on balance, seems best at the time (voluntary behaviour). All these things rely on nerve networks that link sensory and motor systems and on the chemical processes that allow nerve impulses to be transmitted rapidly between different parts of the nervous system and ultimately to the muscles.

Emotion

Our emotions are the area of our experience that, at present, is least well defined. When we talk about emotion in everyday conversation we generally mean that we are talking about how we feel and the kind of mood that we are in. We talk too of what we see of other people's behaviour, whether they appear aggressive or laid back, happy or sad. Emotion seems to involve several systems:

- sensory systems informing us of our experience
- motor systems generating responses both somatically (somatic nervous system) and viscerally (autonomic nervous system)
- other parts of the nervous system influencing our level of alertness.

Memory and learning

Nerve impulses last for only a fraction of a second. Yet we remember skills we have learnt long after we have finished practising. We also recall names and faces, facts and figures. Sometimes just one powerful exposure to a

Nursing practice includes many skills that are both rehearsed and repeated, for example giving injections, taking temperatures, taking blood pressures: when these skills have been used countless times they are seldom forgotten and may become mechanical. Conscious thought about the effect on the patient should always accompany the action.

Table 20.1 Origin and meaning of some anatomical terms*

Origin	Term	Meaning
Latin	Cerebellum	Small brain
	Colliculus	A little hill
	Commissure	A join
	Cortex	Bark, rind
	Fasciculus	A little bundle
	Foramen	A hole
	Limbic	Bordering, edging
	Nucleus	A kernel
	Ventricle	A little cavity
Greek	Arachnoid	Like a spider
	Chiasma	Greek letter 'x'
	Cranium	Skull
	Gyrus	A turn or twist
	Ganglion	Knot or swelling
	Hippocampus	Sea-horse
	Lemniscus	A strip or band
	Thalamus	Inner room
	Hypothalamus	Below the thalamus

* *Source*: Butterworths Medical Dictionary (1978).

set of events will imprint them on our minds, and overrule all others. Usually, for a memory to be formed, rehearsal and repetition of the stimuli will be needed to forge the long-term links between the brain cells concerned. Once firmly stored in the form of connections between nerve cells, a new pattern of thought and action is established.

Memory is a complex function that requires the involvement of a number of discrete brain areas (cortex, cerebellum, hippocampus). What lay-people generally regard as memory is the hippocampal-based function which is lost or impaired in neurodegenerative disorders such as Alzheimer's disease.

STRUCTURE OF THE NERVOUS SYSTEM

TERMINOLOGY

Anatomists describe what they see, and so the various parts of the brain have usually been named according to their appearance rather than their function, rather in the way that in geography names are given to distinctive features in a landscape. Often these names are derived from Latin or Greek words so their ordinariness is not immediately obvious. Pons, for example, means 'bridge' and sulcus is a 'furrow' and so on. Some common terms and their meanings are listed in Table 20.1. Occasionally other, self-evident terms are used: the olive, for example, looks that shape.

Superficial structures

The component parts of the nervous system (brain, spinal cord and peripheral nerves) are shown in Figure 20.1. The central structures, namely the brain and spinal cord, are termed the central nervous system whereas the nerves connecting these parts to the muscles form the peripheral nervous system. The brain consists of three parts:

• cerebrum
• cerebellum
• brain stem.

The surface of the cerebrum is thrown into many folds (gyri and sulci). There are also deep grooves (fissures) dividing the two halves of the cerebrum (the cerebral hemispheres) into subsections (lobes).

Internal structures

Nervous tissue is greyish-white in appearance because much of the nervous tissue consists of nerve axons. Axons contain relatively few organelles. They therefore do not absorb much light and consequently appear white. The whiteness is made more intense where axons are enveloped by myelin.

The cell bodies of the neurones contain the nuclei and other organelles normally found in cells. These do absorb some light. Consequently, where many cell bodies are clustered together within the brain and spinal cord, the tissue appears grey.

Spinal cord

The appearance of the spinal cord in cross-section is shown in Figure 20.2. The grey part (grey matter) consists mostly of cell bodies and their dendrites whereas the whiter areas surrounding this (white matter) consist of the axons of neurones carrying signals up and down the cord.

Brain

Similarly, in sections cut through the brain, some areas appear darker than others. Where cell bodies are

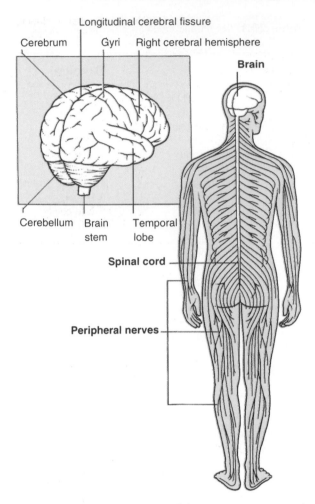

Figure 20.1 Component parts of the nervous system and the names given to some of the major external features of the brain.

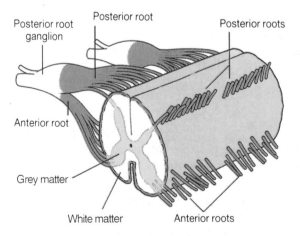

Figure 20.2 A section of the spinal cord showing the roots of the nerves carrying impulses into and out of the central nervous system, and the grey and white matter within the spinal cord. (From Rogers 1992, with permission of Elsevier.)

grouped together to form a rounded cluster of cells, the cluster is usually referred to as a nucleus: some clusters are occasionally termed ganglia (singular = ganglion).

The outer layer (cortex) of the cerebral hemispheres and of the cerebellum differs in appearance from the neural tissue beneath (subcortical structures). The cortex appears greyish because there are many cell bodies, but they are arranged differently from those in the nuclei. A closer look at the cortical tissue under the high power of the microscope reveals that the cells are organized in columns, and that cells differ in size and shape at different levels, giving rise to a layered appearance.

The areas of the brain that appear white consist again of axons. Where axons are grouped into bundles or other structures linking one part of the brain with another they are sometimes described as lemnisci, tracts etc. A large band of nerve fibres (corpus callosum) links the two cerebral hemispheres.

ORGANIZATION

Developmental origins

During weeks 3–4 post-fertilization there is a rapid development of the embryonic plate cells into three separate layers of cells:

- ectoderm
- mesoderm
- endoderm.

The embryonic mesoderm will further differentiate into muscle and connective tissue, and participates in the development of most organs, whereas the embryonic endoderm gives rise to the gut, digestive organs and lungs. The critical embryonic layer, from the point of view of nervous system development, is the ectoderm, or neuroectoderm. Very early in development the primitive cells (neuroectoderm) giving rise to the nervous system form a hollow fluid-filled tube (neural tube) and the neural crest (Fig. 20.3A).

Neural tube

The cell bodies of the neurones in the neural tube are grouped together around the central canal. These cell bodies will form the grey matter, and axons extending from them will form the white matter on the outside of the tube. In the primitive neural tube the grey matter is divided into two layers:

- alar lamina
- basal lamina.

The alar lamina develops into sensory systems, whereas the basal lamina develops into motor systems.

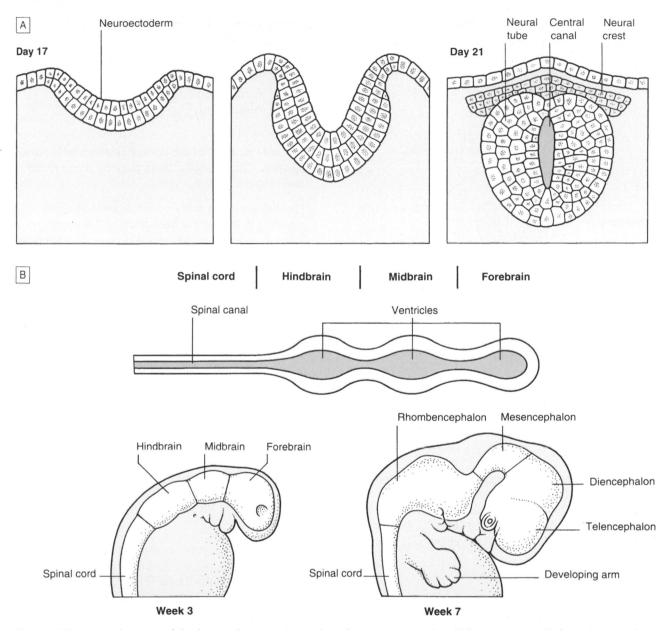

Figure 20.3 Development of the human brain and spinal cord. A, First 3 weeks of life: primitive cells form the neural tube and neural crest. B, First 2 months of life: part of the neural tube develops into the primitive brain.

Early in development, the front part of the neural tube becomes noticeably different from the rest (Fig. 20.3B). Three enlargements appear, the forebrain, midbrain and hindbrain. Each develops into different parts of the mature brain:

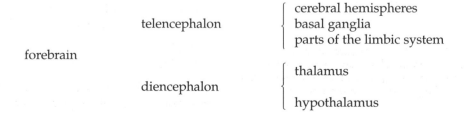

| midbrain | mesencephalon | superior and inferior colliculi
midbrain reticular formation
cerebral peduncles |
| hindbrain | rhombencephalon | pons
medulla oblongata
cerebellum |

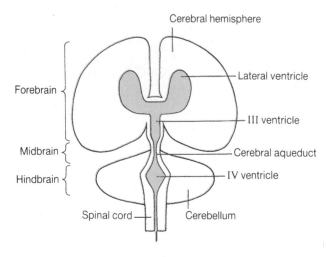

Figure 20.4 Diagrammatic representation of the four ventricles of the brain and their position in relation to other structures. (From Rogers 1992, with permission of Elsevier.)

The rest of the neural tube becomes the spinal cord. The hollow part of the primitive neural tube persists as the central canal in the spinal cord, and as the ventricles of the brain, of which there are four (Fig. 20. 4). The fluid inside is cerebrospinal fluid, formed by cells lining the ventricles.

Spina bifida

Failure of caudal neuropore of the neural tube to close results in a disruption of the lumbar and sacral segments of cord, with structures superficial to the cord also being involved (i.e. meninges, vertebral arch, paravertebral muscles, skin) since their development relies on closure of the neural tube. This will lead to malformations of vertebral arch and cord of the kind seen in spina bifida.

Spina bifida means cleft spine, or incomplete closure of the spinal column. There are three main types:

- spina bifida occulta
- meningocele
- myelomeningocele.

Spina bifida occulta is a common but relatively minor defect of one or more spinal arches. It is a condition usually only found incidentally through a radiological examination for another disease. The spinal cord is normally formed, in the normal position with normal function. Occasionally, there may be some minor neurological defects.

Meningocele is a fairly common form of spina bifida, resulting in the simple herniation of the meninges through a defect in the neural arches. The condition, which carries the risk of infection, may have some accompanying neurological disability. Myelomeningocele causes the herniation, into a skin-covered sac, of the meninges and spinal cord through a defect in the neural arches. Most recent figures suggest that it occurs in approximately 2 out of 1000 pregnancies. The nerve roots are abnormally situated, because of the herniation, often causing paralysis below the level of defect. Meningitis is a complication that may lead to further central nervous system damage.

Neural crest

Neural crest cells migrate to form dorsal root ganglion cells, sympathetic ganglion cells, Schwann cells, melanocytes and the musculoskeletal elements of head and neck.

Spinal cord

This cord of nervous tissue (Fig. 20.1) is housed within the vertebral canal and consists of collections of nerve cell bodies (grey matter) and bundles of nerve cell axons (white matter) (Fig. 20.2). Axons, carrying nerve impulses to and from the periphery, extend from the cord as the roots of the spinal nerves.

Grey matter

The grey matter occupies the central part of the cord. It is here that synaptic contact is made between different cells. The cells are arranged in an ordered way in the grey matter. On the basis of its appearance the grey matter can be divided into 10 different layers (laminae) (Fig. 20.5A). Incoming sensory nerve fibres make synaptic contact with cells in laminae I to IV, and VI, in the posterior horn of the grey matter, whereas the cell bodies of the neurones conveying impulses to the muscles (motor neurones) are grouped together in the anterior horn in lamina IX. Many of the cells within the cord are interneurones.

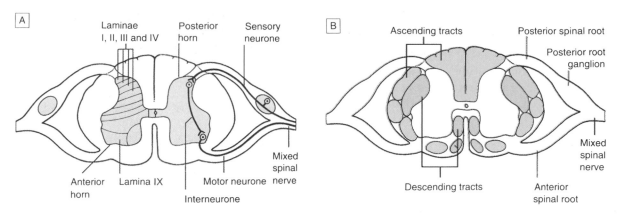

Figure 20.5 Typical structure of the spinal cord in the lumbar region. A, Grey matter: laminae and arrangement of sensory and motor neurones. (Note: the left and right halves of the spinal cord have the same basic structure. In this diagram, laminae are shown on the left and sensory and motor neurones on the right only for simplicity.) B, White matter: ascending and descending tracts.

White matter

The white matter of the cord consists of the axons of nerve fibres carrying impulses up and down the cord. The fibres are grouped into tracts (Fig. 20.5B). Their constituent fibres are either sensory and carry information up the spinal cord towards the brain (afferent neurones, ascending tracts) or they are motor and carry signals from different parts of the brain down towards the muscles (efferent neurones, descending tracts).

Pre-conceptual care

For most women, pregnancy is not confirmed until the fetus is already 2 to 3 months old. Throughout the most vulnerable period of fetal development, the woman may be unaware that conception has taken place if her periods are normally irregular. Until confirmation of pregnancy, she may continue to smoke, take analgesics, drink alcohol, perhaps eat an inadequate diet, and work with pesticides or industrial chemicals, all of which may cause developmental abnormalities. Some women do not know whether they have been immunized against rubella (German measles) which, if contracted during the first 3 months of pregnancy, is likely to cause deformities of the fetus, including total deafness.

Many family practitioner surgeries now provide pre-conceptual clinics. Women are encouraged to take responsibility for the health of their developing babies and advised to work towards optimum health before attempting to conceive. At the clinic the woman will be given a general health check, be immunized against rubella if necessary, and be given all the advice about potential hazards that is normally given on confirmation of pregnancy. Women who are already taking medication for a condition such as epilepsy receive special advice. The anticonvulsants used to control epilepsy are liable to cause fetal abnormalities, and the medication may need to be reduced, or discontinued if the woman has not had a fit for 3 years.

Poliomyelitis (anterior poliomyelitis, polio, infantile paralysis)

Very few children in the UK escape being immunized against poliomyelitis. The drops, administered on a sugar lump or straight into a baby's mouth, are a recognized part of the immunization schedule. The disease, which was prevalent worldwide 30 to 40 years ago, is now well controlled in many countries, although it still causes deaths and distressing physical handicaps in the developing world.

The poliovirus causes a severe influenza-like illness but, if it spreads via the bloodstream to the central nervous system (CNS), it destroys motor cell bodies, particularly those in the anterior horns of grey matter in the spinal cord (anterior poliomyelitis) and in the medulla oblongata.

For those who survived the CNS infection, permanent disability often resulted. This may have been anything from mild weakness of a limb to paralysis of all muscles from the neck down, the person spending the rest of his/her life in an 'iron lung' – a respirator that encased the trunk and limbs.

The severity of the disease has been forgotten by many in the UK and parents are likely to ask whether immunization is really necessary because polio is so rare. Without mass immunization, it is possible that outbreaks would occur again. The virus circulates widely in the environment and can be ingested in drinking water contaminated with sewage and food contaminated with faeces, as well as by inhalation. Sea and river water may also become a source of virus.

Spinal roots

Sensory information enters the cord posteriorly through the posterior roots of the spinal cord, and motor signals leave anteriorly through the anterior roots. Not far from the spinal cord, the two roots merge to form a spinal nerve consisting of both afferent and efferent fibres bundled together. Included as well in this mixed nerve are autonomic fibres of the sympathetic or parasympathetic system.

Spinal nerves

There are 31 pairs of spinal nerves (see Fig. 20.6), which are named according to the level of the vertebral column at which they emerge from the spine:

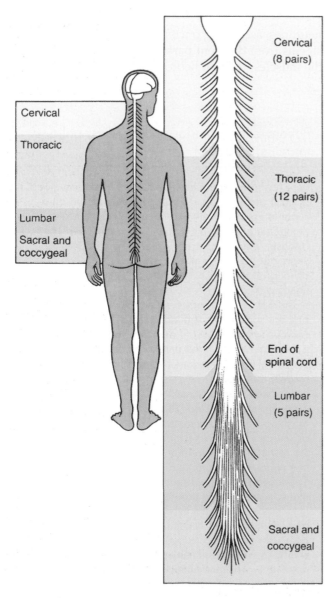

Figure 20.6 The spinal nerves.

- cervical (8 pairs)
- thoracic (12 pairs)
- lumbar (5 pairs)
- sacral (5 pairs)
- coccygeal (1 pair).

Each nerve innervates a group of muscles (myotome), and an area of skin (dermatome). Most also innervate some of the thoracic and abdominal organs.

The spinal nerves are classified as being mixed, in that they have both a sensory and a motor aspect. The motor fibres emerge from the anterior horns of the grey matter, with the sensory fibres terminating in the posterior horns (see Fig. 20.5A). This figure also shows how the sensory and motor neurones come together to form the mixed spinal nerve.

The sensory and motor neurones are established in such a way as to form what is known as a reflex arc. This allows signals to be passed from the sensory to the motor neurones, via interneurones, without first passing to the brain. As a result of this, a reflex motor reaction can occur in response to a specific sensory input, e.g. the rapid withdrawal of your hand from a very hot flame.

The information is still passed on up the appropriate neuronal pathway to the relevant part of the brain which processes pain (thalamus), although there would obviously be a delay of a few milliseconds until the pain would be felt or experienced.

Anterior and posterior rami

Each of the spinal nerves divides to form two branches, the anterior and posterior rami (Fig. 20.7). The posterior rami innervate:

- muscles that extend the spine
- skin at the back of the body (from upper buttocks to the top of the skull)

whereas the anterior rami innervate:

- muscles of the
  - back that flex the spine
  - body wall
  - arms and legs
- skin of the
  - front and sides of the neck and trunk
  - limbs.

Brain

From its external appearance the adult brain consists of three main parts (Fig. 20.1):

- brain stem
- cerebellum
- cerebral hemispheres.

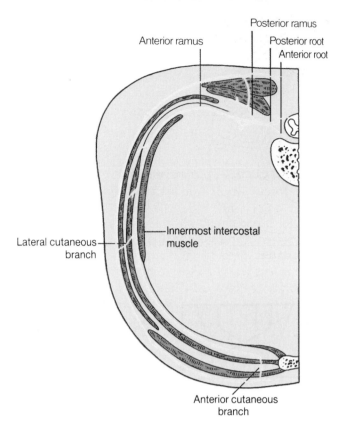

Figure 20.7 Branches of a spinal nerve innervating muscles and skin of the thorax. (From Rogers 1992, with permission of Elsevier.)

Brain stem and related structures

The brain stem is the continuation of the spinal cord (Fig. 20.8A & B). It consists of:

- medulla oblongata
- pons
- midbrain.

The grey matter of the spinal cord continues up through the middle of the brain stem. The central core of this forms the reticular formation. The reticular formation has multiple ascending and descending connections which mediate level of alertness (ability to interact with environment) and arousal (sleep and wakefulness). They regulate activity of spinal motor neurones, regulate and coordinate autonomic function, and modulate transmission of pain through spinal cord. Around this core are groups of cell bodies forming distinct clusters (nuclei). The white matter (nerve fibre tracts of the cord) also continues up into the brain stem. The nerve endings may synapse with cells of the reticular formation, or with the nuclei. Some nerve fibres cross over from one side of the brain stem to the other so that information from each side of the body is transmitted to the brain on the opposite side. A good example of this crossing over (decussation), but for descending rather than ascending fibres, is provided by the tracts that have an important role in controlling the movements of the fingers and toes (corticospinal tracts). These fibres decussate at the boundary between the medulla oblongata and the spinal cord. The appearance of this crossover point has resulted in it being called the 'pyramids'. For this reason the corticospinal tracts are sometimes referred to as the pyramidal tracts.

The brain stem performs sensory, motor and reflex functions. Nuclei in the medulla contain a number of reflex centres. Among the most important of these are the cardiac, vasomotor and respiratory centres. The medulla also contains the centres for other, non-vital reflexes, e.g. vomiting, coughing, sneezing, hiccuping and swallowing. The pons contains centres for reflexes mediated by cranial nerves V, VI, VII and VIII. The pons also contains the pneumotaxic centres involved in the regulation of respiration.

Beyond the structures of the midbrain, which include the inferior and superior colliculi, is the hypothalamus. The hypothalamus is part of the forebrain. It consists of several nuclei. The hypothalamus has connections both with the spinal cord below the brain stem and with the cerebral hemispheres above. It is an important link between the somatic and the autonomic nervous systems and the nervous systems and the endocrine system. Much of the internal environment is controlled from here (see Ch. 11). It is involved in motivational and emotional aspects of behaviour.

Cerebellum

Straddling the pons and attached to it by the cerebellar peduncles (i.e. cerebellar feet) is the cerebellum (Fig. 20.9), which has an important role in the control of movement. The cerebellum also consists of grey matter and white matter, but the grey matter is subdivided into:

- cerebellar cortex
- nuclei.

> Knowledge of which structures are innervated by each nerve provides an estimation of the level at which damage has occurred.

> When the motor cortex of either of the cerebral hemispheres is damaged by injury, disease or pressure, the person is likely to have impaired movement on the opposite side of the body because of the decussation of nerve tracts.

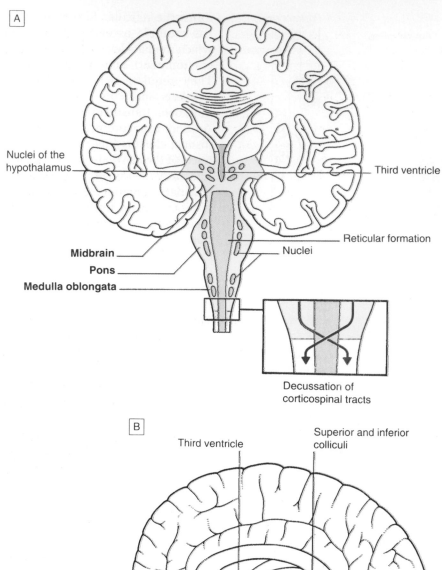

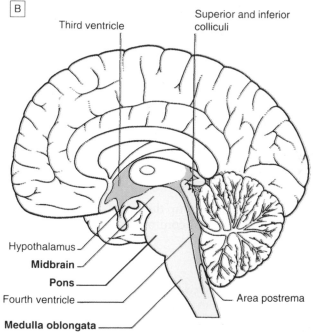

Figure 20.8 The brain stem – component parts. A, Brain cut in half: front view of back half. B, Brain cut in half, separating the left and right cerebral hemispheres: side view of right half.

The nuclei are embedded deep within the cerebellum, and the much-folded cortex completely envelops them. The cerebellar peduncles consist of bundles of nerve axons linking the cerebellum with other parts of the brain.

Although the cerebellum and the cerebrum are separated from each other by a fissure (cleft) they are both anatomically and structurally very similar. Both gross structures have a grey matter cortex, with white matter at the core. The internal white matter layout resembles the vein patterns found in a leaf, hence the name, arbor vitae, sometimes given to the cerebellum. Not only do the cortical surfaces of both the cerebellum and the cerebrum exhibit sulci and gyri (troughs and peaks), they are also both divided into hemispheres.

The cerebellum plays an important role in three movement-related functions. Firstly, it is involved in the process of equilibrium via the control of skeletal muscle. Secondly, it plays a key part, subconsciously, in the maintenance of proper posture. It is this role that makes our movements smooth, steady and co-ordinated rather than trembling, disjointed and ineffective. Thirdly, and perhaps most importantly, the cerebellum acts with the motor cortex to produce accurate, co-ordinated movements by 'comparing' actual movements with intended movements.

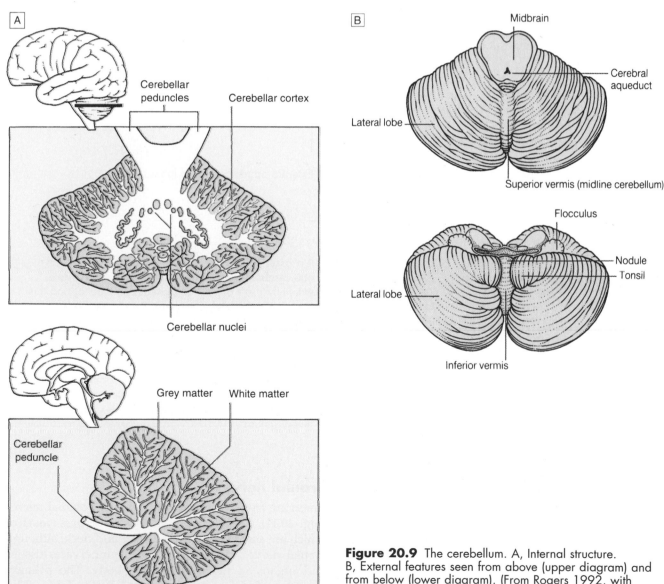

Figure 20.9 The cerebellum. A, Internal structure. B, External features seen from above (upper diagram) and from below (lower diagram). (From Rogers 1992, with permission of Elsevier.)

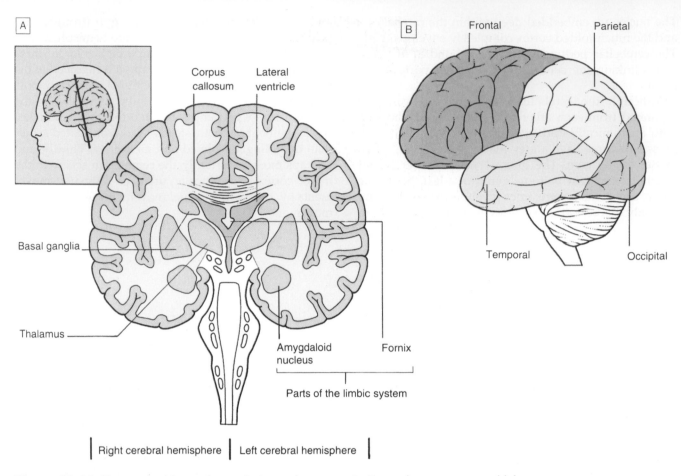

Figure 20.10 The cerebral hemispheres. A, Internal structure. B, External appearance and lobes.

Cerebral hemispheres

The two cerebral hemispheres, like the cerebellum, contain discrete clusters of cells (nuclei) enveloped by a much-folded layer of cortex and traversed by numerous nerve fibre tracts (Fig. 20.10A). The nuclei include the basal ganglia, which are involved in controlling movement, and the thalamus, which has both sensory and motor functions. Buried deep within the cerebral hemispheres are the structures forming the limbic system, which, together with the hypothalamus, is involved in motivation and emotion. The two hemispheres are linked by a massive bundle of fibres (corpus callosum).

The extensive folding of the cortical surface gives the brain a wrinkled appearance (Fig. 20.10B). Some of the folds dip deeply into the tissue, dividing the hemispheres into several lobes:

- frontal
- temporal
- parietal
- occipital.

It is asserted that the majority of the population have one cerebral hemisphere that develops to a greater extent than the other (hemisphere dominance) and this is normally the left hemisphere. People whose left hemisphere is dominant are right-handed and the speech centres will develop in this hemisphere in early childhood. Damage to the left hemisphere of the brain from a stroke or haemorrhage may result in dysphasia. Many left-handed people also have a dominant left cerebral hemisphere. Ascertaining true right cerebral hemisphere dominance involves complex neurological investigations.

Cranial nerves

Emerging from the brain are 12 pairs of cranial nerves (Fig. 20.11). These supply various structures, most of which are associated with the head and neck, although cranial nerve X (the vagus) chiefly innervates tissues and organs in the trunk of the body. The primary functions of each of the nerves are listed in Table 20.2.

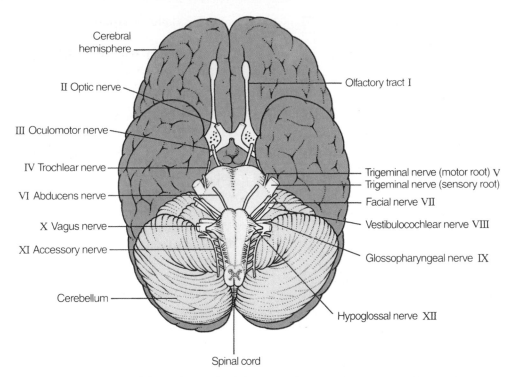

Figure 20.11 View of the underneath of the brain showing the 12 pairs of cranial nerves. (From Rogers 1992, with permission of Elsevier.)

Table 20.2 The cranial nerves

| Number | Name | Functions | |
		Sensory	Motor
I	Olfactory	Nose	–
II	Optic	Eye	–
III	Oculomotor	–	Muscles moving eyeball Ciliary muscle, iris
IV	Trochlear	–	Muscles moving eyeball
V	Trigeminal	Face, tongue, teeth	Muscles of mastication
VI	Abducens	–	Muscles moving eyeball
VII	Facial	Tongue, soft palate	Muscles of face
VIII	Vestibulocochlear	Balance organs, ear	–
IX	Glossopharyngeal	Taste buds, pharynx	Salivary glands
X	Vagus	Tissues and organs of throat, thorax, abdomen	Tissues and organs of throat, thorax, abdomen
XI	Accessory	–	Muscles of head, neck, shoulders
XII	Hypoglossal		Tongue

SUPPORTIVE STRUCTURES

Glial cells

About 90% of the cells within the central nervous system (CNS) are not neurones but glial cells or neuroglia (Fig. 20.12). Glial cells occupy only about 50% of the brain volume, and differ from neurones in that they do not branch as much, nor do they initiate or conduct nerve impulses. At first they were thought to act like 'mortar', but, as more research has been carried out, other varied and important roles for the glial cells have become apparent. These include an action not unlike connective tissue, plus roles in both physical and

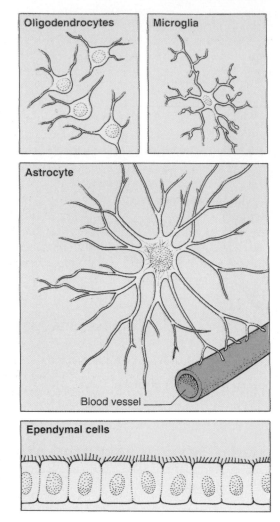

Figure 20.12 Glial cells.

metabolic support. There are four major types of glial cells:

- astrocytes
- oligodendrocytes
- ependymal cells
- microglia.

Much has been learnt recently about the functions of the astrocytes. These star-shaped cells seem to have an important role in regulating the composition of the brain interstitial fluid. They remove some neurotransmitters (glutamate and GABA (γ-amino butyric acid)) and take up potassium from the vicinity of cells. This results in the maintenance of the correct extracellular fluid (ECF) concentration of K⁺, thereby sustaining normal neuronal excitability. Astrocytes are also believed to act as a scaffold during the development of the nervous system. Membrane receptors have been identified on them, making it clear that their function can be regulated. Defective function of these cells is likely to give rise to some neurological disorders.

In a similar way to the Schwann cells of the peripheral nervous system, the oligodendrocytes form the myelin sheath around the axons of central nervous system neurones. The internal cavities of the brain (3rd, 4th and lateral ventricles) are lined with ependymal cells which produce cerebrospinal fluid (CSF; see later). Microglia are derived from the same cell line as the monocytes, which helps to explain the 'immune response' role they carry out in the central nervous system. Under normal circumstances the microglia are stationary and inactive, releasing low levels of nerve growth factor (NGF). NGF is one of the family of substances referred to as neurotrophins, which play an important role in neuronal development and maintenance. When activated by infection or injury the microglia transform into macrophages which remove any debris via the process of phagocytosis. It may be the case that in certain degenerative disorders there is an over-proliferation of these potentially destructive cell types.

Types of brain tumour

The individual brain cell types are sites of specific tumours within the cranium.

Oligodendrocytes give rise to oligodendromas (sometimes known as oligodendrocytomas). These are rare, slow-growing tumours of middle age and are relatively benign.

Astrocytes give rise to astrocytomas grades I–IV, grade IV (known as glioblastoma multiforme) being the most rapidly growing and extremely malignant. The tumour infiltrates surrounding tissues extensively and therefore can seldom be totally removed.

Ependymal cells give rise to ependymomas, which are rare and slow-growing tumours of children and young adults.

The meninges give rise to meningiomas from the arachnoid villi. They are benign in that they do not infiltrate other tissues or show malignant change, but may be life-threatening due to size and site causing difficulty in removal. The commonest malignant brain tumour of childhood is the medulloblastoma arising from the medulla oblongata or the central part of the cerebellum (the vermis).

The acoustic neuroma arises from the myelin sheath of the eighth cranial nerve. It is benign and usually unilateral. An acoustic neuroma may vary in size; therefore the time and symptoms may vary before the patient seeks medical advice.

Brain blood supply

A continuous, uninterrupted blood supply to the brain is critical to maintain normal brain function. As with all cells in the body, the cells of the brain are dependent upon both oxygen and glucose to generate the energy necessary to support normal function. Since the brain has no intrinsic store of glucose, it requires a continuous supply of the nutrient and any interruption of the blood supply will cause a resultant loss of energy substrate supply. Such an interruption in supply can occur as a result of a stroke (haemorrhagic or ischaemic).

The circulation of blood to the brain (cerebral circulation) has several distinctive features that are important in preserving a constant environment for the nerve cells:

- control mechanisms
- capillary function
- venous sinuses.

Control mechanisms

The circulation to the brain is preserved at times when blood flow to other organs is threatened. The baroreceptors located within branches of the carotid arteries are important in registering any drop in pressure and in bringing about corrective changes in the circulation that maintain the pressure of blood to the brain (see Ch. 12).

Sympathetic nerves sparsely innervate the arterioles of the brain. Thus when vasoconstriction occurs elsewhere in the body there is little or no vasoconstriction in the brain. However, local factors, such as the concentration of CO_2, act as powerful vasodilators of the cerebral arterioles. Blood flow to different parts of the brain increases during different activities. It appears that if blood flow increases at one site it is reduced at another (though not to a pathological level) so that the total blood flow to the brain hardly changes. The only notable exception is during an epileptic seizure when significant increases in total cerebral blood flow can occur.

Neurosurgery and trauma cause insults to central nervous system tissue. Following an insult to the brain it is important that the oxygen supply is maintained at a constant level. Hypercapnia and hypoxia both cause cerebral vasodilation. If the cerebral structures are swollen due to surgery or trauma, then vasodilation will increase the intracranial pressure further and reduce the oxygen supply to the cerebral tissue.

Following neurosurgery or trauma to the central nervous system a patient's respiratory system may be controlled through a ventilator in order that their CO_2 and O_2 levels may be maintained at constant levels.

Capillary function

Cerebral capillaries are much less permeable to many constituents of blood than are any other capillaries in the body. Molecules such as glucose that have free access to the interstitial fluid in other tissues have to be transported across cerebral capillaries by carrier mechanisms in order to get through to the brain interstitial fluid in adequate amounts. Many other molecules of this size and greater have difficulty diffusing passively from the blood into the brain tissue fluid. As a result, the nerve cells are not exposed to as high a concentration of many potentially harmful substances as they might be. The unusual restrictiveness of the capillary barrier led scientists to coin the term blood–brain barrier. Substances that can cross this barrier easily are either very small molecules (e.g. water) or they are liposoluble (e.g. alcohol). Gases, such as ammonia, oxygen and carbon dioxide that are both small and liposoluble, cross very easily (Table 20.3).

In a few small areas, including the posterior pituitary and parts of the hypothalamus, the blood capillaries are much more permeable. This permits hormones secreted by these neurones to get into the blood and gives blood-borne substances, such as glucose and fatty acids, freer access to the neurones there.

Drugs and the blood–brain barrier

When central nervous system infections occur, the antibiotic to which the organism is sensitive may not be able to cross the blood–brain barrier. It then becomes necessary to administer it directly into the subarachnoid space. This is done via a lumbar puncture needle, which is inserted between the 3rd and 4th or 4th and 5th lumbar vertebrae – the intrathecal route.

Patients may find this treatment distressing and, apart from the normal reassurances given in such circumstances, some may require an explanation of why 'tablets won't work'. Use your local drug information sources, including your pharmacist, to find out the normal dose of an antibiotic for injection via the intrathecal route. Compare this with the intravenous dose.

Why does the dose of an intravenous antibiotic vary so greatly from the intrathecal dose?

Some drugs do cross the blood–brain barrier. Those that are liposoluble, such as hypnotics, sedatives, analgesics and antidepressants, can diffuse across the lipid component of the membranes. L-dopa, used in the treatment of Parkinson's disease, is transported on a protein carrier. Others cross but do so less easily, for example insulin (a water-soluble polypeptide) crosses only very slowly.

Table 20.3 Permeability of the blood–brain barrier to various substances

Very high	Intermediate	Very low
Water	Glucose	Proteins
Carbon dioxide	Amino acids	Dopamine
Oxygen	Electrolytes (e.g. Na$^+$, K$^+$, Cl$^-$, HCO$_3^-$)	Bilirubin
Ammonia	Urea	Bile salts
Gaseous anaesthetics (e.g. halothane, nitrous oxide)	L-dopa	
Alcohol		

The blood–brain barrier can be disrupted by infection and irradiation, and is abnormal in tumours. Because of this, if an injection of a radiolabelled marker is given, it is possible to identify areas of brain disease, as only these areas will allow the marker to get through.

Venous sinuses

Another distinctive feature of the cerebral circulation is the way in which the venous sinuses are supported by and anchored to adjacent tissue. This prevents them from collapsing even though the pressure of blood here may be sub-atmospheric when someone is standing upright.

Categories of stroke

There are two main categories of stroke (ischaemic and haemorrhagic), both of which prevent the flow of blood, oxygen and key nutrients to the area of the brain normally supplied by the damaged vessel.

Ischaemic strokes occur following the occlusion of a blood vessel by either a thrombus or an embolus. When blood vessels are damaged by atherosclerosis, fatty deposits build up on the wall and project into the blood stream. As these deposits build up, they narrow the vessel and are put under more and more pressure by the arterial blood flow. If the surface of the plaque is damaged a clot can form and narrow the vessel, sometimes to the point of occlusion. This results in a thrombotic stroke and is the most prevalent type. Alternatively, a clot can form somewhere else in the body and a part of it (an embolus) break off and travel through the bloodstream. If this embolus is carried to the brain it can eventually become lodged in a vessel of a smaller diameter, thereby producing an embolic stroke.

Rather than flow being disrupted by the blockage of a vessel, it is also possible that the rupturing of an artery in the brain can cause the disruption. The end result of this haemorrhage is that those areas of the brain normally supplied by the vessel are similarly

Stroke

Someone who has suffered a stroke usually experiences a short period of flaccidity followed by the onset of spasticity. The effects are usually most severe in the muscle groups that flex the leg and extend and lift the arm. This is the result of an exaggeration of normal spinal reflexes. The pattern of spasticity is directly related to the reflexes which normally dominate posture. For example, without appropriate care, the shoulder of the affected side will become fixed lower than the unaffected one, with the elbow joint flexed and the fingers clawed. The nurse should therefore ensure proper positioning and support to maintain correct body alignment and prevent abnormal patterns of posture developing.

Passive exercises should be carried out three or four times a day to maintain mobility and prevent contractures. Importantly, nothing should be placed in the patient's hand or under the sole of the foot, for this would stimulate reflexes and make the situation worse. Untreated spasticity leads to contractures, so, to maximize recovery, physiotherapy needs to be complemented by good nursing care and encouragement from relatives.

deprived of their essential nutrients and oxygen. The clotting of the haemorrhaged blood exacerbates the damage caused by this type of insult. The presence of this clotted mass can cause further displacement of normal brain tissue or the compression of neighbouring vessels.

Pathologic changes during stroke

Cell death occurs due to the failure of the affected cells to synthesize ATP, which is required to support the resynthesis of macromolecules in the normal course of cell maintenance. Cell survival is threatened by this inadequate energy source. Since the cell is unable to use the normal aerobic metabolic processes, it switches to anaerobic metabolism.

However, intracellular acidosis occurs due to this enhanced anaerobic glycolysis. The resultant fall in pH produces depression of mitochondrial respiration and enhanced free radical formation. The increased levels of oxygen radicals lead to lipid peroxidation and the disruption of normal ion homeostasis. Calcium, sodium and chloride ions flow into the cell (with water) and the increased cellular water content causes further cellular damage. The regional brain swelling which occurs causes the neighbouring blood vessels to be compressed and blood supply to the injured area is further reduced.

Meninges

In the same way that other organs and tissues are enveloped by a double layer of membranes (e.g. the pleurae surrounding the lungs, and the peritoneum around the abdominal organs), the brain and spinal cord are enveloped by meninges. The layer in contact with the brain and spinal cord is the pia mater, while that doubled over on top of it is the arachnoid mater (Fig. 20.13). The arachnoid mater is covered in turn by a tough layer called the dura mater. The dura mater enveloping the spinal cord is separated from the adjacent bone tissue (periosteum) by epidural tissue (sometimes known as the epidural space).

The space between the pia mater and the arachnoid mater (subarachnoid space) is filled with cerebrospinal fluid. These membranes extend a little below the end of the spinal cord, forming the lumbar sac. When a lumbar puncture is performed to obtain a sample of CSF, it is this sac that is punctured. Arteries run in the subarachnoid space and branch to form vessels extending into the brain tissue.

Cerebrospinal fluid (CSF)

The CSF (Table 20.4) is secreted by the layer of cells (ependyma) lining the walls of the ventricles, especially those cells covering the out-pouchings of blood vessels (choroid plexus) in each ventricle (Fig. 20.14). About 500 ml of CSF is formed per day. It flows out from the ventricles into the subarachnoid space and thence through the arachnoid villi (or granulations) into the venous sinuses between the dura mater and the skull. The pressure of the CSF in someone lying flat is normally about 130 mmH$_2$O (13 cmH$_2$O; 10 mmHg). This is low compared with arterial blood pressure (100 mmHg). If there is obstruction anywhere in the system, fluid is dammed back, and pressure rises. In the newborn, in whom the bones of the skull are not yet firmly joined, the head swells (hydrocephalus).

The CSF, like the brain interstitial fluid, provides a closely regulated environment shielding most of the central nervous system from the fluctuating concentrations of hormones and other chemicals in the

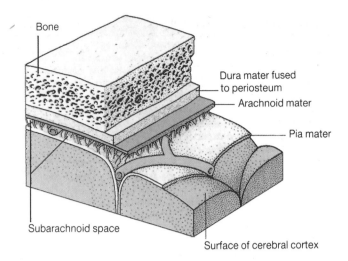

Figure 20.13 Section through part of the skull and cerebral cortex to show the meninges. (From Rogers 1992, with permission of Elsevier.)

Labels: Bone; Dura mater fused to periosteum; Arachnoid mater; Pia mater; Subarachnoid space; Surface of cerebral cortex

Calcium channel blockers

Following a subarachnoid haemorrhage, when the response of the cerebral blood vessels is to constrict, vasoconstriction of cerebral blood vessels may result in a diminished supply of oxygen to cerebral tissue and result in cerebral ischaemia (stroke). Nimodipene is an example of a calcium channel blocking agent. This drug is administered to patients routinely after a diagnosis of a subarachnoid haemorrhage in order to maintain the cerebral blood flow and therefore the supply of oxygen to injured brain tissue.

Table 20.4 Composition of the cerebrospinal fluid (CSF) and plasma

Component (concentration)	CSF	Plasma
Na$^+$ (mmol/l)	147	150
K$^+$ (mmol/l)	3	5
Cl$^-$ (mmol/l)	113	99
HCO$_3^-$ (mmol/l)	25	25
Glucose (mmol/l)	3	5
Urea (mmol/l)	5	6
Protein (g/l)	0.2	70
pH	7.33	7.4

bloodstream. However, substances diffuse freely between the CSF and the brain interstitial fluid, through the ependyma of the ventricles and the pia mater. Consequently, substances injected directly into the CSF can reach brain tissue.

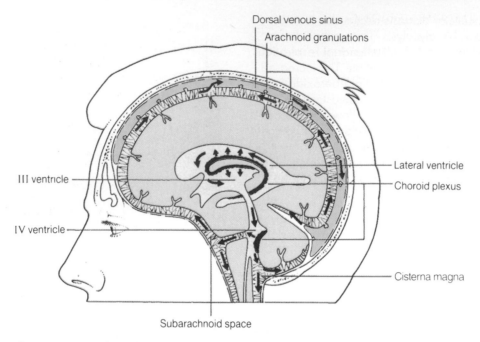

Dorsal venous sinus
Arachnoid granulations

III ventricle

IV ventricle

Lateral ventricle
Choroid plexus

Cisterna magna

Subarachnoid space

Figure 20.14 Flow of CSF from the ventricles via the subarachnoid space into the venous sinuses. (From Rogers 1992, with permission of Elsevier.)

Lumbar puncture

Examination of CSF is diagnostic of a wide range of neurological conditions, including haemorrhage into the subarachnoid space, infection of the central nervous system, e.g. meningitis, and conditions involving demyelination. The pressure of the CSF is also measured during lumbar puncture.

It is the lumbar sac that is punctured during this procedure, and extreme care is required as damage to a small area of the spinal cord may cause widespread disability. The patient is normally positioned on their left side with the spine parallel to the edge of the bed. The patient then flexes knees and hips while bending the head forward. This position opens the spaces between the lumbar vertebrae making the passage of the needle fairly easy. After a specimen of CSF has been obtained, other substances, such as drugs or contrast medium, can be introduced. The latter will clarify the subarachnoid space on X-ray.

Epidural anaesthesia is introduced by the same route but the anaesthetic is injected into the epidural tissue outside the subarachnoid space. Injecting local anaesthetic into the CSF is known as spinal anaesthesia but is rarely used because of the risk of a sudden fall in blood pressure and other complications.

Raised intracranial pressure

After the bones of the skull have become firmly joined, raised CSF pressure usually causes severe headache and other symptoms, e.g. vomiting. If, as the result of a head injury, there is a fracture through the base of the skull, a CSF leak may occur. CSF drips from a nostril or oozes from an ear (CSF rhinorrhoea and otorrhoea). To reduce the risk of organisms entering the skull and brain, the patient should avoid sniffing, blowing the nose or attempting to clean the ear.

If the patient requires enteral feeding following a new diagnosis of a base of the skull fracture, then this is a contraindication to the passage of a nasogastric tube. An alternative method of delivering enteral feeding must be found.

REFERENCES AND FURTHER READING

Carpenter R 1997 Neurophysiology, 3rd edn. Oxford University Press, Oxford

Critchley M (ed) 1980 Butterworths medical dictionary, 2nd edn. Butterworths, London

Diamond M C, Schiebel A B, Elson L M 1985 The human brain coloring book. Harper Collins, New York

Gertz D 1999 Liebman's Neuroanatomy made easy and understandable, 6th edn. Aspen Publishers, Maryland

Hillman H, Jarman D 1991 Atlas of the cellular structure of the human nervous system. Academic Press, London

Kiernan J A 1998 Barr's 'The Human Nervous System'. Lippincott/Williams & Wilkins, Baltimore, MD

Lasserson D, Gabriel C, Sharrack B 1997 Crash course! Nervous system and special senses. Mosby, St Louis

Longstaff A 2000 Instant notes in neuroscience. Bios, Oxford

Rogers A W 1992 Textbook of anatomy. Churchill Livingstone, Edinburgh

Roland P E, Freiberg L 1985 Localisation of cortical areas activated by thinking. Journal of Neurophysiology 53: 1219–1243

Sanes D H, Reh T A, Harris W A 2000 Development of the nervous system. Academic Press, San Diego

Shepherd G M 1994 Neurobiology, 3rd edn. Oxford University Press, Oxford

Williams P L 1995 Gray's Anatomy, 38th edn. Churchill Livingstone, Edinburgh

Sensory systems: an overview

Our sensory systems enable us to detect, analyse and respond to some of the many different forms of energy to which we are exposed. The selection is made by our sensory receptors. These are set up to respond to some forms of energy much more readily than others.

Impulses generated by the receptors are transmitted along a variety of nerve pathways to several destinations in the central nervous system. Some sensory pathways (specific sensory systems) link up the receptors to cells of the cerebral cortex in a point-to-point way, so that 'maps' of sensory information are created in the brain. These pathways mediate specific sensations like those of vision, hearing, touch, taste, smell and pain. Other nerve pathways (non-specific sensory systems) channel sensory signals to the cerebral cortex via the reticular formation of the brain stem. Part of these non-specific systems, the reticular activating system, controls our level of alertness and consciousness.

All sensory information arrives at the cerebral cortex in the form of action potentials. From these impulses our minds create the impressions we have of our surroundings and ourselves. The impressions created depend upon the destination of the information in the brain, the number and blend of signals arriving there, and how they have been analysed en route. If sensory systems are disordered then our impression of reality alters and our responses change.

SENSORY RECEPTORS

TYPES

Sensory receptors are specialized neurones that detect and respond to changes occurring in their vicinity. These changes may be:

- mechanical (e.g. stretch, compression)
- chemical (e.g. concentration of kinins, histamine etc.)
- electromagnetic (e.g. radiation from the sun)
- thermal.

Although any receptor can be excited by any form of stimulus, provided it is strong enough, each receptor responds best to a particular type of stimulus. Thus receptors can be classified as:

- mechanoreceptors
- chemoreceptors

- photoreceptors
- thermoreceptors.

Within each group, receptors are specialized to respond to a particular form of that stimulus. For example, in the skin there is a variety of mechanoreceptors. Some are very sensitive and respond to the lightest of touches. Others respond only when pressure is applied. In the eye too there are four different types of photoreceptor (red rods, green rods, blue rods and cones), each of which responds best to a slightly different range of wavelengths of electromagnetic radiation, allowing us to have both day and night vision.

SENSITIVITY

The specific sensitivity of the receptor depends in part on the specialization of the receptor itself. For example, the four different photoreceptors in the eye each contain a different pigment. Each pigment absorbs electro-magnetic radiation of a different range of wavelengths.

But sensitivity can also depend on the accessory structures associated with the receptor because these determine the kind of stimuli that actually get through to it. For example, the receptors both in the ear and in the balance organs (vestibular apparatus) are hair cells that are excited when their cilia bend (Fig. 21.1). In the

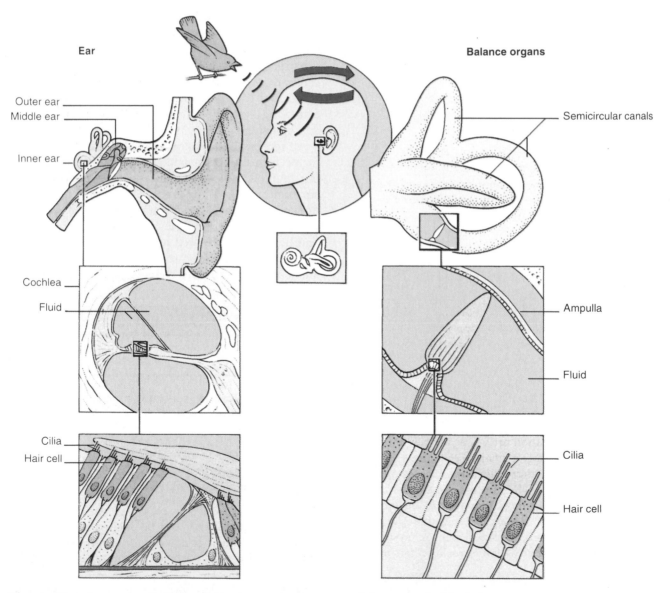

Figure 21.1 Receptor cells (hair cells) and accessory structures of the ear and of the balance organs. Note the similarities and differences between the two sense organs.

ear, however, the bending is caused by vibrations (produced for example by a musical instrument), which are transmitted through the outer and middle ear to the fluid of the inner ear, whereas in the semicircular canals of the balance organs, bending of the cilia results from fluid movement within the canals caused by turning, lifting or lowering the head (Fig. 21.1).

STRUCTURE

Some receptors consist simply of the endings of a sensory neurone (unspecialized nerve endings). Other receptors have endings that are visibly adapted to form specialized structures (Fig. 21.2). If the endings are walled off from the surrounding tissues they are termed encapsulated endings (e.g. Pacinian corpuscles, Meissner's corpuscles in the skin).

Some receptor cells (such as photoreceptors in the eye and hair cells in the ear; Fig. 21.2) are separate from the sensory neurones transmitting signals into the central nervous system. In these cases the sensory neurones are excited by neurotransmitters released by the receptor cells.

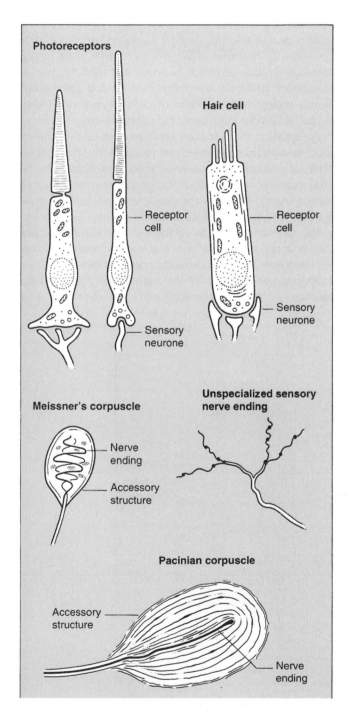

Figure 21.2 Examples of several different sensory receptors.

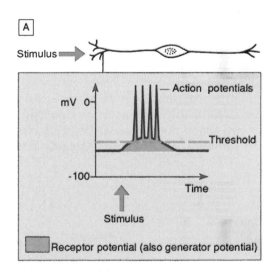

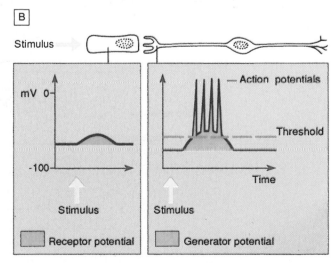

Figure 21.3 Electrical events recorded in response to a stimulus from: A, a sensory nerve ending; B, a receptor cell (e.g. a hair cell) and its sensory neurone.

EXCITATION

Sensory receptors of any kind convert the energy of a stimulus into a change in the voltage (receptor potential) of the receptor cell membrane (Fig. 21.3A). If the change in voltage is big enough it will generate one or more action potentials which are then conducted along the sensory neurone.

In the systems in which receptor cells and sensory neurones are separate (Fig. 21.3B), excitation is passed from cell to cell by the release and action of neuro-transmitters until a cell is reached that is able to generate an action potential and carry the signal in that form into the central nervous system.

The change in voltage actually giving rise to the action potential is termed the generator potential. Unlike an action potential, it can be large or small depending on the strength of the original stimulus. Also it develops more slowly and lasts longer, as can be seen in Figure 21.3A & B. Because of this, a single stimulus can produce more than one action potential. As long as the membrane voltage remains over the threshold level (say at $-50\,mV$ if threshold was $-60\,mV$) action potentials will keep on being generated. If the initial stimulus was small, the membrane at the ending will return to its unexcited state very quickly and only one or two action potentials will be generated. However, if the stimulus was large, the generator potential will be bigger and will stay over threshold level for longer, and consequently more action potentials will be fired. In this way the strength of a stimulus is translated into the frequency of action potentials (number of action potentials per second) in a sensory neurone.

ADAPTATION

If the stimulus is maintained, the receptor begins to get used to it. It adapts to the stimulus. The frequency of action potentials (number of impulses per second) in the sensory neurone gradually decreases even though the size of the stimulus has not changed (Fig. 21.4). Receptors differ in the degree to which they adapt. Some adapt very quickly (phasic receptors). Others adapt only very slightly (tonic receptors).

Adaptation is useful in that it reduces the amount of information that has to be processed by the brain at any time. If our minds have registered and stored the fact that a change has occurred in our environment, then the next thing that is important to know is when there is a further change. While all remains steady there is little point in continually receiving exactly the same, very detailed report. A note of what is going on (from tonic receptors) will do. But when circumstances change it is important to know fully the nature and extent of that change.

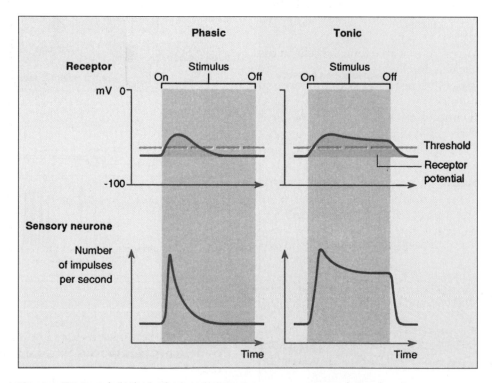

Figure 21.4 Adaptation of sensory receptors to a maintained stimulus. Some receptors (phasic receptors) adapt quickly and completely whereas others (tonic receptors) hardly adapt at all.

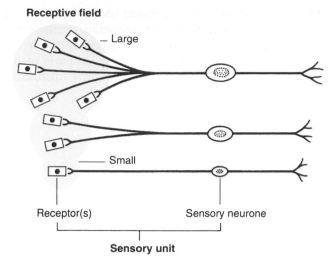

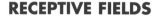

Figure 21.5 Sensory units and receptive fields. A sensory unit consists of one sensory neurone together with all the sensory receptors to which it is linked.

RECEPTIVE FIELDS

A sensory neurone may have several endings, or be connected to several receptor cells (Fig. 21.5). The result of this arrangement is that a stimulus that activates any of the endings or receptors will generate impulses in the same sensory neurone. The area covered by the sensory neurone in this way is termed its receptive field. If there are many receptors or endings spread over a wide area then the receptive field is large. If there is only one receptor per ending (as for example for cone cells in the eye) the receptive field is small.

The size of the receptive field makes a difference to the accuracy with which stimuli can be located and to the sharpness of the impression gained by our minds. If the receptive field of a sensory neurone is large, our impression of the stimulus will be vague. A good example is the difference between vision at night and in broad daylight. In the daytime when the cones are used for vision, the picture is much sharper than at night, when the rods are used. The neurones carrying information to the brain from the rods have large receptive fields, whereas those from the cones are small.

ROUTING OF SENSORY SIGNALS

Impulses generated in the sensory neurones follow several different routes to arrive at various destinations in the nervous system (Fig. 21.6). Impulses are transmitted to:

- motor neurones via interneurones to activate muscles (reflex pathways)

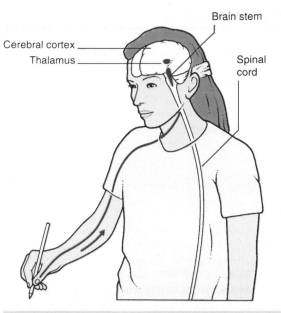

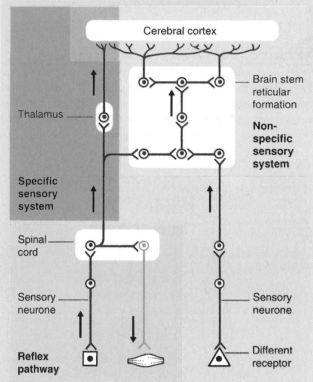

Figure 21.6 Where impulses from sensory receptors travel to within the central nervous system and how they get there.

- chains of neurones carrying impulses to the cerebral cortex (specific sensory systems, e.g. visual, auditory etc.)
- neurones that transmit impulses to the cerebral cortex via the reticular formation (non-specific sensory system).

REFLEX PATHWAYS

When you pick up something painfully hot, and then drop it without thinking, your instinctive response is caused by the sensory impulses generated by the nociceptors in your hand that reflexly excite muscles of your arm. Much that we do is powered by reflex responses of this kind.

Syringomyelia is the development of a space (syrinx) within the spinal cord. The syrinx acts like a space-occupying lesion. The patient may report a loss of temperature sense and consequently protective reflexes are impaired. Therefore patients with this type of sensory loss need special consideration when, for example, being served with extra-hot drinks, sitting next to very hot radiators or being provided with unprotected hot water bottles.

SPECIFIC SENSORY SYSTEMS

The impulses that pass to the cerebral cortex follow relatively direct routes in which there are few intervening synapses. The main relay stations en route are in the spinal cord and brain stem, and the two thalami (one thalamus in each cerebral hemisphere). There are very ordered relationships between the sensory receptors and neurones in these parts of the central nervous system resulting in three distinctive features of specific sensory systems:

- sidedness
- mapping
- proportional representation.

Sidedness

The primary sensory fibres synapse first in the central nervous system on the same side of the midline as the receptors are located. Subsequently, with only a few exceptions, the second order nerve axons cross over the midline. Thus information from one side of the body is transmitted to parts of the brain on the opposite side (i.e. contralaterally) (Fig. 21.7A). The second order fibres carry the impulses to the thalami. From here the impulses are transmitted to specific regions of the cerebral cortex (primary sensory receiving areas). Thus information from the right side of the body (about touch, warmth, sight etc.) is registered in the left cerebral hemisphere, and information from the left side goes to the right cerebral hemisphere. For our sense of vision it is important to be aware that the information

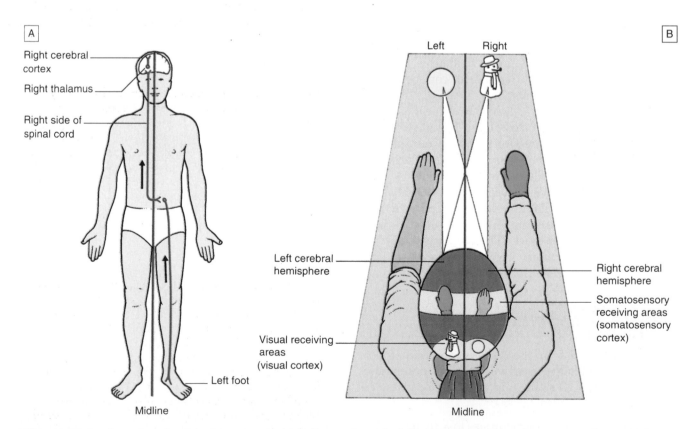

A
Right cerebral cortex
Right thalamus
Right side of spinal cord
Left foot
Midline

B
Left   Right
Left cerebral hemisphere
Visual receiving areas (visual cortex)
Right cerebral hemisphere
Somatosensory receiving areas (somatosensory cortex)
Midline

Figure 21.7 The right side of the brain receives information from the left side of the body and vice versa, for example information about: A, pressure on the skin; B, objects to the left of the midline.

that is registered in each hemisphere is not what is seen by the eye on the opposite side of the body, but all those things, seen by both eyes, that lie to one side or the other of the midline (Fig. 21.7B).

'Maps' of the body

Each of the neurones in the chain between the receptors and the cerebral cortex (Fig. 21.6) may be likened to a team member in a relay race. Just as the baton gets passed between consecutive members of the team, but not between members of different teams, so sensory signals get directed in an ordered way to specific places in the thalamus and then in the cerebral cortex. The relationship of adjacent neurones to one another is preserved faithfully so that adjacent areas of the cerebral cortex register information from receptors that were next to one another (in the skin or eye for example) in the same way that a geographer's map faithfully records the relative positions of different features on the land.

Scale of representation

If part of the body is richly supplied with sensory receptors, then this is matched within the central nervous system by the number of cells devoted to that part of the body. This is seen clearly in the part of the cerebral cortex receiving information from receptors in the skin and muscles (somatosensory cortex) (Fig. 21.7B). Large parts of the somatosensory cortex deal with information from the hands and from the face (Fig. 21.8). Both of these places are richly supplied with sensory receptors. In contrast, very much smaller areas of the somatosensory cortex are devoted to the trunk and limbs, where there are fewer receptors. You can get some impression of this fact of physiology if you close your eyes, try to forget what you look like and consider how big you would think different parts of your body are just from the way that they feel. Usually one is very aware of face and hands and less so of trunk and legs.

THE NON-SPECIFIC SENSORY SYSTEM

Sensory impulses are transmitted to the reticular formation of the brain stem via branches (collaterals) of the neurones in the specific sensory systems. The reticular formation is a network of neurones (hence its name – reticulum means 'little net') extending through the brain stem. Impulses are passed from cell to cell across many synapses. Eventually excitation is passed on to the cerebral cortex but it is not restricted to discrete areas of the cortex (such as the somatosensory cortex and the visual cortex) and it is no longer identifiable as coming from specific receptors.

What appears to happen is that information from different senses is pooled in the reticular formation (Fig. 21.6). This pooled activity generates impulses that are chiefly transmitted to the association areas of the cerebral cortex. This sensitizes these cortical cells so that they respond easily to the identifiable signals reaching them via the specific sensory systems. The non-specific sensory system thus arouses cortical cells and determines how responsive they are to incoming signals.

Reticular activating system

The cells in the reticular formation and the pathways carrying the excitation on to the cerebral cortex are collectively termed the reticular activating system (RAS). When activity in this system is high, we are

---

When a limb is amputated the axons of the sensory neurones are cut across, but the cell bodies remain intact in the dorsal root ganglion. Consequently the nerves do not degenerate. The cut ends may sprout (see Ch. 25) and the nerves can still transmit impulses. If the nerves are irritated and therefore excited, impulses will be transmitted to the brain, giving rise to an impression that the limb is still there.

The presence of a cerebral tumour, degeneration of the cerebral cortex, or other disease processes may stimulate cortical cells to produce abnormal sensations. The sensations might include a feeling of hot or cold water trickling down limbs, insects crawling over the skin or excessive heat. Visual disturbances occur in the form of hallucinations, including the bright, shimmering fortifications and flashing lights experienced by migraine sufferers. It is also possible to experience smells (usually unpleasant) and tastes in the absence of external stimulation.

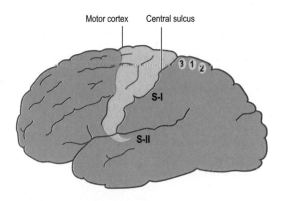

Figure 21.8 The sensory cortex. (After Davies et al 2001, with permission of Elsevier.)

awake and alert. When activity is low, we fall asleep. The level of activity depends in part upon the amount of sensory information that is being fed into the system. On a very hot, bright, sunny day, with the noise of traffic, voices and daily activities outside, it may not be easy to get to sleep even after a tiring spell of night duty. The reason for this is the raised level of activity in the RAS. Conversely, sitting in a darkened classroom listening to a monotonous voice talking dully about physiology may well have the opposite effect!

Anaesthesia, sleep and coma

Because sensory signals are passed between so many synapses in the reticular formation, this pathway is particularly susceptible to the blocking action of some drugs. If transmission at each synapse is reduced even slightly, the cumulative effect, after many synapses have been traversed, will be large. So it is possible to produce anaesthesia by damping down the activity of the RAS, without blocking the transmission of nerve impulses everywhere else (see Ch. 29).

General anaesthesia is not the same as sleep in that someone cannot be aroused easily from it. This marks the difference between a state of unconsciousness (not arousable) and sleep (arousable). Unconsciousness may be temporary, as in a faint or under anaesthesia, or it may be prolonged or even permanent, as in cases of damage to the RAS. It is then termed coma.

Electroencephalogram (EEG)

Different levels of consciousness are associated with different patterns of electrical activity in the brain as recorded from electrodes placed on the scalp. The pattern of activity changes as an awake person gradually drifts off to sleep. In the awake state, the electroencephalogram (EEG) gives a series of low voltage, fast frequency waves. As someone drifts off to sleep, the waves become bigger but there are fewer of them. In the awake but relaxed state with eyes closed, the pattern seen is described as the alpha rhythm. In deep sleep the waves are bigger and occur less frequently. In brain death no waves are seen at all.

REFERENCES AND FURTHER READING

Bloch G J 1985 Body and self: elements of human biology, behaviour and health. W H Freeman, Oxford

Bryan J 1993 Smell, taste and touch: the sensory systems. Prentice Hall, Upper Saddle River, NJ

Clarke K A 1989 Neurophysiology: application in behavioural and biomedical sciences. Ellis Harwood, Chichester

Davies A, Blakeley A G H, Kidd C 2001 Human physiology. Churchill Livingstone, Edinburgh

Lasserson D, Gabriel C, Sharrack B 1997 Crash course! Nervous system and special senses. Mosby, St Louis

Penfield W, Rasmussen T 1968 The cerebral cortex of man: a clinical study of localisation of function. Macmillan, New York

Salter M (ed) 1997 Altered body image – the nurse's role, 2nd edn. Baillière Tindall, London

Smith C U M 2000 Biology of sensory systems. John Wiley, Chichester

22 Body senses, proprioception, taste and smell

The sensations which we perceive are created in our minds as a result of the activation of a variety of sensory receptors, many of which are situated in the skin. Information from these and other receptors is carried into the central nervous system via spinal and cranial nerves, and is then routed to the cerebral cortex via specific pathways in the spinal cord and brain stem.

Awareness of the position and movement of our bodies is specifically termed proprioception. It is derived from sensory information flowing from receptors in muscles and joints, and the balance organs, as well as the skin. Proprioception is very important in posture and movement.

The sensations of taste and smell, vital to our enjoyment of food as well as our protection, are mediated by receptors in the mouth and nose.

BODY SENSES

RECEPTORS

Skin

Types of receptor

There are a variety of receptor endings in the skin (Fig. 22.1). Some are free nerve endings, while others, such as Meissner's corpuscles, Merkel's discs, Ruffini endings and Pacinian corpuscles (all of which are mechanoreceptors), have characteristic structures determining the stimuli that are most effective in exciting them. For example, the layers enveloping the nerve ending in the Pacinian corpuscle act as a filter so that only certain mechanical stimuli will get through.

Most cutaneous receptors are situated in the dermis (Fig. 22.1). Meissner's corpuscles and Merkel's discs are situated at the boundary between the epidermis and the dermis. The nerve terminals of Ruffini endings intermingle with collagen fibres in the dermis, and Pacinian corpuscles are found in deeper layers of the skin and in the subcutaneous tissue (see Ch. 16).

The position of the receptors influences the kind of stimuli that excite them. Receptors situated deeper in the skin may require a larger external stimulus to excite them whereas some receptors, such as Ruffini endings, can be excited by stimuli at a distance as a result of the forces tugging on fibres, such as collagen, in the skin.

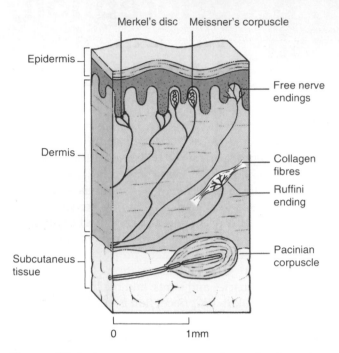

Figure 22.1 Sensory receptors in non-hairy skin (e.g. skin of the palms of the hands and soles of the feet).

Sensory units

Most cutaneous receptors do not have their own 'private line' to the brain. Usually receptors of the same type are grouped together into sensory units, each unit being innervated by a single nerve fibre. For example, several Meissner's corpuscles, each tucked up in one of the papillary ridges of the dermis, are grouped together and served by the same sensory neurone (Fig. 22.1).

The sensory units differ in their characteristics (Table 22.1). Some have small receptive fields whereas others have large ones. Some units adapt rapidly to a maintained stimulus whereas others do not. All these features affect the quality of the sensations we experience.

Hairy and non-hairy skin

The sensory innervation of the skin is not the same all over the body. Differences exist in the numbers and types of receptor present. Some differences between hairy and non-hairy (glabrous) skin are listed in Table 22.2.

The glabrous skin of the palmar surface of the hand is especially richly endowed with sensory units. The total number of mechanoreceptive sensory units has been estimated to be about 17 000. The number per unit area is very high, especially on the fingertips (about 240 per cm^2).

Similarly, the skin of the soles of the feet differs from that on the top of the feet, and the skin of the trunk and limbs differs from that of the hands and feet.

Sensations

The different sensations that we identify, namely touch, pressure, pain, itch, heat, cold etc., do not correspond exactly to the different types of receptor seen under the microscope. Information from more than one receptor type is usually combined in our minds to create different feelings. Some of the receptors that are believed to contribute to the different sensations we experience are listed in Table 22.3. It is interesting that free nerve endings are believed to mediate a variety of sensations, which suggests that there are differences in the structure of the endings not revealed by histology.

Organs and tissues of the body cavities

All tissues and organs of the body are innervated by sensory receptors but not all of these contribute to the sensations we experience. For example, baroreceptors and chemoreceptors detect changes in the internal

Table 22.1 Characteristics of sensory units in the glabrous skin of the hand*

Type[†]	Constituent receptors	Rate of adaptation	Breadth of receptive field (mm)	Usefulness
SA I	Merkel's discs	Slow	2–8	Outlining and locating the texture and shape of objects in contact with the skin
FA I	Meissner's corpuscles	Fast		
SA II	Ruffini endings	Slow	40–80	Broadly registering forces exerted on and in the skin (e.g. when holding an object or moving the finger and thumb)
FA II	Pacinian corpuscles	Fast		

* Compiled from Johansson & Vallbo 1983.
† Defined by characteristics of the units, such as rate of adaptation (SA, slow adapting; FA, fast adapting).

Table 22.2 Hairy and non-hairy human skin: distinguishing features

	Hairy	**Non-hairy**
Structure	'Thin' epidermis* Not ridged	'Thick' epidermis* Ridged
Sensory units	Less numerous	Very numerous
Sensory receptors	Many sensory endings close to hair follicles Ruffini endings Free nerve endings	Merkel's discs Meissner's corpuscles Pacinian corpuscles Ruffini endings Free nerve endings
Glands	Sebaceous (associated with hair follicles)	Sweat glands numerous

* Epidermal thickness ranges between 0.1 mm (thin) and 0.5 mm (thick). Total thickness of the skin ranges between about 1 and 5 mm in different parts of the body.

Table 22.3 Cutaneous receptors and sensations

Receptors	Sensation(s)
Nerve endings associated with hair follicles	Touch
Free nerve endings	Warmth, cold, pain
Merkel's discs	Pressure
Meissner's corpuscles	Tapping
Pacinian corpuscles	Vibration (high frequency) Tickle

environment but we are not consciously aware of the fluctuations in blood pressure and blood composition that they detect. But there are other receptors that do give rise to a variety of different sensations, including pain, 'fullness' (of the stomach for example) and warmth.

The majority of these receptors are unspecialized nerve endings. They are found in various places, including the walls of:

- blood vessels
- the gastrointestinal tract
- the bladder.

Effective stimuli for these receptors include ischaemia and distension.

In addition, free nerve endings and specialized mechanoreceptors like some of those in the skin (such as Pacinian corpuscles) are found in the epithelia and connective tissue enveloping organs in the thoracic, abdominal and cranial cavities (pleurae, peritoneum, meninges). Cutting, as in a surgical operation for example, excites some of these receptors.

Muscles, tendons and joints

Sensory receptors in muscles, tendons and joints are very important in the control of movement. They also contribute to our bodily sense, especially proprioception. These receptors include:

- joint receptors
- Golgi tendon organs
- muscle spindles.

Joint receptors

The sensory receptors found in the lining surfaces of the joints include:

- Ruffini endings
- receptors similar to, but smaller than, Pacinian corpuscles
- free nerve endings.

Excitation of these cells contributes to our awareness of the angle at which joints are held and of movement. If there is inflammation, as in arthritis for example, irritation of some of the receptors contributes to the sensation of pain.

Golgi tendon organs

Golgi tendon organs are relatively simple in structure (Fig. 22.2). They consist of a set of branching nerve terminals lodged between the collagen fibres of the tendons attached to muscles. When a muscle contracts, it pulls on the collagen fibres, compresses the nerve endings and excites them. Golgi tendon organs monitor the amount of tension developed in the motor unit attached to their bundle of collagen fibres (see Chs 4B, 25).

Muscle spindles

Muscle spindles provide information about the length at which muscles are held and how that changes as we move.

Each spindle consists of a group of tiny modified muscle fibres (intrafusal fibres) surrounded by a connective tissue capsule (Fig. 22.2). These tiny fibres lie

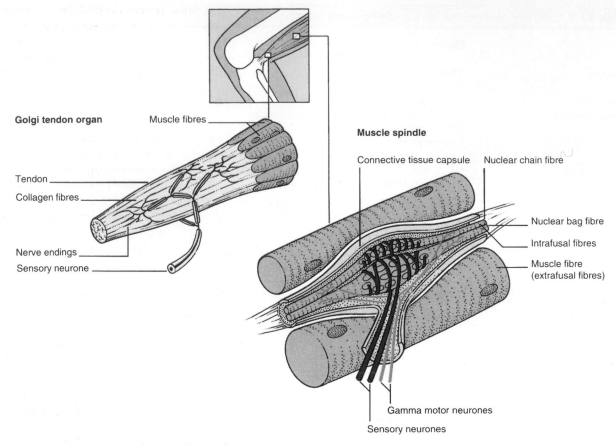

Figure 22.2 Structure of a Golgi tendon organ and a muscle spindle.

in between the much larger true muscle fibres (extrafusal fibres). The sensory part of the spindle is in the middle portion of the intrafusal fibre. When it is stretched, impulses are triggered (Fig. 22.3A) and conducted along the sensory neurone. Thus, whenever a muscle is lengthened (for example when you extend your arm the biceps lengthens), the spindles are excited. When the muscle is made shorter, there is less stretch and fewer impulses are fired.

The sensitivity of the spindle to stretch is adjusted by varying the contraction of the muscular part of the intrafusal fibre (Fig. 22.3B). When the muscular part contracts it makes the sensory portion of the spindle tauter and more sensitive to further stretch. If, however, the muscle fibres of the spindle are completely relaxed then the sensitive part is not under tension and the spindle is not very responsive.

Contraction of the muscular part of the intrafusal fibres is controlled by the somatic motor neurones innervating them (gamma motor neurones) (Fig. 22.2) and these in turn are influenced by the systems in the brain and spinal cord controlling posture and movement.

There are at least two types of intrafusal fibre (Fig. 22.2):

- nuclear bag
- nuclear chain.

Each has slightly different characteristics. The bag fibres respond best to a sudden stretch (a change in length), and adapt quickly to a stretch if it is maintained, whereas the nuclear chain fibres do not adapt very quickly. Consequently, it is the chain fibres that provide information continuously to the brain about the length at which the extrafusal fibres are being held, while the bag fibres signal abrupt changes (see also Chs 4B, 25).

SENSORY NEURONES

Size and properties

The sensory neurones innervating all the receptors described so far in the skin, muscles, joints and tendons differ in size and properties. Neurones range in size from tiny unmyelinated nerve axons of the free nerve endings mediating the sensations of pain, heat and cold, to large myelinated axons innervating the muscle spindles and the Golgi tendon organs (Table 22.4). The transmission of impulses in the large myelinated fibres is much faster than that in the small unmyelinated

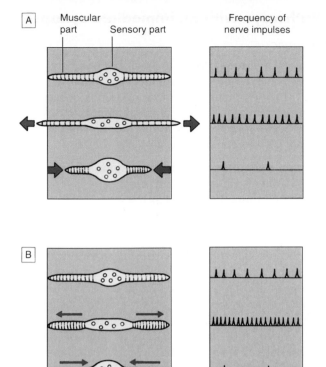

Figure 22.3 How the frequency of action potentials in the sensory neurone from a muscle spindle varies with: A, the length of the intrafusal fibre; B, contraction and relaxation of the muscular part of the intrafusal fibres.

fibres. The fibres also differ in their susceptibility to the effects of an anaesthetic block, such as a local anaesthetic, and to ischaemia.

Sensory neurones innervating different receptors from one part of the body are grouped together to form a mixed nerve. This mixed nerve also includes the axons of motor neurones supplying that region. If this mixed nerve becomes ischaemic, and therefore hypoxic (for example as a result of pressure compressing the blood vessels), transmission of impulses in some of the fibres will be blocked more readily than in others. The consequence is that an unusual blend of sensory information will be received by the brain from that area and the part of the body served by the nerve will feel odd (paraesthesia). The most familiar example of paraesthesia is the curious and usually painful feelings following the numbness of a limb 'gone to sleep'. Another relatively common clinical example is the altered sensation experienced by someone with carpal tunnel syndrome.

Dermatomes and myotomes

Each spinal or cranial nerve carrying somatic sensory information transmits that information from particular areas of the body. The area of skin innervated by one spinal nerve is termed a dermatome (Fig. 22.4) and the muscles innervated are referred to as a myotome. Injury to a particular spinal nerve or to a nerve root therefore produces a predictable pattern of sensory loss.

Somatic and autonomic fibres

Sensory receptors in the skin, joints and muscles are innervated by somatic nerves, whereas those mediating bodily sensation from internal organs and other tissues, including blood vessels everywhere, are mostly innervated by autonomic nerves. The axons of somatic sensory neurones and autonomic neurones are bundled

Table 22.4 Characteristics of sensory neurones innervating somatic receptors

| Receptors | Sensation | Sensory neurones | | Susceptibility to blockage by: | |
		Diameter (μm)*	Classification	Ischaemia	Local anaesthesia
Muscle spindles Golgi tendon organs	Proprioception	13	A alpha	Average	Below average
Cutaneous mechanoreceptors	Touch Pressure	11	A alpha		
Thermoreceptors Nociceptors	Cold Pain	4	A delta		
Thermoreceptors Nociceptors	Cold Heat Pain	1	C	Below average	Above average

* Typical values.

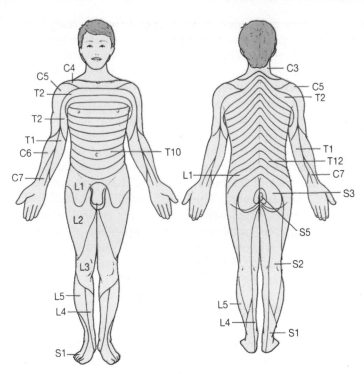

Figure 22.4 The dermatomes: areas of the skin innervated by each of the spinal nerves. (From Rogers 1992, with permission of Elsevier.)

together with the axons of motor neurones to form the spinal and cranial nerves.

Autonomic nerves are associated only with certain of the spinal and cranial nerves. Thus sensory information from internal organs and tissues converges with that from the skin and muscles, entering the spinal cord and brain stem at particular levels (for example segments S2 to S4). This convergence of information affects the impression we have of the source of sensations originating from internal organs and tissues.

PATHWAYS IN THE SPINAL CORD AND BRAIN STEM

Sensory axons entering the central nervous system may:

- synapse immediately with interneurones in the grey matter of the cord or brain stem
- continue up the spinal cord or brain stem before synapsing further on.

The following description focuses on the pathways in the spinal cord carrying information from the spinal nerves, but the same principles apply to pathways in the brain stem carrying information from the cranial nerves.

Pathways with an immediate synapse

Somatic

Sensory neurones that synapse immediately include those mediating the sensations of touch, pain, heat and cold. In the spinal cord these neurones synapse with interneurones in several of the laminae that, in turn, give rise to long axons carrying the information up the spinal cord to one of three sites (Fig. 22.5):

- brain stem reticular formation (spinoreticular tracts)
- thalamus (spinothalamic tracts)
- cerebellum (spinocerebellar tracts).

Sensations of touch, pain, heat and cold are mediated by the spinoreticular and spinothalamic tracts. The spinocerebellar tracts carry proprioceptive information used in the control of movement, from mechanoreceptors in the joints, muscles and the skin overlying them, to the cerebellum.

The spinoreticular and spinothalamic tracts run up the spinal cord on the opposite side of the body (contralaterally) to that from which the sensory signals have come. Interneurones connect the primary sensory fibres with ascending tracts, which carry the signals up the opposite side of the spinal cord (Fig. 22.6). Because of this crossover of information in the spinal cord, sensory signals mediating touch, pain, heat and cold from the left side of the body are transmitted up spinal tracts on the right side of the cord and vice versa.

The spinocerebellar tracts differ from this. Some carry impulses up the same side of the cord as their point of entry (ipsilaterally) whereas others carry them up the opposite side (contralaterally).

Autonomic

Autonomic nerves also synapse with interneurones in the laminae of the cord. Some of the interneurones with which they synapse are the same as those used by some somatic fibres. Where this happens sensory signals from autonomic and somatic fibres converge on to the same neurones. The consequence is that from that point onwards the brain cannot distinguish impulses originating in an internal organ from those originating in somatic structures such as the skin. As the more usual source of sensation is the somatic one, any signals are interpreted as having originated from the skin and not from the internal organ. This is one explanation of referred pain, the pain caused by injury or disease of an internal organ or tissue that is felt to be coming from another part of the body such as the arm or the back.

Pathways without an immediate synapse

Some primary sensory neurones, having entered the central nervous system, continue for a distance up the

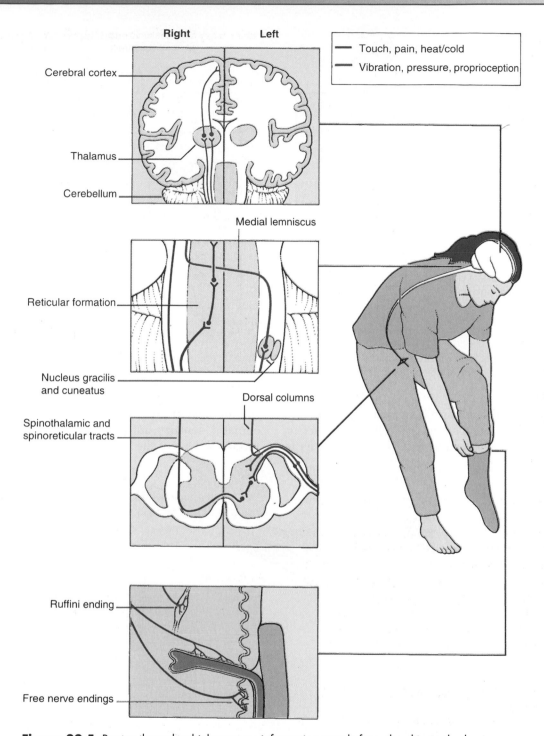

Figure 22.5 Routes through which sensory information travels from the skin to the brain.

spinal cord as very long axons before synapsing. This applies to neurones mediating the sensations of pressure, vibration and proprioception. In the spinal cord, these nerve fibres form bundles of fibres (dorsal columns) running up the cord on the same side as their point of entry (Fig. 22.5). The left dorsal column carries sensory information from the left side of the body and the right dorsal column from the right side. The primary sensory neurones giving rise to the dorsal columns do, however, also give off branches (collaterals) that synapse in the laminae of the grey matter. These collateral fibres are involved in influencing the transmission of signals through other pathways, for example the spinoreticular tracts, which mediate the sensation of pain.

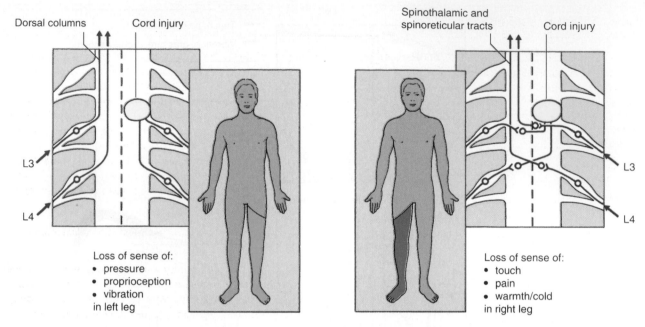

Figure 22.6 Effects of an area of injury on one side of the lumbar region of the spinal cord on sensation in the legs. Note that both legs are affected but in different ways.

Axons of the dorsal column neurones synapse first in the medulla of the brain stem with cells of the nucleus gracilis and the nucleus cuneatus. These two nuclei in

the medulla are the first level in this pathway where somatic sensory information can be analysed or modified. One of the functions of interneurones in the

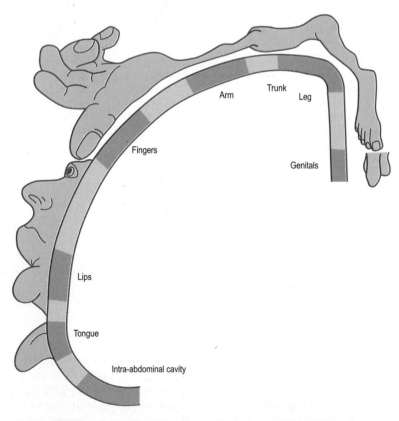

Figure 22.7 The sensory cortex. (After Davies et al 2001, with permission of Elsevier.)

How sensation is tested

A full neurological examination cannot be carried out properly when time is at a premium. If the patient is to give reliable answers to the tests, he must feel relaxed and reassured. To gain some idea of how a patient feels during the specific assessment of sensation, ask a colleague to carry out the tests described below on you, under two conditions:

- with the tester in a hurry and urging the 'patient' to make quick decisions
- with the tester relaxed and assuring the 'patient' that there is plenty of time.

Then decide which you felt was the most accurate assessment.

Before commencing the examination, it is usual for the neurologist to enquire whether the patient suffers from any abnormal spontaneous sensation (paraesthesia), such as pain, numbness, tingling, 'pins and needles', 'electric shocks'. During the tests, the patient is asked to close his eyes so that sensations from the body surface are experienced without visual perception of their cause.

The integrity of the following sensory pathways is tested:

- the lateral spinothalamic pathway – chiefly mediating pain and temperature sense
- the anterior spinothalamic pathway – chiefly mediating touch and pressure sense
- the posterior (dorsal) column pathway – light touch, proprioception and vibration.

The results of these tests, though somewhat crude, indicate where a lesion might be sited and, hence, which more specific investigations are required. The development of sophisticated scanning has reduced the need for many neurological investigations, for example lumbar air encephalography and arteriography, but the crude tests are still used to indicate to the neurologist and radiologist where to look for a lesion. The tests outlined below are all performed with the patient's eyes closed.

Pain and temperature – lateral spinothalamic pathway

- Pain is tested by lightly pricking the skin with a sterile needle. The patient is asked whether he can feel anything and, if so, to describe the feeling (is the experience sharpness, pain, or both?) and its location. Areas of cutaneous numbness, for example, can be mapped by dragging a needle across the skin, the

patient being asked to indicate when the sensation changes. Deeper pain is often assessed by squeezing the Achilles tendon or a muscle.
- The test for temperature sensitivity requires two tubes. They should preferably be metal (a better conductor of heat than glass) but test tubes are often used. One is filled with ice or very cold water and the other with hot water. Care must be taken not to have the water too hot because a sensation of pain may be elicited rather than heat. Again the patient is asked to describe and locate the sensation.

Crude touch and pressure – the anterior spinothalamic pathway

- This test is carried out by touching the patient's skin with the fingers or a blunt object, such as the end of a pen. The patient is asked whether he can feel anything and, as pressure is increased, to describe what he feels.

Light touch, proprioception and vibration – the posterior column pathway

- Light touch is tested by using a wisp of cotton wool on the patient's skin. Two-point discrimination of touch should be tested with an instrument called a two-point discriminator, but ordinary dividers are often used. The two-point discriminator has blunt ends and is calibrated to measure the distance of discrimination between two points. As dividers have sharp points and no calibration, care must be taken not to elicit pain rather than touch. The patient is touched randomly with one or two points to find out whether he can appreciate the two sensations rather than interpreting them as one. Normal separation between points on the palmar surface of the thumb and fingers is 0.5 cm and much wider on, say, the back of the neck where there are fewer receptors.
- Proprioception or joint position sense. The examiner moves the patient's fingers or toes and asks him to say whether the digit is pointing up or down. Again care must be taken not to confuse sensation; if the digit is held incorrectly, the patient may guess its position from the pressure of the examiner's fingers, rather than from joint sensations.
- Vibration. A tuning fork is struck and, while vibrating, is placed on a bony prominence, such as the ankle or wrist. The patient should be able to feel the vibrations, usually described as a tingling sensation.

nuclei is to sharpen up the impression of the stimuli transmitted to the brain through this route by the process of lateral inhibition.

The neurones in the nucleus cuneatus and nucleus gracilis give rise to axons (medial lemniscus) that cross over the midline of the brain stem and run to the thalamus on the opposite side of the body. Eventually, therefore, sensory information from different receptors in the same part of the body, which has travelled up the cord on different sides in the spinothalamic tracts and the dorsal columns, is brought back together on the same side of the brain (Fig. 22.5).

In areas of the body where innervation is sparse, for example on the back, it is sometimes difficult to locate the precise place of, say, an itch. Armed with a back scratcher, knitting needle or ruler, you attack the place where the itch seems to be only to find that, for relief, you have to scratch an inch or so either way. It is often more difficult to locate an itch for a patient – on occasions you may end up rubbing the whole back, having given up on the 'down a bit', 'to the left a bit' instructions.

DESTINATIONS IN THE BRAIN

Only sensory information reaching the thalamus and cerebral cortex gives rise to conscious sensations. Information transmitted to the cerebellum via the spinocerebellar tracts is almost entirely involved in controlling movement. Much of that which travels to and through the reticular formation contributes to our general state of arousal. But that which gets to the thalamus and cortex via the spinal tracts, or by the equivalent routes through the cranial nerves and brain stem, creates specific 'feelings' of touch, pressure, warmth, cold and pain.

Somatosensory cortex

The area of the cerebral cortex to which the signals are transmitted is the somatosensory cortex in the post-central gyrus of the parietal lobe (Fig. 22.7). Much of the somatosensory cortex is concerned with sensory information derived from the hands and the face. Both these areas of the body are very richly supplied with sensory receptors, and the large number of cortical neurones devoted to these areas matches this.

CHARACTER OF SENSATIONS

The character of somatosensory sensations may be:

- discrete and well localized
- diffuse and disturbing.

The quality perceived depends upon the route through which nerve impulses have reached the somatosensory cortex.

Discrete and well localized

The sensory information reaching the cerebral cortex via pathways such as the dorsal columns and spinothalamic tracts (specific sensory pathways) is recognized by us as having come from discrete parts of our bodies. The location of the stimulus can be quite accurately defined. This is because of the highly ordered arrangement of the neurones and because

the process of lateral inhibition operates at some of the synapses. At each level, in the spinal cord, the medullary nuclei, the thalamus and the cortex, the body is 'mapped out' in the relative positions of the neurones. If the density of innervation is high and if there is lateral inhibition, the map is very detailed and precise (as it is for the skin of the hands and face). If, however, innervation is sparse, then the map is less detailed and more like a sketch (as it is for the skin of the back).

Diffuse and disturbing

Sensory information reaching the thalamus and the cerebral cortex via the reticular formation (spino-reticular tracts) is less well ordered. This is because the transmission of the signals is not rigidly restricted to particular pathways and because lateral inhibition does

Awareness of proprioception

We all make use of proprioception but some activities rely more heavily on it than others. A typist used to one keyboard may well take some time to get used to another. Nursing skills, in the main, require visual input, speech therapists require auditory input and a physiotherapist proprioceptive and sensorimotor input. With the increase in the need for keyboard skills, we may all need to develop more proprioception. Prodding a keyboard with two fingers and visually searching for letters is both frustrating and time-consuming.

Some people are normally less aware than others of the position of their limbs in relation to their surroundings. These are the people who are dismissed as clumsy, hamfisted, accident prone. The mug of coffee lands on the table with a resounding crash, chairs are knocked over, feet hit the stairs so heavily that the house shakes. The development of clumsiness, or an increase in awkwardness that is not normal for the person requires investigation. Messages from the proprioceptors, via the posterior (dorsal) column pathways, are interpreted at a conscious level in the parietal area of the sensory cortex of the brain. If a tumour or other lesion develops in one of the parietal lobes of the brain, one of the first symptoms noticed by the patient may be clumsiness, a tendency to knock things over and misjudge distances.

When proprioceptive information does not reach the cerebellum, varying degrees of ataxia become evident. Ataxia is lack of coordination of movement. A person with ataxia is, for example, unable to walk heel to toe along a straight line or to touch the tip of the nose with the index finger while the eyes are closed.

not occur at all. Consequently, our sensory impressions are more diffuse though no less disturbing. Indeed because the signals tend to be more widely dispersed, they may be more likely to disturb and distract us. The sensation of burning pain is mediated by this route.

PROPRIOCEPTION

When our eyes are closed, the sense we have of the position and movement of our bodies (proprioception) is created by sensory information derived from a variety of different receptors including the balance organs (vestibular apparatus) as well as receptors in the skin, the joints, the muscles and tendons already described. All these receptors are said to have a proprioceptive function. However, the term proprio-

ceptors is most often applied to the receptors present in joints, muscles and tendons (muscle spindles, Golgi tendon organs and joint receptors).

All proprioceptive information is important in the control of posture and movement. Consequently, much sensory information from these receptors is directed to regions of the brain, such as the cerebellum, that are specifically concerned with motor control. Some signals do reach the sensory cortex. These are the ones that make us aware of our position and movement.

THE BALANCE ORGANS (VESTIBULAR APPARATUS)

The balance organs specifically monitor the position and movement of the head. They consist of a pair of

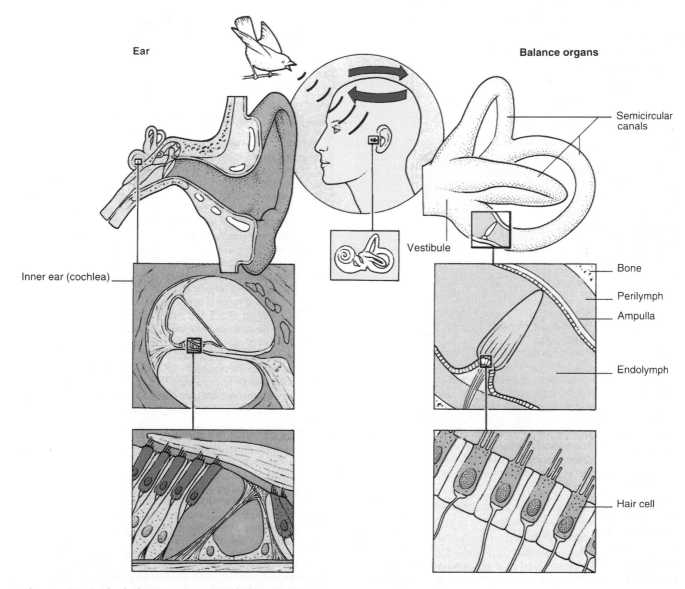

Figure 22.8 The balance organs (vestibular apparatus).

fluid-filled labyrinths, one on either side of the head, containing receptors influenced by movement or by gravity. The system is linked with the cochlea of the ear, and contains similar receptors (hair cells), but the way in which the receptors are excited differs (Fig. 22.8).

Structure

Each balance organ (Fig. 22.9) consists of:

- three semicircular ducts
- two sacs (utricle and saccule).

The ducts and sacs form part of the membranous labyrinth, which lies inside the bony (osseus) labyrinth consisting of:

- semicircular canals
- vestibule
- cochlea.

The ducts and sacs are lined by a secretory epithelium and are filled with endolymph and surrounded by perilymph.

The sensory receptors (hair cells) are grouped into two different types of sensory organ (Fig. 22.10A & B):

- crista
- macula.

There is one crista in the ampulla of each of the semicircular ducts. The two maculae of each balance organ are in the utricle and saccule.

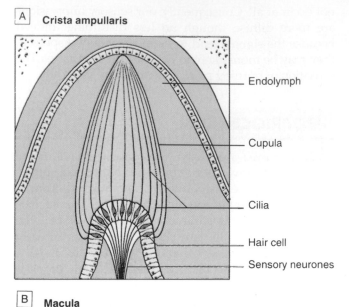

A   **Crista ampullaris**

Endolymph

Cupula

Cilia

Hair cell

Sensory neurones

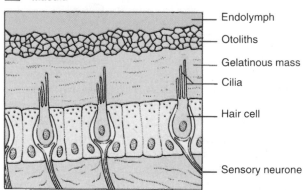

B   **Macula**

Endolymph

Otoliths

Gelatinous mass

Cilia

Hair cell

Sensory neurone

Figure 22.10 The two different types of sense organ in the vestibular apparatus.

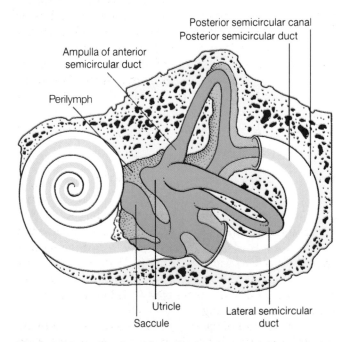

Posterior semicircular canal
Posterior semicircular duct

Ampulla of anterior
semicircular duct

Perilymph

Utricle

Saccule

Lateral semicircular
duct

Figure 22.9 The three ducts and two sacs of the vestibular apparatus, lying within the canals and chambers formed of bone. (From Rogers 1992, with permission of Elsevier.)

Cristae

The hair cells of the cristae possess very long cilia enveloped in a gelatinous mass known as the cupula (Fig. 22.10A). This plume-like structure is fixed to the top of the ampulla, but otherwise it is free to move. If the fluid in the ducts moves, then the cupula bends like seaweed moving with the current and this in turn bends the cilia.

Maculae

The cilia of the maculae are shorter but they too are embedded in a gelatinous mass (Fig. 22.10B). Stuck on to the surface of this jelly-like layer are small crystals of calcium carbonate (otoliths). These weigh the jelly down if they are on top, or tend to exert a pull on it if they are underneath. In either case the cilia are bent and this alters the number of action potentials generated in the sensory neurones.

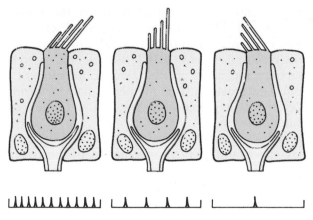

Frequency of action potentials in sensory neurone

Figure 22.11 Relationship between the bending of the cilia on the hair cell and the frequency of action potentials in the sensory neurone.

Excitation of the sensory receptors

When the cilia are upright (Fig. 22.11) the cells fire quite spontaneously at a steady rate. If they are then bent in one direction, the cell increases its firing rate, but if they are bent in the opposite direction, the firing of impulses is inhibited. As can be seen from the diagram (Fig. 22.12), the two maculae in each balance organ are oriented at different angles in the utricle and the saccule. Consequently each fires impulses at a different rate. If the head is moved to a different position, the maculae alter their firing rate. The pattern of impulses from the maculae thus differs for each position of the head.

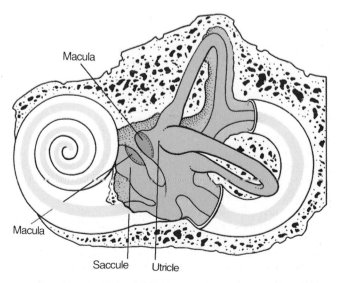

Figure 22.12 Position of the maculae in the utricle and the saccule. Notice that they are differently oriented. (From Rogers 1992, with permission of Elsevier.)

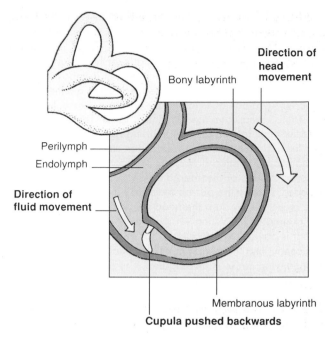

Figure 22.13 How the cupula of the crista ampullaris is disturbed by head movement.

The cristae differ from the maculae in that they are best at detecting sudden movements of the head up and down, to the left and to the right, and so on. When the head is moved, the fluid in the ducts does not immediately move with it. It lags behind and so the cupula is dragged in the opposite direction to that in which the head moved (Fig. 22.13). This is just the same as the jerk backwards that you experience on a bus or train when it begins to move. When the cupula is jerked backwards the cilia bend and the cells are excited.

The different orientation of the three semicircular ducts allows us to detect swivel movements of the head in any direction. The most horizontally oriented duct canal is best at picking up turns of the head to the left and the right, while the other two are better at detecting movements up and down.

False impressions of movement

Whenever and however fluid moves within the ducts, signals are generated that are interpreted by the brain as movement. It is possible to create convection currents in the endolymph of the balance organs by syringeing ears with fluid that is colder or warmer than core temperature. The convection currents displace the cupula and the person having his ears syringed is likely to feel as if the room is 'swimming'.

The same kind of feeling is often voluntarily induced by children who have discovered that by whirling around very rapidly several times and then stopping, eyes closed and backs pressed safely against a wall,

That dizzy feeling

Dizzy, giddy, light headed – what exactly do we mean when we use these and similar terms? It is impossible to experience the sensations generated within another's body, so careful questioning by a doctor is essential to establish what form the 'dizziness' takes. The example in the main text of children whirling round to experience a feeling of continued movement on stopping is a realistic description of vertigo. Vertigo is the consciousness of disordered orientation of the body in space. Usually the person feels very insecure, frightened to move quickly, turn the head or, perhaps, look at flickering lights. When vertigo occurs without a cause that is obvious to the sufferer, for example too much alcohol, then the symptom will be treated while the underlying cause is investigated. The doctor will wish to know the nature of the dizziness and sometimes the patient may give a better description to a nurse in the course of conversation because he feels that the nurse has more time to listen. The sensations are described in the following ways:

- movement of the surroundings, rotating or oscillating
- movement of the body, rotating or a sense of falling – sometimes it is just the head that feels as if it is moving
- unsteadiness of the limbs and movement not well coordinated.

There are many known causes of vertigo and much research has been carried out, but often the underlying cause in a particular patient is not found. However, by investigation, the more worrying causes are eliminated. Not all vertigo is associated directly with the balance organs, but the causes of aural vertigo are the most numerous and probably the easiest to diagnose. It is not difficult to think of the obvious causes, such as wax in the external meatus, infection of the middle ear (otitis media), sudden changes in atmospheric pressure. Less obvious perhaps are drugs (salicylate (aspirin) and quinine in particular), impairment of blood supply, head injury, inflammation of the balance organs. These are additional to Ménière's disease, referred to in the main text. Vertigo is a very distressing and frightening symptom; the experience is actually far worse than the simulated sensation experienced by a child whirling just for fun.

they experience curious feelings of movement. The reason for these feelings is that, when you stop abruptly after a period of spinning, the fluid in the ducts continues to flow around for several seconds and the cilia of the cristae are displaced.

Impressions of movement and position are also built up from comparisons made by the brain of sensory information from the balance organs on each side of the head. A difference in signal between the sensory receptors on each side is interpreted either as movement (cristae compared) or as a different head position (maculae compared). If there is damage to the vestibular apparatus on one side or impairment of impulse transmission, as in Ménière's disease, then the sufferer will experience feelings of dizziness and apparent movement.

These unpleasant feelings are often complicated by reflex effects triggered by stimulation of the balance organs. These include nystagmus (a characteristic pattern of eye movements) and postural adjustments.

TASTE AND SMELL

The taste of food depends as much on its texture and its smell as it does on chemical stimulation of the taste buds. Think of how food tastes when you have a cold (sense of smell dulled) and how texture alters your appreciation of food. Receptors sensitive to the chemicals in food are found in the mucosal lining throughout the digestive tract, but only those in the mouth and nose contribute to the sensation of taste (see Ch. 9).

MOUTH

Receptors

A variety of different receptors are present in the mouth:

- mechanoreceptors
- thermoreceptors
- nociceptors
- chemoreceptors.

Receptors mediating the sensations of touch, pressure, pain, heat and cold are found in the mucosa lining the oral cavity and the tongue. The mucous membranes towards the back of the mouth are especially sensitive to touch.

Chemoreceptors

The chemosensitive cells are grouped together within taste buds (Fig. 22.14) most of which are found on the tongue, but some are also present elsewhere in the mouth and throat (pharynx). These gustatory cells within the taste buds respond to a great variety of chemicals. Tastes have been categorized into at least four types:

- sweet
- sour
- salt
- bitter.

Tongue

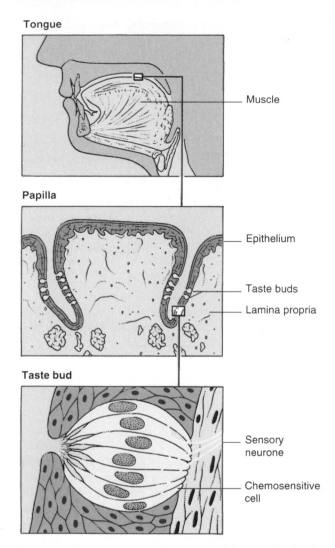

Muscle

Papilla

Epithelium

Taste buds

Lamina propria

Taste bud

Sensory neurone

Chemosensitive cell

Figure 22.14 Position and structure of the taste buds of the tongue.

In *coryza* (common cold) the mucous membranes become swollen and the flow of air through the olfactory cleft becomes obstructed. As a result the sense of smell (and taste) is dulled.

Sour tastes tend to be produced by acids, whereas salty tastes are produced by inorganic ions such as sodium and potassium, and their associated anions. Other than this, little correspondence has been found between the chemical structure of a molecule and the taste it produces. Most taste buds tend to be better at mediating one type of taste than another. Consequently, different parts of the mouth are best at detecting different constituents in food.

Sensory neurones, pathways and destinations

Impulses generated by receptors in the mouth are transmitted along cranial nerves V, VII, IX and X to the medulla of the brain to synapse with neurones carrying signals via the thalamus to the somatosensory cortex. Impulses transmitted to the limbic system and the hypothalamus affect appetite. Stimulation of receptors in the mouth also evokes reflex responses via centres in the medulla, such as the secretion of digestive juices and vomiting.

NOSE

The sense of smell (olfaction) is not as important for humans as it is for some other creatures, but its loss, temporarily or permanently (anosmia), does affect our appreciation of food. The olfactory receptors are tucked away high up in the nasal cavity (Fig. 22.15). Nerve impulses generated by them are transmitted to parts of the brain involved in emotion and motivation, as well as in the control of food intake and its digestion.

Receptors

Structure and location

The olfactory receptors consist of specialized nerve endings embedded in the mucosa of the olfactory cleft (Fig. 22.15). In gentle breathing, very little air reaches the receptors whereas, in sniffing, the airflow around the conchae becomes turbulent and more molecules are wafted into the cleft. The receptors possess many cilia presenting a very large surface area for airborne molecules to contact.

Sensitivity

The receptors are amazingly sensitive to airborne molecules. Only a couple of odorous molecules need to be present in a whiff of air for them to be detected. No

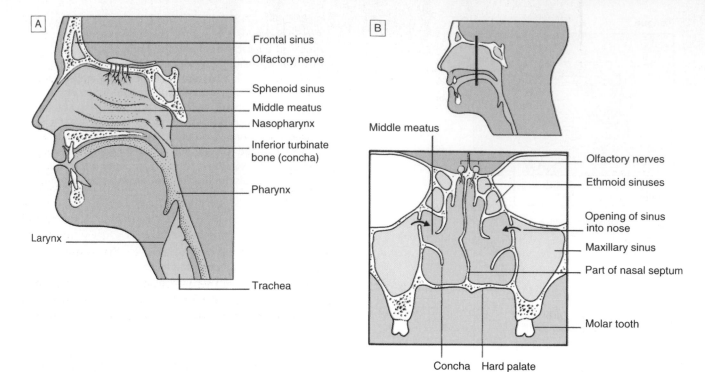

Figure 22.15 Position of the olfactory receptors in the nasal cavity.

distinguishing features have yet been found between the receptors, and little is known about the way in which different chemicals give rise to the patterns of information interpreted by the brain as up to 4000 different odours.

Sensory neurones, pathways and destinations

Nerve fibres extend from the receptors, through the cribriform plate, and pass to the olfactory bulb. Here, the neurones synapse with the next neurones in the system. There is much convergence of information at this level (receptor : neurone ratio of about 250:1), which probably accounts for much of the high sensitivity of the olfactory system.

From the olfactory bulb, nerve fibres pass to the frontal lobes of the brain and to the prepyriform cortex of the limbic system. Both of these areas are involved in our emotional and motivational drives and connect with the hypothalamus and the autonomic nervous system, thus affecting appetite and the digestion of food.

REFERENCES AND FURTHER READING

Davies A, Blakeley A G H, Kidd C 2001 Human physiology. Churchill Livingstone, Edinburgh

Ferguson D B 1988 Physiology for dental students. Butterworth Heinemann, Oxford

Finger T E, Silver W L, Restrepo D 2000 The neurobiology of taste and smell. John Wiley & Sons, New York

Johansson R S, Vallbo A B 1983 Tactile sensory coding in the glabrous skin of the human hand. Trends in Neuroscience 6(1): 27–32

Junquiera L C, Carneiro J, Kelley R O 1998 Basic histology, 9th edn. Appleton & Lange, East Norwalk, CT

Lephart S M, Fu F H (eds) 1999 Proprioception and neuromuscular control in joint stability. Human Kinetics Europe, Champaign, IL

McMahon S B 1992 Itching for an explanation. Trends in Neuroscience 15(12): 497–501

Penfield W, Rasmussen T 1968 The cerebral cortex of man: a clinical study of localisation of function. Hafner

Rogers A W 1992 Textbook of anatomy. Churchill Livingstone, Edinburgh

Wright A 1988 Dizziness. Croom Helm, Beckenham

Our ears are sensitive to the tiny pressure changes occurring in air when objects vibrate. These pressure changes (sound waves) cause the eardrum to vibrate, and the vibrations are passed on through the structures in the ear to the auditory receptors (hair cells) (Fig. 23.1) which convert the vibratory energy into nerve impulses. Nerve impulses travel along central pathways to the auditory areas of the cerebral cortex, giving rise to the sensation of sound.

Deafness occurs if there is either a physical blockage in the transmission of vibrations through the ear or if there is damage to the auditory receptors or pathways.

SOUND WAVES

When objects vibrate, they cause the molecules in the air next to the object to be alternately pushed together (compressed) and then moved apart (rarefied) (Fig. 23.2). This alternating pressure is transmitted to the next layer of air and so on. The alternating wave of pressure in the air caused by a vibrating body is described in terms of its amplitude and its frequency. The amplitude relates to the loudness of the sound and the frequency to its pitch. Of special importance are the frequencies of sound that are crucial to an understanding of speech.

CHARACTERISTICS

Amplitude and loudness

The amplitude of a sound wave refers to the difference in air pressure between the greatest compression and the greatest rarefaction (Fig. 23.3). The bigger the amplitude of the wave, the greater is its intensity in terms of energy and the louder the sound. The intensity of a sound is measured in bels.

Bels and decibels

The quietest sound that is just audible to a normal ear under ideal conditions is used as a reference level against which the intensity of all other s compared.

$$\text{Intensity (bels)} = \log_{10} \frac{\text{Intensity of the so}}{\text{Intensity of the referen}}$$

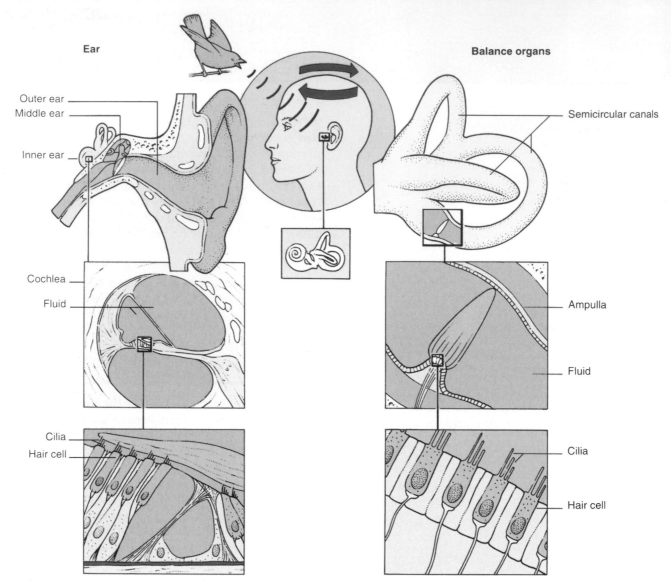

Figure 23.1 The ear: receptor cells and accessory structures.

As logarithms are used in the calculation, if the intensity of the sound being measured is exactly the same as the reference sound (0.0002 dynes/cm^2) then:

$$\text{Number of bels} = \log_{10} \frac{0.0002}{0.0002} = \log_{10} 1 = 0$$

The intensity of sound waves in everyday conversation is about one million times (10^6) greater than the reference level. As the log of 10^6 is 6, the number of bels is 6. As 1 bel = 10 decibels, this is 60 decibels (dB).

The intensity of everyday sounds ranges between 0 and about 100 dB (Table 23.1). Sounds of greater intensity may be painful and can cause permanent damage. An increase in decibels from 80 to 100 may not seem very much but, since the bel system uses the log scale, it represents a 100-fold increase in sound intensity. An increase to 120 dB at a very loud band concert represents an increase of 10 000 times.

Frequency and pitch

The frequency of sound waves is the number of cycles of compression and rarefaction occurring per second.

One cycle per second   = 1 hertz (Hz)
1000 cycles per second = 1000 Hz
                       = 1 kilohertz (kHz)

The frequency of the waves determines the pitch we hear (Table 23.2). Waves of low frequency are heard as

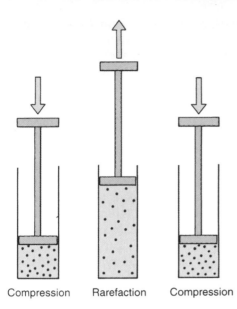

Figure 23.2 Meaning of the terms 'compression' and 'rarefaction'.

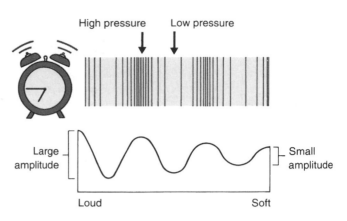

Figure 23.3 Amplitude of a sound wave.

Awareness of environmental noise pollution

Occupational health nurses in industries where there is prolonged intense noise should alert workers to the potential danger of progressive and permanent hearing loss, and encourage the use of special protective earmuffs or earplugs. Where the noise is greater than 90 dB, employers are obliged by law to provide appropriate protection.

Health educators should target groups who may be exposed regularly to loud music in discos or on personal stereos as this causes sensorineural deafness in a significant number of young people. Disco music can be as high as 120 dB.

It is an interesting exercise to compare noise levels in different everyday settings. Why not record noise levels for a 10-minute period in a hospital ward, a college canteen, a city street with road works in progress and your own home, and discuss your findings.

Table 23.1 Intensity of some sounds

Sound	Intensity (decibels)
Jet plane	140
Very loud band music	120
Pneumatic drill	110
Power tools	100
Noisy restaurant	80
Busy traffic	75
Conversational speech	66
Whisper	30

Table 23.2 Range of frequencies detected by the human ear

Frequency (Hz)	
20	Lowest detectable sound*
120	Male voice†
250	Female voice† (about middle C)
4000	Top notes on piano†
20 000	Highest detectable sound*

* In young people.
† Fundamental frequency.

---

sounds of low pitch (someone with a deep voice, a motorcycle); waves of high frequency are heard as sounds of high pitch (squeak, dental drill).

Speech sounds

The sounds we hear are usually complex ones made up of a mixture of different frequencies rather than pure notes such as those produced in an audiometer or by a tuning fork. Each sound has a fundamental frequency, but in addition to this there are harmonics and other components that add 'colour' or 'depth' to the sound.

THE EAR

The ear consists of three sections (Fig. 23.4A):

- outer
- middle
- inner.

The outer part funnels sound waves down to the tympanic membrane (eardrum) which then vibrates.

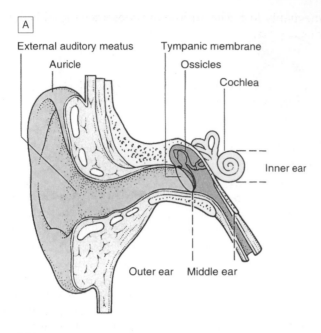

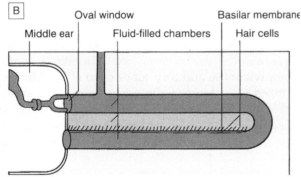

Figure 23.4 Structure of the ear. A, Component parts: outer, middle and inner. B, Diagrammatic representation of the cochlea (uncoiled) showing its various parts.

The vibrations are transmitted through an interconnected set of three small bones (ossicles) in the middle ear to the inner ear. The inner ear consists of a small spiral tunnel (cochlea) in the bone of the skull, divided internally into three fluid-filled chambers (Fig. 23.4B). Set into the membrane (basilar membrane) which divides two of the chambers are the auditory receptors (hair cells). When the vibrations are transmitted from the middle ear through the oval window to the fluids of the inner ear, the basilar membrane vibrates, and this excites the hair cells.

OUTER EAR

The auricle (pinna) of the outer ear (Fig. 23.4A) helps to gather sound waves and direct them along the external auditory meatus to the eardrum (tympanic membrane). The shape of the auricle causes sound waves coming from in front of us to be picked up better than those from behind. This helps us to locate the source of a sound. When we turn our heads in response to a sound, we are testing out that sound from different directions and in effect taking bearings on it. From this information, derived from both ears, our brain works out the direction from which the sound has come.

The external auditory meatus is the tube leading to the eardrum. The outer third is formed of cartilage and lined by hairy skin possessing sebaceous and wax-secreting glands. The rest is formed of bone and is lined by non-hairy skin. The meatus is not completely straight but is constricted part of the way along. The size and shape of the auditory meatus affects the blend of sounds received by the eardrum. Just as sounds appear different when listened to through a long tube, so the tiny tube of the auditory meatus modifies the blend of sound waves reaching the eardrum.

The eardrum is pearly white in appearance and consists of fibrous tissue. It is covered externally by skin and internally by a mucous membrane.

MIDDLE EAR

The middle ear is a small air-filled cavity that has an opening into the pharynx through the auditory tube (eustachian tube) (Fig. 23.5). Bridging the gap between the eardrum and the oval window are three tiny bones (ossicles), which transmit the vibrations from the eardrum to the inner ear. Vibrations can be damped by the contraction of two tiny muscles, which protect the ear, to some extent, against the damaging effects of loud sounds. Normally the pressure in the middle ear is the same as that in the pharynx, but if the auditory tube is blocked, pressures differ and sounds become muffled.

Ossicles

The three bones of the middle ear are the:

- malleus (hammer)
- incus (anvil)
- stapes (stirrup).

These bones act as a lever system so that when the eardrum vibrates the vibrations are transmitted to the oval window. In fact the pressures produced are magnified in the process because of the lever action of the bones and because the area of the oval window is much smaller than that of the eardrum. This magnification (+30%) of the pressure changes is important because at the next stage, when the vibrations are passed on to the fluid of the inner ear, some energy is

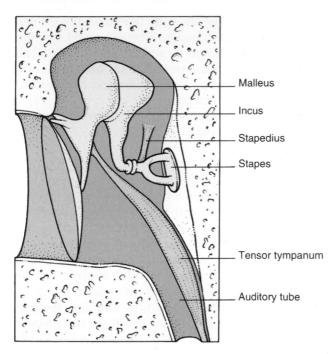

Malleus

Incus

Stapedius

Stapes

Tensor tympanum

Auditory tube

Figure 23.5 Structure of the middle ear.

Otitis media (inflammation of the middle ear)

Acute otitis media
In infections which involve the upper respiratory tract, the inflammatory response can cause swelling of the mucous membrane lining the middle ear, and exudates may collect in what is normally an air-filled cavity. If untreated, the swelling and fluid will together block conduction, cause severe pain and may eventually rupture the eardrum.

The acute condition is treated with antibiotics and analgesics.

Chronic serous otitis media
This is an accumulation of fluid in the middle ear accompanied by loss of hearing and discomfort, and is common in young children. It is usually a result of blockage of the auditory (eustachian) tube by enlarged adenoids or swollen mucous membrane due to allergy or chronic infection.

The specific cause is identified and treated. The main aim is to ensure that the auditory tube is patent and can fulfil its role of ventilating the middle ear. In addition, it may be necessary to perform a myringotomy (opening into the eardrum from the external auditory meatus) to drain the fluid from the middle ear space. A plastic tympanostomy tube (grommet) may be inserted into this opening to permit continuous drainage and ventilation of the middle ear. The grommet usually stays in place for 2 or 3 weeks and then dislodges into the external auditory meatus and is discarded. By which time the cause of the original problem should be resolved.

inevitably lost. The middle ear boosts the signal before this happens.

Muscles

The action of the bony lever system is adjusted by two muscles (Fig. 23.5):

- tensor tympanum
- stapedius.

Both muscles are anchored at one end to the wall of the middle ear, and at the other end, to one of the ossicles. The tensor tympanum is fixed to the malleus and controls tension in the eardrum, whereas the stapedius is fixed to the stapes and pulls this bone away from the oval window. In both cases, contraction of the muscles stiffens the system and reduces transmission of vibrations, muffling the sound. This is a protective response, shielding the delicate structure of the inner ear from vibrations that may be damaging. Contraction of the muscles occurs reflexly in response to loud sounds.

Pressures

Sounds also become muffled when the pressure of air in the middle ear differs from that outside. This can happen when the auditory tubes close or are blocked. The tubes close temporarily when there is an abrupt change in atmospheric pressure (as on take-off or landing of an aircraft). The sweets sometimes offered to airline travellers at the beginning and end of a flight are not just a social gesture. Sucking the sweets increases the flow of saliva, and encourages swallowing. Swallowing opens up the auditory tube. Yawning has a similar effect. Once the pressures are equal again, normal hearing is restored.

INNER EAR

The inner ear consists of a membranous tube (cochlear duct) lying in a small coiled tunnel in the bone of the skull (cochlea). Within the cochlear duct is the basilar membrane that vibrates when the ear is excited by sound waves.

Cochlea

The cochlea is divided into three chambers (Fig. 23.6A):

- scala vestibuli
- scala media
- scala tympani.

The fluid (perilymph) in the outer two chambers differs in composition from the fluid (endolymph) in the scala media. The chamber containing perilymph has a small opening linking it with the fluid in the vestibular apparatus (Fig. 23.6A).

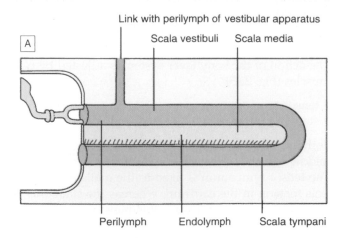

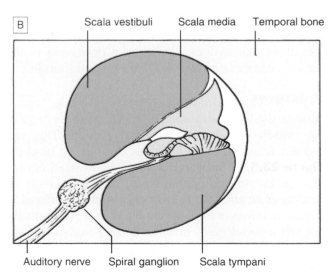

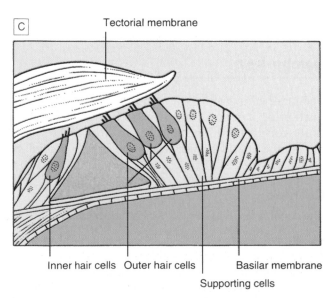

Figure 23.6 The inner ear (cochlea). A, Diagrammatic representation (uncoiled). B, Histological structure in cross-section. C, The spiral organ (of Corti).

The tissue dividing the scala tympani from the scala media consists of the basilar membrane and the spiral organ (of Corti), flanked by supporting cells (Fig. 23.6B & C). The basilar membrane extends from one end of the cochlear duct to the other. If it could be unrolled it would be about 35 mm long.

The auditory receptors (hair cells) are in the spiral organ. They are arranged in two sets (Fig. 23.6C):

- inner
- outer.

They are ciliated cells innervated by sensory neurones of the auditory nerve (cranial nerve VIII). The tips of the cilia of the outer hair cells are embedded in another membranous structure, the tectorial membrane, lying on top of them. The outer hair cells are arranged in three rows and each cell has some 50–100 stereocilia. When the basilar membrane vibrates, the cilia are bent first one way and then the other in time with the vibrations. Bending in one direction excites the cells (depolarization) whereas bending in the opposite direction inhibits them (hyperpolarization). The inner hair cells have approximately 50–60 stereocilia, but they are not embedded in the tectorial membrane.

Basilar membrane

The way in which the basilar membrane vibrates differs according to the frequency and amplitude of the sound waves. If the sound is of low frequency (e.g. 100 Hz), the whole membrane vibrates in time with the alternating pressure wave. Whereas, if the sound is of high frequency (e.g. 2000 Hz), then the part of the basilar membrane furthest away from the oval window does not move at all (Fig. 23.7). The higher the frequency the smaller is the length of membrane that vibrates.

The frequency of a sound wave therefore affects the pattern of impulses in the auditory neurones in two ways:

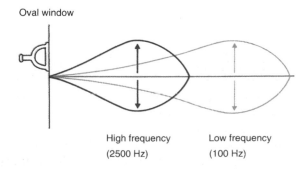

Figure 23.7 Patterns of vibration of the basilar membrane in response to sound waves of high and low frequency.

- by determining the frequency of nerve impulses
- by selecting which neurones are excited.

Both are important in coding the pitch of the sound we hear.

The frequency code is best for sound waves of low frequency (<1000 Hz). This is because the theoretical maximum frequency of impulses that neurones can transmit is 1000/second (i.e. 1000 Hz).

At frequencies greater than 1000 Hz, it is the position of the vibrations on the basilar membrane that matters most. Because of this, selective degeneration of auditory neurones, as in presbyacusis, tends to affect the detection of high frequency sounds more than those of low frequency.

Differences in the amplitude of the sound waves produce corresponding differences in the amplitude of vibration of the basilar membrane. The larger the amplitude, the greater the number of receptors excited, and the louder is the sound we hear.

SENSITIVITY OF THE EAR

The human ear is sensitive to frequencies of sound ranging from about 20 to 20 000 Hz (20 kHz), but it is most sensitive between 1000 and 4000 Hz (1–4 kHz).

The sensitivity of the ear to sounds of different frequencies is measured by finding the minimum number of decibels needed for someone to just hear the sound under conditions in which there is very little or no background noise. The results obtained are plotted on a chart to give an audiogram.

If the ear is obstructed, for example by wax, or if transmission of sound through the middle ear is impaired, then the intensity of the sounds that can just be heard is greater than normal. This is typical of conductive deafness. In other cases of deafness only part of the audiogram may be abnormal. This indicates selective loss of auditory function, for example through damage to receptors on part of the basilar membrane, or to nerves in the auditory pathway. This is typical of sensorineural deafness.

AUDITORY PATHWAYS

The nerve pathways between the ear and the cerebral cortex (auditory pathways) are complex. There are many places at which synapses occur, and therefore at which analysis and modification of the information can occur. The main parts of the auditory pathway (Fig. 23.8) include the cochlear nucleus, inferior colliculus, superior olive and thalamus. Each

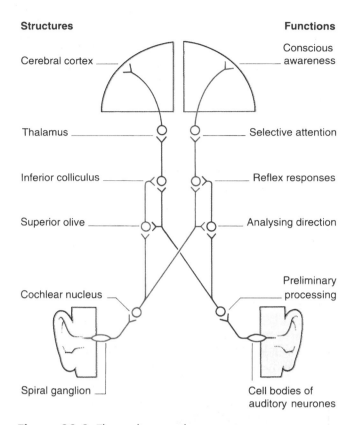

Figure 23.8 The auditory pathway.

part plays a different role in enabling us to become aware of, analyse and respond to, sound waves detected by the ear.

HAIR CELLS AND SENSORY NEURONES

The majority of neurones in the auditory nerve (about 90%) are associated with the inner row of hair cells. Each of the inner cells is innervated by several sensory neurones, whereas several outer hair cells are all innervated by the same neurone. The cell bodies of all the sensory neurones are gathered together in the spiral ganglion.

An unusual feature of the auditory system is that the auditory receptors and sensory neurones are innervated by efferent neurones that control their sensitivity. These efferent neurones (olivocochlear bundle) originate in the superior olives, two nuclei in the medulla oblongata of the brain stem. The olivocochlear bundle is believed to play a part in enabling us to tune in to some sounds and to blot out others, for example when listening to conversation at a party.

COCHLEAR NUCLEUS

Nerve axons extend from the spiral ganglion to the cochlear nucleus on the same side of the head. The organization of cells in this nucleus is related to the placing of the receptors along the basilar membrane and to the frequency of the sound (tonotopic representation). Cells responding best to a sound of high frequency are situated in one part of the nucleus whereas those responding best to another frequency are at a different place.

INFERIOR COLLICULUS

From the cochlear nuclei, the information is passed to the opposite side of the brain either directly or indirectly to the inferior colliculi. These two clusters of neurones form part of the system enabling us to turn reflexly in response to a sudden sound. For example if someone cries out, you turn instinctively, to face the source of the sound.

SUPERIOR OLIVE

One of the indirect pathways between the cochlear nucleus and the inferior colliculus is via the superior olive. This group of cells, one on each side of the medulla oblongata, receives an input from both ears. The superior olive probably makes some of the comparisons of sound from each ear that enable us to locate the source of a sound, as well as enabling us to turn in response to a sudden sound.

Pathways originating in the cochlea of both ears innervate the majority of the neurones in the superior olive. Since the information is provided in such a way, comparisons can be made on the signal received from both the right and left side of the auditory field. By 'comparing' this differential input the superior olive is able to localise the sound i.e. identify which direction it is coming from. Depending on the direction of the sound source the input received by both ears will be different in terms of both time and intensity.

The superior olive is subdivided into 2 regions, namely the lateral and medial nuclei. The lateral nucleus receives input from both the right and left cochlear nuclei, with the cells being excited by the ipsilateral input and inhibited by the contralateral input. This lateral area uses intensity differences to aid with the localisation of predominantly high frequency sounds. On the other hand, the medial nucleus receives input from a subdivision of the ventral cochlear nucleus and uses time differences to aid with the localisation of predominantly low frequency sounds. In this way the brain is able to localise the full frequency range of sounds.

THALAMUS

From the inferior colliculi, impulses pass to the medial geniculate nucleus of the thalamus. The thalamus is thought to act as a filter for sensory signals and may play a role in selecting the sounds to which we pay attention. Some cells in the medial geniculate nucleus are known to have the property of responding less and less well to a sound that is repeated (habituation). In this way we become oblivious to familiar sounds while remaining alert to those that are new.

AUDITORY CORTEX

Nerve impulses reach the auditory areas in the temporal lobes of the cerebral hemispheres (Figs 23.8 and 23.9). The primary auditory cortex is the area which first receives the incoming impulses. Here the cells are still organized tonotopically to some extent but they possess more specialized and interesting features. For example, each cell is sensitive to a much narrower band of frequencies than the neurones before it on the pathway, and some cells respond best to sounds that change in pitch, either up or down.

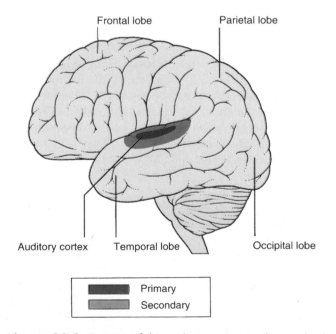

Figure 23.9 Position of the auditory cortex in the cerebral hemispheres. (Only the left hemisphere is shown; the right auditory cortex in the right cerebral hemisphere is similar.)

Adjacent to the primary auditory cortex are secondary auditory areas in which cells are even more selective in their responsiveness. Some respond best to clicking sounds whereas others even respond selectively to one voice and not to another.

Next to these areas are the auditory association areas that play an important role in the understanding and interpretation of sounds.

Descending control of auditory pathways

Given the fact that our environment contains a constant barrage of auditory stimuli, it makes perfect sense that we should have an overarching control mechanism which limits the amount of information that actually reaches our consciousness. This ability to limit the information can occur at either a conscious or a subconscious level. Selective suppression is used to allow us to identify one person's voice over another's in a crowded room, and we can subconsciously switch off information in the background e.g. the hum of an air-conditioner or traffic noises outside our window.

A number of neurones descend from the higher areas of the auditory cortex down to the aforementioned lower levels of the auditory pathway, including the medial geniculate and the inferior colliculus. These descending neurones can even descend from the cochlear nucleus down as far as the cochlear nerve and the associated hair cells. These downward projections are very precisely organized and many of the pathways involve inhibitory interneurones, which utilise the neurotransmitters *gamma*-aminobutyric acid (GABA) and glycine. It is probably the case that similar inhibitory influences can impact on all levels of the auditory pathway from the cochlea to the cortex.

Auditory reflexes

Up to this point we have discussed the ascending pathways involved in the perception of sound. It should also be noted that there are 'branching' pathways which are involved in the control of some reflex actions. The reticular formation of the brain stem receives this branching input from the main auditory pathway and utilises it to control sudden muscle activity e.g. the startle response that occurs, causing you to jump, when you hear a sudden loud noise. Similarly, if a noise is perceived as being too loud, signals are sent via cranial nerves V and VII (trigeminal and facial) to the muscles surrounding the ossicles in the middle ear. These muscles then contract, thereby limiting the vibration of the malleus, incus and stapes, reducing the stimulation of the cochlea and, as a result, preventing potential cochlear damage. These are relatively simple reflex pathways, however, it should be noted that more complex pathways also exist which are involved in aspects of eye, head and body movement.

DEAFNESS

There are many causes of deafness, some of which are easily treated, and some of which are not. The two main forms are conductive deafness and sensorineural deafness. They may be distinguished by simple tests.

CONDUCTIVE DEAFNESS

Conductive deafness results when there is obstruction to the transmission of vibrations through the outer and middle parts of the ear. This may be due to a build-up of wax, or it could be due to damage to or disease of the lever system in the middle ear.

With conductive hearing loss, the sound waves are not able to stimulate the sensory cells of the inner ear (i.e. cause a fluid wave within the cochlea). This may be due to atresia, a perforation of the tympanic membrane, ossicular discontinuity, otosclerosis or serous otitis media.

As a result, the sound waves cannot be transformed into a fluid wave within the cochlea and the sensory cells receive decreased or no stimulation. Many conductive hearing losses are amenable to surgical correction; e.g. in serous otitis media, the fluid in the

Characteristics of impaired hearing

Many people find hearing impairment embarrassing and are reluctant to admit to deafness, but the following behaviour patterns should alert family or healthcare professionals to its presence:

- failure to respond when spoken to and lack of response to sounds that warn of danger in the environment (e.g. approaching traffic)
- straining towards the speaker and turning the better ear to catch what has been said, or requesting that it be repeated
- speaking more softly or more loudly than before
  - a person with conductive deafness will usually speak more softly than normal because he can hear himself through the vibrations from within
  - someone with sensorineural deafness will speak more loudly because damaged nerves cannot transmit sound waves and therefore he cannot hear himself
- developing a flat toneless voice
- a drop in the level of job performance in adults, and social withdrawal.

Table 23.3 Some causes of sensorineural deafness

Cause	Examples	
	Circumstance	**Person(s) affected**
Microorganisms	Infection with the rubella virus during early pregnancy	Embryo and fetus
Hypoxia	Asphyxia at birth	Neonate
Antibiotics	Treatment with streptomycin, kanomycin or quinine	Anyone
Intense sounds	Very loud music	Anyone
	Personal stereos played at high volume	
	Industrial machinery	
Uncertain*	Growing older	The elderly

* Cells degenerate and die but why is not known. It may be the result of accumulated exposure to noise throughout life.

middle ear space can be removed by performing a myringotomy, or, in otosclerosis, the stapes bone can be replaced with a prosthetic bone.

SENSORINEURAL DEAFNESS

In sensorineural deafness, conduction is normal but the generation and transmission of nerve impulses is impaired. Injury can occur at any level of the auditory pathway. Some common causes of sensorineural deafness are listed in Table 23.3.

The deafness associated with ageing (presbyacusis) is due to loss of neurones. These losses are greater if there has been repeated exposure to very loud sounds earlier in life, such as using a pneumatic drill, or listening to or playing amplified music at high volume. Unfortunately, the serious effects of such exposure are not immediately obvious to the listener. Acute exposure to very loud sounds does cause an immediate decrease in the sensitivity of the ear to sound, but then hearing recovers. However, repeated exposure has cumulative, irreversible effects.

In sensorineural deafness it is often the high frequency components of sound that are lost. This seriously affects the intelligibility of speech because hearing words properly depends crucially upon consonants. Consonants have many high frequency components. For example, the word 'soar' would be heard as 'oar' if the ear became relatively insensitive to frequencies above about 4 kHz, and would be confused easily with words like it, such as bore, core, door, store etc.

REFERENCES AND FURTHER READING

Carpenter R H S 1984 Neurophysiology. Edward Arnold, London

Emslie-Smith D, Paterson C R, Scratcherd T, Read N W (eds) 1988 Textbook of physiology, 11th edn. Churchill Livingstone, Edinburgh

Ehret G, Romand R 1997 The central auditory system. Oxford University Press, Oxford

Fletcher H 1929 Speech and hearing. Macmillan, London

Freeland A 1989 Deafness: the facts. Oxford University Press, Oxford

Jahn A F, Santos-Sacchi J 1988 Physiology of the ear. Raven Press, New York

Lasserson D, Gabriel C, Sharrack B 1997 Crash course! Nervous system and special senses. Mosby, St Louis

Loeb M 1986 Noise and human efficiency. John Wiley, Chichester

Pickles J O 1988 An introduction to the physiology of hearing, 2nd edn. Academic Press, London

Royle J A, Walsh M (eds) 1992 Watson's Medical–surgical nursing and related physiology. Baillière Tindall, London

Rubel E W, Popper A N, Fay R R (eds) 1997 Development of the auditory system. Springer-Verlag, New York

Sataloff R T, Sataloff J 1993 Hearing loss, 3rd edn. Marcel Dekker, New York

24 Vision

Vision is the sensation created in our minds as a result of the stimulation of sensory receptors in our eyes. The stimulus exciting the receptors is electromagnetic radiation.

The quality of the picture formed depends upon:

- the optics of the eye
- the photoreceptors in the retina
- the processing of information in the nervous system.

These things affect the detail we can see, how much illumination we need to be able to see, and whether the picture is in colour or in black and white.

ELECTROMAGNETIC RADIATION

Electromagnetic radiation is the energy given out by excited atoms. The energy released depends on the nature of the atoms and on the level of excitation.

Forms of electromagnetic radiation range from low energy radio waves (long wavelength and low frequency) to very powerful cosmic rays (very short wavelength and high frequency). However, our eyes are sensitive only to a narrow band of radiation in the middle of this range (400–700 nm in wavelength). This is the visible part of the electromagnetic spectrum.

All forms of electromagnetic radiation travel at the same speed (about 1100 million kilometres per hour), and in straight lines, unless they are deflected by a surface (reflection) or slowed down by entering a medium that is denser than space or the atmosphere, in which case they bend (refraction). Short wave radiation is refracted more than long wave. This is why sunlight striking raindrops, and being refracted as it passes through them, gives rise to the rainbow. The electromagnetic radiation radiated by the sun contains a mixture of rays including those of the visible spectrum. Each of these is refracted to a different extent.

Radiation can pass straight through tissues or be absorbed by molecules within them. For example, X-rays penetrate soft tissues but are absorbed by bone, whereas microwaves and infrared rays are easily absorbed by soft tissue and do not penetrate very far. The radiation of the visible spectrum is also absorbed by skin and underlying tissues but passes straight through

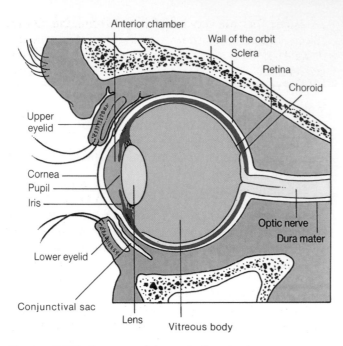

Figure 24.1 Structure of the eyeball and orbit. (From Rogers 1992, with permission of Elsevier.)

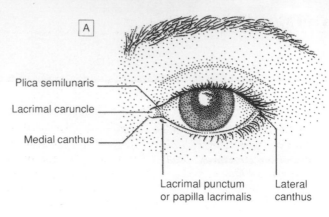

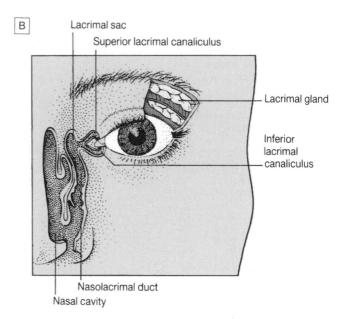

Figure 24.2 Protective structures of the eye. A, Eyelids. B, Lacrimal glands and drainage system. (From Rogers 1992, with permission of Elsevier.)

tissues that are crystalline in structure, such as the cornea and lens of the eye.

THE EYE

The eye (Fig. 24.1) is housed within the orbit of the skull, protected by the eyelids, and kept moist by the fluid secreted by several glands, including the lacrimal glands. The optical structures of the eye, the cornea, the lens and the fluid-filled chambers in front of and behind the lens, are all normally transparent. Electromagnetic radiation is refracted as it passes through them to be focused on the light-sensitive surface (retina) at the rear of the eyeball.

PROTECTIVE STRUCTURES

Eyelids

The eyelids consist of two folds of tissue, which meet at the medial canthus and lateral canthus (Fig. 24.2A). Each eyelid consists of connective tissue, muscle and small glands, and bears two or three rows of hairs (eyelashes). The inner side of each lid is covered by mucous membrane (conjunctiva) that extends over part of the eyeball. The space between the eyelids and the eyeball is the conjunctival sac (Fig. 24.1).

Lacrimal glands

The lacrimal glands lie under the upper eyelids (Fig. 24.2B) and secrete a watery solution containing antibacterial substances, including lysozyme. Secretion is increased by irritation of the cornea and conjunctiva, by a parasympathetic reflex. Fluid is swept over the cornea regularly by reflex blinking of the eyelids. Irritation provokes blinking and helps to protect and moisten the delicate tissue of the eyeball.

The fluid swept across the eyeball drains away through two small openings, close to the medial canthus, one in each eyelid (lacrimal punctum) (Fig. 24.2A). From the lacrimal punctum the fluid flows through a series of small vessels into the nasal cavity (Fig. 24.2B), which is why you need to blow your nose when you cry.

OPTICAL STRUCTURES

Cornea

The cornea (Fig. 24.1) is a transparent structure which forms the front one-sixth of the surface of the eye. It consists almost entirely of orderly collagen fibres, the even size and arrangement of which, coupled with a lack of blood vessels, give it a transparent appearance. The fibres in one layer run at 90° to those in the next, forming a regular structure. The frontal surface of the cornea is continuous with the conjunctiva, a mucous membrane covering the sclera and reflected back to line the eyelids. The conjunctiva secretes mucus which lubricates the eye surface.

The inner corneal surface is lined by a thin endothelium. The requirements of the cells in the epithelium and endothelium for nutrients and oxygen are met simply by the diffusion of these substances from the fluids of the eye or from the atmosphere.

The outer corneal surface is kept moist by the secretions formed by several glands:

- lacrimal glands – watery secretion
- tarsal glands of the eyelids – sebaceous secretion
- mucous glands of the inner lining of the eyelid – mucus.

Lens

The lens (Fig. 24.3), unlike the cornea, is composed entirely of cells, the overwhelming majority of which are dead. They are very long (about 1.0 cm), thin (2 μm) fibres, stacked in an orderly way like very thin wafers in a packet. The fibres are packed full of proteins (crystallins). These fibres were formed originally from the living epithelium at the front of the lens. Cells at the ends of the epithelium assemble into long thin fibres which are added to the fibres already there. New fibres go on being added throughout life, but increasingly slowly. In the centre of our eyes we still have the fibres that were formed long before we were born.

The very regular arrangement of the fibres, and the nature of the proteins inside them, makes the lens transparent. Opaque patches (cataracts) form when the nature and arrangement of the proteins change. Later on, calcium sometimes accumulates in the same area and this increases the opacity. The whole of the lens and the epithelium is covered by a thin elastic covering of connective tissue (capsule).

The lens is held under tension by the suspensory ligament which encircles it and which is anchored to the ciliary muscle (Fig. 24.4). When the ciliary muscle contracts, the tension on the lens decreases and the lens accommodates by rounding up in shape. This alteration in shape changes the focal length of the lens. With age, the lens becomes less flexible and is less able to thicken when the tension on the ligament is slackened. Consequently the focal length cannot be altered to allow focus on near objects to the same extent.

Iris and pupil

Just in front of the lens is the iris (Figs 24.4 and 24.1). This is a ring of tissue that includes pigment cells and smooth muscle, and is responsible for giving the eye

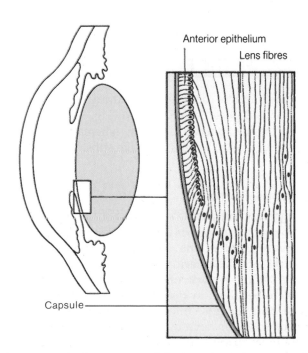

Figure 24.3 The structure of the lens. (From Rogers 1992, with permission of Elsevier.)

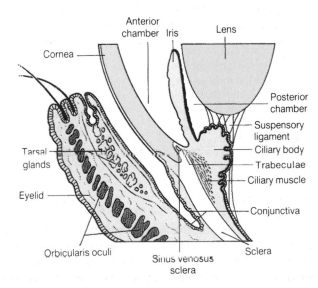

Figure 24.4 The sclerocorneal junction. (From Rogers 1992, with permission of Elsevier.)

Drugs affecting the autonomic nervous system and their uses in ophthalmology

This group of drugs either potentiates or blocks the action of normal chemical transmitter substances in the body and is used to control dilation of the pupil, lens accommodation and the production and flow of aqueous humour.

Sympathetic system
The postganglionic fibres of the sympathetic system supply the dilator pupillae, the trabecular meshwork and the blood vessels of the eye. The chemical transmitter is noradrenaline.

Drugs mimicking the action of the chemical transmitter (sympathomimetics) will therefore produce dilation of the pupil (mydriasis), decrease production of aqueous humour, lower outflow resistance and constrict conjunctival vessels. Examples are adrenaline (epinephrine) and phenylephrine.

Parasympathetic system
Here the postganglionic fibres innervate the constrictor pupillae and ciliary muscles as well as sending branches to the lacrimal gland and the trabecular meshwork. The chemical transmitter is acetylcholine.

Parasympathomimetics (which mimic the action of acetylcholine) may work directly or indirectly. Examples of direct action are:

- pilocarpine, which causes miosis (constriction of the pupil), accommodation and increased outflow of aqueous humour
- Miochol, which produces rapid constriction of the pupil and is particularly useful during some kinds of intraocular surgery.

An example of a drug that produces incorrect action by acting on enzymes that potentiate the action of acetylcholine is phospholine iodide, which is used in glaucoma.

Parasympathetic antagonists block the action of acetylcholine and cause pupil dilation and varying degrees of cycloplegia (paralysis of accommodation). Atropine is the most powerful long-acting agent. Tropicamide is a short-acting drug which dilates the pupil but has limited effect on accommodation. Cyclopentolate dilates the pupil and causes cycloplegia for up to 24 hours.

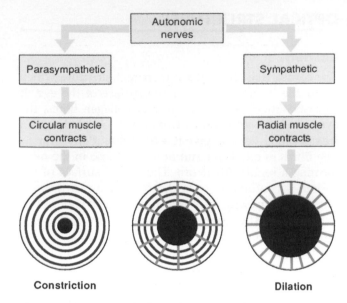

Figure 24.5 Control of pupillary size.

- parasympathetic fibres constrict the pupil
- sympathetic fibres dilate it.

These autonomic nerves form part of the reflex system controlling the amount of light passing through the pupil to the retina. If the light reaching the retina increases, the pupil reflexly constricts (pupillary light reflex), thereby reducing the amount of light entering; if it decreases, the pupil dilates, allowing more light in (see Ch. 5).

FLUIDS OF THE EYE

The small spaces between the cornea and the lens (anterior and posterior chambers) (Fig. 24.4) are filled with a liquid, aqueous humour, whereas the rest of the eyeball is filled with a jelly-like substance, vitreous body.

Aqueous humour

The aqueous humour is secreted continuously at the rate of about 2 ml per day by cells of the ciliary body. It flows up out of the posterior chamber, through the pupil into the anterior chamber and is reabsorbed through a meshwork of tiny bands of connective tissue (trabeculae), in the angle formed between the cornea and the iris, into a thin-walled vein (sinus venosus sclera or canal of Schlemm) (Fig. 24.4). If this drainage system is obstructed, the fluid pressure (normally 12–20 mmHg) increases. This happens in glaucoma.

colour. The pigment absorbs light rays. The more pigment present, the darker the colour of someone's eyes. Some of the smooth muscle is arranged radially and some encircles the hole in the centre (pupil). Contraction of the smooth muscle is controlled by the autonomic nerves (Fig. 24.5):

Damage to the vitreous body

Loss of substance from the vitreous body through trauma is serious because, unlike the aqueous humour, it is not renewed and loss may result in collapse of the eyeball or retinal detachment with resultant blindness. The vitreous body has a tendency to liquefy and contract in the elderly, making them more susceptible to retinal detachment.

If there has been vitreous loss, the patient may experience flashing lights because the pull on the retina of what remains of the vitreous body can stimulate the discharge of random impulses.

The vitreous body may become clouded by blood or other exudates from the retina, thus obstructing vision. This can be experienced as 'shreds of curtaining' impairing the visual field.

Vitrectomy (surgical removal of a damaged vitreous body) and replacement with infusion fluid, air or silicone oil, may be performed in an attempt to preserve retinal function.

Vitreous body

The vitreous body (or vitreous humour) consists of a jelly-like substance formed largely of hyaluronic acid, some collagen fibrils and water. The surface of the jelly is slightly firmer than the rest (rather like skin on custard) and is termed the vitreous membrane. This membrane is attached to the inside of the eyeball at two sites. At the front it is attached to the membrane covering the ciliary body, and at the rear to the rim of the optic disc.

FOCUSING THE IMAGE

Normal vision

For a clear image to be formed, the rays of light from an object must be focused on the retina in the same way that the lens of a camera focuses light rays on to a film. The cornea and the lens are the focusing system of the eye. They refract light rays because of their density and their shapes. The greater their density and their curvature, the greater is their focusing power, measured in dioptres.

Cornea

The cornea alone, due to its curved shape, has a focusing power of about 43 dioptres, but this is not enough to focus the light rays sharply on the retina.

Lens

The lens contributes about another 17 to 31 dioptres depending on its shape. At its flattest it contributes an

Glaucoma

Glaucoma is a pathological condition in which raised intraocular pressure can cause irreparable damage to the retina and optic nerve head by restricting essential capillary blood supply. It is a major cause of blindness.

There are several different types of glaucoma depending on the specific cause, but basically they all relate to either:

- an increase in intraocular content, such as over-production of aqueous fluid, bleeding or products of infection; or
- an obstruction in the trabecular drainage mechanism.

Glaucoma may be acute or chronic. An acute onset is accompanied by severe pain, but in chronic glaucoma, where onset is gradual, the condition is initially painless and may be difficult to detect before considerable damage has been done.

Prevention of the effects of glaucoma can best be achieved through:

- regular screening of high-risk individuals and people over the age of 40 years
- meticulous monitoring of postoperative or traumatized patients.

Early detection means that treatment can be started sooner to reduce intraocular pressure.

Treatment depends on the cause, the principle being to reduce the amount of fluid secreted into the eye, or to improve the drainage of fluid out of the eye.

If the cause relates primarily to a defect in the drainage system:

- eyedrops may be used to constrict the pupil and so stretch and open up the trabecular meshwork (e.g. pilocarpine)
- the trabecular meshwork may be opened up by various surgical procedures, creating additional drainage channels (e.g. trabeculectomy)
- laser treatment to the trabecular meshwork causes scarring which stretches the tissue between the laser burns and opens the spaces in the trabecular meshwork, thus allowing quicker drainage (trabeculoplasty).

If the cause relates primarily to over-production of aqueous humour, the treatment will be medical, using either eyedrops, such as timolol, or oral medication to inhibit production.

If the cause is trauma or surgery, then a combination of measures will be used.

extra 17 dioptres, which is sufficient to create a sharp image of a distant object on the retina in a normal eye (emmetropic eye). By shortening and thickening when the ciliary muscle contracts, another 12 to 14 dioptres is

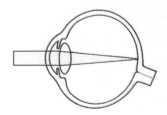

Myopia

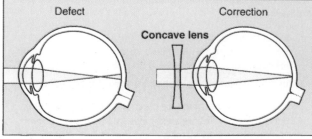

Hypermetropia

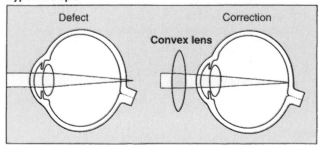

Figure 24.6 Optical problems and their correction.

added, enabling near objects (up to about 10 cm from the eye) to be seen clearly.

Myopia and hypermetropia

In some people, the focal length of the cornea and lens is not well matched to the length of the eyeball. Consequently light rays are brought to a focus either in front of or behind the retina (Fig. 24.6). In either case the image formed is blurred. In myopia (short-sightedness) the system is more powerful than normal, i.e. the focal length is shorter. Consequently objects can be brought closer to the eye than normal and are seen in more detail but objects at a distance are out of focus. Conversely in hypermetropia (long-sightedness), the system is less powerful than normal, the focal length is longer. As a result, distant objects can be seen clearly but close work becomes a problem.

Myopia can be caused by either an 'over-curved' cornea or, more frequently, an eyeball that is too 'long'. If the eyeball is overly long, the light rays emanating from a distant object are brought to a

focus too soon, and the focus has been lost by the time the light hits the retina.

Alternately, hypermetropia occurs as a result of either an 'under-curved' cornea or, more frequently, an eyeball that is too 'short'. If the eyeball is too short, the rays of light can not be brought to a focus in time. This results in an area of the retina being stimulated instead of a fixed point. This is perceived as blurred vision.

Both myopia and hypermetropia can be corrected by lenses of the right optical form and power (Fig. 24.6): concave lenses for myopia and convex lenses for hypermetropia.

Ophthalmoscopy

Usually an optometrist or an ophthalmologist will look at the structures inside the eyeball using an ophthalmoscope. This instrument enables a small beam of light to be shone into the eye. The rays reflected off the structures inside are focused by a series of lenses in the head of the instrument. By altering the focus, different parts of the eye, including the retina, and the surfaces of the cornea and lens can all be inspected.

RETINA

The retina (Fig. 24.7) is a thin film of tissue lining most of the inside of the eyeball. It contains:

- blood vessels
- nerve cells
- photoreceptors
- pigment cells.

Viewed through an ophthalmoscope, the retina looks an orangey-red colour. This is because of its blood supply and pigments, together with those of the choroid beneath it. In one part, a whitish patch can be seen (optic disc). This consists of axons of the optic nerve, and is the site where these axons leave the eyeball. The disc appears white because the axons here are myelinated.

From the optic disc, blood vessels extend outwards over the surface of the retina. The arteries are narrower than the darker veins. One area does not have any large blood vessels crossing it and appears slightly different in colour (macula lutea meaning 'yellow spot'). In its centre is a small depression, the fovea.

Photoreceptors

There are two types of photoreceptor: rods and cones (Fig. 24.8). A distinctive feature of both is the multiple layers of membrane stacked closely one on top of the other at one end of the cell. These membranes contain a

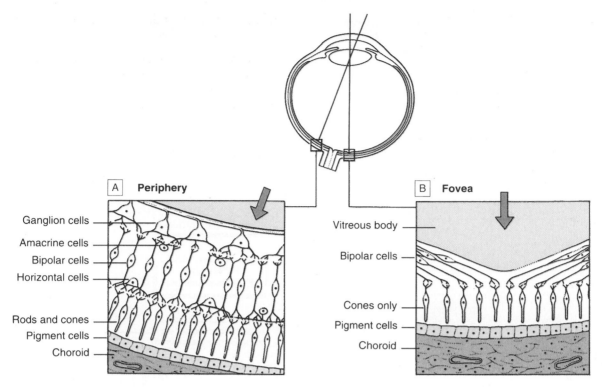

Figure 24.7 The retina and its structure. A, Periphery. B, Fovea.

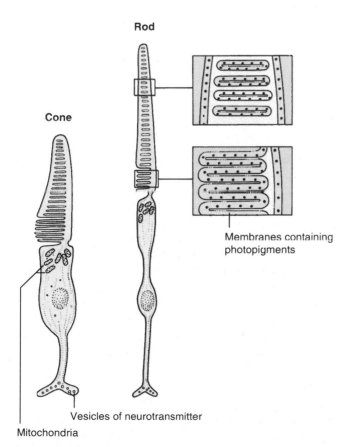

Figure 24.8 Structure of cones and rods.

photopigment that absorbs electromagnetic radiation and activates the receptor.

Rods

There are approximately 100 million rods per retina and they are responsible for 'shades of grey' vision and night vision. They have a high level of sensitivity and a low level of acuity. In terms of their location in the retina, the rods are more numerous in the periphery.

Cones

There are approximately 3 million cones per retina and they are responsible for 'colour' vision and day vision. They have a low level of sensitivity and a high level of acuity. In terms of their location in the retina, the cones are concentrated in the region of the fovea, the area of clearest and most detailed vision.

Photopigments

Photopigments consist of retinal, a derivative of vitamin A, coupled to one of several lipoproteins (opsins). In the human eye there are four different lipoproteins creating four different photopigments:

- rhodopsin in the rods
- erythrolabe, chlorolabe and cyanolabe in the cones (i.e. red sensitive, green sensitive and blue sensitive respectively).

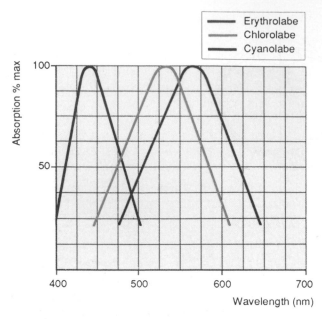

Figure 24.9 Spectral sensitivity of cone pigments. (After Marks et al 1964, and Brown & Wald 1964.)

Only one type of photopigment is present in each cone.

Each pigment is best at absorbing light rays of a particular range of wavelengths (Fig. 24.9). These ranges overlap. Consequently, rays of one wavelength are absorbed by more than one photopigment, but to differing extents. For example, 580 nm rays are absorbed by both erythrolabe and chlorolabe, but not by cyanolabe.

The sensation of colour is created by the blend of signals generated by the three different types of cone. If one or more types of cone are absent from the retina or lack photopigment then our perception of colour changes (colour blindness). Some colours may not be seen at all; others are confused.

Activation

Absorption of light rays by the photopigment changes the shape of the opsin, which in turn affects ion channels in the membrane, and alters the membrane voltage. This triggers the release of neurotransmitter from tiny vesicles in the receptor cells. The neurotransmitter diffuses across the synaptic cleft to activate the adjacent bipolar cell (Fig 24.10).

Innervation

Rods and cones are innervated by bipolar cells but whereas a large number of rods may all be innervated by the same cell, cone cells are sometimes individually innervated (Fig. 24.11). This is characteristic of the cones in the fovea. This difference in innervation is one of the reasons why objects that we look at directly (using the fovea) appear much more detailed than

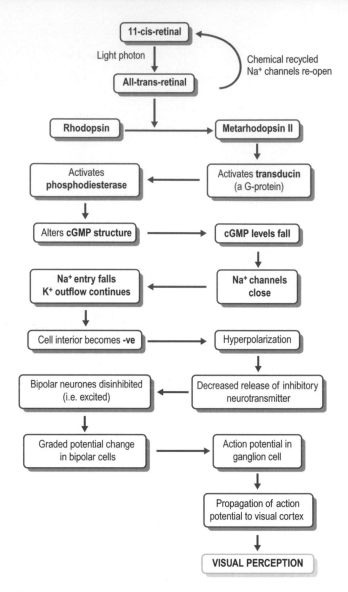

Figure 24.10 Sensory processing at the retina.

objects seen out of the corner of our eyes (peripheral field of vision).

The bipolar cells pass on the signal to the ganglion cells. These generate action potentials which are transmitted in the nerve fibres of the optic nerve.

Distribution

There is an uneven distribution of rods and cones in the retina (Fig. 24.11). The fovea has cones only, most of which are of the red or green type. Away from the fovea the number of cones decreases dramatically and the number of rods increases. There are no receptors of any type at the optic disc. As explained earlier, this part of the eye just contains the axons of the optic nerve. The absence of receptors here creates a small blind spot in the field of vision.

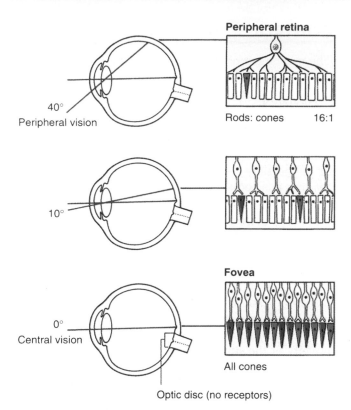

Rods: cones   16:1

Fovea

0°
Central vision

All cones

Optic disc (no receptors)

Figure 24.11 Differences in the innervation and distribution of rods and cones at the fovea compared with two peripheral areas of the retina.

You can demonstrate this if you close your right eye and look straight at the patient in Figure 24.12. Now move the book gradually backwards and forwards, whilst still keeping your eye on the patient. You should find a point where the bedpan disappears!

Nerve cells

The nerve cells in the retina form quite a complex system (Fig. 24.7). At least four different types of cell are present:

- ganglion cells
- bipolar cells
- amacrine cells
- horizontal cells.

The ganglion cells are the cells whose axons form the optic nerve (cranial nerve II). The axons lie on the surface of the retina, and are bundled together to form the optic nerve at the optic disc.

The bipolar cells are beneath the ganglion cells. They link the ganglion cells with the photoreceptors below. Running horizontally across the retina, the amacrine cells and horizontal cells allow some communication between adjacent receptors and also between ganglion cells.

Fovea

At the fovea, the structure of the retina looks slightly different (Fig. 24.7B). All the components are present, but the bipolar cells and ganglion cells appear to be pushed away from the centre, leaving the photoreceptors more exposed than at any other part of the retina.

Pigment cells and choroid

Beneath all these layers of cells is a pigment cell layer. This absorbs electromagnetic radiation that passes through the photoreceptor layer, and limits the amount of radiation that gets through to the choroid beneath.

The choroid also contains many pigment cells as well as blood vessels and connective tissue. It performs an important role in nourishing and maintaining the photoreceptors and the pigment cell layer.

The degree of pigmentation of the pigment cell layer and the choroid varies between people and is normally related to skin colour.

EYE MOVEMENTS

Movement of each eyeball is controlled by three pairs of muscles (Fig. 24.13), innervated by cranial nerves III, IV and VI:

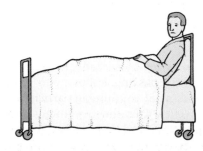

Figure 24.12 The blind spot!

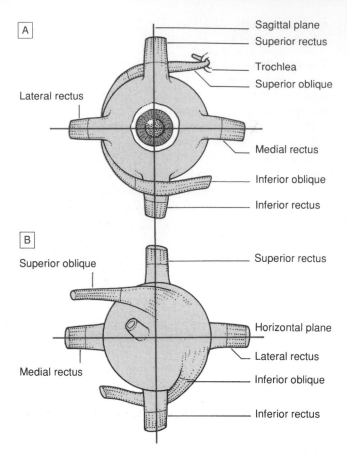

Figure 24.13 Muscles of the eyeball seen from in front and from behind.

- superior and inferior rectus
- superior and inferior oblique
- lateral and medial rectus.

These muscles enable us to look around as well as swivel our eyes inwards in order to view a near object (convergence).

There are two kinds of movement:

- pursuit
- saccadic.

In a pursuit movement, the eyeballs turn slowly and steadily in one direction, keeping track of the object in view, until the eyeballs have turned as far as they can. At this point the pursuit movement stops and the eyeball flicks back to its centre position. This rapid flick is a ballistic movement (saccade). The combination of movements, pursuit followed by saccade, is seen in rail travellers as they view the passing scenery.

When we are not looking at anything in particular but just looking around, we use saccadic movements too, to fix our eyes first on one point and then on another. From these several snapshots, we build up in our minds a full picture of the scene.

CONTROL

The movement of our eyes is controlled:

- reflexly
- voluntarily.

Reflexes make us look at a new object of interest and keep it in view regardless of whether we, or the object, are moving. Voluntary control enables us to look around or deliberately focus on an object of our choice, as in reading this book, for example.

Reflex control

Noticing a new object

When a novel object suddenly appears in our field of view we usually feel impelled to turn and look at it. Depending on where it is, we may simply turn our eyes, or we may turn our heads and bodies too. These movements are entirely reflex. They are triggered by the novelty of the stimulus, and their purpose is to enable us to bring the image of the novel stimulus on to the foveal part of the retina, which provides us with the clearest and most detailed vision.

We do not have to be conscious of the stimulus to react to it. We respond automatically because the parts of the brain that coordinate these responses are in the brain stem and not the thalamus and cerebral cortex, which are involved in consciousness. Consequently, a person who has sustained cerebral injury involving the visual cortex may still respond to an abrupt change in his surroundings, such as a flash of lightning, even though he cannot actually see it.

Similar reflexes enable us to turn our heads and bodies to face a new stimulus when we are startled by a sound, such as breaking glass, or by an unexpected tap on the shoulder. Again, the purpose of the reflex movement is to enable us to face and look at the novel stimulus.

Fixing on an object while you move

When walking down the road looking at the scenery, although your body goes up and down at each step, the picture in your mind's eye of the buildings or trees and bushes does not. However, if you attempt to take a photograph while walking the resulting picture is usually blurred.

The picture we see with our eyes is not blurred but remains steady chiefly because reflex movements of our eyes and head compensate for the movement of the body. The displacement of our bodies is rapidly detected by sensory receptors in the vestibular apparatus, and this sensory information reflexly triggers contraction of the appropriate muscles of the eyeball (vestibulo-ocular reflex) and of the neck (vestibulocollic

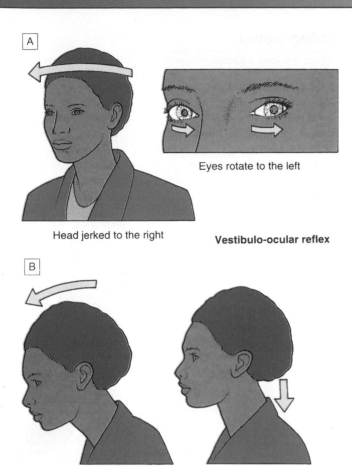

A

Eyes rotate to the left

Head jerked to the right **Vestibulo-ocular reflex**

B

Head tipped forwards | Neck muscles pull head back
Vestibulocollic reflex

Figure 24.14 Reflexes stabilizing eye position.

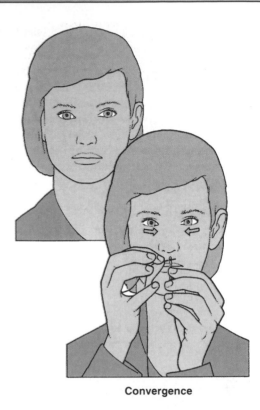

Convergence

Figure 24.15 Movement of the eyeballs for near vision.

reflex) (Fig. 24.14). As a result, the image of the object we are looking at is kept centred on the foveal part of the retina.

Tracking a moving object

Keeping our eyes fixed on a moving object, such as a bird or a car, depends upon a different reflex (opto-kinetic reflex). The movement of the object of interest is registered by cells in the visual areas of the cerebral cortex. Impulses from these cells are used to power a pursuit movement of the eye which is used to track the moving object and keep the image of it on the foveal region of the retina for as long as possible.

Viewing a near object

When we glance from a distant object to a near object, our eyeballs turn towards one another (converge) so that both point directly at the new object of interest (Fig. 24.15). This binocular movement is powered by a cortical reflex, which forms part of the near response.

Nystagmus

Nystagmus is a distinctive pattern of involuntary eye movement occurring sometimes in neurological disorders. An observer looking at someone's eyes would see that they do not remain steady but track rapidly and repeatedly in one direction. The pattern consists of a pursuit movement followed by a recentring saccade. There are two main sources of nystagmus:

- vestibular
- cerebellar.

Vestibular nystagmus

Vestibular nystagmus is provoked by signals originating from the vestibular system. Normally, movements of the eyes are reflexly triggered when movement of the body is sensed by the balance organs (vestibulo ocular reflex) (Fig. 24.14). This reflex depends partly on a comparison, made by cells of the vestibular nuclei, of the signals received from the balance organs on each side of the head.

If the vestibular system on one side is defective, the difference in signals from the balance organs on each side of the head is noted by the vestibular nucleus. This difference gives someone the impression that movement is occurring when it is not, and also triggers the reflexes normally associated with that movement, such as the vestibulo-ocular reflex. Consequently the eyes move as if pursuing an object and then recentre and begin the pursuit again, and keep on doing this.

Vestibular nystagmus is often accompanied by vertigo and nausea. The condition can be frightening for the sufferer, but reassurance and rest in a quiet darkened room can help.

Vestibular nystagmus can be evoked temporarily in healthy people by the simple manoeuvre of spinning someone around in a rotating chair, and then stopping the chair abruptly. The fluid in the subject's semicircular canals continues to spin for several seconds and, while it does, the vestibular receptors are stimulated, the impression of movement is created, and the vestibulo-ocular reflex is triggered, giving rise to nystagmus.

Cerebellar nystagmus

Nystagmus of cerebellar origin differs from vestibular nystagmus in that it happens only when movement is attempted. It is a form of intention tremor occurring when the gaze is shifted from one object to another. It disappears once the new object has been fixated.

Convergence is guided by the difference in the images of the object viewed through each eye. Convergence stops when the two images (formed by right eye and left eye) fit together best in the 'mind's eye'. These two images of a near object can never be exactly the same, but they are near enough for our minds to form an apparently single image.

The slight differences that continue to exist produce the three-dimensional view of objects (stereoscopic view) that we normally enjoy. This three-dimensional view helps us to form an impression of the relative distance of objects from us.

If there is weakness in one or more of the ocular muscles of either eye, it may become impossible for the two eyes to work together. Because they no longer point at the same object (strabismus or squint) the result is double vision (diplopia). If this occurs in young children, one of the two images may be suppressed. This can lead to irreversible changes in the visual cortex so that sight from one eye is permanently impaired.

Voluntary control

Voluntary control of eye movements, for example in looking around or reading, depends upon normal function of regions of the motor cortex and the cerebellum.

Looking around

When we look around, we scan the scene around us and fix our eyes briefly on different objects. This provides us with a number of snapshots of the scene from which we may choose one to inspect. Once something has caught our attention, the vestibulo-ocular, vestibulo-collic, and optokinetic reflexes maintain the position of the object of interest on the fovea, until we are

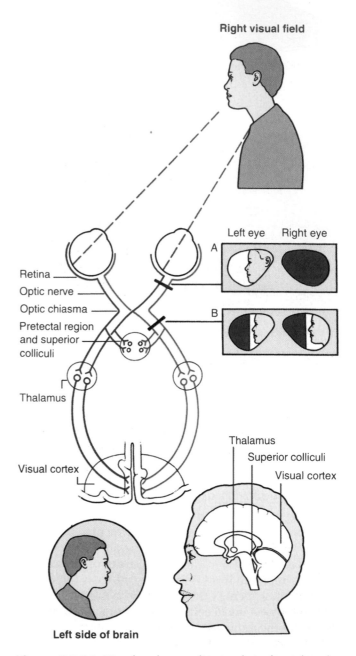

Figure 24.16 Visual pathways showing how the right side of our field of view is represented in the left visual cortex and the resulting effects of lesions of the pathway on vision in each eye: A, lesion of right optic nerve – loss of vision in right eye; B, lesion of the right optic tract beyond the chiasma – loss of vision in left visual field of both eyes.

The optic chiasm (Fig. 24.16) describes the union of the right and left optic nerves. Anatomically, this structure lies slightly anteriorly to the hypophyseal fossa.

When a patient has a pituitary tumour, they often describe symptoms of the loss of a field of vision.

Describe a possible field deficit in a patient who has a pituitary tumour.

distracted by something else or choose voluntarily to look at a different object.

Reading

When we read a book or a letter, our eyes do not move steadily across the page but jump from one point to the next in a series of saccades. Some techniques designed to improve reading speed do so by reducing the number of saccades necessary to read a page of text. Reading difficulties may sometimes be caused by disordered control of eye movements.

VISUAL PATHWAYS

The optic nerves from each eye meet up at the optic chiasma (Fig. 24.16). Here the nerve fibres carrying signals from the nasal half of the retina cross over to the other side, so that information about objects on the right-hand side of the scene we are looking at (right visual field) is carried over to the left side of the brain and vice versa. If injury occurs to the visual pathway on one side of the brain after the chiasma, there will be loss of vision in one half of the visual field of both eyes (Fig. 24.16B).

From the chiasma, impulses are transmitted to the midbrain to evoke several visual reflexes and to the thalamus and the visual cortex in the cerebral hemispheres to give rise to the sensations of light, colour and movement.

MIDBRAIN

After the optic chiasma, some fibres branch off the optic tract to go to parts of the pretectal region and to the superior colliculi. These areas are concerned with several visual reflexes including the pupillary light reflex, and reflex eye and head movements.

Pupillary light reflex

When light is shone into either or both of the two eyes the pupils normally constrict. Because this reflex is coordinated in the midbrain and not further along the visual pathway, it can be evoked in someone who has cortical brain damage. If the visual cortex itself is damaged, someone is unable to see even though the pupillary light reflex is present.

CEREBRAL HEMISPHERES

Axons of the retinal ganglion cells pass to the thalamus in each cerebral hemisphere. From there another set of nerve fibres carry the signals to the visual cortex in the occipital lobe of each hemisphere.

Visual cortex

The visual cortex is made up of a number of different areas, each of which plays a different role in the processing of impulses from the eyes. Each area receives information from both eyes (binocular vision) creating a three-dimensional (3D) mental picture of what we see.

Areas and their functions

One area of the visual cortex, referred to as V4, creates the sensation of colour, another creates an awareness of movement, and yet another, the primary visual cortex or striate cortex, is primarily concerned with the shape of objects. Normally these areas are interlinked, and so the features they represent are fused in our minds. However, if they become disconnected, or if one area is damaged, there can be curious disturbances of perception, such as seeing objects but not properly following their movement.

In each of the different areas, adjacent cells receive signals from adjacent areas of the retina, so that each area of the visual cortex is like a map of the retina (retinotopic representation). However, the map is not to scale, because it relates to the number of receptors in the retina and the way they are innervated. As the fovea is richly innervated with nerve fibres, a disproportionately large area of the visual cortex is devoted to it.

Binocular vision

When we look at an object close to us, the image of it seen by each eye is not exactly the same. Although the differences are minimized by the way in which our two eyes are caused to swivel inwards, as part of the near response so that the image falls on the fovea in each eye, they are not eliminated because each eye views the object from a slightly different perspective.

We actually see both pictures although we think we are only looking at one, and as a result we gain the impression of depth and perceive three dimensions rather than two.

VIEWPOINT

All that has been described begins to reveal how an image is created in our minds, but it does not explain how we know what we are looking at. The black and white picture shown in Figure 24.17 makes this clear. What do you see? Your retina and visual cortex analyse the pattern of light and dark, and create a mental image of it. But did you see a young person or an old lady when you first looked at the picture? Your answer will depend on the links (associations) formed in your mind between that pattern of black and white and other images remembered from the past.

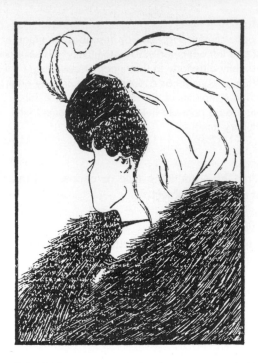

Figure 24.17 Drawing made by the cartoonist A. E. Hill in 1915.

REFERENCES AND FURTHER READING

Brown P K, Wald G 1964 Visual pigments of single primate cones. Science 144: 45–82

Davson H 1990 Physiology of the eye, 5th edn. Macmillan Press, Basingstoke

Elkington A R, Khan P T 1988 ABC of eyes. British Medical Association, London

Gaston H, Elkington A 1986 Ophthalmology for nurses. Chapman & Hall, London

Hill W E 1915 My wife and mother-in-law. Puck, Week ending 6 November 1915 (The original publication of this now very familiar cartoon)

Marks W B, Dobelle W H, MacNichol E F 1964 Visual pigments of single primate cones. Science 143: 1181–1183

Parr J 1989 Introduction to ophthalmology, 3rd edn. Oxford University Press, Oxford

Perry J P, Tullo A B (eds) 1990 Care of the ophthalmic patient: a guide for nurses and health professionals. Chapman & Hall, London

Remington L A, McGill E 1997 Clinical anatomy of the visual system. Butterworth-Heinemann, Oxford

Rogers A W 1992 Textbook of anatomy. Churchill Livingstone, Edinburgh

Tovee M J 1996 An introduction to the visual system. Cambridge University Press, Cambridge

25 Motor systems: an overview

When skeletal muscle contracts it causes movement of parts of the skeleton (e.g. lifting a leg or bending the neck), or it stiffens and supports different structures (e.g. tensing the abdominal wall or holding the head up).

Movement usually involves the coordinated activity of different muscles. The simplest form of coordination occurs in reflex movements. These are chiefly mediated via the spinal cord and brain stem. The more complex movements we make when we choose to perform various actions involve other parts of the central nervous system including the motor cortex and basal ganglia of the cerebral hemispheres, and the cerebellum (Fig. 25.1).

REFLEX MOVEMENTS

A reflex is an automatic response triggered by a stimulus. It happens without our thinking about it. It can be simple, like a knee jerk, or more complicated, such as maintaining your balance if you are pushed. Simple reflexes involve just a few sensory receptors and a few muscle groups. Complex reflexes draw upon sensory information from several sources and coordinate activity in many different muscles.

ORGANIZATION AND TERMINOLOGY

The basic components of a reflex are shown in Figure 25.2. A reflex arc consists of a sensory component and a motor component, linked usually by connecting neurones (interneurones). When the sensory receptor is excited, impulses are transmitted to the motor neurones exciting the muscle and causing it to contract.

Muscles that, on contraction, cause extension of a limb are termed extensors whereas those that cause flexion are termed flexors. Hence some reflexes are referred to as 'extensor', for example the plantar reflex, whereas others are termed 'flexor', for example the withdrawal reflex.

Muscles acting in opposite ways at a joint are referred to as the agonist and antagonist respectively. For example, the biceps and triceps muscles of the arm operate as an agonist/antagonist pair. Contr of the biceps flexes the arm; contraction of the extends it. The agonist muscle is defined as which by contraction causes movement. Thus v

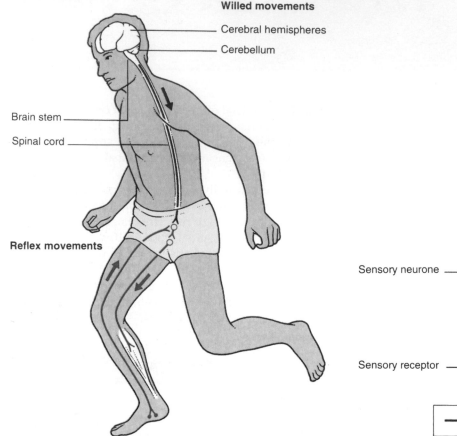

Figure 25.1 Voluntary and reflex control of movement.

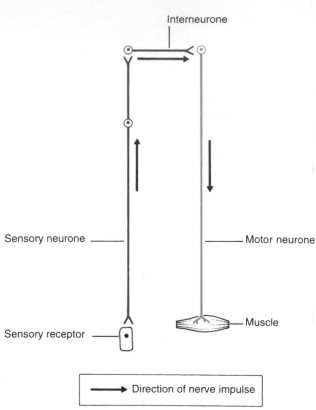

Figure 25.2 Basic components of a reflex arc.

arm is flexed the agonist is the biceps; when the arm is extended the agonist is the triceps.

When the agonist is excited, contraction of antagonist muscles is often, but not always, inhibited. The way in which agonist and antagonist muscles are linked into the reflex arc (reciprocal innervation) enables them to react in opposite ways to the same stimulus (Fig. 25.3).

SIZE OF THE RESPONSE

Order of recruitment of motor units

When a muscle, such as the biceps, is activated, all its motor units (Fig. 25.4) are not usually active at the same time. If the stimulus is small only the smallest motor units are excited. As the stimulus increases in size larger motor units are co-opted (recruited). Eventually, at maximum contraction, all motor units are participating. This set order of recruitment of the units is determined by how closely packed together the synaptic contacts are on the motor neurones. The smallest motor units are innervated by motor neurones with the smallest cell

bodies. In these cells the synapses are very close to one another on the cell body in the central nervous system (Fig. 25.4). This makes it easy for the motor neurones to be excited. On the larger cell bodies of the motor neurones of the large motor units, the synapses are more spaced out, and many more stimuli are needed to excite the motor neurone.

Spread of excitation

The nerve terminals of the sensory axons and of the interneurones make many synaptic contacts in the brain and in the spinal cord, some of which connect with motor neurones supplying other muscles. If the original stimulus is weak, then only a few muscles are reflexly excited and the movement evoked is small. If the stimulus is stronger, other interneurones and motor neurones are recruited and more muscles are activated. This is known as irradiation of the stimulus. For example, if you touch something hot you may simply withdraw your hand. Only muscles of the arm are excited. But if the stimulus was very large, you would probably react by pulling your whole body away. In this

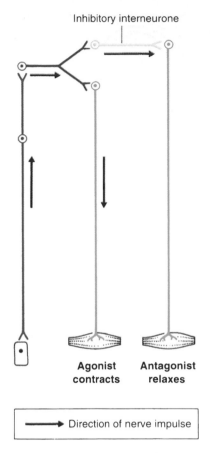

Figure 25.3 Reciprocal innervation of agonist and antagonist muscles.

Agonist contracts

Antagonist relaxes

→ Direction of nerve impulse

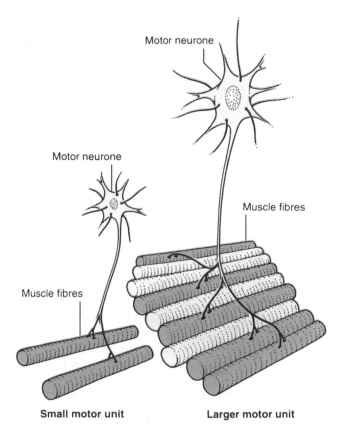

Figure 25.4 Motor units of different size (a motor unit is a motor neurone plus all the muscle fibres it innervates).

case muscles of the trunk and legs would be reflexly excited as well.

MUSCLE TONE AND THE STRETCH REFLEX

Definition and basis

If you lift someone's arm or leg and gently flex and extend it, you should feel a very slight resistance. This resistance to movement is termed muscle tone. It is due to the reflex contraction of the muscles of the limb flexed and extended (stretch reflex), in response to the excitation of sensory receptors (muscle spindles) embedded in the muscle.

A stretch reflex can be elicited if the patellar tendon is tapped just below the kneecap (Fig. 25.5). For this reason stretch reflexes are sometimes referred to as tendon jerks. When the tendon is tapped, the muscle of the thigh, quadriceps femoris, is briefly stretched, and this stretch excites the muscle spindles. This provokes reflex contraction of the same muscle. Similarly, when

Recruitment of neurones and irradiation of the stimulus are particularly evident in Jacksonian fits. These are focal epileptic seizures which may be caused by cerebral tumours, vascular lesions or an abscess. The 'fit' progresses in a stereotyped manner; for example jerky, spasmodic movements (clonic spasms) starting in the thumb and index finger may spread to the hand and arm and perhaps to the rest of the body. The individual may also lose consciousness depending on the extent of the cerebral cortex involved.

Protecting the patient from harm during a seizure is an essential role of the nurse and allied health professional staff. While maintaining a safe environment for your patient during their seizure activity, what observations would you note in order to report these to the medical team?

the leg is flexed, the spindles in the thigh muscles are stimulated. This causes a small reflex contraction of these muscles, and the slight resistance to movement that can be felt.

The degree of resistance felt depends upon the sensitivity of the muscle spindles. If their sensitivity to

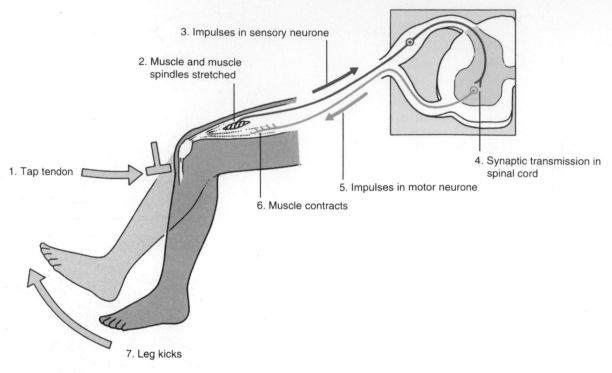

3. Impulses in sensory neurone

2. Muscle and muscle
spindles stretched

1. Tap tendon

4. Synaptic transmission in
spinal cord

5. Impulses in motor neurone

6. Muscle contracts

7. Leg kicks

Figure 25.5 The knee jerk (stretch reflex).

stretch is high, they respond much more vigorously and evoke a much stronger reflex contraction of the muscle; consequently resistance to passive movement is high (hypertonia). Conversely, if the sensitivity of the spindles to stretch is low, very little if any resistance will be felt. As a result, the limb will feel limp (hypotonia).

Sensitivity of muscle spindles

The sensitivity of the muscle spindles is controlled by small motor neurones (gamma motor neurones) that innervate the muscular part of the intrafusal fibres of the muscle spindle. The cell bodies of the gamma motor neurones are intermingled in the anterior (ventral) horn of the spinal cord with the motor neurones supplying the muscle itself. The latter are classified, and often referred to, as alpha motor neurones.

If the frequency of impulses in the gamma motor neurones increases, the muscle spindle becomes more sensitive to stretch, whereas if the gamma motor neurones fire less frequently the spindles become less sensitive.

Changes in tone

If the spindles are more sensitive to stretch, or if alpha motor neurones are more excitable, at least two things occur:

- exaggeration of stretch reflexes
- hypertonia.

This means that when stretch reflexes are elicited by tapping the tendon of a muscle, the muscle jerk is produced much more easily and is bigger, and when the limbs are moved passively, increased resistance to movement is felt by the examiner.

Exaggerated reflexes and hypertonia occur when there is a reduction in impulses from the areas of the cerebral hemispheres involved in the control of movement. This can happen as a result of a spinal injury or a stroke. As the effect of these impulses from the brain is usually inhibitory, their withdrawal makes alpha and gamma motor neurones more excitable. The result is either:

- spasticity, or
- rigidity.

In spasticity, reflexes are exaggerated, and there is increased resistance to passive movement of the limbs. In rigidity, however, it is noticeable that muscles are tensed even when there is no movement, either active or passive. Also, when an examiner attempts to move the limbs passively, the resistance felt does not feel the same as in spasticity. These differences in tone are related to the specific parts of the brain which are injured or abnormal, and may involve increased sensitivity to stretch of different types of intrafusal fibres (nuclear bag and nuclear chain).

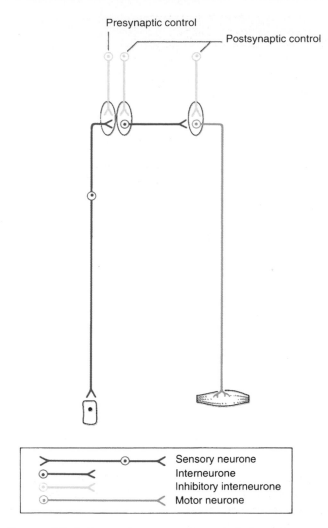

Presynaptic control
Postsynaptic control

→——————⊙——<	Sensory neurone
⊙——————<	Interneurone
⊙——————<	Inhibitory interneurone
⊙——————<	Motor neurone

Figure 25.6 Pre- and postsynaptic control of neurones forming a reflex arc.

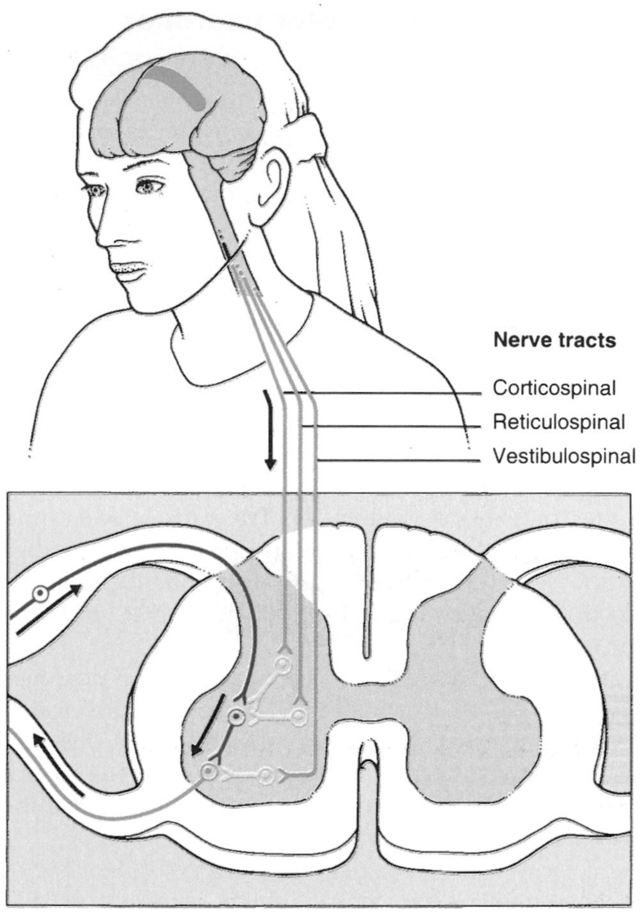

Nerve tracts

Corticospinal
Reticulospinal
Vestibulospinal

Figure 25.7 Major spinal tracts controlling the movement of the trunk and limbs.

CONTROL OF REFLEXES

Any reflex can be prevented or exaggerated through the influence of impulses from elsewhere in the nervous system. The excitability of interneurones and motor neurones is affected by transmitters released from other nerves making synaptic contact pre- or postsynaptically either with the interneurones or with the motor neurones of the reflex arc (Fig. 25.6). For example, knee jerks are sometimes easier to elicit if someone is feeling tense. This is because the excitability of the motor neurones (alpha and gamma) is increased by a change in the balance of the excitatory and inhibitory inputs. Conversely, if someone is feeling very 'laid back', reflex responses may be smaller because synaptic transmission of impulses is depressed by inhibitory neurotransmitters.

Control by different brain areas

When we choose to perform more complex movements, reflexes are allowed or disallowed through the release of neurotransmitters triggered by impulses from several parts of the brain. These areas include:

- cerebral cortex (specifically, motor cortex)
- brain stem (reticular formation and vestibular nuclei).

Impulses are transmitted from these areas to the interneurones and motor neurones of the basic reflex loops through several nerve tracts (Fig. 25.7). The tracts are named according to their origin and their destination. Thus the corticospinal tracts link the motor cortex with the spinal cord whereas the vestibulospinal tracts connect the vestibular nuclei in the brain stem with the neurones in the spinal cord. Corticobulbar tracts (not shown in the figure) link the cerebral cortex with the brain stem.

Upper and lower motor neurones

As neurones forming these tracts carry impulses from the brain towards the muscles, they are classified as motor neurones. However, a distinction is made between the motor neurones actually contacting (innervating) skeletal muscle (lower motor neurones) and those coming from the brain (upper motor neurones) that influence the lower motor neurones. Injury to lower and upper motor neurones produces different sorts of disability. Lower motor neurone injury produces:

• paralysis
• flaccidity
• atrophy.

Paralysis occurs because the muscle cannot be excited either reflexly or voluntarily. The muscle feels limp (flaccid) because impulses from muscle spindles cannot get through to it and consequently there is no tone. Because the muscle is not used it gradually atrophies.

In contrast, damage to the upper motor neurones alters the ease with which different reflexes are elicited (either increasing or decreasing them) but it does not usually abolish them. What does change is the control that can be exerted over voluntary movements and the way that they are executed.

Spinal shock

If impulses from the brain are cut off completely, because of injury to the spinal cord, the muscles controlled by motor neurones below the level of injury are initially temporarily paralysed (spinal shock). Both voluntary and reflex activity is lost. After a time spinal reflexes return, but when they do they are more powerful than normal. This is because many of the reflexes are normally held in check by the effects of inhibitory neurotransmitters released as a result of activity in the upper motor neurones. If the release of these transmitters is prevented because of injury to the upper motor neurones, reflex responses are unrestrained.

WILLED MOVEMENTS

When we choose to sit or stand, turn over the pages of a book, look around, run after someone, or perform some other more complicated activity, muscle contraction is coordinated and refined by three parts of the brain:

• motor cortex of the cerebral hemispheres
• basal ganglia
• cerebellum.

Spinal injury

If there is complete transection of the spinal cord causing *paraplegia* (loss of movement and sensation in the lower extremities), the lack of signals to the muscles of the lower limbs results in flaccid paralysis. Once the patient's condition is stable, the flaccid limbs should be put through a full range of movements every day to prevent atrophy and disuse contractures. A *contracture* is a deformity caused by shortening of muscle and an associated thickening of surrounding connective tissue.

The physiotherapy programme will also aim towards building the unaffected parts of the body (i.e. neck, shoulders, arms and trunk) to optimal strength for eventual weight-bearing activities. Such programmes are designed according to each individual's specific neurological deficit.

However, in many patients with paraplegia, spasticity follows the initial flaccidity because the normal balance between excitatory and inhibitory nerve impulses has been upset. Exaggerated reflexes can result in joints becoming flexed and fixed, and painful flexor and extensor spasms occur – often triggered by touch. The position of the limbs is important. The knees must be kept almost straight and the feet supported in dorsiflexion, or standing will become impossible.

Antiembolic stockings will help prevent pooling of blood in the legs. Hospital guidelines will provide guidance regarding deep vein thrombosis prophylaxis. Whilst positional changes need to be minimized to prevent further trauma, a variety of pressure relieving aids and special nursing beds are available to prevent the formation of pressure sores.

Spinal shock is the term given to the loss of all reflex, motor, sensory and autonomic activity below the level of the spinal lesion/injury. It may last several weeks. In addition to being paralysed, patients in spinal shock lack vasomotor tone in their lower extremities and consequently will become hypotensive in an upright position (see Ch. 6).

Each part differs in its functions. The motor cortex receives impulses from parts of the brain, including the basal ganglia, that link our awareness of ourselves and our environment with appropriate actions. Movements are refined by the cerebellum, with the help of sensory feedback from receptors in the muscles and tendons (proprioceptors), to achieve actions that are as close as possible to those intended. Injury or disease produces different forms of disability depending on the part of the brain affected.

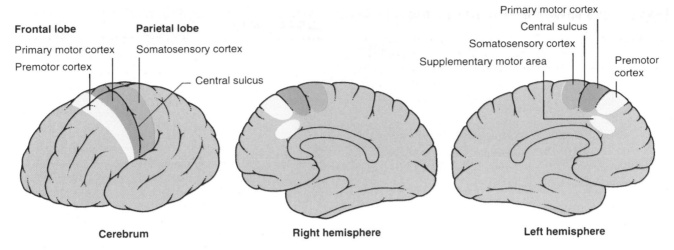

Figure 25.8 Regions of the cerebral cortex involved in the control of movement.

ROLE OF THE MOTOR CORTEX

Specific areas and their functions

The primary motor area of the cerebral cortex lies in the frontal lobes of the cerebral hemispheres just in front of the central sulcus (Fig. 25.8). If cells in this area are stimulated, specific movements of different parts of the body occur. A map can be drawn of the parts of the body affected by stimulation of different cells (Fig. 25.9) just as it could for the cells of the somatosensory cortex. It can be seen from the diagram of the homunculus ('little man') that most of the cells of the primary motor area are concerned with movements of the hands, face and lips.

At least two other areas of the cerebral cortex also have a major role in the control of movement. These are the premotor area and the supplementary motor area (Fig. 25.8). The homunculi in these areas differ from that of the primary motor area. For example, most of the cells of the supplementary area are concerned with movements of the limbs, and less are involved with the hands, face and lips.

The cortical cells are normally excited by stimuli transmitted to them from:

• the thalamus
• the somatosensory cortex
• some areas of the association cortex.

The cells of the motor cortex represent one of the later stages in the process by which thoughts are translated into actions. Signals from the association areas of the cerebral cortex that are involved in perception and thinking are transmitted to cells of the motor cortex which pass on the information to appropriate upper motor neurones.

Upper motor neurones

Cells of the motor cortex exert control over muscle contraction through either direct or indirect routes. The direct routes begin in the primary motor area and end on interneurones and/or lower motor neurones in the brain stem (corticobulbar tracts) or spinal cord (corticospinal tracts). The corticobulbar tracts control muscles of the face and jaws, whereas the corticospinal tracts control muscles of the limbs and trunk.

Many of the lower motor neurones innervating muscles controlling the fingers, lips and tongue are directly innervated by neurones originating in the cerebral cortex. Thus the cerebral cortex is particularly important in the control of activities such as handling objects, writing and speaking.

The indirect routes pass from the premotor and the supplementary motor areas of the cerebral cortex to the interneurones in the brain stem and the spinal cord, via nuclei in the reticular formation. The nerve tracts originating from the nuclei in the reticular formation that innervate interneurones in the spinal cord are termed the reticulospinal tracts. These tracts have a major role in the control of voluntary changes in posture and in moving arms and legs.

Effects of injury

Damage to the motor cortex (e.g. in a stroke) impairs voluntary movement. Muscles can still be activated reflexly. In other words, they are not paralysed, but voluntary movements are weak (paresis). Some reflexes, for example stretch reflexes such as the knee jerk, are exaggerated. This is because the upper motor neurones have a predominantly inhibitory effect on these reflexes, so that, if their influence is

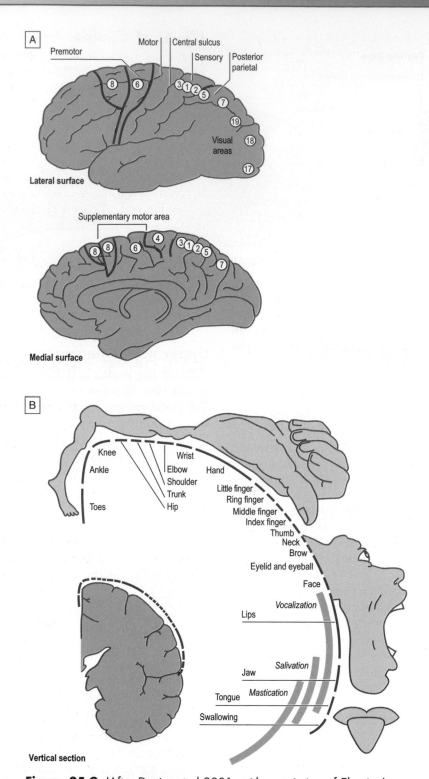

Figure 25.9 (After Davies et al 2001, with permission of Elsevier.)

withdrawn, reflexes are elicited much more easily. Stretch reflexes are enhanced and muscle tone is increased (spasticity).

ROLE OF THE BASAL GANGLIA

Nature and organization

The basal ganglia consist of several clusters of cell bodies (nuclei) deep within the cerebral hemispheres. The nuclei are interconnected, and are linked also to the thalamus (Fig. 25.10).

The basal ganglia receive impulses from different parts of the association areas of the cerebral cortex. They are thus supplied with information about our thoughts. The command signals sent out from the basal ganglia pass first to the thalamus and from there to many different areas of the cerebral cortex including the motor cortex, particularly the premotor and supplementary motor areas.

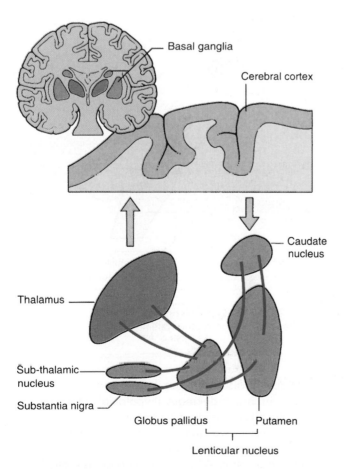

Figure 25.10 The basal ganglia and their relationship to and with the cerebral cortex.

Effects of disorder

Much of the understanding that has been gained over the years about the role of the basal ganglia in the control of movement has been deduced from studies of patients with movement disorders.

A characteristic feature of all disorders of the basal ganglia is that unsolicited movements occur even when someone is not intending to move. The magnitude and nature of these movements differ according to which group of cells is affected and how their function has become disordered. Some examples are listed in Table 25.1.

Another characteristic feature of disorders of the basal ganglia is that muscle tone is often increased, but the character of the change (rigidity) is different from that characteristic of injury to the motor cortex (spasticity).

ROLE OF THE CEREBELLUM

Organization and functions

The cerebellum sits astride the back of the brain stem linked to it by the cerebellar peduncles, which consist of afferent and efferent nerve fibres. There are extensive links between the cerebellum and the balance organs (vestibular system), and also with other nuclei in the brain.

One part of the cerebellum (flocculo-nodular lobe) (Fig. 25.11) is specifically concerned with balance. Other areas (vermis and paravermal regions) are associated chiefly with walking and gait. The lateral hemispheres are involved with the performance of highly skilled movements such as drawing, speaking, and pointing to and placing objects accurately.

The cerebellum receives nerve impulses from all the other areas of the brain involved in the control of movement, as well as from sensory receptors including muscle proprioceptors, via the spinocerebellar tracts, and the balance organs, via the vestibular nuclei (Fig. 25.12). It is therefore able to compare information about the intended movement with the actual movement occurring. If there is a difference between intent and performance, corrective adjustments are made by the cerebellum to the movement while it is being performed. Signals from the cerebellum are passed back to the other motor areas with the result that the command signals issued via the upper motor neurones are modified. As a result, the movement is made more accurate.

In this way the cerebellum controls and coordinates movements that have been initiated elsewhere.

Table 25.1 Disorders of the basal ganglia

Disorder	Characteristic features	Site of defect
Athetosis	Involuntary slow writhing movements (mostly distal muscles)	Lenticular nucleus
Ballismus	Involuntary violent flailing movements	Sub-thalamic nucleus
Chorea	Involuntary rapid jerky movements	Caudate nucleus
Parkinson's disease	Poverty of movement (akinesia) Rigidity Involuntary tremor	Substantia nigra

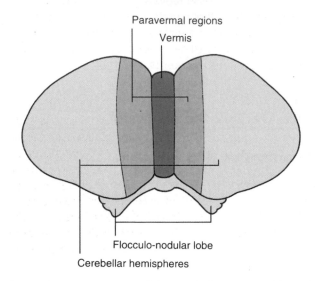

Figure 25.11 Structure of the cerebellum (viewed from the back).

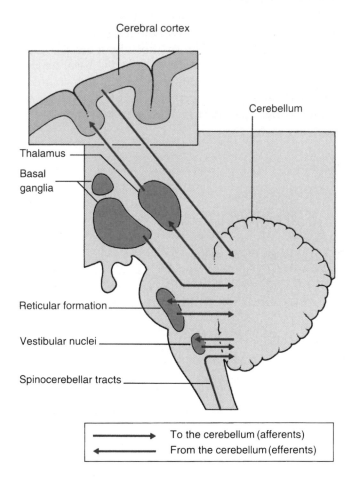

Figure 25.12 Functional connections of the cerebellum with other parts of the motor system.

Effects of disorder

Cerebellar disorders are characterized by inaccurate and uncoordinated movements (ataxia) (Table 25.2). For example, a person with cerebellar disorder may not be able to reach straight towards an object and pick it up accurately. He will over- or undershoot, then over- or undercorrect and so on until eventually the object is secured. Also, movements that are normally coordinated and performed smoothly may be broken down into their separate parts. The ordinary movement of raising a hand may only be achieved by first moving the shoulder, then the upper arm, and finally the forearm.

As movements in general are less accurate, a different stance may have to be adopted in walking to reduce the likelihood of falling over. Changes in muscle tone are not a prominent feature of cerebellar disorders, but if they do occur the effect is usually a decrease (hypotonia). Many of the signs of cerebellar impairment, namely unsteadiness in walking, slurred speech and clumsiness, are also seen in someone who has drunk too much alcohol. All parts of the brain are affected by alcohol but the impairment of skilled activities is most noticeable.

Table 25.2 General features of cerebellar disorder

Feature	Technical term
Incoordination of movement in general	Ataxia
Drunken gait	Locomotor ataxia
Inaccuracy in positioning hands and feet (as when reaching out to pick up an object)	Dysmetria (past pointing)
Tremor when making a movement	Intention tremor
Inability to perform rapidly alternating movements	Adiadochokinesia

MUSCLES AND MOVEMENT

PRINCIPLES

Movements

When one part of the skeleton is moved by muscle contraction, related parts have to be steadied by other muscles for the movement to be effective. The muscle which pulls on the moving bone (movable point) has to be anchored to another bone which is steadied (fixed point). The joint between them acts as the fulcrum or pivot of the system (Fig. 25.13A).

Usually there are at least two opposing muscles (agonist and antagonist) acting on a joint, one causing it to flex (flexor), and the other causing it to extend (extensor) (Fig. 25.13B). If the joint allows rotation, other muscles inserted in slightly different places can twist the bone in one direction or the other when they contract.

Supporting forces

Maintaining an upright posture, whether sitting or standing, requires energy. However, there are efficient and inefficient ways of doing this. If for example someone stands erect, with legs slightly apart, the body is well balanced, and the force of gravity acts straight down the weight-bearing line of the body (Fig. 25.14). Relatively little energy is required to sustain this posture and, if the body sways, only minor additional effort is needed to recentre it. If someone slouches, however, more energy is needed and extra strain is placed on ligaments and joints.

Lever systems

The least stable part of the body is the head, perched on top of the spine. It is balanced on top of the atlas but the weight of the front part, which tends to make the head fall forward, has to be counteracted by a steady downward pull of the neck muscles to the rear (Fig. 25.15A). This is an example of one of several lever systems used in the body that maximize the efficiency of the movements that are made and minimize the energy required to sustain certain postures. Other examples are shown in Figure 25.15B & C.

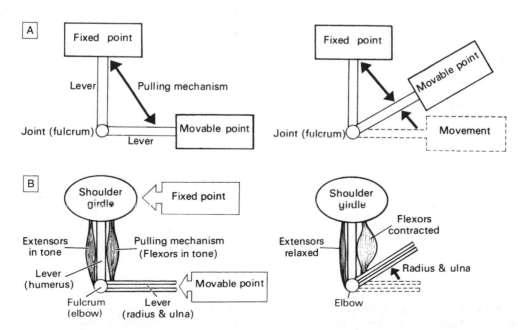

Figure 25.13 Principles of movement. A, Theoretical components. B, Relation to movement of the forearm. (From Chilman & Thomas 1987, with permission of Elsevier.)

TYPES OF MOVEMENT

The types of movement, flexion, extension, abduction, adduction and so on that are possible for different parts of the body are illustrated in Figure 25.16.

MUSCLES AND NERVES

Superficial muscles of the trunk and limbs, and their relation to major nerves, are shown in Figures 25.17 and 25.18. The major muscles involved in some of the movements shown in Figure 25.16 are listed in Tables 25.3 and 25.4.

CONTROL AND COORDINATION

MAINTAINING AN UPRIGHT POSTURE

Body

The natural upright posture is maintained by a number of different reflexes that excite extensor muscles of the lower limbs, trunk and neck.

The plantar reflex is evoked by excitation of low threshold mechanoreceptors in the skin of the soles of the feet. When excited these reflexly excite the extensor muscles of the leg.

The balance organs play their part in maintaining balance by detecting movement and reflexly evoking contraction of the extensors through impulses passing along the vestibulospinal tracts. If the balance organs are impaired, a person will have difficulty staying upright, particularly with the eyes closed. With eyes open, visual reflexes also help to maintain balance.

Stretch receptors in the muscles (muscle spindles) also maintain contraction of the extensor muscles. Swaying slightly to one side, muscles of the leg and trunk of the opposite side are stretched, this reflexly excites their contraction and pulls the body back to the centre line.

If, in response to a painful stimulus, we reflexly lift one foot off the ground, the crossed extensor reflex will at the same time cause increased contraction of the extensor muscles of the other leg to maintain balance.

Head

Keeping the head up requires strong and maintained contraction of the neck muscles. This is sustained by tonic neck reflexes and righting reflexes powered by excitation of receptors in the muscles and joints of the neck, and by the vestibulocollic reflex excited by stimulation of the balance organs.

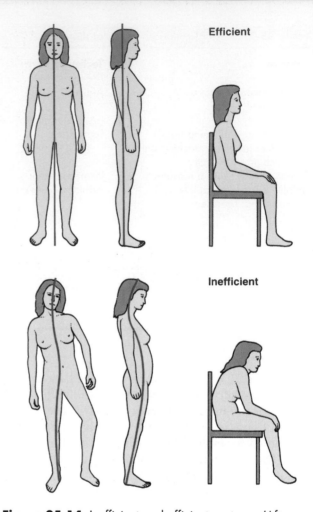

Figure 25.14 Inefficient and efficient postures. (After Chilman & Thomas 1987, with permission of Elsevier.)

MOVING: ROLE OF DIFFERENT BRAIN AREAS

Moving from one posture to the next requires some reflexes to be inhibited while others are facilitated. Some complex patterns of movement, such as those involved in walking, are pre-programmed in the nervous system. Others are acquired only by experience. Brain areas involved include:

- motor cortex of the cerebral hemispheres
- basal ganglia
- cerebellum.

Motor cortex

Cells in the motor cortex of the cerebral hemispheres exert direct control over the interneurones and motor neurones of the reflex arcs in the brain stem and the spinal cord via the corticobulbar and corticospinal tracts. The cells in the motor cortex receive impulses

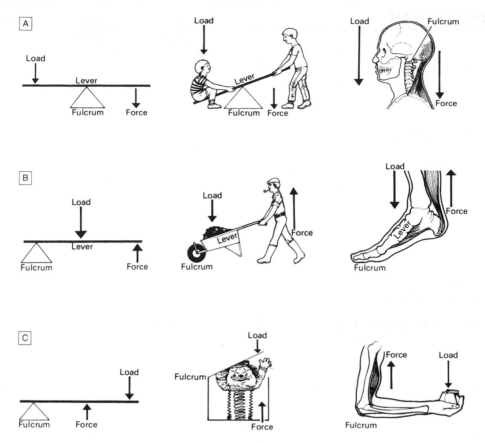

Figure 25.15 Lever systems. A, Head and neck. B, Foot. C, Arm. (From Chilman & Thomas 1987, with permission of Elsevier.)

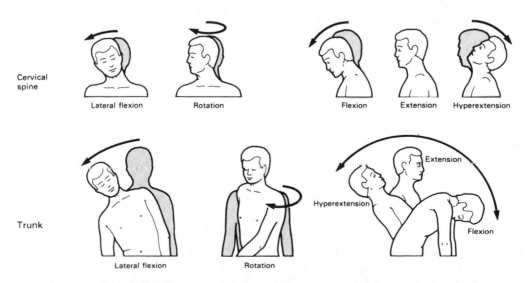

Figure 25.16 Range of motion exercises for joints: cervical spine, trunk, shoulder, hip, elbow, knee, wrist, ankle, fingers and toes. (From Boore et al 1987, with permission of Elsevier.) (Continued overleaf)

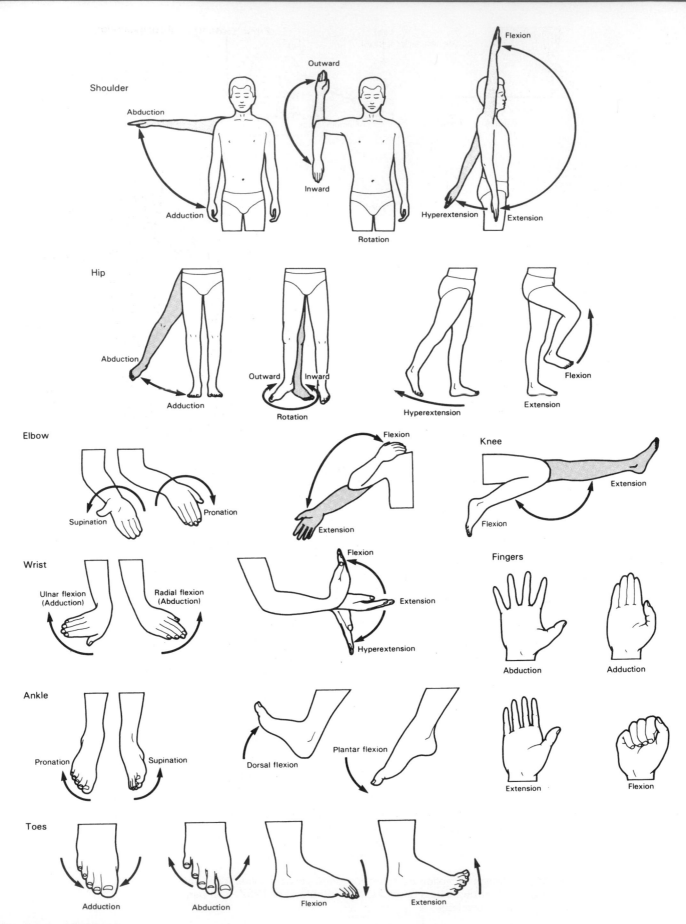

Figure 25.16 (Continued).

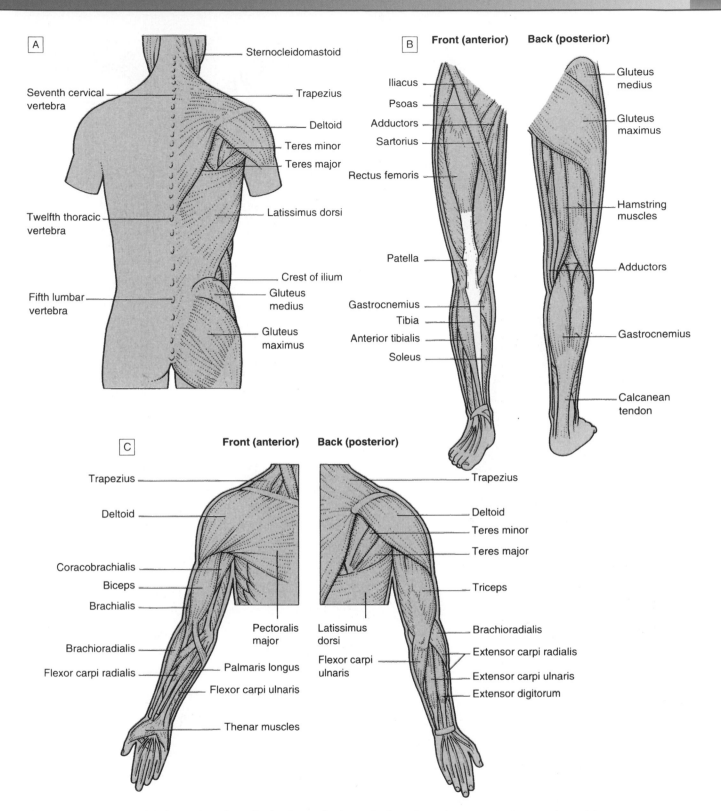

Figure 25.17 Superficial muscles of (A) the back, (B) the lower limb and (C) the upper limb. See also Table 25.4. (After Wilson 1990, with permission of Elsevier.)

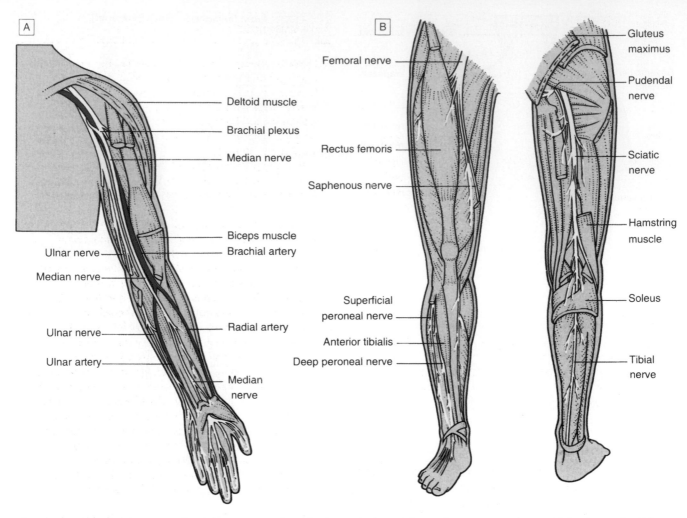

Figure 25.18 Major nerves of (A) the upper and (B) the lower limb and their relation to muscles and blood vessels. (After Williams et al 1989, with permission of Elsevier.)

Table 25.3 Muscles involved in movements of different parts of the body*

	Movement			
	Flexion	**Extension**	**Abduction**	**Adduction**
Cervical spine	Sternocleidomastoid	Trapezius Sacrospinalis[†]	–	–
Trunk	Abdominal muscles	Sacrospinalis[†]	–	–
Shoulder	Coracobrachialis Deltoid (anterior fibres) Pectoralis major	Teres major Deltoid (posterior fibres) Latissimus dorsi	Deltoid	Pectoralis major Latissimus dorsi
Hip	Psoas, iliacus Rectus femoris Sartorius	Gluteus maximus Hamstrings	Gluteus medius Gluteus minimus	Adductor group

* See Figures 25.16 and 25.17.
[†] These lie underneath the latissimus dorsi and the trapezius muscles and run up the vertebral column from the sacrum.

Table 25.4 Muscles involved in movements of the limbs*

	Movement	
	Flexion	**Extension**
Elbow	Biceps Brachialis	Triceps
Knee	Hamstrings Gastrocnemius	Quadriceps femoris
Wrist	Flexor carpi radialis Flexor carpi ulnaris	Extensor carpi radialis (longus and brevis) Extensor carpi ulnaris
Ankle	Gastrocnemius Soleus (plantar flexion)	Anterior tibialis Toe extensors (dorsiflexion)

* See Figures 25.16 and 25.17.

Impulse conduction in peripheral nerves can be blocked by pressure. Prolonged pressure on a nerve will cause a leg, for example, to 'go to sleep'. Sensation, and often movement, is impaired until nerve function and blood circulation return to normal.

from the association areas of the cerebral cortex and from the basal ganglia via the thalamus. They are also influenced by impulses coming from the cerebellum.

Basal ganglia

The role of the basal ganglia in movement control is still not well understood but evidence suggests that these brain areas play a role in allowing or disallowing different patterns of movement.

For example, in Parkinson's disease, the commonest disorder of the basal ganglia, patients may have difficulty in starting and stopping chosen sequences of activity. Walking is not a problem once the individual has got going, but making the initial moves is difficult. Likewise, stopping this activity may be a problem. Consequently, a person may find little difficulty in walking outdoors where movement is relatively unobstructed, whereas moving around the house, where continual adjustments need to be made to avoid obstructions, is much more difficult.

One of the other features of this and other disorders of the basal ganglia is that the patient may have unwanted movements while at rest. This suggests that programmes of activity are being allowed that have not been chosen.

Another observation that points to the function of the basal ganglia in posture and movement is that the spon-

Demyelination

In some diseases the myelin sheath is destroyed with the result that the nerve axon loses ability to conduct impulses quickly. Little is known about why the myelin sheath degenerates but research shows that demyelination is responsible for the symptoms of many neuropathies (-*opathy* = something is wrong but exactly what is not known).

In *multiple sclerosis*, patchy demyelination occurs within the spinal cord and brain, followed by damage to nerve fibres and the formation of plaques of scar tissue. The disease is characterized by remissions and relapses, which are unpredictable. The relapses may be very distressing for the patient. Initially, the person experiences sensations related to abnormal impulse conduction – tingling, numbness, weakness in one or both arms or legs. Visual disturbances are also common. The disease is progressive and the person eventually becomes confined to a wheelchair.

The Guillain–Barré syndrome develops rapidly following an often mild, pyrexial illness. Although marked demyelination of spinal nerve roots and peripheral nerves (see Ch. 20) occurs, the nerve fibre is not damaged. The myelin sheath gradually regenerates and normal function returns. The affected person suffers severe motor impairment and the muscles are very tender. It is an alarming condition due to the rapidity and severity of onset. The patient requires very careful observation, nursing and much reassurance.

What observations would you record and document on a patient with a diagnosis of Guillain–Barré syndrome?

Why are the observations important in monitoring the status of a patient with Guillain–Barré syndrome?

Symptoms of inadequate transmission of nerve impulses, such as numbness, are also experienced by some people suffering from *diabetes mellitus*. Research shows that these symptoms are caused by demyelination and axonal degeneration. When numbness affects one or both feet the risk of infection, following unfelt injury, is high. The cutting of toenails must be carried out with great care, if necessary by a chiropodist, and the feet should be inspected daily. It is advisable for the person to wear shoes that provide adequate protection. It has been known for an affected person to walk long distances with a sharp object embedded in the foot.

taneous movements that are made usually relate more to the muscles involved in posture and limb movement than those which are concerned with the intricate movements of the fingers (see below). This suggests that the basal ganglia may have a key role in determining the postures adopted and how we move between them, and less to do with the intricate movements of the hands.

Drug treatment of Parkinson's disease

The principal features of Parkinson's disease are tremor, rigidity and akinesia. It is thought that these signs and symptoms are the result of an imbalance between two neurotransmitters, acetylcholine and dopamine, and that improvement might be expected if the effects of the neurotransmitters could be modified. Currently, drug treatment is aimed at either decreasing cholinergic excitatory activity or increasing dopaminergic inhibitory activity.

Cholinergic activity in the basal ganglia can be blocked by atropine, and the synthetic anticholinergic drugs have a similar action. Such drugs include benzhexol, orphenadrine and procyclidine. They reduce rigidity but do not improve tremor or akinesia. The drug dose is increased gradually until optimum benefit is achieved or toxic effects occur. Toxicity is indicated by the atropine-like effects of dry mouth, blurred vision, constipation and urinary retention.

Dopaminergic activity can be enhanced by the administration of levodopa. Maximum improvement may take up to 6 months, but some 75 to 80% of patients obtain some benefit. Adverse effects include postural hypotension, nausea and vomiting, and involuntary movements, such as jerking of limbs (myoclonus), abnormal restlessness (akathisia) and facial grimacing. However, in the long term, the benefits of the drug often disappear and, after 5 years, only one-third of the patients prescribed levodopa still show improved function.

Cerebellum

This part of the brain is involved in the development of skilled programmes of activity for rapid targeted movements. As the cerebellum coordinates a mass of information from both sensory and motor areas of the nervous system, it is able to refine movements so that they are performed efficiently and accurately. Without this function, movements of all kinds become much more clumsy. For example, an upright posture can still be maintained but with more difficulty and only by adopting a physically more stable stance: legs placed wide apart to widen the base. Walking is still possible but in a staggering fashion and not in a straight line.

USING OUR HANDS: ROLE OF DIFFERENT BRAIN AREAS

We use our hands to pick up and hold objects, to feel their shape and explore their texture, and to perform skilled actions such as writing and drawing. All these actions require considerable coordination of visual, somatosensory and motor activity.

Primary motor and sensory cortex

The primary motor area of the cerebral cortex has a dominant role in the control of these highly skilled activities. The corticospinal tracts directly innervate many of the lower motor neurones supplying the muscles that control the movements of the hands and fingers.

Several cortical reflexes are involved in grasping and holding on to an object. For example, if the object begins to slip through the hands, this is detected by mechanoreceptors in the skin of the palm and grasp of the object is reflexly strengthened. Similarly, when feeling and exploring the surface of an object that we are touching, the exploratory movements of the fingers are guided partly by the sensory information detected by cutaneous receptors and transmitted to the somatosensory cortex which lies right next to the motor cortex.

The hands and the muscles that control them are extremely well represented in both the primary motor cortex and the adjacent somatosensory cortex. The two areas are linked by interconnecting nerve fibres, so that the neurones in the motor cortex can be controlled by the sensory information arriving at the adjacent sensory area.

If there is damage to these parts of the brain it is possible for someone to experience difficulty in handling objects and in writing, without necessarily having difficulty in walking or other movements.

Other areas

The kinds of tasks that require a considerable degree of hand–eye coordination involve other parts of the brain too, including the visual cortex. Picking up a small object between finger and thumb, or placing the correct finger on the right place on a keyboard, requires knowledge of the position of the target, calculation of the amount of movement required, as well as selection of an appropriate course of action to achieve the task. Feedback of information from sensory receptors may also be used to refine the movement as it is being performed so that it is achieved with the highest degree of accuracy. Here again the cerebellum, particularly the neocerebellum, plays its part. If function is disordered, movements are performed with much less accuracy. Highly skilled learned activities such as writing and drawing, through which we express our thoughts and communicate with others, depend not only on the skill with which we can actually execute the individual movements involved but also on our ability to string together a whole series of different movements in a meaningful and purposeful way. These activities rely on the function of the association areas of the brain in the parietal and frontal lobes of the cerebral hemispheres.

REFERENCES AND FURTHER READING

Alberts B, Bray D, Lewis J, Raff M, Roberts K, Watson J D 1983 Molecular biology of the cell. Garland Publishing, New York

Boore J R P, Champion R, Ferguson M C 1987 Nursing the physically ill adult. Churchill Livingstone, Edinburgh

Chaffin D B, Anderson G B J 1991 Occupational biomechanics, 2nd edn. John Wiley, Chichester

Chilman A M, Thomas M 1987 Understanding nursing care, 3rd edn. Churchill Livingstone, Edinburgh

Davies A, Blakeley A G H, Kidd C 2001 Human physiology. Churchill Livingstone, Edinburgh

Galley P M, Forster A L 1987 Human movement: an introductory text for physiotherapy students, 2nd edn. Churchill Livingstone, Edinburgh

Ger R, Abrahams P 1989 Essentials of clinical anatomy. Churchill Livingstone, Edinburgh

Goodwill C J, Chamberlain M A 1997 Rehabilitation of the physically disabled adult, 2nd edn. Nelson Thornes, Cheltenham

Gunn C 1992 Bones and joints: a guide for students. Churchill Livingstone, Edinburgh

Hayward J, Boore J R P 1994 Information: a prescription against pain/Prescription for recovery. Scutari Press, London

Henderson V, Nite G 1978 Principles and practice of nursing, 6th edn. Macmillan, New York

Humphrey D R, Freund H J (eds) 1991 Motor control: concepts and issues. John Wiley, Chichester

Jenkins D B 1991 Hollinhead's Functional anatomy of the limbs and back, 6th edn. W B Saunders, Philadelphia

Lumley J S P 1990 Surface anatomy: the anatomical basis of the clinical examination. Churchill Livingstone, Edinburgh

Murray P D F 1985 Bones: a study of the development and structure of the vertebrate skeleton. Cambridge University Press, Cambridge

Oliver J 1993 Back care: a teaching manual. Butterworth-Heinemann, London

Oliver M, Zarb G, Silver J R et al 1988 Walking into darkness: the experience of spinal cord injury. Palgrave Macmillan, New York

Penfield W, Rasmussen T 1968 The cerebral cortex of man: a clinical study of localisation of function. Hafner

Rogers A W 1992 Textbook of anatomy. Churchill Livingstone, Edinburgh

Rothwell J C 1993 Control of human voluntary movement. Kluwer Academic Publishers, Dordrecht

Williams P L, Warwick R, Dyson M et al 1989 Gray's Anatomy, 37th edn. Churchill Livingstone, Edinburgh

Wilson K J W 1990 Ross & Wilson Anatomy and physiology in health and illness, 7th edn. Churchill Livingstone, Edinburgh

26 Communicating

COMMUNICATION

We communicate with one another in many different ways by vocal and non-vocal means. We use sounds to express our thoughts in words, and the intonation of our voices to express how we feel. We also use facial expression and body language to convey messages and display our moods and attitudes.

VOCAL COMMUNICATION

We produce sounds using the vocal apparatus of the larynx and associated structures of the oral cavity, throat and pharynx. Many different muscles are involved. Their activity is controlled by cells in several parts of the brain, including the brain stem and limbic system as well as the cerebral cortex, cerebellum and basal ganglia. The production of clear speech involves many brain areas. If the function of any part is disturbed, speech is impaired (dysarthria).

Mechanics of sound production

Sounds are produced by the vibration of parts of the vocal apparatus, shown diagrammatically in the form of a musical instrument in Figure 26.1. The vocal folds in the larynx vibrate when air is forced past them through the glottis (the gap between the folds). Other vibrations are added by structures such as the lips, tongue and soft palate often when airflow is abruptly altered. The pitch of a sound (high or low) depends upon the length and tension of the vibrating structures whereas the form of the sound (e.g. aaah, eee, ooo) depends upon the shape and size of the chambers, such as pharynx, nose and oral cavity into which it is projected.

Vibration

The normal sounds of breathing are caused by vibration of structures within the respiratory system as air flows in and out of the lungs through the airways. If there is narrowing of airways or presence of fluid, other abnormal sounds may be produced such as wheezing in asthma, or the crepitations heard in pneumonia.

In speaking and singing (see below), the respiratory muscles are used to produce a prolonged expiration, and air is forced through the narrowed glottis causing the vocal folds to vibrate.

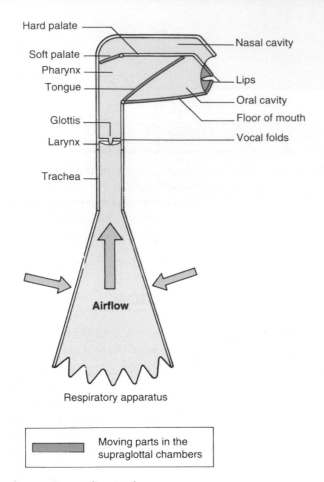

Figure 26.1 The vocal instrument.

Cleft lip or palate

During the tenth week of fetal life, the maxillary bones and the palatal processes fuse as the beginning of human face construction. Sheets of skin and muscle start to organize themselves around the landmarks of the mouth, nose and eyes. A single flap grows symmetrically down the middle to form the forehead, the upper eyelids, the front of the nose and the web that links the inside of the upper lip and the gum. If the bones fuse normally, but the overlying skin does not close, the result is a cleft lip, sometimes called a 'harelip' because it looks like the lip of a hare. This abnormality may appear on either the right or left side of the lip, the cleft running down from the nostril.

Sometimes, there is imperfect fusion of the underlying bones leaving a large gap in the hard palate, in which case the nasal cavity opens into the mouth and the nasal septum and vomer bone are often absent. Such an abnormality is called cleft palate and often, but not always, occurs in conjunction with cleft lip.

In infancy, cleft palate and cleft lip both limit the child's ability to suck and may lead to malnutrition. Cleft palate may later lead to the development of speech difficulties. Both abnormalities can be corrected by surgery.

Facial paralysis

Paralysis or paresis of the facial muscle served by the seventh cranial nerve is called Bell's palsy. It is most common in persons between 20 and 40 years of age. The condition is characterized by a vague sensation of muscle tension on the affected side, in which there is flaccidity, and drooping of the mouth. There may also be watering of the eye. The paralysis is conspicuous in that the person fails to smile, whistle or grimace.

Nursing principles focus on keeping the patient comfortable, helping him to cope with a changed body image and preventing complications. Since patients are self-conscious about their appearance, their desire for privacy should be respected, especially during meals. Families are warned not to show surprise at the patient's appearance or make comments that may embarrass him or remind him of the change. The condition may sometimes be relieved within a week or a month without treatment other than rest, a nutritious diet and vitamins. In other cases, the disorder may persist for months or years.

Pitch and form

The fundamental pitch of the sounds produced when the vocal folds vibrate depends largely on the length and tension of the folds. On average, the vocal folds are longer in men than in women and for this reason the pitch of a man's voice is lower.

The shape of the cavity into which the sound is projected determines which harmonic frequencies will resonate best. This alters the blend of frequencies in the sound and determines its form and character. As the relative dimensions of the structures of the pharynx, nose and oral cavity differ slightly from person to person, voices sound different too.

The action of the resonating cavities in the head is illustrated by the change in quality of the voice when a person has a severe cold and the nose and sinuses are congested.

Neural control of sound production

We use our voices to cry out when we are hurt, to laugh when we are amused, and to sing and speak. The neural control mechanisms range from the simple reflex of the cry of alarm, to the complexity of cerebral and cerebellar control of speech.

The cry of alarm

The cry or scream of alarm is the most primitive of sounds we make. It is basically the result of a simple brain stem reflex triggered by pain or danger. Neurones in the vicinity of brain areas associated with pain pathways, such as the peri-aqueductal grey matter, are involved.

Crying and laughing

The more complicated patterns of sound characteristic of crying, moaning and laughing etc. involve the limbic system and the hypothalamus. The motor cortex, cerebellum and thalamus exert relatively little control over the production of these sounds. Thus, patients who have suffered injury to the cerebral cortex leaving them unable to speak may still be able to laugh and cry.

Speaking and singing

Speaking and singing involve the coordinated contraction of over 100 different muscles controlled by the motor areas of the cerebral cortex, the basal ganglia and the cerebellum, acting through the lower motor neurones of the pons, medulla and spinal cord in the cranial and spinal nerves.

Speaking

The processes involved in speaking and singing can be divided into several components:

- producing an airstream
- producing sounds
- modifying sounds by resonance
- smooth transitions between one sound and the next (articulation).

Producing an airstream

The pattern of breathing is altered when we speak or sing. Instead of the usual regular pattern of inspiration and expiration, sharp inspirations are interspersed with periods of steady expiration. In speech and singing, expiration is not a passive process but is controlled by muscle contraction. Both internal and external intercostal muscles are involved, acting to brake the usual recoil-powered expiration, and to maintain airflow at an appropriate rate when the recoil force lessens or would have ceased (see Ch. 7).

When we speak, the automatic inspiratory–expiratory cycle, set by the respiratory centres in the pons and medulla, is overruled by impulses from the motor cortex. The intercostal nerves are controlled directly by impulses in the corticospinal tracts rather than by impulses originating from the brain stem.

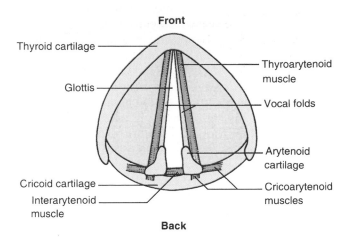

Figure 26.2 Position of the vocal folds in relation to other laryngeal structures.

Producing sounds

When breathing without speaking, the glottis is open. When we speak, the glottis is narrowed by the contraction of several laryngeal muscles including the cricoarytenoid and interarytenoid muscles (Fig. 26.2). Air forced out through this narrow opening causes the cricovocal ligaments (vocal folds) to vibrate. This vibration compresses and rarefies the air and produces sound waves. Contraction of the muscles sets the length and tension in the folds and thus determines the pitch of the sound. Muscle spindles monitor the length of the muscle fibres, helping to maintain them at the length required. The motor neurones innervating the laryngeal muscles form part of the laryngeal nerves, which are branches of cranial nerve X (vagus).

The consonants of speech, such as 't', 'p', 'k' and 'd', are produced by briefly closing off the oral cavity in a variety of different ways using the muscles of the jaws, lips and tongue. The sudden release of air causes other structures, such as lips, to vibrate, adding further frequencies of vibration to those originating from the vocal folds.

The sounds 'p', 'b' and 'd' consist of vibrations produced by the vocal folds, as well as vibrations produced by other structures. In sounds like 'sss' and 't', however, the vocal folds are not used at all. The vibrations are created by air flowing through the narrow openings formed by the lips and tongue. A whisper hardly uses the vocal cords at all.

Resonance

The primary sound formed by the vocal folds is modified by the shape of the chambers within which it resonates. For the human voice, the chambers include the pharynx, the oral and nasal cavities, and the air-filled sinuses. We change the shape of several of the chambers by opening and closing our mouths, including or excluding the nasal cavity by elevating the soft palate, and altering the relative positions of lips, tongue, teeth and cheeks (Fig. 26.1). Different vowel sounds are produced in this way.

To produce 'a', 'e', 'i', 'o' and 'u', we normally use the oral cavity alone and block off the nasal cavity with the soft palate. If the nasal cavity is used as well, nasal vowel sounds are formed. These are used a lot in some languages, such as French. If the nasal cavity is open when the oral cavity is closed, then nasal consonants like 'm', 'n' and 'ng' are produced.

Articulation

Speech consists of a series of different sounds linked together to form words, and words linked together to form phrases. It is a highly skilled motor activity requiring smooth transitions, in a short space of time, from one pattern of muscle activity to the next. The movements required have to be exceedingly precise. Very small differences in the position of the lips and teeth alter the sounds produced. The differences made to speech by the loss of teeth or the acquisition of dentures are well known. Considerable coordination of activity is required to ensure that the correct sequencing of sounds is achieved easily and crisply. Without this, speech becomes slurred or laboured. This precision is achieved by the control exercised by the motor cortex and the cerebellum.

The lips, tongue and the soft palate play an important role in articulation. However, if damage occurs at higher levels, as it does in strokes, the patient may suffer from one of the various forms of aphasia, which means the inability to express oneself linguistically. The neuromuscular apparatus of the voice and tongue may be intact, but the patient cannot put his thoughts into words.

Dysarthria

Defects in the motor control of speech lead to characteristic speech impairments (dysarthrias). Speech is disordered if there is impairment of (Fig. 26.3):

- the muscles of speech: respiratory, pharyngeal, facial etc.
- lower motor neurones: cranial nerves – V, VII, IX, and XII; spinal nerves – phrenic, intercostal
- upper motor neurones: e.g. corticospinal and bulbar tracts
- brain areas: motor cortex, basal ganglia and cerebellum.

There are four main types of dysarthria:

- flaccid
- spastic

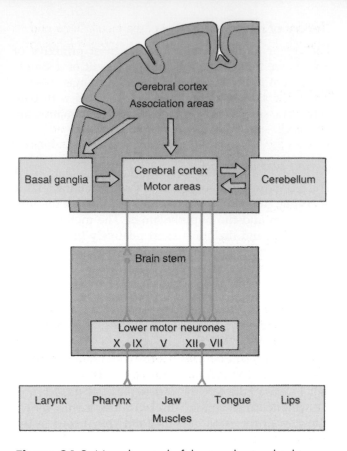

Figure 26.3 Neural control of the muscles involved in speech.

- ataxic
- hypokinetic.

Flaccid dysarthria

Flaccid dysarthria results from injury to one or more lower motor neurones. The effects on speech depend upon which lower motor neurones are affected. The effects may include breathiness in phonation, nasal emission of air, and audible inspiration.

The tone of the affected muscles is reduced, as in any lower motor neurone lesion, which is why this form of speech disorder is termed a flaccid dysarthria. A temporary dysarthria can result from dental anaesthesia.

Spastic dysarthria

The lower motor neurones of the lips, tongue and cheeks are directly innervated by neurones from the motor cortex (corticobulbar tracts) (Fig. 26.3). If there are lesions of these tracts, or of the cerebral cortex, speech becomes slow and words are articulated imprecisely and with difficulty. If there is extensive cortical damage then speech becomes impossible, as will any voluntary movement of the mouth, face and tongue. In addition, muscle tone is increased, hence the term 'spastic' dysarthria.

Ataxic dysarthria

Speech is also imprecise and not well articulated if there is damage to the cerebellum. Words can still be formed but with much less precision, and they are not as smoothly articulated in sentences. The slurred speech resulting from alcohol intoxication is a good example of the results of cerebellar dysfunction.

Hypokinetic dysarthria

One example of altered speech associated with defective function of the basal ganglia is the hypokinetic dysarthria that may appear in Parkinson's disease. The articulation of speech is normal and words are properly formed, but there is a monotony of pitch and loudness. This makes speech seem dull because many of the usual stresses that are normally added in saying words and sentences are absent. Another feature sometimes present is difficulty in actually beginning to speak. These features parallel the difficulties that people with Parkinson's disease tend to have in making other movements (akinesia).

NON-VOCAL COMMUNICATION

Much communication occurs without a single word being spoken. The way we look at another person, and the way he or she looks at us, conveys a lot of information, as does the body language of posture and gesture. We convey feelings and attitudes such as those of happiness, expectancy and welcome, or of hostility, anger and withdrawal. We study one another's faces and read facial expressions.

Facial expression

The facial expressions adopted in emotions such as fear, anger, disgust, sadness, surprise and happiness are similar in different cultures and countries, suggesting that they are pre-programmed reflex patterns of muscle contraction triggered by our emotional state.

When we are surprised we raise our eyebrows; when we are angry we lower them. When we are happy we pull up the corners of our lips by contracting the zygomatic muscles in order to smile and we screw up our eyes by contracting the outer part of the orbicularis oculi (Fig. 26.4). We can pretend various emotions by voluntarily contracting the same muscles but it is interesting that most people do not seem to be able to contract the outer part of the orbicularis oculi voluntarily. Only genuine happiness seems to act as the trigger.

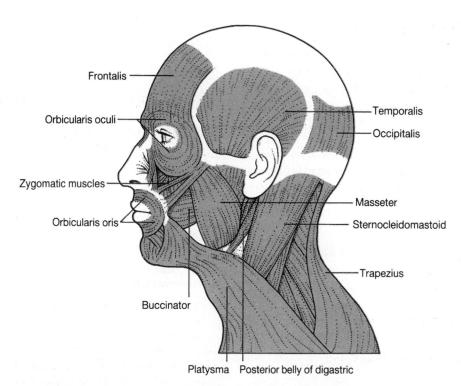

Figure 26.4 Muscles of the head and neck. (From Rogers 1992, with permission of Elsevier.)

If there is impairment of motor function, some of these natural forms of expression may be affected too, and the cues that tell us how that person is feeling may be lacking. A face may be expressionless but that does not necessarily mean that the person behind the face has no feelings. In Parkinson's disease, for example, a patient may have an expressionless ('dead-pan') face. This is because of the patient's difficulty in putting motor programmes into action.

LANGUAGE

The spoken and written word is very important to us as humans. Without it, our ability to communicate with one another would be much more limited.

At its simplest, language involves associating a symbol or sound with an object or activity. But in addition to this, we communicate a much richer understanding of our experience by the way in which we bring those symbols together to form sentences. In order to communicate fully, we need to be able to do both those things. The first concerns our vocabulary (chiefly nouns and verbs); the second relates to syntax (the construction of sentences).

THE SPOKEN WORD

Two areas of the cerebral cortex that have a major role in vocabulary and in syntax are:

- the posterior speech area (Wernicke's area)
- the anterior speech area (Broca's area).

The posterior speech area lies at the junction of the temporal and parietal lobes of the cerebral cortex whereas the anterior area lies just in front of the primary motor cortex (Fig. 26.5). These areas were identified many years ago by Wernicke and Broca who noticed that specific disorders of spoken language (aphasias)

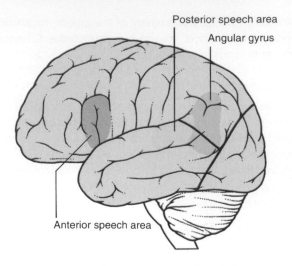

Figure 26.5 Major language areas of the left cerebral hemisphere.

exhibited by some of their patients were associated with damage to these two parts of the brain.

Damage to the posterior area chiefly created problems with vocabulary and comprehension of the spoken word (Wernicke's aphasia), whereas damage to the anterior area resulted mainly in difficulty in constructing sentences and in actually speaking (Broca's aphasia). Other types of aphasia, including global, conductive and anomic, have since been described (Table 26.1). Global aphasia usually results from extensive damage to both speech areas, whereas conductive aphasia is thought to be due to impaired impulse transmission between the two areas. Anomic aphasia is a more selective language impairment often seen in patients who have recovered from other, more severe, forms of aphasia.

Vocabulary and comprehension

In Wernicke's aphasia, which is sometimes referred to as a form of sensory or receptive aphasia, an individual

Table 26.1 Several different forms of aphasia and their key features

Type of aphasia	Fluency of speech	Comprehension	Ability to name objects	Ability to repeat spoken words
Broca's	*	*****	*	***
Wernicke's	*****	***	***	***
Global	*	*	*	*
Conductive	*****	*****	***	***
Anomic	*****	*****	***	*****

Key: ***** = moderate to good; *** = impaired to a greater or lesser degree; * = severely impaired.

has difficulty in selecting the correct word for different objects and activities. This is one form of anomia (difficulty in naming objects). Words do come to mind and are used but they are the wrong ones. Sentences are formed from the words found and are articulated and spoken, often very fluently, but what is said may make little sense. Not surprisingly, there is also poor understanding of what other people say.

Wernicke's aphasia is a very distressing disorder causing frustration, anxiety and anger. Imagine sharing a conversation with someone who speaks an obscure language, without being able to share words for objects and activities because they change frequently! Extreme patience and understanding are required by all.

Forming sentences and speaking

Conversely, in Broca's aphasia, which is sometimes referred to as a motor or expressive aphasia, understanding of speech is much better. The correct nouns and verbs are chosen to describe objects, but there is difficulty in saying them and in forming sentences. Prepositions and conjunctions tend to be left out, so that sentences are often reduced to a bare minimum. A sentence such as, 'I am feeling very tired and I would be glad if I could go home soon,' might be reduced to 'tired . . . go home'. People who display Broca's aphasia can have difficulty in understanding sentences whose meaning crucially depends on the order of words. A sentence such as, 'The patient that the nurse was helping was tired,' could leave them wondering who was helping whom, and who was tired!

As the anterior speech area is close to the primary motor cortex, injury to this general area usually also results in features characteristic of damage to the motor cortex such as slowness of speech and difficulty in articulation (dysarthria).

THE WRITTEN WORD

Other areas of the cerebral cortex are specifically involved in creating the associations enabling reading and writing. Adjacent to the posterior speech area is the angular gyrus (Fig. 26.5). The angular gyrus performs the same sorts of function as the posterior speech area but is concerned more with the written rather than the spoken word. Injury to this area leads to an inability to read (alexia) or to difficulties in reading (dyslexia).

Translating thoughts into written symbols is different from translating them into spoken words. Writing depends on a slightly different set of associations involving control of finger and hand movements. It can be impaired (agraphia) independently of other aspects of language.

REFERENCES AND FURTHER READING

Blakemore C 1990 The mind machine. BBC Books, London

Bradshaw J L 1989 Hemispheric specialisation and psychological function. John Wiley, Chichester

Carpenter R H S 1984 Neurophysiology. Edward Arnold, London

Graham R B 1990 Physiological psychology. Wadsworth Publishing, Belmont, CA

Murdoch B E 1990 Acquired speech and language disorders. Chapman & Hall, London

Paul R 2001 Language disorders from infancy through adolescence, 2nd edn. Mosby, St Louis

Rogers A W 1992 Textbook of anatomy. Churchill Livingstone, Edinburgh

27

Sleep, emotion and behaviour

Sleep is important. Without it we become irritable and concentration suffers. When awake, we may feel alert or drowsy, responsive to events or sluggish. These different levels of consciousness are set by neural systems that influence the cerebral cortex. Their activity can be modified by drugs.

Closely linked to our level of arousal, but different from it, is the experience of how we feel. We talk about being happy, or sad, angry or afraid. Emotional experiences are complex. They draw together many different aspects of brain function: a specific sensory experience, for example passing an examination, triggers distinctive patterns of behaviour, such as surprise, and laughter; and this includes both somatic control (e.g. of facial expression) as well as autonomic responses (e.g. the increased heart rate of excitement).

Many different parts of the brain are involved in emotions but a central role is played by the limbic system, which acts as an interface between the somatic and visceral components of the nervous system. The somatic components include the association areas of the cerebral cortex, whereas the visceral control areas comprise the hypothalamus, the pituitary gland and the autonomic nervous system.

Brain injury can result in changes of mood. Conversely, moods can affect the body and its state of health.

SLEEPING AND WAKING

We become drowsy and go to sleep when activity in cells of the cerebral cortex becomes synchronous. Synchrony is achieved by regular pulsing of the cortex by impulses from particular groups of cells in the thalamus (non-specific nuclei). The result of this pulsing is that impulses reaching the brain from sensory receptors are no longer registered properly in the cerebral cortex, and as a result we are unaware of them.

When we are awake, pulsing of the cerebral cortex by the thalamus is prevented by excitatory activity reaching the thalamus from groups of cells within the reticular formation of the brain stem (Fig. 27.1). These cells form part of the system that produces the regular sleep/wake cycle and determines the characteristics of sleep, such as its depth and episodes of dreaming. The neurotransmitters involved include serotonin, noradrenaline and acetylcholine.

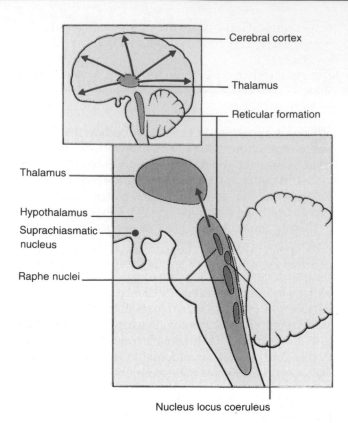

Figure 27.1 Parts of the brain involved in determining the level of consciousness.

SLEEP/WAKE CYCLE

The activity of groups of cells within the reticular formation of the brain stem, such as the raphe nuclei and the nucleus locus coeruleus (Fig. 27.1), waxes and wanes daily, driven by a 'biological clock' in the hypothalamus. Activity is also affected by impulses in sensory systems, allowing us to be aroused from sleep, or conversely prevented from sleeping.

Biological clock

The cells in the hypothalamus acting as a clock are those in the suprachiasmatic nucleus (Fig. 27.1). The circadian rhythm set by this clock causes most of us to be awake for about 16 hours and asleep for about 8 hours each day, though the pattern changes from birth to old age and there are individual variations particularly in the duration of sleep. If someone is allowed to go to sleep and get up when he or she wishes, in an environment which provides no clues as to time of day, a regular cycle of sleeping and waking occurs with a period of about 25 hours. The cycle is normally entrained to the 24-hour day by cues such as light, the ringing of an alarm, and social habits. Any routine events can func-tion in this way, and therefore cue us into sleeping and waking.

Arousal

The activity of cells in the reticular formation is also affected by impulses in the sensory systems. Signals from almost all the senses enter the reticular formation along fibres that are branches (collaterals) of the main sensory pathways. These impulses raise the level of excitation in the reticular formation and disrupt the regular bursts of impulses generated by the thalamus. As a result we wake up. This is why it is difficult to get to sleep when we are awake and wanting to sleep, but are being bombarded with information from our senses about sounds and lights around us. Conversely, when stimulation is lacking, perhaps in a darkened, warm classroom or lecture theatre, when listening to a very monotonous voice, there is less to disturb the regular activity of the thalamic cells and we may easily drift off to sleep.

CHARACTERISTICS OF SLEEP

When we fall asleep and stay asleep for a while, our level of consciousness alters, and the state of mind and body alternates regularly between two types of sleep:

- non-REM
- REM.

Each form of sleep is marked by characteristic patterns of the electroencephalogram (EEG), and distinctive changes in muscle tone, mental activity, heart rate and breathing.

Non-REM sleep

When we fall asleep, the pattern of electrical activity recorded in the EEG changes and heart rate and blood pressure fall. Four stages (I–IV) of non-REM sleep have been distinguished by EEG. The last of these, stage IV, is sometimes referred to as deep sleep or slow wave sleep. It is more difficult to arouse someone from this level of sleep than from the other three. Stage IV sleep is also the stage in which sleepwalking and talking, nightmares and tooth grinding may occur in some people, particularly in young people. The amount of stage IV sleep tends to diminish as we grow older, with the benefit that these phenomena tend to disappear.

When we first fall asleep, we progress rapidly through the four stages of sleep, spend a short while at the lowest level reached and then return through them. This cycle recurs at about 90- to 100-minute intervals throughout the night, but with the depth of sleep becoming less as the night progresses.

REM sleep

A different form of sleep, REM sleep, occurs at regular intervals during a period of sleep. It is associated with a number of distinctive features, including:

- rapid eye movements (REM)
- dreaming
- profound muscle relaxation
- increase in blood pressure, pulse and breathing.

When the changeover occurs between non-REM sleep and REM sleep, the EEG pattern alters abruptly to one resembling the awake state. Yet, paradoxically the sleeper is very deeply asleep. For this reason REM sleep has been termed 'paradoxical sleep'. If the sleeper is aroused from REM sleep, he will often report that he has been dreaming. This is why there is movement of the eyeballs, as in his mind he is visualizing and following the events of his dream. There may be occasional twitches of the body, but overall, muscle tone and activity is profoundly reduced. The mind, especially the imagination, is active but the body is relaxed. Blood pressure, pulse and rate of breathing, however, increase and vary much more than during non-REM sleep.

The first episode of REM sleep lasts for only a few minutes, but as the night progresses the episodes gradually lengthen. The transition from REM sleep to non-REM sleep and vice versa is marked by an increase in body movement, and a change in body position. The rest of the sleeping time, whether REM or non-REM, is generally associated with muscle relaxation.

EMOTION AND MOTIVATION

DEFINITION AND BASIS

Emotion and motivation are familiar terms, yet it is not easy to define exactly what each consists of and how each is produced by our nervous systems.

Emotion

Our emotions contribute to the depth of our personal life by giving a unique passion and character to all our actions. Despite the extent to which it pervades our everyday existence, there is, as yet, no precise scientific definition of the term 'emotion'. When we discuss 'emotion' we are usually referring to our 'feelings'. Despite the abstract nature of the terminology, emotion, like perception and action, is controlled by distinct neuronal circuits in the brain.

Any emotion includes:

- particular patterns of behaviour (smiling, shaking fist etc.)
- autonomic effects (racing heart, sweaty hands etc.)
- our conscious perception of these responses (feelings)
- the description we give to our feelings (happy, angry etc.)
- the stimuli acting as triggers (success, a missed bus).

Each of these involves the activity of different parts of the nervous system and the effects produced on the tissues and organs controlled by them. Thus emotional experience and behaviour involve many parts of the brain including:

- cerebral cortex (cognition) and basal ganglia
- limbic system (mood)
- hypothalamus (endocrine and autonomic effects)
- autonomic nervous system and pituitary gland.

In our emotions, activity in the parts of the brain which are chiefly concerned with the control of the internal environment (hypothalamus, pituitary gland and autonomic nervous system) is closely associated with activity in the somatic nervous system (cerebral cortex and basal ganglia). The limbic system acts as the interface between these two.

Motivation

Motivation springs from the need to satisfy basic drives for:

- food
- water
- warmth
- survival (through sex and reproduction).

Satisfaction of these needs depends upon our ability to behave appropriately (go shopping, turn on a tap, put on clothes, date a boyfriend/girlfriend etc.) as well as upon the internal controls of plasma glucose, osmolality and temperature, and gonadal function. We have to work to buy food; we have to consider how best to clothe and house ourselves and our families. To do these things we need to know and understand about shops, materials and money etc., as well as be motivated to make use of them.

Motivation couples the need to satisfy the basic drives, with our perception of the likely results of different courses of action. If a strategy (e.g. going for a hot drink) appears to fulfil a basic need (e.g. for water) it will be attractive to us, whereas if it appears to be harmful (raising body temperature) we will be inclined to avoid it. If there is danger but the possibility of reward (e.g. standing one's ground in a crowd of people all trying to buy a hot drink during the interval at a show), we may react aggressively. These behaviours are intimately interwoven with our different emotions. Things that are attractive and rewarding usually bring pleasure; those that appear harmful make us feel afraid; if our actions are frustrated we may feel anger.

All of this involves a detailed assessment both of our internal bodily state and of our surroundings, and the selection of a pattern of behaviour appropriate to our needs. The limbic system has a central role in this overall process of assessment and decision and therefore plays a key role in motivation as well as in our emotions.

LIMBIC SYSTEM

The limbic system is a complex system, which is very important in determining behaviour. It has links with other parts of the nervous system including:

- neocortex of the cerebrum
- hypothalamus
- olfactory system.

Structure

The main parts of the limbic system and their situation in the brain are shown in Figure 27.2A & B. The limbic system consists of a number of clusters of cell bodies (nuclei) linked together with neural tissue in which the cells are arranged in layers (cortex). The overall appearance is of a ring of neural tissue bordering on the neocortex surrounding it (limbus means border).

The limbic system represents the highest level of brain activity in some animals. In humans, the limbic system has been overtaken by the development of the neocortex (Fig. 27.2A) functionally as well as structurally (the limbic system is buried underneath the cerebrocortical mantle). Consequently our behaviour is much more complex than that of other intelligent creatures.

Functions

It has been difficult to obtain information about the functions of the limbic system in humans, because the various structures are buried deep within the cerebral hemispheres. Some functions have therefore been inferred from the results of studies of animal behaviour. In experimental studies in the 1950s, it was found that rats appeared to enjoy having parts of the limbic system stimulated electrically. If they were enabled to deliver their own stimuli by means of a lever they would go on doing so for hours! It was concluded that, in some way, stimulation was experienced by the animals as

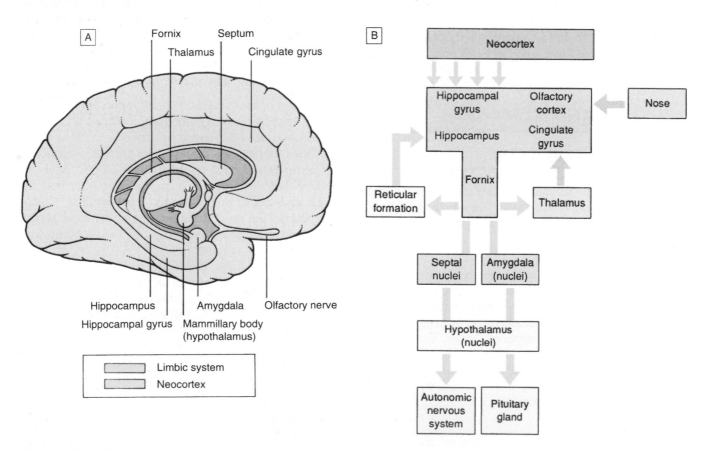

Figure 27.2 The limbic system. A, Position and parts. B, Connections.

rewarding. Conversely, stimulation of other areas led to avoidance of the lever, suggesting that in some way the stimulus was unpleasant.

There have been some studies in humans of the effects of stimulation of parts of the limbic system. Subjects have reported stimulation as evoking feelings of pleasure, relaxation, anger, fear, and even terror. Other information in humans has been derived from the effects of lesions or injury to the limbic system. Damage to the amygdala, for example, has been shown to produce a loss of aggression in men as well as feelings of hypersexuality.

Links with other brain areas

Neocortex of the cerebrum

Links between the limbic system and the neocortex enable information, gleaned from our senses about the outer world, to be received and logged. One region of the limbic system, the hippocampus, appears to play a crucial role in our memory of sensory experiences. This is probably of importance in determining our learned emotional responses to different situations. If an event in the past was associated with unpleasant consequences, when we encounter a similar situation again we will remember the previous experience, and 'relive' its unpleasant associations.

Hypothalamus

The links between the limbic system and the hypothalamus enable our behaviour to be controlled in a way that serves the needs of the internal environment. For example, the control of body temperature involves the choices we make about what clothes to wear, and whether or not to turn up the central heating, as well as autonomic responses such as vasodilation and vasoconstriction of cutaneous blood vessels (see Ch. 17). Choosing to turn up the central heating requires that we have learnt some basic information about heating systems and how to work them. We have to access that information, logged in the neocortex and hippocampus, in order to create a comfortable environment and maintain body temperature.

Another example is the control of the desire to eat. There are two areas in the hypothalamus concerned with feeding and fullness (satiety). These areas are linked with specific regions of the amygdala (Fig. 27.3). It has been shown in animal studies that stimulation or lesions in these areas of the amygdala can cause an animal either to overeat or not to eat at all. Interestingly, these changes in feeding behaviour are associated with changes in emotional behaviour too. The combination of going off one's food and feeling tired and depressed is familiar to most people. Here we see some of the complex links that may be involved in certain behaviours, and the associations between one's state of mind and activities such as eating (see Ch. 9, 15).

Olfactory system

Part of the limbic system is linked directly to the olfactory system (Fig. 27.2). This sensory system is unique in our bodies in that sensory signals do not pass via the thalamus to the cerebral cortex but go instead straight to the limbic cortex. The sense of smell is a powerful regulator of behaviour in animals. It is less obviously important in us, but even so smells are probably more powerful in evoking emotional feelings, whether of pleasure or disgust, than any other sensation.

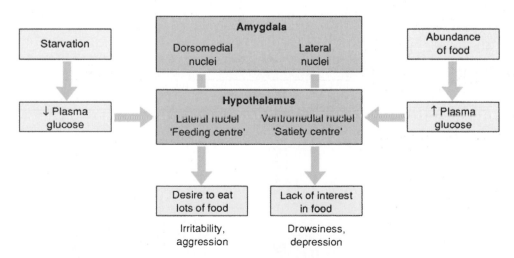

Figure 27.3 Systems involved in controlling the desire to eat.

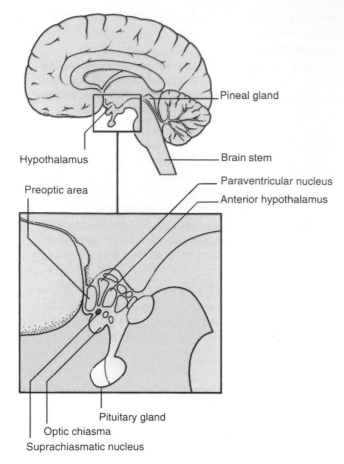

Figure 27.4 Nuclei of the hypothalamus.

THE HYPOTHALAMUS AND VISCERAL CONTROL

The hypothalamus consists of several clusters of neurones (nuclei) (Fig. 27.4) that are concerned with the control of different aspects of the internal environment (Table 27.1). These cells are linked with the somatic nervous system through the limbic system. They

Table 27.1 Functions of nuclei and/or areas in the hypothalamus

Nuclei/area	Functions
Lateral and ventromedial	Feeding/fasting
Supraoptic and paraventricular	Water balance
Anterior/posterior	Temperature regulation
Preoptic area	Reproduction
Suprachiasmatic	Circadian rhythms

control the activity of our internal organs through the autonomic nervous system and the hormones of the pituitary gland (Table 27.2).

Autonomic nervous system and hormones

When we feel excited, whether angry or desperate to run away from a threatening situation, or buoyed up with eager anticipation, the sympathetic nervous system is activated, producing many changes in the activity of the internal organs. We are conscious of many of these changes, a pounding heart, hands feeling damp from the sweat, and the changed tone of the gastric and intestinal muscle making us feel queasy. All these contribute to the emotional experiences of excitement, anger or fear.

Different emotions are thought to be associated with slightly different patterns of activation of the autonomic nervous system and different balances of hormones. Whereas the secretion of adrenaline and noradrenaline is linked with anger and fear, anxiety is associated with raised levels of ACTH and corticosteroids, and aggression can be correlated with the levels of androgens, particularly testosterone in males. Other hormones that have been implicated in changes in mood and behaviour include thyroid hormones, gonadal hormones in women and endogenous opioids.

Table 27.2 Hormones of the pituitary gland

Hormone	Abbreviation	Target gland
Adrenocorticotrophic hormone	ACTH	Adrenal cortex → corticosteroids
Arginine vasopressin/Antidiuretic hormone	AVP/ ADH	
Follicle stimulating hormone	FSH	Gonads → oestrogens
Human growth hormone	HGH	Liver → somatomedins
Luteinizing hormone	LH	Gonads → { oestrogens, progesterone, testosterone }
Oxytocin		
Prolactin		
Thyroid stimulating hormone	TSH	Thyroid → thyroxine, triiodothyronine

REFERENCES AND FURTHER READING

Bloch G 1985 Body and self: elements of human biology, behaviour, and health. William Kaufmann, Los Altoz, CA

Dobbing J (ed) 1997 Developing brain and behaviour. Academic Press, London

Donovan B T 1985 Hormones and human behaviour. Cambridge University Press, Cambridge

Feuerstein M, Labbé E E, Kuczmierczyk A R 1986 Health psychology: a psychobiological perspective. Plenum Publishing, New York

Gloor P 1997 The temporal lobe and limbic system. Oxford University Press, New York

Graham R B 1990 Physiological psychology. Wadsworth Publishing Company, Belmont, CA

Hobson J A 1989 Sleep. W H Freeman, New York

Hughes J 1987 Cancer and emotion: psychological preludes and reactions to cancer. John Wiley, Chichester

Kandel E R, Schwartz J H, Jessell T M 1995 Essentials of neural science and behavior. Appleton and Lange, East Norwalk, CT

Logue A W 1986 The psychology of eating and drinking. W H Freeman, Oxford

McCarley R W, Steriade M 1990 Brainstem control of wakefulness and sleep. Kluwer Academic/Plenum Publishers, New York

Mendelson W B 1987 Human sleep: research and clinical care. Plenum Publishing, New York

Panter-Brick C, Worthman C M (eds) 1998 Hormones, health and behaviour. Cambridge University Press, Cambridge

Learning and memory

The physiological basis of learning is the formation and modification of synaptic contacts between neurones. The physiological basis of memory is the connections existing between neurones. While these persist, we retain the ability to perform learned tasks and to 'relive' past experiences in our imagination.

Brain areas having a key role in learning and memory include the hippocampus of the limbic system, the cerebral cortex and the cerebellum. Neurones in these areas have the potential to form an amazing number of synaptic contacts. The greatest changes in synaptic contact occur in the early years of life, but some flexibility of contact is retained throughout our adult years.

Motor skills, once learned, are largely automatic. We do them 'without thinking'. However, remembering things that we have heard or seen or felt depends upon forming an imprint of the experience in our minds and on bringing that imprint from our subconscious minds to consciousness. If we cannot remember, it may be because long-lasting contacts have not been formed, or because contacts have been lost, or because we cannot gain access to the relevant neural circuits.

DEFINITIONS

LEARNING

When we learn, changes are occurring in the connections between neurones in the nervous system. Some of these changes, such as those in infancy and childhood involved in learning to sit, stand and walk, are genetically pre-programmed. Others, such as learning to speak Japanese, or how to play the clarinet, depend on our specific experiences as individuals. Experience affects the chemistry of the brain through specific changes occurring at well-used and at under-used synapses, as well as through the excitatory and inhibitory effects associated with different states of arousal and emotion.

Thus, we learn as we grow and as our nervous systems develop in utero, through infancy and in childhood, and we go on learning as we continue to be exposed to new stimuli, experiences and circumstances throughout life. The potential for learning is greatest while the nervous system is still developing,

Early development

All aspects of child development have been studied to a greater or lesser degree; some activities lend themselves more readily to investigation than others. The sequence of developmental steps is the same for all infants because it depends on the maturation of motor and visual skills, and the ability to coordinate those skills. Those professionals whose job it is to assess the development of infants use a series of milestones (or stepping stones), which are more detailed than when the infant smiles, sits or crawls, as criteria for normal progress (see Ch. 31). Consider, for example, the ability to reach for and grasp an object. A month-old baby will stare fixedly at an interesting object – grasping with the eyes! By about 2 months the baby will start swiping at objects with a closed fist. By 4 months the baby will be using an open hand and judging the distance by glancing from hand to object. By 5 months the object is reached for and grasped accurately.

It has been found that in families where the infant is given frequent stimulation and encouraged to reach for interesting objects, the developmental milestones for reaching and grasping will be arrived at earlier than the normal age. When a baby is fed, changed and returned to his cot without time being given for 'play' the milestones will be achieved at the normal age. Frequent, appropriate stimulation throughout childhood encourages the formation and maintenance of synaptic contacts and the child tends to progress more rapidly. Health visitors advise mothers and other carers on providing appropriate stimulation during the early years. Not all mothers find it easy to play with babies and young children and so need extra help.

but considerable scope still exists after it has reached developmental maturity.

MEMORY

If learning is defined as the process of forming or modifying contacts between neurones, memory can be defined as the changes in synaptic contact that outlast the period of learning. The new pattern of synaptic contact may consist of links involving our motor systems allowing us to exercise a new skill, such as riding a bicycle, or they may be links between sensory experiences enabling us to remember the word for an object, or recall a past event.

Skills

It is said that once you have learned to ride a bicycle you never forget. After a long spell of not riding, your first attempts may be a little inexpert but you instinctively remember what to do. You don't have to think about it – you just ride. Motor memories (skills) differ from thought memories in that we can make use of them without conscious thought. A skilled pianist can play a complex piece of music 'from memory' without actually having to think about how to play.

Thoughts

Memory of past experiences, however, can be both conscious as well as unconscious. We carry in our minds a complex record of all that has happened to us in our lives, though for most of the time we are unaware of it. When fragments of this record are brought to consciousness, we actually remember. When we cannot bring the record to consciousness, the memory is still there in the connections between neurones, but our recollection of it is impaired.

Having a 'poor' memory

In everyday conversation we talk of having a poor memory, meaning that we have forgotten the name of a new friend or that we find difficulty in remembering what we have done or read recently (how much can you remember now of the chapter you read before this one?). Some people, through injury or disease, experience loss of memory (amnesia). Although in conversation we seem to be talking about the same thing, namely a difficulty with memory, the causes of that problem vary. Memory may be poor because:

- synaptic contacts do not form very easily (a difficulty in learning)
- contacts between cells have not been maintained (actual loss of memories)
- recall of the stored memory is impaired (memory intact but not brought to consciousness).

To understand how learning takes place and memories are formed, we need to begin by looking first at the factors that influence the formation of synaptic contacts, and how, once such contacts are formed, they are maintained.

DEVELOPMENT AND MAINTENANCE OF CONTACTS BETWEEN NEURONES

The number of nerve cells in the brain reaches a maximum early in life. After this no new nerve cells are formed. However, like all nucleated cells, neurones have the ability to grow and develop. Provided the cell body of a neurone is intact there can be:

- growth of axons and dendrites
- formation of new synapses between neurones
- modification of existing synapses.

All these processes are influenced by the chemical environment of the cells as well as by the internal activity of the cells themselves. Both vary as impulses are transmitted through the neurones, and as neurotransmitters and other agents are released and recycled. By these means new links can be forged between neurones, and the effectiveness of existing synapses can be altered. This ongoing flexibility in connections between neurones is termed plasticity. It is greatest in the early years of life but is retained in adulthood. In contrast to many other cells, however, mature nerve cells cannot reproduce. When nerve cell bodies are injured and die they cannot be replaced.

PLASTICITY

Developmental

The total number of synapses in the brain reaches a peak around the age of 5 years and then decreases to a plateau in the adult years. The number of cells and synapses in the brain is affected by our experience. If our senses receive plenty of stimulation in early life, many synaptic contacts are established and maintained. But if relevant experiences are lacking, synapses are less profuse.

During development, synapses that are used are strengthened and retained, whereas those that are inactive deteriorate and are eventually lost. In this way each of us develops a unique pattern of contacts shaped by our unique experience as individuals. No two brains can be exactly alike because no two lives are ever exactly the same.

In adulthood

Plasticity still exists in the adult brain but to a lesser extent. We continue to be able to learn new things, though not with the same facility as in our younger years.

If there is injury to the brain, for example through a cerebral haemorrhage, it is possible for nearby uninjured neurones to sprout and form new contacts, replacing those that have been lost (reactive synaptogenesis). The extent to which this occurs depends on age, the extent to which the neurones are used, and the degree of injury.

In old age, the number of cells and synapses may decrease. In senility there is a big reduction in the number of cells and synaptic contacts in several parts of the brain including the cerebral cortex and the hippocampus.

THE CHEMISTRY OF SYNAPTIC CONTACT

Making contact

Nerve cells are stimulated to grow by trophic factors that promote growth and guide their direction. These factors may be chemicals released from adjacent nerve cells or by glial cells nearby. The trophic factors attract the growing nerve endings. Sometimes cells, such as astrocytes in the brain, act as a framework guiding the direction in which growth occurs.

One of the fascinating things revealed in recent years by sophisticated filming techniques is the dynamic nature of these events. Speeded up film of nerve cells in culture reveals just how active cells really are and how much exploratory activity goes on. Dendrites are seen to move around, extend and retract, contacting other cells and surfaces in the vicinity as they do so. If the chemistry is right when contact is made, a closer association is formed, and synapses develop; if it is not, the dendrite retracts and tests other sites.

The chemistry that matters includes the chemistry of recognition between molecules on the membranes of the cells in contact as well as the chemistry of the local environment. Influential substances include neurotransmitters such as noradrenaline, acetylcholine, dopamine and serotonin.

Some substances are influential during a specific period of development. For example, the hormone thyroxine is necessary for normal brain development in the first few years of life. If this hormone is deficient at that time, profound mental retardation results that cannot be reversed by giving thyroxine later on (cretinism).

Keeping contact

Once contact has been established the maintenance of the synapse depends on its usage. Inactivity and activity produce different local chemical states that, in turn, affect cell function. Modifications in the junction can occur both pre- and postsynaptically.

The neurotransmitter released by the presynaptic terminal is picked up by receptors on the presynaptic membrane as well as binding to receptors on the postsynaptic membrane (Fig. 28.1). These presynaptic receptors regulate the functioning of the nerve ending, and the amount of transmitter released.

At the postsynaptic membrane, long-term changes in the number of receptors inserted into the membrane affect the responsiveness of the cell to the transmitter released by the presynaptic ending. The sensitivity of the receptors is also influenced by regulatory proteins in the membrane adjacent to the receptors, which are themselves affected by local conditions.

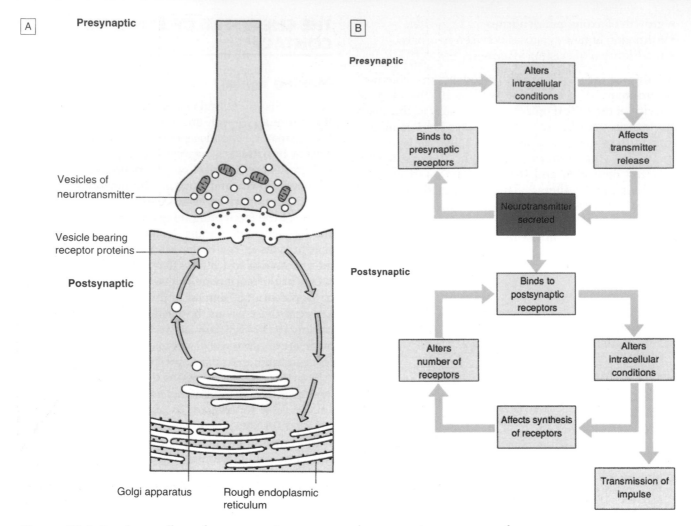

Figure 28.1 Regulatory effects of neurotransmitters at pre- and postsynaptic components of a synapse.

Some of the changes occurring at synapses, such as the changes in concentrations of intracellular ions and second messengers, will be shortlived. But those that involve restructuring of the membranes and organelles of the synapse, through the control of protein synthesis, will result in long-lasting changes.

ASSOCIATIVE LEARNING

INSTINCT AND INTELLECT

The links developing between neurones during growth and development, as a result of genetic pre-programming, create instinctive patterns of behaviour. You touch something hot and instinctively pull your hand away, not because you have learned by experience to do so, but because of the pattern of neural

connections between nociceptors and muscles determined by your genes. What we learn with experience is to recognize hot objects before we touch them. We can then intelligently choose either not to pick them up or, alternatively, aim to do so with great care.

CONDITIONING

It was shown by the Russian scientist Pavlov that responses to certain stimuli could be conditioned. If a bell was regularly sounded at the same time that food was presented to one of his dogs, after a while the dog would salivate in anticipation of the arrival of food whenever the bell was rung, even though there was no smell or sight of food anywhere.

The way in which this association of sensory signals and responses may develop is shown in Figure 28.2. Simultaneous activity in salivatory and auditory path-

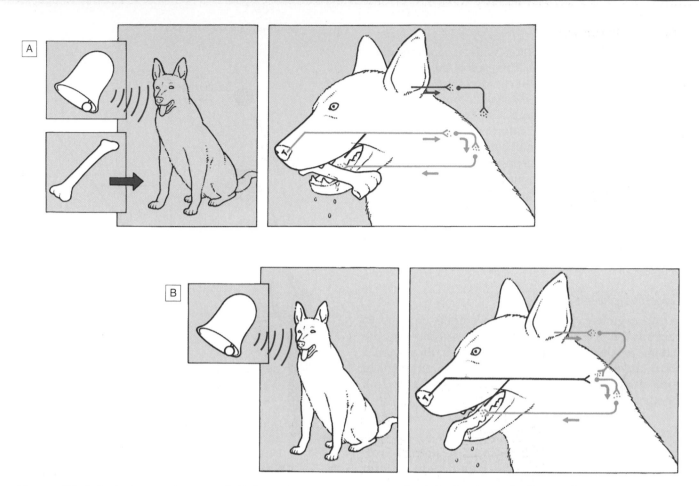

Figure 28.2 Pavlovian conditioning. A, Reflex salivation in response to food. B, Conditioned reflex – salivation in response to a stimulus associated with food.

ways is believed to create the right chemical conditions for the development of synaptic contacts forging links between the auditory system and the salivary glands. This may occur by the strengthening of existing contacts or by the establishment and growth of new ones.

The association created externally by ringing the bell at the same time as presenting food is thus transformed into actual physical connections made between the nerve fibres. Once this has happened the brain has a long-term memory of that association recorded in the connections developed between the neurones. If association is not renewed from time to time, the connections may weaken and eventually be lost.

KEY BRAIN AREAS

The parts of the brain that are believed to have a key role in learning (cerebral cortex, hippocampus and cerebellar cortex) contain cells that have two distinctive features:

- huge dendritic trees
- dendritic spines.

The pyramidal cells of the cerebral cortex and hippo-campus and the Purkinje cells of the cerebellar cortex all possess huge dendritic trees. The dendrites possess tiny spurs, not commonly seen on other nerve cells. Synaptic contacts are made with these spurs. The number of dendritic spines and synapses is affected by experience. For example, visual deprivation in the early years of life decreases the numbers of spines formed on cells of the visual cortex.

DEVELOPING SKILLS AND KNOWLEDGE

Although the principles of associative learning are the same regardless of the nature of what is being learned, there are some differences between the learning of motor skills and the development of intelligence.

Motor skills

The learning of new motor skills is an important function of the cerebellum. This part of the brain has a major role in enabling us to coordinate and refine our movements. It also has extensive connections with many other parts of the brain that are concerned with movement, and receives information from proprioceptors about how the movement is actually being performed. This feedback is important in learning. If the action is successful, associations are strengthened.

The learning of a new motor skill has been divided into three phases:

- cognitive
- associative
- automatic.

Cognitive phase

In the cognitive phase, you concentrate on how to perform the task in hand. This involves knowing the actions needed, the sequence in which they should occur and how quickly they should be performed. In your mind you consciously and deliberately link together all the elements of the task.

Associative phase

In the associative phase these links are strengthened. You then concentrate not so much on how to perform the task, but on refining and improving it, so that it is performed with increasing ease and minimum effort. It is thought that the brain builds up a pattern of associations between the command signals and their outcome, rather in the way that you may plot a graph between two variables (Fig. 28.3). In this way we do not have to learn every possible movement but instead we build up a set of rules (schema) that can be used to determine the command needed for a 'new' task of a similar kind. It may be for this reason that the development of motor skills is often best achieved by practising different but related movements, rather than by repeating exactly the same movement over and over again.

Automatic phase

Ultimately the action being learned becomes automatic. It can be performed without conscious control. A skilled pianist, for example, can play a piece of music without looking at the scripted music or thinking about when, where and how to move his fingers. Most of our day-to-day activity consists of automatic programmes triggered by the routine events of the day.

Skills do not develop overnight. They take time. In the early stages recognizable gains in skill occur quite quickly, but refinement of movement and the establishment of those patterns takes longer. It is said that com-

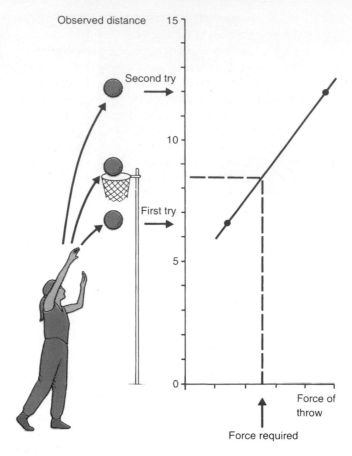

Figure 28.3 Development of rules in our minds (schema) linking actions with outcomes.

plex patterns of behaviour take about 2 years to become properly established.

Learned motor activities, once established, are not easily forgotten. If practice does not continue, performance may deteriorate but the memory remains. Why learned movements should be retained so well is not clear. It may be that some basic components of the activity are common to other tasks, so that 'practice' continues though in a different guise. It may also be that movements learned subsequently interfere less with what has already been learned than is the case for 'thinking' memory.

Knowledge

At its simplest, knowledge is the linking together of inputs from several senses. Learning the meaning of words, for example, involves associating either the sound of a word or its appearance in print with the characteristics of the thing that the word describes. In most people, these linguistic associations develop chiefly in the parieto-occipital and temporal areas of the left hemisphere of the cerebral cortex, whereas visuospatial associations, such as the shape and form of objects, form in the right hemisphere.

Once links have been established, the presentation of one stimulus, such as the spoken word, will be sufficient to call up the associated sensory experiences in our imagination. So having said the word 'apple', in the mind's eye we imagine an apple: we recall something of its appearance, its flavour, its smell and how it feels, even though the relevant sensory receptors are not activated. We know what an apple is like because the memories of its features are fixed in our minds in the pattern of synaptic connections between neurones. This is an example of semantic memory. Another form of memory is termed episodic and relates to the memory of more complex experiences such as events.

Intellectual learning, unlike motor learning, is known to be particularly sensitive to:

- our level of arousal
- our degree of motivation.

Arousal

Moderate levels of arousal are necessary for optimum learning. If someone is either overexcited or drowsy, learning is not as good. The level of activity in the reticular activating system (RAS) creates background conditions that facilitate or depress learning. Raised levels of activity in the reticular formation are associated with the release of noradrenaline, which is known to have a widespread influence on neurones in the brain. It raises the level of excitability and facilitates learning.

Motivation

Things that are well remembered are usually those that arouse our emotions, whether pleasantly or unpleasantly. Activity in the limbic system, part of the brain involved in the elaboration of emotion, is involved in learning. Hippocampal neurones are believed to control the ease with which synaptic contacts are formed in other parts of the brain. Also, the limbic system is known to be involved in determining our choice of behaviour. Stimulation of certain areas of the limbic system has been shown to evoke feelings of either pleasure or displeasure, and behaviour that either seeks to repeat the experience or to avoid it at all costs. As synaptic changes are consolidated by repetition, any system encouraging the repetition of specific actions will play a significant role in learning.

REMEMBERING AND FORGETTING

The development of synaptic contacts can explain how associations between sensory signals become literally

Memory loss and the elderly person

The elderly person who suffers from memory loss usually becomes very irritating to all but the very placid and patient. The type of memory loss varies from individual to individual. It is not like just having a poor memory where retrieval is possible given the right cues. The total blankness and the knowledge that retrieval is impossible, when faced frequently with something that one knows one must have done, is quite unnerving and has to be experienced to be understood fully.

Many elderly people are able to give detailed descriptions of events which occurred decades earlier, but cannot remember what they were told 5 minutes ago. This is why some elderly people manage better in their own homes, with help, than in, say, a home for the elderly. Once moved from the environment that is familiar, the details of which are stored in long-term memory and can still be retrieved, it is difficult either for the features of the new accommodation to be processed and stored or for the information to be retrieved. The elderly person may well wander about trying to find familiar surroundings and the whereabouts of certain people. The label 'confused and disoriented' is often applied. Attempts to sedate the person frequently make matters worse whereas appropriate stimulation and individual attention may help to relieve the anxiety. For some there is no alternative to 'living in the past'.

fixed in our minds as memories, but it does not readily explain how we remember things from moment to moment, such as the number that we have just found in the telephone book, the name of someone to whom we have just been introduced, or what we have just read. This short-term memory (or working memory) differs from long-term memory. Each is the result of different processes and can be disrupted in different ways.

We are unconscious of most of what we have learned. The memories are there in the patterns of synaptic contact that develop over our lives, but we are not conscious of all that is stored in our minds. Most of what we know intellectually is kept below the level of consciousness until such times when it is recalled or 'brought to mind'.

SHORT-TERM MEMORY

It is believed that sensory information is, for a short while, passed around neuronal circuits repetitively so that the experience lingers in our minds. Neuronal circuits of this kind are termed reverberating circuits. It may be that, if neural activity persists for long enough, under the right circumstances it is then converted into physical changes in synaptic contacts so that the memory becomes long term.

If short-term memory processes are disrupted acutely, long-term memories are not formed. For example, an individual who is knocked out by a blow to the head may not remember the events around the time of the injury at all well. The same kind of memory loss is experienced by those who are given ECT (electro-convulsive therapy). Events immediately preceding the shock treatment are not remembered. This is termed retrograde amnesia. However, the remembrance of earlier events is unaffected as is the formation of new memories subsequently.

LONG-TERM MEMORY

The ability to form new long-term memories is affected if there is damage to parts of the temporal cerebral cortex and the limbic system, especially the hippo-campus. Damage to the temporal cerebral cortex is associated with loss of semantic memory whereas injury to the hippocampus gives rise to loss of episodic memory.

When there is damage to the hippocampus, new information is retained only for a very short space of time before it is lost completely. Thus no new long-term memories of events are formed (anterograde amnesia). The person affected remains locked in the past and has great difficulty learning and remembering new experiences. Interestingly, some tasks can be learned but the individual cannot remember having learned them.

RETRIEVING INFORMATION

Remembering involves retrieving information that has been stored and bringing it to consciousness. This process is distinct from those that form memories in the first place. All are needed for us to have a 'good memory' (Fig. 28.4).

We will all have had the experience of trying desperately hard to remember something important and then finding that when we turn to something else, suddenly the answer comes 'out of the blue'. Our conscious minds are oblivious to the 'computer search' in progress until the answer is found. The retrieval of information is assisted by association. It is often the case that a related though different fact will act as the trigger. It helps the search to take place in the relevant 'files' in our minds.

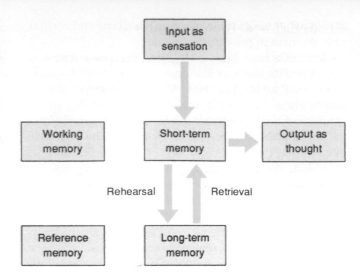

Figure 28.4 Learning and remembering.

The recall of information is influenced by brain chemistry. The concentration of acetylcholine appears to be of especial significance but noradrenaline and adrenaline also affect the process. There is evidence to suggest that the memory loss associated with ageing and senility is caused by a deficiency of acetylcholine within the hippocampus. This part of the limbic system seems to be involved both in the establishment of long-term memories and in their retrieval into consciousness.

THE UNCONSCIOUS

More goes on in our minds below the level of conscious awareness than we ever imagine. We can absorb information subconsciously, process it, store it and make use of it often all without conscious thought.

This buried information influences and directs our behaviour without our knowing. For example, some people suffer from unaccountable phobias in which a particular object, circumstance or set of events produces immediate fear and panic. Some may feel afraid of going out; others may have a fear of lifts; others still may feel panic at the sight of a feather. These reactions may be inexplicable to the person concerned. It may be that inappropriate associations have been formed early in development. If these reactions seriously hamper a person's life, then attempts may be made to decondition inappropriate responses and build more helpful associations.

REFERENCES AND FURTHER READING

Agras W S 1985 Panic: facing fears, phobias and anxiety. W H Freeman, Oxford

Brown M C, Hopkins W G, Keynes R J 1991 Essentials of neural development. Cambridge University Press, Cambridge

Davey G 1987 Cognitive processes and Pavlovian conditioning in humans. John Wiley, Chichester

Freeman Somers M 1991 Spinal cord injury. Appleton & Lange, East Norwalk, CT

Hoyenga K B, Hoyenga K T 1988 Psychobiology: the neurone and behaviour. Brooks/Cole Publishing Company, Pacific Grove, CA

Huttenlocher P R 1979 Synaptic density in human frontal cortex: developmental changes and effects of ageing. Brain Research 163: 195–205

Kidd G, Lawes N, Musa I 1992 Understanding neuromuscular plasticity: a basis for clinical rehabilitation. Edward Arnold, London

Schmidt R 1989 Motor control and learning – a behavioural emphasis. Human Kinetics Publishers, Champaign, IL

Squire L R, Kandel E R 2000 Memory. Scientific American Library, New York

Winlow W, McCrohan C R (eds) 1987 Growth and plasticity of neural connections. Manchester University Press, Manchester

Like vision, hearing, touch, smell and taste, pain is a sensation evoked by the excitation of nerve cells in the brain. It usually occurs when specific sensory receptors are excited, but, like other sensations, it can be experienced whenever and however pain pathways are stimulated. The character (sharp or burning) and perceived location of a pain (discrete or vague) depend on:

- the types and situations of the receptors excited
- the pathways through which the impulses are transmitted
- the ultimate destinations of the signals within the brain.

The main purpose of the sensation of pain is that of protection. It is responsible for giving us the conscious awareness that some form of tissue damage is occurring or about to occur. It elicits both behavioural (withdrawal or defence) and emotional (crying or fear) responses.

THE SENSATION OF PAIN

Damage to tissues is not invariably felt as pain. For example, the small intestine can be cut and cauterized without pain being felt. Likewise, in brain surgery, once a hole has been made in the skull under local anaesthesia, brain tissue can be cut without the patient feeling anything. However, at the other extreme, even slight injury to tissues such as the skin and the peritoneum can produce very sharp and discomforting pain. This shows that receptors sensitive to tissue damage, which mediate the sensation of pain, are not uniformly distributed throughout the body. Lining layers, such as the skin and peritoneum, tend to be more richly supplied with receptors than internal structures, such as the liver and the intestines.

THE EXTERNAL SURFACE: SKIN

Types of sensation

The skin is abundantly supplied with receptors excited by noxious stimuli (nociceptors), most of which are unspecialized nerve endings. When the skin is damaged, two recognizably different qualities of pain can be

In some conditions, such as rheumatoid arthritis, chronic pain may serve a protective function. In others, like back pain, it may have outlived its usefulness as a warning. The back pain sufferer commonly believes that painful movements will lead to further injury. However, after the initial acute phase, lack of exercise leads to muscle wastage and further pain. Patients who suffer from back pain should be encouraged to engage with their employers and healthcare professionals in order to agree a programme of work-related activities that will assist the patient to remain active and prevent muscle wastage.

distinguished. There is the sharp, well-localized pain felt at the time of injury, and the longer-lasting, more diffuse discomfort experienced shortly afterwards. These two types of sensation are sometimes referred to as 'fast' and 'slow' pain. The differences between them are due to differences in the receptors stimulated and in the routes and destinations of the impulses within the nervous system.

Fast pain

Fast pain occurs upon stimulation of mechanical and thermal nociceptors, and the impulses are carried to the brain via myelinated Aδ fibres, which synapse in the spinal cord and brain stem with tracts carrying the signals directly to the thalamus and on to the somatosensory cortex (Fig. 29.1). Fast pain is perceived as a sharp, prickling sensation, which is easily localized due to the direct and discrete routing of the impulses.

Slow pain

When tissues are damaged, a variety of cellular products are released, including bradykinin and prostaglandins. Slow pain occurs following stimulation by these chemicals of a different class of pain receptors, namely the polymodal nociceptors. The name polymodal refers to the fact that this class of receptors will respond to a range of stimuli. Impulses are carried to the brain by small unmyelinated C fibres that synapse within the spinal cord, with fibres carrying the impulses on to the reticular formation of the brain stem, via the spinoreticular tracts, and then on to the thalamus and the cortex. Within the reticular formation, the excitation does not remain discretely localized but spreads out to activate adjacent nerve cells, so that the excitation becomes more diffuse and more areas of the brain are activated, including parts involved in our emotional responses, such as the hypothalamus. Consequently

our perception of the site of injury is more vague and we experience more distress.

Physiological pain control: the pain gate

It is well known that the discomfort experienced when we injure ourselves can be made to feel different: just rubbing the injured part has a soothing effect; courageous rescuers are sometimes unaware of serious injuries they have sustained until after an emergency is over; 'positive thinking' can influence what we feel. None of this is in any way mysterious. The transmission of any signals within the nervous system can be inhibited at synapses. The first place this occurs in pain pathways is within the spinal cord or brain stem.

Melzack & Wall (1965) coined the word 'gating' to describe the way that signals from nociceptors arriving at the spinal cord could be prevented from being transmitted further, thus reducing the sensation of pain and producing physiological analgesia. Disturbances and diseases affecting this pain control system give rise to a variety of abnormal sensations including 'pins and needles' (paraesthesia) and supersensitivity to painful stimuli (hyperalgesia).

Physiological analgesia

The crucial feature in the body's system of pain control is the presence of inhibitory interneurones, which synapse with neurones in the pain pathway (Fig. 29.2). These inhibitory interneurones are activated by:

- simultaneous activity in other sensory neurones (usually large diameter myelinated fibres (Aβ) carrying information about touch and pressure from the skin)
- nerve fibres carrying signals down from the brain.

The axons of sensory neurones conveying signals about touch and pressure from the trunk and limbs become the dorsal columns of the spinal cord. Just before they do, these axons branch in the dorsal horn forming collaterals that synapse with the inhibitory interneurones. Consequently, when the skin in the vicinity of the injured area is gently rubbed (which excites the large diameter fibres), these inhibitory interneurones are activated and this reduces the transmission of signals in the 'pain pathways'.

The nerve fibres coming down from the brain, which have similar effects, include some which originate in two areas of the brain stem (Fig. 29.2):

- peri-aqueductal grey matter
- raphe nuclei.

Some of the nerve cells involved in influencing (modulating) the transmission of pain are cells secreting a different class of neurotransmitters, the endogenous opioids, which include peptides such as:

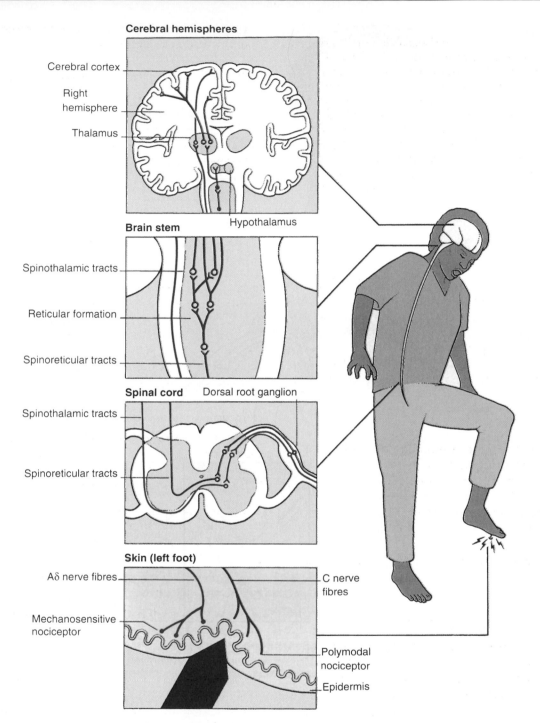

Figure 29.1 Routes through which impulses from nociceptors in the skin are transmitted to the brain, giving rise to the sensations of 'fast' pain (red lines) and 'slow' pain (blue lines). (Note that the skin receptors being excited are on the left side of the body whereas the destination of the nerve impulses in the brain is on the opposite side.)

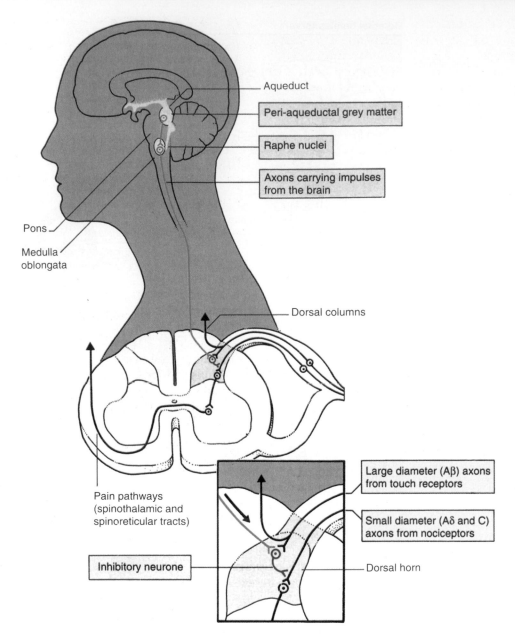

Aqueduct

Peri-aqueductal grey matter

Raphe nuclei

Axons carrying impulses from the brain

Pons

Medulla oblongata

Dorsal columns

Large diameter (Aβ) axons from touch receptors

Small diameter (Aδ and C) axons from nociceptors

Pain pathways (spinothalamic and spinoreticular tracts)

Inhibitory neurone

Dorsal horn

Figure 29.2 Component parts of the body's system of pain control. The transmission of signals in the 'pain pathway' can be inhibited by simultaneous activity in (1) other sensory neurones conducting impulses from the skin and (2) axons conducting impulses from the brain, both of which excite inhibitory interneurones.

- endorphins
- enkephalins
- dynorphin.

The gate control theory highlights the presence of ascending and descending influences on pain perception. Pain is never solely physical or purely psychological. The relative influence of these factors will vary according to the extent of tissue damage, the context in which the pain occurs and individual interpretation.

Paraesthesia and hyperalgesia

The discomfort experienced a short while after a leg or an arm has gone numb when you have been lying on it awkwardly is very familiar. When the limb comes 'back to life' again, a mixture of sensations are felt (paraesthesia) and the pain can be excruciating.

When tissue is compressed and becomes ischaemic, the nerve axons stop transmitting nerve impulses, and sensation is lost. As blood flow recovers, the axons recover too but this takes longer for the large diameter fibres than the smaller ones. Consequently, after a period of numbness, the small diameter unmyelinated nerve fibres, some of which transmit signals from nociceptors in deeper tissues of the limb, begin transmitting signals before the large diameter fibres involved in the gating of pain have recovered. Briefly, activity in the small diameter fibres is uninhibited by gating mechanisms and the affected individual experiences the result! As activity returns to normal in the larger fibres, the transmission of signals from the small diameter fibres is gated again and the discomfort fades.

Other examples of imbalance in transmission giving rise to abnormal sensations include the hyperalgesia that may be experienced for a short time when a severed nerve regrows, and postherpetic neuralgia.

The hyperalgesia occurring some while after a nerve has been severed is caused by the smaller fibres growing fastest and re-innervating their sensory receptors first. As a result, the area of the skin innervated by the regenerating fibres will, for a time, be hypersensitive to painful stimuli. In postherpetic neuralgia, a common sequel to shingles (herpes zoster), prolonged excruciating pain results from the damage caused to large diameter myelinated fibres by viruses.

INTERNAL STRUCTURES

Pain is felt when some but not all internal tissues are damaged or stressed. Tissues and organs are innervated by autonomic and somatic nerve fibres. The quality of the sensations felt and the stimuli that evoke pain differ according to the type of innervation.

Sources of pain

Pain arises if there is:

- local ischaemia (e.g. inadequate skeletal muscle or coronary blood flow)
- chemical damage (e.g. leakage of enzymes in the pancreas)
- spasm of smooth muscle (e.g. of the intestines)
- overdistension of a hollow organ (e.g. bladder)
- irritation of the peritoneum, pleurae or pericardium.

Some tissues, such as the alveoli of the lungs and the liver acini, are insensitive to injury, whereas neighbouring structures, such as the bronchi, the capsule of the liver and the bile ducts, are very sensitive.

Innervation

The sensory nerve axons mediating pain run in:

- autonomic nerves
- somatic nerves.

Autonomic nerves

Many of the axons transmitting signals from nociceptors are unmyelinated C fibres running in the sympathetic nerves. They transmit signals from many internal organs and from tissues, such as skeletal muscle, and include axons innervating the walls of blood vessels.

Somatic nerves

The axons mediating the sensation of pain are small diameter fibres (Aδ and C). They innervate:

- the parietal peritoneum
- the pleurae
- the pericardium
- the connective tissue associated with some organs (e.g. mesentery of the intestines; capsule of the kidney).

Qualities of sensation

The sensations experienced are broadly of two kinds:

- localized and acute
- diffuse and debilitating.

In some cases the pain is actually felt at a different site (referred pain) to that from which it originates.

Localized and acute

The character of the painful sensations arising from excitation of axons in the somatic spinal nerves is similar in some respects to that of cutaneous pain. It can be sharp in character, and is usually localized to the injured area. For example, the sharp stabbing pain of an inflamed appendix that is felt in the lower right hand part of the abdomen is a result of irritation of the overlying parietal peritoneum.

Diffuse and debilitating

The character of the pain felt when sensory axons in the autonomic nerves are stimulated is quite different. It is usually more diffuse, long-lasting and debilitating. For example, the burning pain of gastritis or pancreatitis is of this kind, as is the intense pain of intermittent claudication caused by muscle ischaemia. The cramping quality (colic) of abdominal pain such as 'stomach ache' and period pains (dysmenorrhoea) is due to periodic contraction of the smooth muscle in the affected tissue.

Referred pain

If pain originates from the viscera, it may be felt as coming from the surface of the body at a site distant from the injured organ. The axons running in the autonomic nerves innervating the internal organs are believed to converge in the spinal cord with somatic

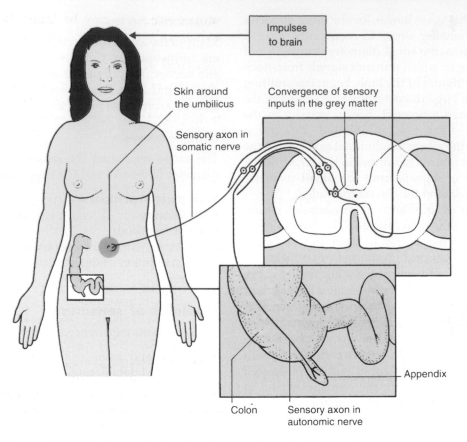

Figure 29.3 The basis of referred pain using the pain of appendicitis as an example: when the appendix is inflamed, some pain is experienced in the region of the umbilicus, although the source of the nerve impulses giving rise to the pain is actually the appendix.

sensory nerve fibres coming from a particular part of the body surface (Fig. 29.3). This convergence arises from the fact that embryologically both parts (viscera and skin) developed from the same primitive tissue. As the brain does not have a 'picture' of the internal organs as it does of the body surface (see Fig. 22.7), signals from internal organs are interpreted as having come from the body surface. They are said to be referred to that surface. Consequently, appendicitis gives rise to a cramping pain around the umbilicus, at a distance from the appendix, as well as the stabbing pain felt in the vicinity of the inflamed tissue itself. Other parts of the body to which pain may be referred as a result of injury to various thoracic and abdominal organs are shown in Figure 29.4.

Effective stimuli

The kinds of stimuli that are effective in evoking pain also differ according to whether autonomic or somatic nerves are involved. Surgeons can make an incision in the intestines (autonomic innervation) without pain being felt, whereas a similar cut in the parietal peritoneum (somatic innervation), stimulating the mechano-sensitive receptors of the Aδ system, is very painful. Conversely, local ischaemia of the intestines caused by muscular spasm or overdistension, which excites polymodal nociceptors and the C fibre system running in the sympathetic nerves, produces great discomfort.

PAIN IN THE HEAD

The principles described so far apply also to the different kinds of pain felt in the head. Damage to surface structures (such as skin of the face and scalp, and mucous membranes of the mouth and teeth) is usually associated with sharp focused pain, whereas stimuli affecting internal structures (such as sinuses, muscles and intracranial structures) tend to produce more diffuse pain that is often referred to other parts of the head.

surface structures may be 'gated' in this nucleus by activity in large diameter fibres.

Internal structures

Irritation of internal structures gives rise to various forms of headache. Some headaches are a result of damage and stresses to tissues of the brain whereas others originate from other structures of the head (Fig. 29.6).

Brain tissue

As in other parts of the body, it is the membranes wrapped around the brain (meninges), and the walls of blood vessels, that are richly innervated with sensory nerve fibres, whereas brain tissue itself is largely insensitive to injury. Pain occurs therefore when there is:

- any tugging on the venous sinuses
- stretching of the dura
- damage to the blood vessels of the dura.

The pain of migraine headaches, for example, is associated with vascular changes. As a result of an abnormal burst of impulses, a short period of local vasoconstriction occurs followed by a prolonged period of vasodilation. The timing of the intense pain tends to coincide with the vasodilation.

Other structures

Headaches may also be caused by stimuli arising in:

- muscles of the neck and temple
- nose and sinuses
- eyes.

In each case the sensory signals are referred to various parts of the head.

Most people have experienced tension headache at some time. In an anxiety state, there is a general increase in muscle tension throughout the body, including muscles in the neck and temple. Increased tension in these muscles probably causes local ischaemia which excites receptors in the blood vessels. The impulses arriving in the sensory cortex from the muscles are interpreted as coming from surface structures of the head with the result that pain is not felt in the tensed muscles but in the head in a vague and discomforting way.

REACTIONS TO PAIN

As well as creating the sensation of pain, activation of nociceptors elicits a variety of reflex responses. Many of these are protective, although they may add to our discomfort. Some contribute to the emotions we feel as a result of injury.

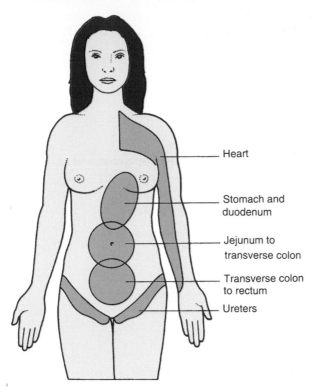

- Heart
- Stomach and duodenum
- Jejunum to transverse colon
- Transverse colon to rectum
- Ureters

Figure 29.4 Parts of the body to which pain may be referred as a result of injury to various organs.

Migraine headache is often preceded by visual disturbances and accompanied by nausea or vomiting. The headache is often unilateral and highly localized. Drug and biofeedback therapies may be effective in avoiding or ameliorating attacks. *Tension headaches* are common among people, such as keyboard operators, who adopt unnatural arm and head postures for long periods. A workplace assessment may assist many sufferers to resolve the problem.

Surface structures

The characteristics of pains originating from surface structures of the head are similar to those originating from surface structures elsewhere in the body. They:

- have 'fast' and 'slow' components
- are relatively well localized
- are mediated by activity in Aδ and C fibres.

Nerves innervating the face, mouth and teeth (Fig. 29.5) converge in the trigeminal nucleus, a large group of cells within the brain stem and top two segments of the spinal cord. The organization of cells within this nucleus resembles that in the dorsal horn of the spinal cord (Fig. 29.2). Signals arising from nociceptors of the

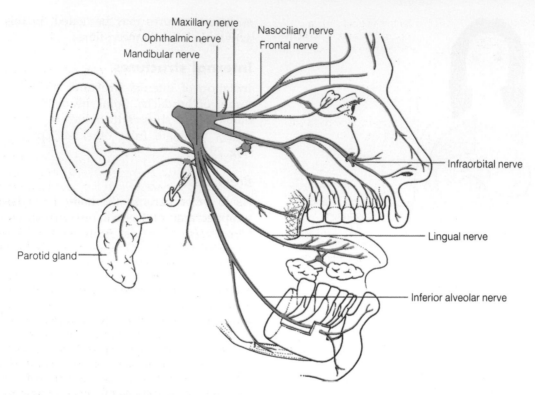

Figure 29.5 Nerves innervating the face, mouth and teeth. The trigeminal nerve (cranial nerve V) contains sensory fibres carrying impulses to the trigeminal nucleus in the brain stem. (From Rogers 1992, with permission of Elsevier.)

In *trigeminal neuralgia* there is hypersensitivity to stimuli delivered to discrete areas of the skin, giving rise to excruciating pain. Examples of some trigger factors may be extremes of hot and cold. One theory is that there is an imbalance of signals between the large and small diameter cutaneous afferents as a result of damage to the larger afferents. Patients who have trigeminal neuralgia may be malnourished due to the anxiety of initiating an attack of pain through eating and drinking.

REFLEXES

The reflexes elicited by excitation of nociceptors may be divided into two groups:

• somatic
• autonomic.

Somatic reflexes

The simple reflex response to the excitation of nociceptors in the skin is the withdrawal reflex, which pulls the injured part of the body away from the source of damage. Excitation of receptors inside the body also evokes characteristic responses. Irritation of the periton-eum, for example, reflexly causes contraction of abdominal muscles overlying the injured area. This is the so-called guarding response.

Impulses giving rise to referred pain can also evoke reflex contraction of the muscles that would ordinarily be stimulated by injury to the skin.

Secondary muscle pain

If the reflex contraction of muscles is prolonged, the muscle tissue itself may become ischaemic. As a result, nociceptors within the muscle are excited, leading to further pain. Consequently muscle pain (myalgia) may be added to the original pain and discomfort increases.

Autonomic reflexes

Activation of pain receptors also excites several autonomic reflexes, producing effects that contribute to a general feeling of malaise and weakness. When you stub your toe on a piece of furniture or suffer from griping pain (colic) due to a stomach upset or painful periods you may well feel weak at the knees and light-headed. This is a result of sympathetic and parasympathetic reflex effects on the circulatory system altering the distribution of blood flow between tissues and lowering blood pressure.

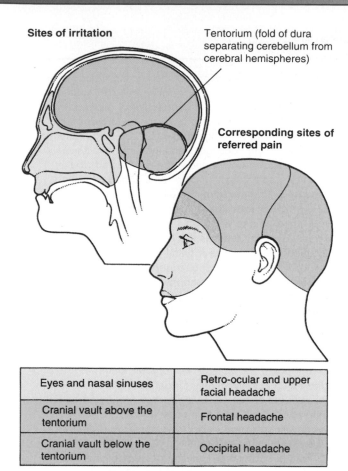

Sites of irritation

Tentorium (fold of dura separating cerebellum from cerebral hemispheres)

Corresponding sites of referred pain

Eyes and nasal sinuses	Retro-ocular and upper facial headache
Cranial vault above the tentorium	Frontal headache
Cranial vault below the tentorium	Occipital headache

Figure 29.6 Headaches: where they originate and where they are felt.

EMOTIONS

Our emotions are complex in that they consist of a blend of feelings, thoughts and behaviour. When we feel pain we also tend to react emotionally with anxiety, alarm or fear. Each of these states is associated with activation of the sympathetic nervous system.

These emotional reactions to injury can be dissociated from somatic reflex responses and the specific sensation of pain. Damage to the frontal lobes of the brain, or the now infrequently performed operation of frontal leucotomy or lobotomy (Fig. 29.7) can result in someone feeling less troubled by pain even though it is still sensed.

PAIN CONTROL

Pain can be controlled by interfering with the transmission of impulses in the nervous system, often with drugs but sometimes by other techniques such as TENS, or even surgery.

Pain as a perceived threat

The onset of pain is usually worrying or alarming. The way in which we interpret and experience pain is influenced not only by the extent of tissue damage but by our expectations of pain. These are based upon our culture, knowledge and past experiences, belief in our own ability (or that of others) to control the pain and the circumstances in which pain occurs. Uncertainty about what is causing the pain and what may happen as a consequence generates anxiety and fear, which intensify the pain. These emotions can be reduced or allayed by giving patients information about what is happening, explaining procedures, and helping patients to learn strategies for coping. This is particularly relevant where a painful process, such as childbirth or surgery, is anticipated or planned. However, many people with chronic pain experience fear and poor pain control because no one has taken the time to explain the likely causes or consequences of the pain nor the rationale for the treatments offered.

Lack of information is a significant cause of worry and even anger for some patients, and most benefit from information which enables them to feel more in control. On the other hand, some become more distressed when confronted with details and prefer not to know. Denial is a way of coping that should be respected but it should never be assumed that those who do not ask do not wish to know. Therefore it is important to assess each patient's needs on an individual basis.

Acute pain is commonly associated with anxiety and fear, while chronic pain may be associated with anxiety, depression, anger or acceptance. Terminally ill patients may experience a wide range of emotions. Some patients express their emotions while others conceal them; a quiet patient may be suffering just as much as one who complains.

Methods that block the transmission of impulses in general within the nervous system reduce our awareness of all sensations (anaesthesia), including pain, whereas those that act more selectively on pain pathways diminish pain sensation (analgesia) without having much effect on other sensations.

ANAESTHESIA

Drugs that produce anaesthesia do so either by blocking the transmission of action potentials along nerve axons (local anaesthetics) or by reducing

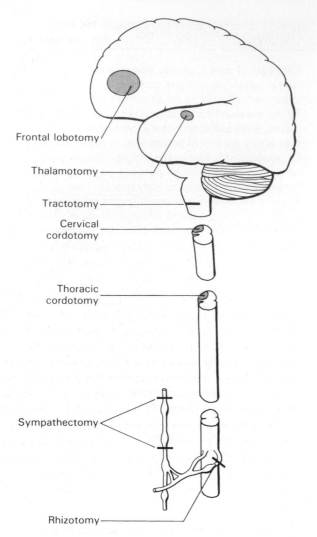

Frontal lobotomy

Thalamotomy

Tractotomy

Cervical cordotomy

Thoracic cordotomy

Sympathectomy

Rhizotomy

Figure 29.7 Sites of some of the surgical operations used in the relief of pain. (From Allen 1988, with permission of Elsevier.)

Pain clinics are available in most health districts to help patients with all types of intractable benign pain (including back pain). In addition to a range of medical and surgical treatment, some offer programmes designed to increase patients' knowledge of their condition, improve levels of exercise and activity, teach relaxation and reduce both dependence on drugs and reliance upon other people.

activity within the reticular activating system (general anaesthetics).

Local anaesthetics

Local anaesthetics, such as lidocaine (lignocaine), work by preventing the generation and conduction of nerve impulses. The primary site of action is the cell

Pain assessment

Assessment is a key aspect of the nursing management of pain. It enhances communication between patient, nurse and doctor. Regular assessment of acute or malignant pain provides a basis for the provision of optimum levels of analgesia (see Ch. 32). Pain intensity, together with the dosage, frequency and effectiveness of analgesia should be individually assessed and monitored to ensure that pain relief is adequate and sustained. Pain measures for all age groups are available, for example numerical scales (0 to 10), word scales (no pain to worst pain imaginable), descriptive scales (physical qualities like burning or aching, emotional qualities like frightful or punishing or evaluative qualities such as miserable or unbearable), colour intensity scales or happy/sad faces. It is necessary to select the method preferred by the particular patient group. Body charts may be used to locate the sources of pain. Assessment frequently reveals discrepancies between the assumptions of health professionals about the patient's pain and the patient's own reports. For patients with chronic pain, the use of a diary may help to identify triggering factors that could be avoided or pain relieving factors that could be better utilized. The patient's own observations provide valuable diagnostic information and help nurses and doctors to understand their feelings.

'Pain is what the patient says it is.' Affective words like 'cruel', 'fearful' or 'vicious' indicate that the patient cannot tolerate the pain. This may be due, in part, to a range of factors which need to be considered in an assessment of the 'whole person'. Unresolved past experiences, family problems, bereavement, employment difficulties, inability to meet commitments or lack of information may all influence someone's ability to tolerate physical pain. The nurse will not necessarily be able to resolve these issues but patients will benefit from knowing that they can, if they wish, share their feelings with someone who understands. The nurse and patient can then plan together a realistic and optimistic strategy for pain control in an atmosphere of mutual trust.

membrane, where they block conduction by decreasing, or preventing, the large transient increase in the permeability of excitable membranes to Na^+, normally produced by the depolarization of the membrane

When injected locally, all nerves in the area tend to be affected, including other sensory axons (e.g. for touch) as well as motor neurones. However, the smaller diameter fibres mediating pain are generally blocked more easily than the large diameter ones involved in touch and movement, due to the high surface area to volume ratio. Anaesthetic injected epidurally locally anaesthetizes the spinal cord and blocks transmission of impulses through that section of the cord.

The duration of action of a local anaesthetic is proportional to the time it is in contact with the nerve. This contact time can be maximized by putting a vasoconstrictor in the local anaesthetic preparation, which reduces local circulation thereby keeping the anaesthetic in the area for a longer period of time.

General anaesthetics

General anaesthetics, such as thiopental, and halothane, have a non-specific effect on all nerve membranes making them less excitable, but the part of the brain whose function is affected first is the reticular activating system (RAS). This system sensitizes much of the cerebral cortex to incoming sensory signals, so that when activity in the RAS is reduced, impulses arriving in the primary sensory areas of the cerebral cortex fail to excite other cortical areas. Consequently, during surgery under anaesthesia, no pain or other sensations are usually experienced even though the surgeon's knife is causing injuries that excite many receptors. Later on, as the effects of the anaesthetic wear off, the usual sensitivity of the cortical cells is restored, consciousness returns and pain is felt.

ANALGESIA

The major classes of analgesics are the opioid analgesics and the non-steroidal anti-inflammatory drugs (NSAIDs). The opioid analgesics (morphine and diamorphine) act on the endogenous system of pain control, whereas the NSAIDs (such as aspirin) reduce the production of the inflammatory mediators that sensitize the nociceptors to bradykinin and serotonin.

It may also be relevant to consider the local anaesthetics as analgesics since they are able to block the conduction of action potentials along the afferent neurones, thereby preventing the pain 'signal' from being processed from the site of damage.

Other miscellaneous drugs which can be used for analgesic purposes include sumatriptan (a $5HT_{1D}$ agonist used in migraine) and carbamazepine (an antiepileptic) which can be used to treat the pain associated with trigeminal neuralgia. The tricyclic antidepressants (including amitriptyline) can also be administered to assist patients in dealing with the long-term effects of chronic pain.

The opioid drugs bind to the receptors of the endogenous opioid transmitters. These drugs block pain information from being transmitted up the spinothalamic tract (anti-nociceptive action), as well as acting centrally to reduce the unpleasantness of the pain state (analgesic action). The main action of the opioid analgesics is mediated via the μ-receptor, causing not only analgesia and anti-nociception but also euphoria, respiratory depression (caused by a reduced sensitivity of the brain stem to PCO_2), miosis and pupillary constriction (caused by the stimulation of the parasympathetic component of cranial nerve III). The opioids can also cause emesis (via stimulation of the chemoreceptor trigger zone, sending signals to the vomiting centre) and constipation (due to increased tone and reduced motility of the gastrointestinal tract).

Problems associated with repeated use of the opioids include tolerance (the gradual reduction in effect) and dependence (both physical and psychological). However, research has suggested that the context in which an opiate is taken can influence whether the 'user' becomes addicted, i.e. if used for removal of severe pain then dependence may not develop.

REFERENCES AND FURTHER READING

Allen D 1988 (ed) Nursing and the neurosciences. Churchill Livingstone, Edinburgh

British Medical Bulletin 1991 Pain: mechanisms and management. British Medical Bulletin 47(3)

Cailliet R 1992 Head and face pain syndromes. F A Davies, Philadelphia

de Dombal F T 1991 Diagnosis of acute abdominal pain, 2nd edn. Churchill Livingstone, Edinburgh

Guyton A C 1986 Textbook of medical physiology. W B Saunders, Philadelphia

Latham J 1991 Pain control, 2nd edn. Austen Cornish Publishers, London

Melzack R, Wall P D 1965 Pain mechanisms: a new theory. Science; 150: 971–979

Melzack R, Wall P D 1991 The challenge of pain. Penguin, London

Rogers A W 1992 Textbook of anatomy. Churchill Livingstone, Edinburgh

Sofaer B 1992 Pain: a handbook for nurses. Chapman & Hall, London

Tiengo M, Paladini V A, Rawal N 1999 Regional anaesthesia, analgesia and pain management. Springer-Verlag Italia Srl, Milan

Wall P D, Melzack R 1989 Textbook of pain, 2nd edn. Churchill Livingstone, Edinburgh

Wood J N (ed) 2000 Molecular basis of pain induction. John Wiley, New York

SECTION 3
The life span

The chapters in this section are wide-ranging and consider the life span as reproduction, birth, maturation and death.

The topics include the physiological aspects of the male and female reproductive systems and the development of the new individual from fertilization of the egg to birth. The events during the course of pregnancy and the process of birth are examined in some detail.

The chapters then follow the individual through growth and development to maturity.

The final chapter considers the process of dying and the circumstances and events which surround death. This chapter has included current information on palliative care of the dying, for example, on programmes of analgaesia.

30 Sex, reproduction and pregnancy

The physiological processes involved in human beings' capacity to reproduce offspring never fail to inspire awe at what nature (and at times what scientists) can achieve. The male and female reproductive organs have the capacity to:

- produce the germinal cells (spermatozoa and ova) from which a new individual is created
- provide a means for the transport of both spermatozoa and ova inside the respective male or female body system and a means for spermatozoa and ova to meet through sexual union (coitus)
- create the right environment for the development of spermatozoa and ova, and later the fertilized cell as it grows into an embryo and then fetus
- a means by which the fetus is physiologically expelled from the body in labour and the childbirth event.

A sound knowledge of these physiological processes enables development of understanding of important aspects in health care:

- health education aspects for optimum reproductive and sexual health in both men and women

- malfunctions or diseases in male and female reproductive processes and therefore your involvement in prevention and treatment of these malfunctions/diseases
- planning for both pregnancy and contraception
- new technological advances in the treatment of infertility and related challenges for the infertile couple.

REPRODUCTIVE ORGANS AND TISSUES

MALE

Overview

The male reproductive system consists of those organs whose functions are to produce, transport and finally introduce mature sperm into the female reproductive tract, where fertilization can occur. The male reproductive organs and their situation in the adult are shown in Figure 30.1.

In both sexes the essential organs of reproduction which produce sex cells or gametes (sperm or ova) are called gonads. The gonads in the male are the testes. In addition, there are a number of genital ducts, glands and supporting structures whose function is to aid the transport of sperm from the gonads to the outside of the body. The ducts include:

- a pair of epididymides (singular: epididymis)
- a pair of vas deferens
- a pair of ejaculatory ducts
- the urethra.

Glands within the reproductive system provide exocrine secretions, which aid in the nourishment, transport or maturation of sperm. These glands are a pair of seminal vesicles, one prostate and a pair of bulbo-urethral glands. Supporting structures include the penis, the scrotum and spermatic cords.

Testes

The testes are suspended outside the abdomen in the scrotum, which is divided externally into two sacs, one for each testis. Both testes are suspended in the scrotal sac by attachment to the scrotal tissue and spermatic cords. During early fetal life the testes are situated in the abdomen but during the seventh month of intrauterine life, they descend through the inguinal canals into the scrotum. Because the higher temperature inside the abdominal cavity will inhibit sperm

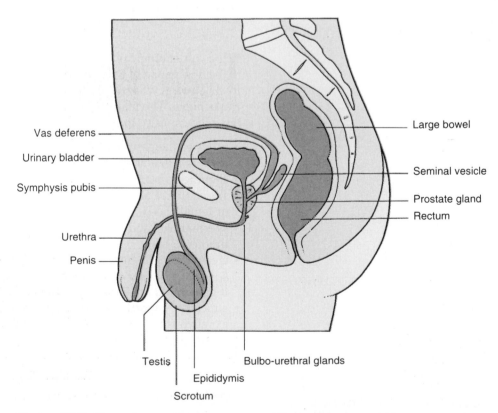

Figure 30.1 The male reproductive organs and their relation to neighbouring structures in the pelvis. (After Bancroft 1989, with permission of Elsevier.)

production, the descent of the testes into the scrotum is essential for normal sperm production to occur.

Each testis is encased in a dense white fibrous capsule called the tunica albuginea which envelops each testis and then enters each gland, dividing each gland into approximately 200 lobules (Fig. 30.2).

Each lobule of the testis comprises two functional components: a network of seminiferous tubules, tiny coiled tubules involved in the production and transport of sperm to the ejaculatory-excretory ducts, and a system of Leydig cells (also called interstitial cells) which occupy the small connective tissue spaces between the tubules, these being the cells which contain the enzymes for the secretion of androgens (mainly testosterone).

Each seminiferous tubule is bounded by a membrane and a layer of smooth muscle cells that effect peristaltic movements of the tubules. In the centre of each tubule is a fluid-filled lumen containing spermatozoa. The tubular wall is composed of differentiating germ cells and Sertoli cells (Fig. 30.3).

The Leydig cells lie in connective tissue between the tubules and are responsible for the synthesis of testosterone (from esterified cholesterol). The amount of testosterone stored within the Leydig cell is small due to newly synthesized testosterone diffusing rapidly into the plasma.

Sperm production (spermatogenesis)

Sperm production involves three integrated processes: mitosis, meiosis and spermiogenesis. Sperm are produced continuously throughout adult life from puberty onwards. Primitive germ cells (spermatogonia) in the wall of the seminiferous tubules begin to divide mitotically (see Ch. 1) at puberty, followed by meiotic cell division cycles producing spermatids (which contain half the number of chromosomes in each cell (see Ch. 1). The final phase of spermatogenesis is a differentiation of spermatids into millions of spermatozoa (spermiogenesis). The entire maturation process takes about 2 to 3 months. Sertoli cells are a key element to spermatogenesis because there are no blood vessels inside the seminiferous tubules. Sertoli cells control the chemical environment of the seminiferous tubules and provide nutrients and chemical stimuli that trigger the production and differentiation of the spermatozoa.

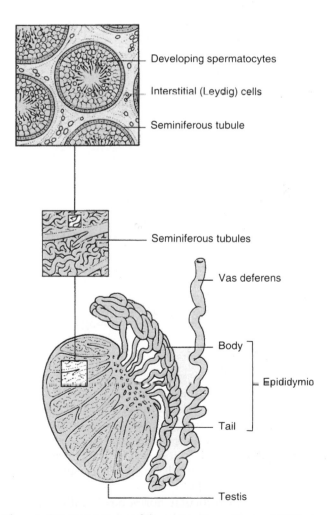

Figure 30.2 Structure of the testis. (From Rogers 1992, with permission of Elsevier.)

Labels: Developing spermatocytes; Interstitial (Leydig) cells; Seminiferous tubule; Seminiferous tubules; Vas deferens; Body; Epididymio; Tail; Testis

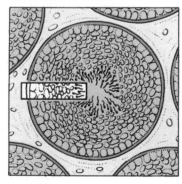

Seminiferous tubule

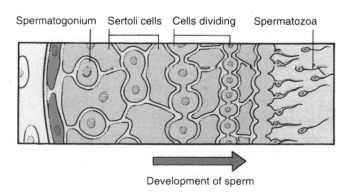

Spermatogonium   Sertoli cells   Cells dividing   Spermatozoa

Development of sperm

Figure 30.3 Development of sperm within a seminiferous tubule.

Structure of mature spermatozoa

Each spermatid matures into a single spermatozoon or sperm cell. The head of the sperm consists of a nucleus containing densely packed chromosomes. The tip of the nucleus is covered by the acrosomal cap, which contains enzymes essential for penetration of the ovum. A short neck attaches the head to the middle piece which mainly consists of mitochondria providing the energy for moving the tail. Most of the tail is a flagellum (group of contractile filaments), capable of propelling the sperm at a velocity of 4 mm/min. The sperm does not contain glycogen stores or other energy reserves and thus derives nutrients from the surrounding fluid environment.

Transport of sperm

The spermatozoa detach from the seminiferous tubules and move through a network of ducts termed the rete testis, followed by a single duct, the epididymis and from there into the vas deferens. The vas deferens and the part of the epididymis closest to it act as a reservoir for the spermatozoa, until they are ejaculated, leak out in the urine or die and are phagocytosed. Movement of the sperm to the epididymis is caused by some fluid current arising from the Sertoli cells in the seminiferous tubules and peristalsis of the tubules, smooth muscle in the epididymis and thence into the vas deferens. The next stage in sperm transport is ejaculation, normally preceded by erection, which enables the insertion of the penis into the vagina.

Hormonal control of male reproductive functions

The hormonal control of the testes functions through the hypothalamic–pituitary–testicular axis (see Fig. 30.4 and Ch. 11) and involves the secretion and inhibition of two hormones:

- follicle stimulating hormone (FSH)
- luteinizing hormone (LH).

Gonadotrophin-releasing hormone (also called luteinizing hormone-releasing hormone) is secreted by hypothalamic neurones in pulsatile bursts approximately every 2 hours. The GnRH acts on the anterior pituitary, triggering the secretion of both FSH and LH, amounts of which are dependent upon age and hormonal status. There is a clear division of the actions of FSH and LH within the testes:

- FSH targets the Sertoli cells (in the seminiferous tubules) to stimulate production of paracrine agents which influence spermatogenesis and other Sertoli cell functions.
- LH acts on the Leydig cells to stimulate the synthesis of testosterone, which acts locally (on Sertoli cells)

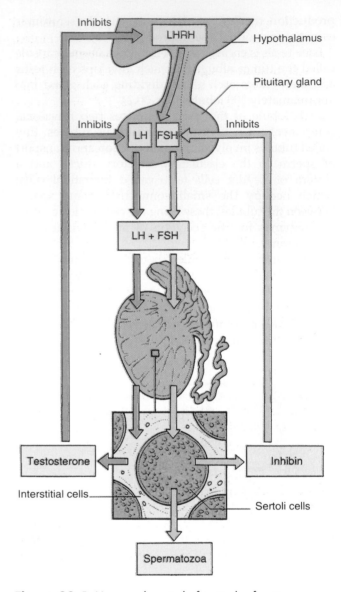

Figure 30.4 Hormonal control of testicular function.

and in addition has other systemic effects. Testosterone is essential for maintaining spermatogenesis.

Testosterone

Testosterone is mainly excreted via spermatic venous blood and testicular lymph drainage. An average of 5 to 10 mg of testosterone is excreted daily, with approximately 25 µg testosterone being present in the testes at any one point in time. Testosterone is transported in the plasma mainly bound to plasma proteins (sex hormone binding globulin (SHBG)).

The control of testicular hormones is influenced by negative feedback signals exerted by the testicular hormones. Rising levels of testosterone exert a negative feedback inhibition on both the hypothalamus and anterior pituitary to reduce LH secretion. A protein hormone, inhibin, secreted by the Sertoli cells produces a major inhibitory signal on the anterior pituitary in relation to rising levels of FSH, thereby reducing FSH secretion. The secretion rates of both FSH and LH can be altered to different degrees by these negative feedback signals.

Testosterone is a steroid hormone (see Ch. 11). It:

- promotes the functional maturation of spermatozoa
- maintains the accessory organs of the male reproductive tract
- influences the secondary sexual characteristics in the male: distribution of facial hair, increased muscle mass and body size, deposits of adipose tissue
- stimulates metabolic processes throughout the body, particularly protein synthesis and muscle and bone growth
- influences brain development and sexual behaviours and drive.

The penis

Penises vary in length, being between 5 and 10 cm long when flaccid, and extending to about 15 cm when erect. The penis consists mainly of blood vessels and supporting connective tissue, covered by skin (Fig. 30.5).

The arteries supplying the penis empty into three rods of tissue (corpora cavernosa and corpus spongiosum) that expand with blood in an erection. Each rod of tissue is surrounded by connective tissue supporting the engorged blood vessels. Running through the centre of the corpus spongiosum is the urethra. At its tip, the corpus spongiosum forms the glans penis which is encircled by a flap of skin (prepuce or foreskin).

The skin of the penis is hairless but contains many sensory nerve endings which are important in sexual arousal. The most sensitive areas are the glans penis and the frenulum on the underside of the penis. The double fold of skin, which forms the prepuce or foreskin, is usually mobile and can be easily retracted over the glans. Secretions (called smegma) can accumulate under the foreskin causing infection; therefore it is advocated that this area should be kept clean. Some consider that removal of the foreskin (circumcision) is preferable to leaving it in place.

Ducts and glands involved in the transport of spermatozoa

There are several different glands in the male reproductive tract (see Fig. 30.1), the chief of these being:

- seminal vesicles
- prostate gland
- bulbo-urethral glands (Cowper's glands).

The secretions from these glands mix with testicular secretions to form semen. The glands and related duct system are important in the onward journey of spermatozoa from the testis to the urethra at the point where ejaculation occurs.

The epididymis draining each testis connects to a vas deferens, a large thick-walled tube which extends toward the abdominal cavity. The vas deferens and blood vessels, nerves and lymphatics are bound together in a connective tissue sheath called the spermatic cord, which passes through the inguinal canal in the abdominal wall. After entering the abdomen, the vas deferens

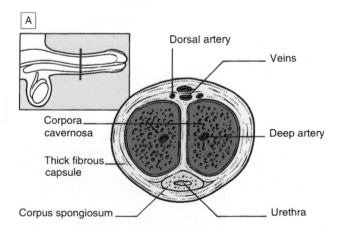

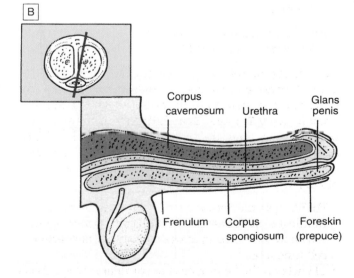

Figure 30.5 Structure of the penis. A, in cross-section. B, Sectioned along its length. (After Bancroft 1989, with permission of Elsevier.)

curves downwards to the back of the bladder base, towards the prostate gland.

Peristaltic contractions in the muscle wall of the vas deferens along with some fluid propel spermatozoa along the length of the duct. Here spermatozoa can be stored in an inactive state for some months. Two large glands, the seminal vesicles lying behind the urinary bladder, drain into the vas deferens. The junction of the vas deferens with the duct draining the seminal vesicles forms the ejaculatory duct that then enters the muscle wall of the prostate gland and joins with the ejaculatory duct leaving the other side of the prostate, before emptying into the urethra.

Semen

The volume of semen released at ejaculation (called an ejaculate) is 2 to 6 ml. Semen contains:

- Seminal fluid – glandular secretions with a characteristic ionic and nutrient composition (Fig. 30.6). The seminal fluid contains the combined secretions of the Sertoli cells and epididymis, seminal vesicles, the prostate, and the bulbo-urethral glands.
- Spermatozoa – semen contains about 300 million sperm cells (100 million/ml). If the sperm count is less than 20 to 40 million/ml the chances of conception are slim.

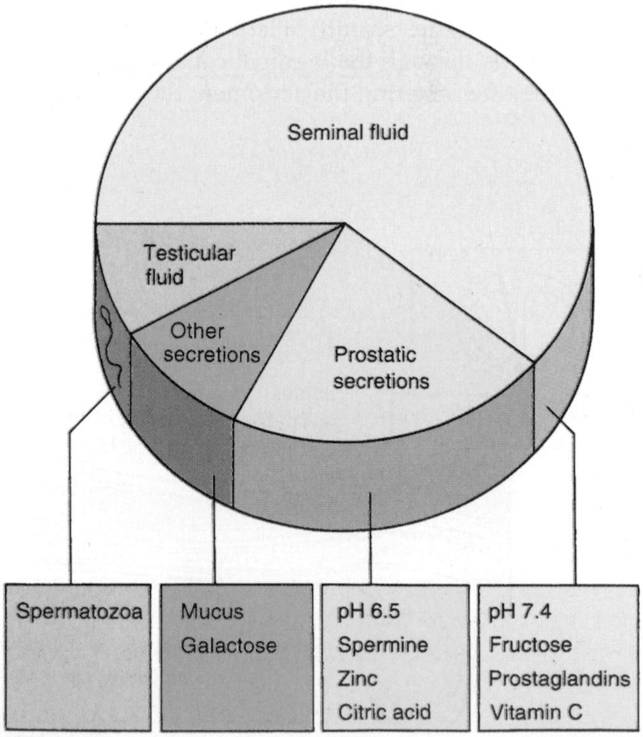

Figure 30.6 Composition of semen.

- Enzymes – some important enzymes are contained in seminal fluid whose functions vary between facilitating the dissolution of vaginal mucus to aiding sperm transport.

Male sexual and reproductive health

Previously, there has been a dominant trend in raising awareness of problems affecting the sexual and reproductive health of *women*, e.g. in infertility, cervical and ovarian carcinomas. Currently, an increase in the public's awareness of issues affecting the sexual and reproductive capacity of men has been noted. The focus on improving men's health aims to reduce fear and ignorance and acknowledge physical and psychosocial needs which are important to men in order to promote sexual and reproductive health with associated quality of life.

An example of this trend can be seen in testicular carcinoma, a condition which is highly treatable and curable but one where still too many young men succumb to this disease. Surgery and platinum-based chemotherapy remain the main treatment modes currently although ongoing research is beginning to focus on alternatives. Other examples of important androgynous issues are infertility, impotence and male contraceptives.

Infertility in men

In attempting to diagnose causes of infertility in men, two aspects figure in investigations:

1. *Can the semen be ejaculated?* Obstructions to seminal fluid flow are excluded such as congenital causes, acquired trauma, infection or carcinoma. The production of semen is also assessed.

2. *Are sufficient live, normal spermatozoa being produced?* Samples of semen will provide information on whether the constituents of semen fall within the normal range. There may be abnormalities of the testes congenital (e.g. cryptorchidism – undescended testes) or acquired (e.g. bilateral inflammation of the testes (orchitis), caused by viral infection (mumps) which can (rarely) cause sterility. Working in excessive heat or wearing tight clothing can affect sperm production. Medical conditions such as diabetes mellitus, coeliac disease and endocrine disorders may lead to defective spermatogenesis. Neurological problems such as dysfunction of the anterior pituitary gland or hypothalamus may prevent GnRH, FSH or LH, thus affecting testicular function and the maturation of healthy sperm. Lastly, occupational or environmental elements (e.g. chemicals and pollutants) may influence male reproductive capacities.

FEMALE

The structures of the female reproductive tract and their positions within the pelvic cavity are shown in Figures 30.7 and 30.8. The main structures are:

- ovaries
- uterus (womb)
- uterine tubes (fallopian tubes)
- vagina
- vulva (external genitalia).

The other part of a woman's body that is specifically adapted to support reproduction is breast tissue (mammary glands).

From puberty until the menopause (see Ch. 31), reproductive organs and associated tissues undergo cyclical monthly changes (menstrual cycle) resulting in the release of an egg (ovum) and the preparation of the woman's body for the implantation and growth of an embryo. Usually one ovum is released each month, wafted into a uterine tube and then propelled through it to the uterus. If sperm have been deposited in the vagina, some will swim up into the uterus and one may fertilize the ovum. If fertilization does not occur, the prepared richly vascularized lining of the uterus breaks down, and blood and cell debris (menstrual fluid) drains out of the uterus for a few days, leaking out of the body through the cervix and vagina. The whole cycle then begins again.

Ovaries

There are two ovaries. Each lies within the peritoneal cavity (Fig. 30.8) up against the wall of the pelvis, one on either side. The ovaries are supplied with blood by the ovarian arteries (branches of the abdominal aorta) and are anchored to the uterus by connective tissue (ovarian ligaments) and by a layer of peritoneum forming part of the broad ligament The ovaries house the ova and manufacture and secrete oestrogens.

The ova are formed during fetal life. At birth a female child possesses about 1 to 2 million ova. By the time she reaches reproductive years at adolescence, numbers have fallen to about half a million, and go on decreasing during adulthood until, by the age of about 50 years, there are none left (see Ch. 31).

Uterine tubes

Each uterine tube is about 12 cm long, extending from the uterus towards the ovary. The end next to the ovary is fringed with finger-like projections (fimbriae) wafting fluid from the peritoneal cavity into the tube. The wall of the tube consists of muscle and is lined internally by a ciliated secretory epithelium. Contractions of the muscle and beating of the cilia help to propel the fluid in the tube towards the uterus.

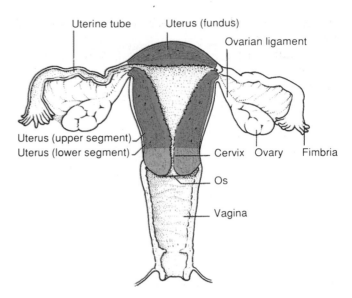

Figure 30.7 Female reproductive organs. (From Rogers 1992, with permission of Elsevier.)

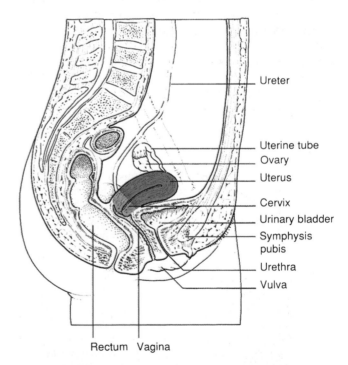

Figure 30.8 Position of the reproductive organs in the female pelvis. (From Rogers 1992, with permission of Elsevier.)

Uterus

The uterus is a small hollow pear-shaped organ lying just behind the urinary bladder (Fig. 30.8). The bulbous part is the body and the narrower part is the cervix, part of which protrudes into the vagina (Fig. 30.7). The uterus is normally in an anteverted position, meaning that it is at an angle in the pelvis, leaning forward with the cervix pointing backwards.

Body

The body of the uterus consists largely of muscle (myometrium) lined internally by a glandular layer (endometrium). Part of this layer is shed at menstruation. New cells grow from the remaining tissue to replace those that are lost.

Cervix

The cervix consists mostly of connective tissue and has few muscle cells. It too is lined by a secretory epithelium which includes many glands (cervical glands). However, unlike the endometrial layer, this secretory epithelium is not shed during menstruation although its secretory activity changes during the menstrual cycle.

Vagina

The vagina is an expandable muscular tube consisting mostly of longitudinally arranged bundles of smooth muscle cells. The vagina is lined internally by tissue that has a rich blood supply but relatively few sensory nerve endings, and no mucous glands. Some of the epithelial cells synthesize and store large amounts of glycogen. When these cells die, bacteria in the vagina (*Lactobacillus acidophilus*) digest the glycogen, producing lactic acid.

Cervical smear test (Papanicolaou or PAP smear test)

Early malignant disease of the cervix can be detected by examination of cells obtained directly from the cervix. Globally, cervical cancer is a major health problem, with a yearly incidence of 371 000 cases and annual death rate of 190 000. Research has evidenced likely causes to be linked to sexually transmitted organisms such as the human papilloma virus and others, e.g. *Trichomonas vaginalis* and *Chlamydia trachomatis* (Wright et al 2002). The cervical smear test is available for all women and is generally a painless procedure. It should be repeated at regular intervals depending on age, health and the results of previous tests. The cells are obtained by gentle scraping of the cervix using a specially shaped cervical spatula. Microscopic examination will indicate if any suspected malignant cells are present. Management may consist of:

- punch biopsies which, if positive, are followed by laser ablation
- a diathermy loop excision biopsy following a positive smear test
- radiotherapy combined with cisplatin-based chemotherapy may be used with hysterectomy if malignancy is extensive.

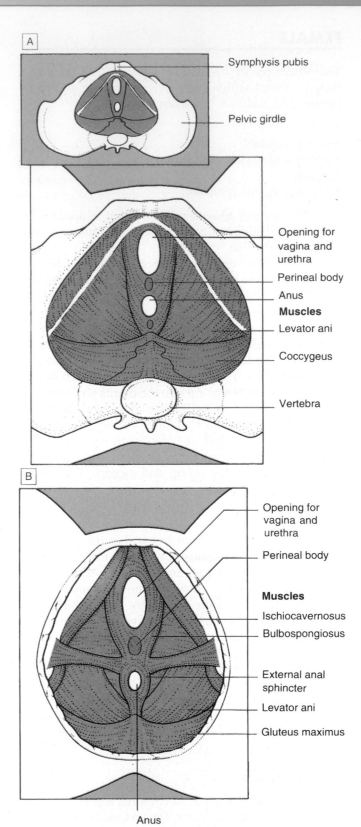

Figure 30.9 Muscles of the pelvic floor and perineum in women. A, Pelvic floor viewed from above. B, Muscles of the perineum viewed from below. (Part A after Chamberlain & Dewhurst 1986, with permission of Elsevier; part B after Williams et al 1989, with permission of Elsevier.)

> Douching of the vagina reduces the numbers of lactobacilli present and consequently raises the vaginal pH. Contrary to popular expectation therefore, douching may promote infection rather than prevent it.

The lactic acid makes the pH of the fluid in the vagina acidic (about pH 4) and this discourages the growth of other bacteria that are not acid loving. This environment and the many lymphocytes and neutrophils (see Ch. 16) present in the vaginal epithelium provide defence against infection.

The vagina and the urethra pass through the layer of muscles that form the pelvic floor (levator ani) and then through another layer of tissues (perineum) which consists of connective tissue and more striated muscle.

> An intact hymen was considered to be a sign of virginity, and its tearing, with associated bleeding, at intercourse was believed to be confirmation of virginity. The now common use of tampons results in the hymen being stretched, so that it is no longer torn during the first sexual intercourse. Gentle stretching, with the fingers, of a tight hymen is recommended if this is the cause of painful intercourse (dyspareunia). Rarely, the hymen completely closes the vagina. This condition (imperforate hymen) is usually discovered when menstruation begins. The hymen is then opened surgically.

When they contract, the pelvic and perineal muscles act like a sphincter around the opening of the vagina (Fig. 30.9A & B).

In the perineum to either side of the vaginal opening are two small masses of erectile tissue (bulb of the vestibule) similar in origin and tissue structure to the corpus spongiosum of the penis. The external opening of the vagina may be partially covered by a thin flap of connective tissue (hymen).

Vulva

The external genitalia (vulva) (Fig. 30.10) consist of several folds of tissue (labia majora and minora) surrounding the vaginal and urethral openings together with more erectile tissue equivalent to that of the penis in the male (see Fig. 30.5). The corpora cavernosa and corpus spongiosum together form the clitoris, the glans of which (just above the urethral opening) is the most sensitive part erotically. The vulva has both sebaceous and sweat glands and a number of mucus-secreting glands around the urethral and vaginal openings. It is also well supplied with sensory nerve endings.

Breasts

The breasts consist of glandular tissue. Each mammary gland consists of about 20 separate tubulo-alveolar glands each of which possesses a separate duct opening out at the nipple (Fig. 30.11). In the female the glandular tissue undergoes further development at puberty (see p. 536), whereas in the male it normally remains immature.

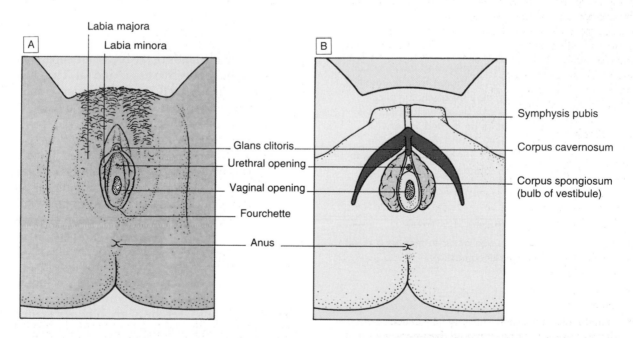

Figure 30.10 Female external genitalia (vulva). A, External features. B, Internal features (compare these with Fig. 30.5, which shows equivalent tissue in the male). (After Bancroft 1989, with permission of Elsevier.)

Genital infections

When sexually transmitted diseases are mentioned, most people think of diseases given frequent media coverage, such as AIDS, gonorrhoea, syphilis and herpes, but there are other infections of the genital tract, such as candidiasis and trichomoniasis, that can be transmitted by sexual intercourse.

Candidiasis (thrush)

Candida albicans is a widespread yeast-like organism which is normally present in nose, mouth, bowel and on the skin. If conditions in the vagina predispose to the organism becoming pathogenic (disease producing), for example loss of normal vaginal bacteria during antibiotic therapy, reduced resistance to infection, increased humidity (wearing tights with closed gusset or tight jeans), then uncomfortable symptoms arise. There is usually pruritus (itching), watery or thick and cottage-cheese-like discharge and discomfort when passing urine (dysuria). When the condition occurs in the male, there are small curd-like plaques or red spots on the glans penis and sometimes dysuria. Both men and women may be asymptomatic but still pass on the organism to partners.

Vaginal thrush is fairly common during pregnancy because the urine often contains some sugar which encourages the growth of *Candida albicans* in the vulval area.

Trichomoniasis (trike)

Trichomonas vaginalis is a protozoon (unicellular animal) possessing flagella. It is capable of surviving for short periods outside the body in most conditions and therefore can be transmitted on shared towels, after swimming for example. Infection results in an unpleasant discharge that is often profuse and fishy smelling, and may be yellow/green, frothy and watery. It is usually accompanied by pruritus and inflammation. In the male there is a similar discharge from the urethra, and dysuria. The condition may be asymptomatic.

Because these infections can be asymptomatic, it is important for both partners to be treated; otherwise there is always the possibility of one reinfecting the other. The regular and correct use of condoms helps to prevent the spread of such infections.

Enlargement of the breasts can occur in men as a result of endocrine disorder (gynaecomastia).

In a radical mastectomy the axillary lymph nodes are removed in an attempt to eradicate cancerous cells that may have spread to the nodes from the primary tumour in the breast.

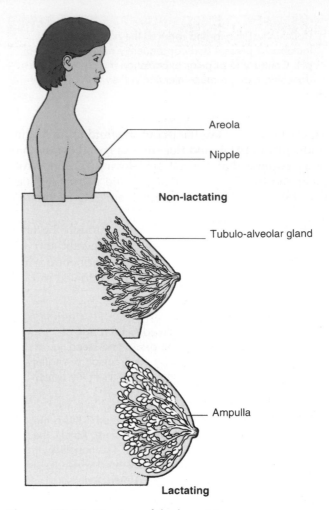

Figure 30.11 Structure of the breast in women.

The individual glands of the breast are separated from one another by connective tissue and fat. The glands are supported by ligaments (Cooper's ligaments) anchoring them to the skin and to the underlying covering (fascia) of the muscles of the chest wall.

There is an enlargement of each duct (ampulla or sinus) just before it passes through the nipple. These sinuses are surrounded by smooth muscle fibres. The ducts too have contractile cells (myoepithelial cells) in their walls which contract reflexly in response to suckling (see p. 509) expelling the milk contained within them.

The skin around the nipple is the areola. It darkens during pregnancy due to the production of extra melanin. The areola has many glands, including tiny mammary-type glands (Montgomery's tubercles) and sebaceous glands secreting an oily substance that creams and protects the nipple during suckling.

About 75% of the lymph draining from the tissues of the breast drains through the lymph nodes of the armpit.

SEXUAL ACTIVITY

Human sexual experience is complex. It involves minds and emotions as well as genitalia. In a sexual response there are:

- changes in the reproductive organs
- experiences of pleasurable erotic sensations
- an altered state of arousal.

At its most basic level, stimulation of sensory receptors in the genital region evokes spinal reflexes which cause changes in male and female genitalia, including vasocongestion and increased secretion. The vasocongestion of erectile tissue firms up the genitalia in both sexes, enlarging the penis in the male and the coital canal in the female ready for sexual union. The experience of pleasurable sensations together with associated attractive stimuli provides the motivation for the sexual behaviour which brings two people together. The sensations evoked by sexual intercourse have a positive feedback effect in this system leading ultimately to a climax (orgasm) in which there is a sudden increase in the intensity of erotic sensations coupled with muscular contractions and, in men, the ejaculation of sperm. This intense but pleasurable experience is rapidly followed by a period of profound relaxation.

> When a woman fails to conceive and the couple seek advice, the initial counselling must establish that sexual intercourse is taking place. Occasionally marriages are not consummated and, even with increased emphasis on sex education, some couples remain ignorant of what sexual intercourse entails.

SEXUAL AROUSAL

Sexual arousal may be provoked by stimulation of receptors locally in the genitalia, as well as by psychic factors, some conditioned by experience. These stimuli evoke many changes in the genitalia and increase the general state of arousal.

Local stimuli and reflex effects

The skin covering the glans penis and the glans clitoris is richly supplied with sensory receptors. There are also other receptors close by especially at the back of the penis and in the vulva. Stimulation of these receptors evokes spinal reflexes (sacral spinal cord) causing several effects including:

- vasocongestion in reproductive organs
- fluid secretion
- muscle contraction.

Vasocongestion

Vasocongestion occurs in the penis and in the equivalent vessels of the clitoris caused by dilation of blood vessels. The penis and the clitoris become engorged with blood and therefore expand. The increasing tissue pressure increases stimulation of the cutaneous receptors, thus increasing the intensity of sensation and the reflex responses. Vasodilation is due to increased efferent activity in the parasympathetic nerves.

In men, the swelling compresses the penal veins, thus reducing the outflow of blood from the penis. As a result pressure increases within the organ and it lengthens and becomes hard. At full erection the pressure of blood within the penis is only just below systolic arterial blood pressure (see Ch. 6). The throbbing sensed is due to arterial pulsations. Additional stiffening is due to reflex contraction of the ischiocavernosus and bulbospongiosus muscles (striated muscles at the base of the penis; Fig. 30.12).

In women, expansion of the vulva creates a firmer cuff of tissue at the opening to the vagina and lengthens the coital canal. Vasocongestion also occurs in the uterus. Contraction of smooth muscle in the tissues supporting the uterus and the vagina causes the upper part of the vagina to elongate and enlarge.

Fluid secretion

In women, as sexual arousal proceeds, fluid is secreted by the walls of the vagina, and there is secretion of

> Erections also occur in men and boys in the absence of sexual stimulation, for example during sleep and on waking, and in arousing but non-sexual situations.

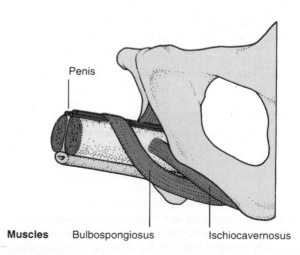

Figure 30.12 Muscles of the penis. (After Bancroft 1989, with permission of Elsevier.)

mucus by the vestibular glands (Bartholin's) at the vaginal opening. Both fluids help to lubricate the movement of the penis within the vagina. The vaginal fluid may also provide a more favourable environment for the survival of ejaculated sperm.

In men too, there is increased glandular secretion during sexual arousal. The amount varies between men but can be great enough to drip from the penis.

Muscle contraction

In men contraction of muscles in the genitalia also causes elevation of the testes and contraction of the scrotum. In women there may be erection of the nipples.

Psychic factors

The spinal reflexes producing these various genital effects are influenced by impulses from the brain such that the sight of a person or an object, or internal imagery in fantasy, also excites or inhibits sexual responses. These responses are mediated by the limbic system which plays a central part in determining mood and emotion (see Ch. 27). Specific areas of the hypothalamus (medial, preoptic/anterior) may be involved. The effectiveness of stimuli in evoking responses depends also on the pre-existing general level of arousal.

General arousal

The effects of sexual arousal on the rest of the body are similar to those produced by other forms of excitement and activity, and reflect a general increase in activity within the sympathetic nervous system. Thus there are increases in:

Impotence

Primary impotence is rare – that is for a man never to have attained and maintained an erection for sufficient time to perform normal sexual intercourse. Secondary impotence may have organic causes or may result from taking certain medications or alcohol. Psychological factors are important too; stress, tiredness, guilt and depression are all possible causes. A man may worry so much about his failure that he is liable to fail again – and again. Adverse comments from his partner about his performance may bring about impotence or prolong it if it has already occurred. There may be something about his current partner that acts as a 'turn-off' (this does not imply lack of love) and, should he be able to perform satisfactorily with someone else, the original problem can be exacerbated by guilt.

Frigidity

Sexual desire varies considerably from person to person. Some women are not particularly interested in sexual activity. If such a woman's partner makes more demands on her than she feels able to enjoy then she will probably label him 'oversexed' and he will label her 'frigid'!

Frigidity suggests unbending coldness and has been used to cover many aspects of female psychosexual problems. Sexual activity is not absolutely essential to a happy and loving relationship. Like any other activity it is fine if it is enjoyed, but it should not become so important that emotional distress results for either or both partners. There may, however, be physical causes for lack of enjoyment of the sexual act, such as pain due to infection or following suturing of the perineum.

Other causes of frigidity may be fear of pregnancy or of contracting a disease, a recent stressful life event or tiredness. Some women with a new baby find that the mother/baby relationship is totally satisfying. For others, there may be something about their partner's behaviour or demands which act as a 'turn-off', for example boredom with the same ritual foreplay. Deep feelings about sex are sometimes instilled during childhood (e.g. sex is dirty), which prevents enjoyment later in life. Some women never experience an orgasm, approximately 10% of women are physically incapable of orgasm (Edwards & Bouchler 1991). Concern about this may cause physical or mental ill-health, the woman thinking that she is frigid. It does not matter what labels are used, if emotional distress is present in either partner then counselling is required.

- blood pressure
- heart rate
- rate of breathing.

The pupils dilate, and there are changes in blood flow and secretory activity in the skin.

ORGASM

This intensely pleasurable experience is one of the least well understood aspects of sexual physiology. It is characterized in both sexes by a peaking of sexual tension followed by a rapid release. In men, this climax is marked by emission and ejaculation of semen, whereas in women there are rhythmic contractions of muscles in and around the vagina.

Somatic sensation and responses

Orgasm is characterized by an explosion of sensory feeling that may simply be localized to the perineal region or may spread out from there to other parts or even the whole of the body. The experience differs from person to person, the only common features seeming to be the mounting intensity, and peaking of feeling which suddenly dies away. In some instances, the extreme change in feeling suggests an altered level of consciousness, bordering even on loss of consciousness.

The sensations of orgasm are accompanied by involuntary contractions of many muscles of the body which can include those of the limbs, abdomen, neck and face. In extreme instances these contractions may resemble convulsions. Very quickly, this brief period of muscular spasms is followed by profound muscular relaxation coupled with a sense of calm.

Genital organs

Propulsion of semen from the male reproductive tract occurs in two stages:

- emission
- ejaculation.

Emission

In emission, contraction of the smooth muscle in the vas deferens, seminal vesicles and prostate gland causes the secretions there to be expelled into the urethra. Muscle contraction is evoked by a sympathetic reflex mediated via nerves leading to (pudendal) and from (hypogastric) the upper lumbar parts of the spinal cord.

Ejaculation

The semen within the urethra is then expelled from it by contractions of the striated muscle at the base of the penis (bulbospongiosus and bulbocavernosus muscles). Simultaneously there is contraction of the internal sphincter of the bladder coupled with relaxation of the external sphincter. The whole process involves several different reflexes coordinated in the sacral part of the spinal cord.

If all goes to plan, the events of emission and ejaculation occur at the climax of sexual excitement. In men, especially those who are older, it can take a little while for the whole system to recover. Consequently another erection cannot be produced immediately after orgasm.

Female responses

In women the climax of sexual excitement is usually marked genitally by repeated contraction of the ring of muscles at the opening of the vagina and the muscle of the vaginal walls. Contraction of the muscle in the uterus is believed to occur too. In contrast to men, once orgasm has occurred re-excitement can be achieved in women quite quickly.

Cardiovascular and respiratory effects

Just before orgasm there is a sharp increase in respiratory rate, and often in women and in some men a flushing of the skin overlying the trunk. At orgasm, heart rate and blood pressure both increase sharply and then fall. Heart rate increases by between 20 and 80 beats per minute, the size of the increase depending on the level of anxiety, as well as the sexual response and physical activity. The same applies to blood pressure. Increases range from 25 to 120 mmHg for systolic pressure and 25 to 50 mmHg for diastolic pressure. In non-stressful situations the demands placed on the cardiovascular system by sexual activity have been estimated to be similar to modest physical exercise.

SPERM TRANSPORT AND VIABILITY

Sperm deposited in a woman's vagina move through the genital tract quite rapidly and reach the uterine tubes within an hour. The spermatozoa have to negotiate the mucus of the cervix before swimming through the fluids in the uterus. At the time of ovulation, when the mucus is thin (see p. 496), penetration by sperm is easier than at other times.

Sperm survive for up to 2 days in a woman's reproductive tract. During this time they change (capacitation) in ways that enable them to adhere better to an ovum. Of the millions of sperm deposited in the vagina less than 100 actually reach the ovum. Of these, normally only one will penetrate the membrane to fertilize the egg.

Sperm cells are foreign to a woman's body and therefore should be recognized and attacked by her immune system just like any other foreign body. However, they are protected by substances secreted in semen that inhibit local immune responses.

PREGNANCY

During her reproductive years a woman's body goes through a series of changes each month preparing her to conceive and bear a child. If conception does not occur, preparations are abandoned, the materials produced are scrapped and a fresh cycle begins. This regular sequence of changes is termed the menstrual

The immunosuppressive effect of substances in semen is believed to contribute to the increased incidence of cervical cancer in sexually active women. Cancerous cells are not destroyed as readily because immune mechanisms locally are suppressed.

Contraception

Contraception or family planning is the means by which conception may be prevented. The only 100% effective contraceptive is abstention from sexual intercourse (even sterilization has a failure rate). Failure rates for other methods are calculated per 100 women years of use (HWY) – this is the number of women who would become pregnant if 100 women used the same method for 1 year. There are five groups of contraceptive methods.

Natural methods

- Coitus interruptus involves withdrawing the penis before ejaculation takes place. The failure rate is high (17 per HWY) because semen leakage often occurs before ejaculation.
- Abstaining from sex during the time of ovulation is a method that involves establishing, by various means, when ovulation is taking place. Changes in early morning body temperature (see p. 497) and the consistency of cervical mucus are two indicators of ovulation. The failure rate for these methods varies from 1 to 11 per HWY.
- Breast feeding in developing countries provides effective contraception because ovulation does not occur while the baby is sucking regularly (see p. 509). If supplementary bottle feeds are given instead of suckling the baby, or the night feed is missed, ovulation is likely to recommence.
- Vaginal douching is used by some women, but as the very motile sperm can reach the internal cervical os within 90 seconds the method is ineffective. There is also the added risk of increasing susceptibility to vaginal infection (see p. 489).

Barrier methods

These methods provide a physical barrier between the semen and the cervix. Spermicides give additional protection. For men, there is the sheath or condom, and for women, the diaphragm. The failure rate for both is 2 to 15 per HWY.

Vaginal sponges are gaining popularity for older women or those who are breast feeding, and at other times when fertility may be reduced. There has been controversy about the failure rate – it may be as high as 25 per HWY.

Intrauterine contraceptive devices (IUCDs)

These devices (there are several types) are inserted into the uterine cavity by a doctor using a special applicator. The IUCD is thought to act in three ways:

- the endometrium is rendered less suitable for implantation
- prostaglandin production may be increased, causing expulsion of the fertilized ovum
- uterine tubal motility may be increased, again causing expulsion of the ovum.

The failure rate is 0.3 to 4 per HWY.

Hormonal methods

These are known collectively as 'the pill'. The combined pill contains oestrogen and a synthetic form of progesterone – progestogen; there is also a progestogen-only pill. They act by suppressing the production of FSH and LH. Consequently, the ovarian follicles do not mature and ovulation does not take place (see p. 496). The failure rate for the combined pill is 0.1 to 1 per HWY, and for the progestogen-only pill, 0.3 to 5 per HWY.

Sterilization

In women, the uterine tubes are divided and clipped to obstruct the passage of the ovum to the uterus. The effect is immediate and reversal is possible. There is an increased risk of ectopic pregnancy following reversal (see p. 499). The failure rate for clips is 2 per 1000 cases.

In men, each vas deferens is divided (vasectomy) and sutured. The effect is not immediate because sperm remain viable in the vas deferens distal to the occlusion for up to 4 months. Other contraceptive methods should be used until two consecutive sperm counts have been negative. Reversal is possible but fertility does not always return. The failure rate is 0 to 0.2 per HWY. Further information about contraceptive methods can be found in Bennett & Brown (1999).

Pharmacological male contraception

New male contraceptive options are being currently explored. An effective male hormonal contraceptive that could be implanted or injected as a long-acting formulation every 3–6 months would be beneficial, particularly in countries where limiting population growth is a priority. Exogenous gonadotrophin-releasing hormone analogues and sex steroid hormones such as testosterone and progestins suppress gonadotrophins and spermiogenesis. Current research focuses upon refining the dosage and the efficacy of these new contraceptives whilst minimizing side effects.

cycle because of the discharge of fluid (menses) occurring via the vagina at regular intervals.

If, however, the ovum is fertilized, many tissues swing into action driven by hormonal signals gearing the woman's body, as well as her womb, to house, nourish and protect the developing new individual. A key structure which forms from the conceptus not the mother, is the placenta, the lifeline between her and her offspring. Through this organ the fetus gains all it needs and disposes of its waste. Extensive changes occur in almost all systems in a woman's body in pregnancy. Some developments such as lactation support the baby after its birth but all are designed to nourish and protect the new life.

PRELUDE: THE MENSTRUAL CYCLE

All the ova that a woman will ever have were produced right at the beginning of her life when she herself was a fetus. They are stored in her ovaries until, at puberty, hormones released by the anterior pituitary (FSH and LH), begin the cycle of changes resulting in the final maturation of a single ovum each month and its release from the ovary (ovulation). Simultaneously other organs of the reproductive tract undergo cyclical changes in activity, preparing the tract for the implantation of a fertilized ovum and the nurturing of the developing embryo.

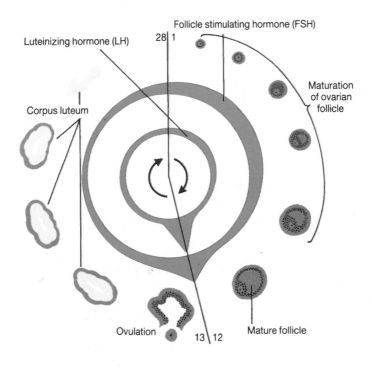

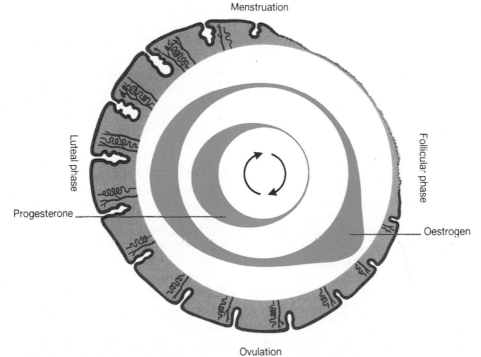

Figure 30.13 The menstrual cycle: hormonal, ovarian and uterine changes. (From Rogers 1992, with permission of Elsevier.)

The events of the cycle may be divided into four stages (Fig. 30.13):

1. menstrual
2. follicular
3. ovulatory
4. luteal.

Menstruation

The beginning of the menstrual cycle is by convention timed from the first day of menstruation. At this time the rich vascular lining of the uterus breaks down and bleeding occurs for about 3 to 5 days. Simultaneously the secretion of FSH and LH from the anterior pituitary begins to increase. These hormones promote the maturation of several ovarian follicles each of which contains a single ovum.

Follicular phase

On about the sixth day of the cycle one follicle overtakes the others in its development and continues to grow while the others regress. As the follicle enlarges it produces increasing quantities of oestrogens. Oestrogens have widespread effects upon a woman's body. In the reproductive organs important changes occur in:

• the endometrium
• the cervical mucus
• the vaginal epithelium.

The endometrium grows thicker and the glands grow. The cervical mucus becomes thinner and more alkaline. These changes favour the survival of sperm and their movement through the female reproductive tract. The vaginal epithelium becomes cornified.

Toxic shock syndrome

Toxic shock syndrome (TSS) may occur in both males and females as a result of the toxins released by some strains of *Staphylococcus aureus*, a microorganism commonly present in skin and lung infections. However, the syndrome is more commonly associated with menstruating females who use tampons. This is because some high-absorbency tampons provide a substrate on which the bacteria multiply and produce large amounts of toxin.

TSS can become a life-threatening illness. It usually presents with very high fever (40.6°C) and associated symptoms: erythematous rash, vomiting, diarrhoea and abdominal pain. Deterioration results in circulatory shock and renal failure. It is advisable to change tampons regularly, and some authorities suggest that an ordinary sanitary towel should be used at night.

Ovulatory phase

Oestrogens also promote the growth of the follicle from which they have come (positive feedback). Simultaneously, together with inhibin (also produced by the developing follicle), they depress the secretion of FSH from the anterior pituitary. Nearing mid-cycle, when the output of oestrogen increases greatly, the oestrogens provoke a surge in the secretion of LH from the anterior pituitary which results in bursting of the follicle and the release of its contents, including the ovum, into the peritoneal cavity (ovulation).

Luteal phase

In the luteal phase the cells of the ruptured follicle begin to proliferate, resulting in the formation of a yellowish looking body (corpus luteum – literally 'body yellow'). The cells of the corpus luteum produce the steroid hormone progesterone as well as oestrogens. Together, these hormones produce further changes in the uterus, cervix and vagina all of which prepare the woman's body for the possibility of pregnancy.

The blood vessels and glands of the endometrial lining develop further and the cells begin to secrete a fluid containing sugars, amino acids and mucus. The cervical mucus now becomes thick and contains many cells. The vaginal epithelium proliferates.

Oestrogens and progesterone inhibit the secretion of FSH and LH from the anterior pituitary. About 1 week after ovulation, if fertilization has not occurred, the corpus luteum begins to regress, and the secretion of oestrogens and progesterone declines. Withdrawal of hormonal support affects the endometrial lining, resulting in breakdown of some tissue. Release of prostaglandins from the necrotic tissue accelerates the process and promotes the flow of menstrual blood.

As the concentration of oestrogen and progesterone in the blood decreases, the secretion of FSH and LH from the anterior pituitary increases again and a new cycle begins.

Associated changes

The cyclical change in hormone levels also brings about other changes including alterations in:

• breast tissue
• body temperature
• mood.

Breast tissue

During the proliferative phase of the cycle, the rising oestrogen concentration causes proliferation of the ducts of the mammary glands. When progesterone is added in the secretory phase there is growth of the lobules and alveoli. Blood flow to the mammary glands increases coupled with increased tissue fluid formation.

Table 30.1 Features of the premenstrual syndrome*

Symptoms and signs

Feeling bloated
Increased abdominal girth
Breast tenderness
Mood changes (e.g. irritability, depression, aggression)

* Compiled from Elder 1988.

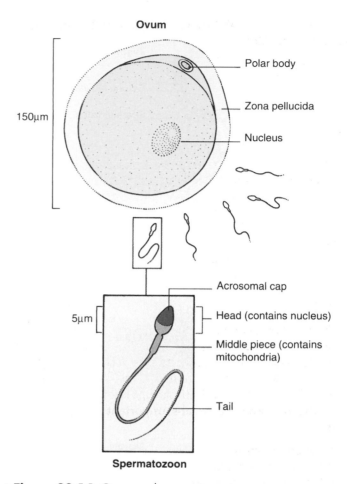

Figure 30.14 Ovum and spermatozoon.

All these changes cause some enlargement of the breasts, which can make them feel tender, and begin to prepare the breasts for lactation.

Body temperature

The change in progesterone levels during the menstrual cycle alters the sensitivity of the temperature regulating systems such that core body temperature rises by about 0.5°C in the secretory phase of the cycle. If ovulation does not occur, the secretion of progesterone does not increase and body temperature does not rise.

Mood

Many women experience changes in mood during the cycle, particularly in the days just prior to menstruation (premenstrual syndrome; Table 30.1). At this time the levels of oestrogens and progesterone are changing quite sharply. In some women the symptoms are associated with a relative lack of progesterone.

CONCEPTION

If the ovum is fertilized by a spermatozoon (Fig. 30.14), the fertilized egg (zygote) divides to form a growing mass of cells (Fig. 30.15) some of which will form the new embryo, and some the placenta. Cells within this mass begin to secrete the hormone HCG (human chorionic gonadotrophin) which maintains the corpus luteum so that it continues to secrete oestrogens and progesterone. As a result, the various changes in the reproductive organs are maintained and breakdown of the uterine lining does not occur. Instead the blastocyst burrows into the endometrium of the uterus and becomes fixed there (implantation) and both embryo and placenta develop from it.

The first days of development

The ovum released from the ovary is transported along the uterine tubes. It is here that fertilization of the ovum by the spermatozoon normally occurs. Some of the sperm reaching the uterine tube adhere to the layer of glycoproteins enveloping the ovum (zona pellucida) to which some nutrient cells (corona radiata) are also attached. The binding of sperm to the glycoproteins triggers a reaction leading to the breakdown of the acrosomal cap in the spermatozoon (Fig. 30.14) and the release of proteolytic enzymes contained within it. These enzymes digest the glycoproteins in the zona pellucida and enable the spermatozoon to penetrate to the cell membrane of the ovum itself.

The fertilized egg (zygote) now begins the process of cell proliferation and differentiation that continues throughout pregnancy as the new individual grows and develops. The zygote divides mitotically to form a clump of cells (morula). The morula develops into a blastocyst as fluid accumulates in the centre of the clump (Fig. 30.15). As cell division and differentiation proceed, an outer layer of cells (trophoblast) can be distinguished from a group of cells that bulge into the fluid-filled cavity (inner cell mass). Cells of the trophoblast are destined to become the placenta, whereas the inner clump of cells becomes the embryo. This stage of development is reached about 4 to 5 days after

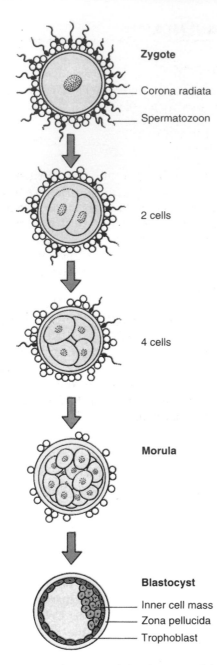

Figure 30.15 Early stages of development of the fertilized ovum (zygote).

fertilization the developing embryo is completely enclosed by endometrial tissue and the cells that will develop into the placenta are in place. At this stage the embryo is nourished by the transfer of materials across the cells of the trophoblast, by diffusion and pinocytosis.

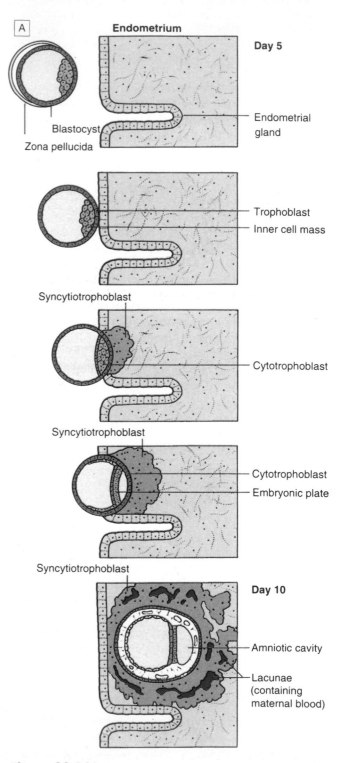

Figure 30.16A

ovulation. By this time the mass of cells has usually reached the uterus.

Implantation

Five days after fertilization, the blastocyst 'hatches' from the zona pellucida, allowing the cells of the trophoblast to directly contact the endometrial wall. When this happens the cells of the trophoblast multiply, and work their way into the endometrium (implantation) (Fig. 30.16A). By about the tenth day after

Female infertility

The first questions to be answered when seeking the cause of female infertility are whether the ovum can reach the uterus and whether the sperm can reach the ovum. There may be obstruction of the uterine tubes due to infection or previous surgery, for example for tubal pregnancy (see Ectopic Implantation on p. 500) which may also cause adhesions of the fimbriae. The uterus may be tilted backwards (retroverted), preventing the collection of semen around the cervix. The cervix itself may be infected, the pus and infected mucus forming a barrier to sperm.

If regular normal ovulation does not occur, conception is less likely to take place. There are many causes of amenorrhoea; severe physical or mental illness: anorexia nervosa; obesity. Lack of, or infrequent, ovulation without amenorrhoea may be due to disorders of the ovaries caused by cysts, tumours or endometriosis. Endocrine disorders affecting the production of FSH and LH may also prevent ovulation.

Finally, it may not be possible for the fertilized ovum to implant in the uterus. The endometrium may not be receptive due to hormonal imbalance (oestrogen and progesterone), there may be congenital abnormalities such as a bicornuate uterus, fibroids may be present – or a forgotten IUCD (see p. 494) may still be in position!

THE PLACENTA

Development

During implantation, the cells of the trophoblast differentiate into two layers (Fig. 30.16):

- syncytiotrophoblast
- cytotrophoblast.

The syncytiotrophoblast burrows further into the endometrium, digesting maternal tissues and resulting in the formation of blood-filled spaces (lacunae) which will form part of the maternal circulation of the placenta (Fig. 30.16B). Extensions consisting of both syncytiotrophoblast and cytotrophoblast cells form and extend into the endometrium and into the spiral arteries which supply maternal blood.

Simultaneously some cells on the embryo side develop, and together with the cells of the trophoblast form the chorionic villi of the placenta which expand into the maternal blood-filled spaces created by the extravillous trophoblast. Cells within the villi develop into blood vessels and join with other vessels originating from the embryonic cells to form the fetal circulation to the placenta.

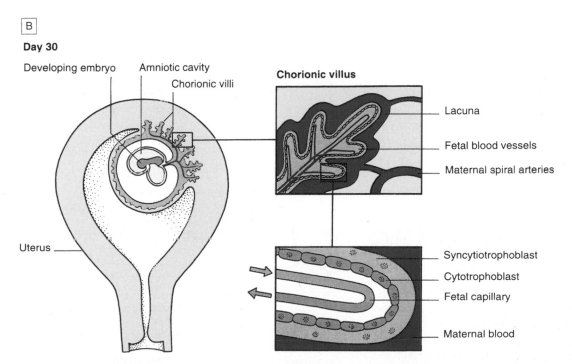

Figure 30.16 Implantation of the conceptus and development of the placenta. A, Implantation. B, Early development of the placenta.

Ectopic implantation

Under normal circumstances, the fertilized ovum embeds in the wall of the uterus, but in about 1 in 50 conceptions the ovum embeds outside the uterus, in a uterine tube, in the abdomen or, rarely, in an ovary. Ectopic implantation may be due to narrowing of the uterine tube as a result of infection or previous surgery.

Tubal pregnancies are not viable. If the implantation is at the end of the tube that is furthest from the uterus (i.e. the distal end), it is possible that a tubal abortion will occur; the developing trophoblast becomes separated from the wall and is extruded into the peritoneal cavity where it is eventually absorbed. If this does not happen, the pregnancy continues until either it is terminated surgically or the tube ruptures (a ruptured ectopic tubal pregnancy). The latter causes severe haemorrhage into the peritoneal cavity resulting in sudden collapse of the mother.

Viable abdominal pregnancy is rare because the fetus usually dies and is calcified. Occasionally the pregnancy reaches term and the baby is delivered by laparotomy. The placenta is not removed because it is attached to the outer wall of the uterus, the abdominal organs or an ovary. Removal would cause uncontrollable haemorrhage.

Functions

The placenta is the life-support system for the developing embryo (Fig. 30.17). It:

- delivers oxygen and nutrients required for growth
- disposes of the waste products of embryonic metabolism
- is a protection against some constituents of maternal blood
- manufactures several hormones important in pregnancy.

Surprisingly, although the cells of the placenta are partly foreign to a woman's body they are not rejected by her immune system (see Ch. 16).

Transport and barrier functions

Oxygen and carbon dioxide passively diffuse across the placenta, whereas substances such as glucose, amino acids, electrolytes and minerals are taken across by specific transport mechanisms.

Most proteins cannot cross the barrier very easily because they are too large, but the IgG class of immunoglobulins is transferred by receptor-mediated endocytosis at one membrane of the syncytiotrophoblast and by exocytosis at the other. In the early stages of pregnancy the amounts transferred are small but by the third trimester concentrations in maternal and fetal blood are similar.

Liposoluble substances, such as alcohol, diffuse passively across the placenta from the mother to the baby. Similarly bilirubin, a waste product of haemo-

Rhesus anti-D antibodies are of the IgG class (Ch. 16). They cross the placenta from mother to baby where they may cause destruction of fetal red cells if the baby's blood group is Rhesus positive.

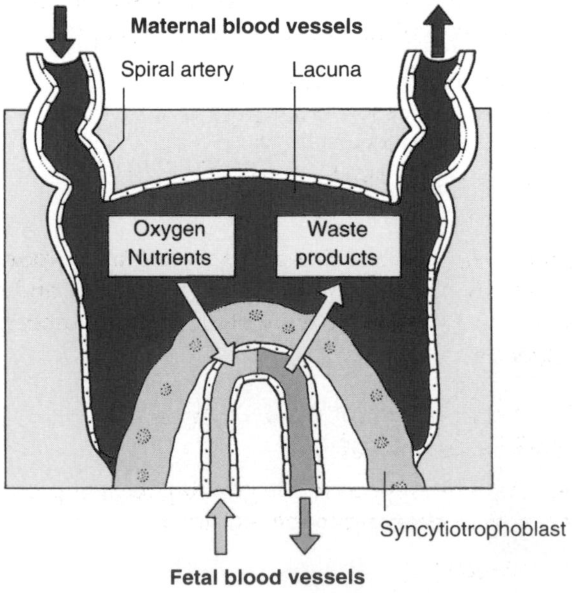

Figure 30.17 Functional organization of the placenta.

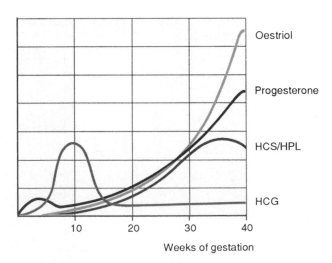

Figure 30.18 Pattern of hormone secretion during pregnancy. The scale used for oestriol and progesterone is the same, but differs from that for HCS/HPL and for HCG which are measured in i.u. (international units) instead of mmoles per litre. (After Hytten & Chamberlain 1991.)

globin breakdown, diffuses in the opposite direction from the fetal to the maternal blood.

Hormones

The cells of the syncytiotrophoblast manufacture several hormones and continue this function throughout pregnancy (Fig. 30.18). These hormones include:

- human chorionic gonadotrophin (HCG)
- human chorionic somatomammotrophin (HCS) (also known as human placental lactogen or HPL)
- progesterone
- oestrogens (principally oestriol).

HCG appears very early in pregnancy, secreted by the outer cells of the blastocyst even before implantation. Its identification by immunoassay (a method which allows very tiny amounts to be detected) in maternal blood is proof of pregnancy. HCG maintains the steroid-secreting function of the corpus luteum until this is taken over by the placenta itself after about the first 3 months of pregnancy.

HCS/HPL, like HCG, is mainly secreted into the maternal circulation. It brings about many of the maternal adjustments necessary to support the growth of the fetus (see below).

Progesterone is synthesized by the placenta from cholesterol. The formation of oestrogens, however, is a cooperative process involving the fetus as well as the placenta (Fig. 30.19) (fetoplacental unit). Consequently, the urinary excretion of oestriol by the mother can be used as an index of fetal well-being.

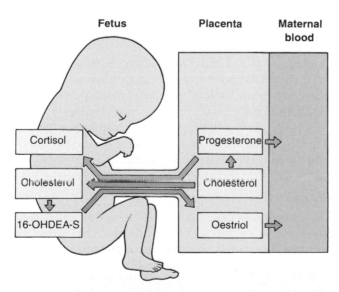

Figure 30.19 Formation of steroid hormones by the fetoplacental unit (16-OHDEA-S – 16-hydroxydehydroepiandrosterone).

Immune mechanisms

Placental and fetal cells are partly foreign to a woman's body because of the paternal component in their make-up. Yet they are not normally rejected but instead grow and develop alongside maternal cells and tissues.

The cells that ought to be in the front line for attack and destruction by maternal immune mechanisms are those of the syncytiotrophoblast that burrow into the uterine lining. However, these cells are unusual in that they lack proteins of the major histocompatibility complex (MHC). MHC proteins have to be present in the membrane of a targeted cell for many T cells to recognize them and act (see Ch. 16). Consequently the cells of the syncytiotrophoblast are not attacked.

In addition, the growth and survival of the placental cells is probably promoted by substances produced by the endometrium that stimulate growth and suppress local immune responses.

MATERNAL CHANGES AND ADJUSTMENTS

During pregnancy, adjustments are made in many systems of the mother's body designed to prepare her to accommodate and support the growing fetus. In the first 2 months of pregnancy, when the fetus is relatively tiny and the placenta is at an early stage of development, the changes are largely produced by the hormones secreted by the corpus luteum of the ovary under the action of HCG. Thereafter the placenta becomes the major source of the hormones involved. These are responsible for promoting the growth of maternal tissues, and for re-adjusting her physiological systems so that the mother can accommodate and maintain the fast growing fetus, whilst maintaining her own internal environment. The systems involved include those determining:

- O_2 supplies and CO_2 disposal
- fluid and electrolyte balance
- nutrient balance
- defence and waste disposal
- temperature regulation.

In addition, there are changes in structural components of the body affecting posture and locomotion, and consequences for the nervous system affecting mood and behaviour.

Oxygen supplies and carbon dioxide disposal

The supply of oxygen to the growing fetus is protected by changes occurring in the mother in:

- ventilation
- numbers of red cells
- circulation.

Antenatal clinics

As soon as pregnancy is confirmed, usually at 2 to 3 months but it may be later, the mother is invited to attend a booking clinic. This is when she meets the midwife who will be caring for her in the community or hospital and sometimes the health visitor as well. The first meeting of mother and midwife should not be rushed; an important relationship is to be developed and subsequent visits to the antenatal clinic should, as far as possible, be enjoyed.

The history taken by the midwife is divided into five parts:

- social history
- family history
- general health
- menstrual history
- obstetric history (if appropriate).

Then follows a physical examination, the purpose of which is to record baseline measurements for future comparison:

- height and shoe size – a height of 5 feet or over with shoe size 3 or above usually indicates a pelvis that is big enough for childbirth
- weight
- blood pressure
- urinalysis
- a blood sample is taken for ABO grouping and Rhesus factor, haemoglobin estimation, rubella antibody titre and alphafetoprotein, syphilis and HIV (possibly) screening.

The mother's breasts are examined and feeding methods discussed. Many women are sensitive about having their breasts examined and may find the thought of breast feeding repugnant. The abdomen is examined, though at early visits the uterus may not be palpable; at later visits, the midwife will assess the height of the uterus and palpate the position of the baby. The mother's legs are examined for signs of oedema and varicose veins.

During this lengthy visit, the midwife is also giving advice, reassuring, answering questions and establishing a baseline for this mother so that any changes at subsequent visits will be recognized quickly.

Subsequent visits to the antenatal clinic always include urinalysis, recording of blood pressure, examination of breasts, and abdominal examination to check the growth of the fetus, its position and heart rate. The mother is always given the opportunity to discuss problems and the midwife will require detailed information about fetal movements; regular movements are normal and indicate that the fetus is well.

Parentcraft and preparation for parenthood classes are usually organized in conjunction with antenatal clinics. One method is for the session to be divided between the midwife and the health visitor. The midwife teaches relaxation and explains what is to be expected when labour commences. The health visitor teaches baby care – from bathing a baby and changing a nappy to the techniques of breast and bottle feeding. Fathers enjoy the opportunity to attend some sessions and ask their own questions.

Ventilation

The need for oxygen increases progressively during pregnancy with the growth of the fetus and of maternal tissues (uterus and breasts). At term, resting oxygen consumption is up by about 15% over non-pregnant levels.

More oxygen is needed also for the extra energy expended in daily activities because of the mother's weight gain (total 12.5 kg on average; approximately 20% of body weight).

Ventilation (see Ch. 7) increases progressively in pregnancy (Fig. 30.20). This is caused by progesterone increasing the sensitivity of the respiratory control system to CO_2 so that ventilation is greater at any particular level of arterial CO_2 than in the non-pregnant state. The depth of breathing increases but the number of breaths per minute does not change.

As a result of the increased ventilation, the partial pressure of oxygen in alveolar air increases and that of carbon dioxide decreases, with the result that maternal alveolar PO_2 increases and PCO_2 falls by about 10 mmHg. The changes increase the rate of diffusion of gases across the placenta, facilitating fetal oxygen uptake as well as carbon dioxide excretion.

Red cell numbers

Production of red cells by the bone marrow is stimulated by erythropoietin and human chorionic somatomammotrophin leading to a 20% increase in the total numbers of red cells in the circulation. However, as the volume of plasma increases by an even larger amount (Fig. 30.20), the number of red cells per litre of blood actually falls (physiological anaemia of pregnancy).

Circulation

The growth of maternal tissues causes an increase in the number of blood vessels in the circulation. In addition, hormonal changes cause relaxation of some vascular smooth muscle, leading to a fall in total peripheral resistance. For example, relaxation is produced by increased levels of progesterone and decreased responsiveness to angiotensin II. Circulatory pressure is maintained by:

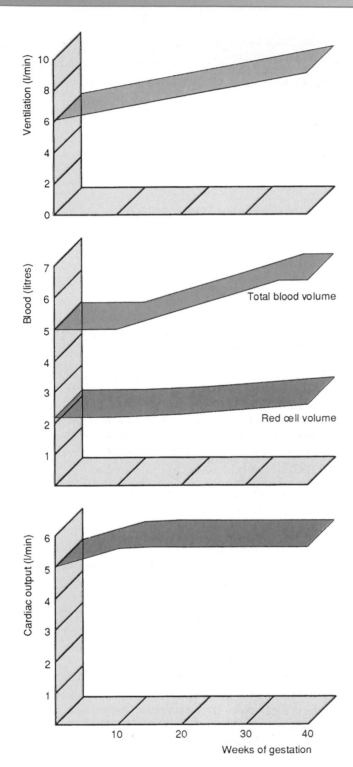

Figure 30.20 Respiratory and circulatory changes in pregnancy. (After Hytten & Chamberlain 1991.)

- expanding blood volume (see Ch. 14 and below)
- increasing cardiac output (see Ch. 12).

The expansion in blood volume is made up of an increase in plasma volume of about 1 litre and by the

The expected weight gain during pregnancy is 2 kg in the first 20 weeks and 0.5 kg per week thereafter, amounting to approximately 12 kg in total. Increased blood volume accounts for about 1.5 kg and interstitial fluid for another 1 kg. The remaining weight increase is accounted for as follows:

- breasts 0.5 kg
- fat 3.5 kg
- placenta 0.6 kg
- fetus 3.4 kg
- amniotic fluid 0.6 kg
- uterus 0.9 kg.

(Bennett & Brown 1999)

progressive increase in total numbers of red cells which occurs throughout pregnancy (Fig. 30.20).

Cardiac output increases early in pregnancy, reaching about 40% above the non-pregnant state by 3 months and remaining that way until term (Fig. 30.20). Heart rate and stroke volume both increase by about 15 to 20%.

As a result of all these changes in volume and cardiac output, arterial blood pressure normally hardly changes although there is usually a small decrease (about 10 mmHg) in diastolic pressure.

Fluid and electrolyte balance

The expansion of blood volume in pregnancy is associated with an expansion also of interstitial fluid volume resulting in an increase of extracellular fluid volume by about 2 to 3 litres. The changes underlying this retention of salt and water are complex and involve:

- altered renal function
- altered sensitivity of control mechanisms.

Renal function

Many changes occur in renal function including alterations in:

- blood flow
- glomerular filtration rate (GFR)
- tubular transport.

Renal blood flow and GFR (see Ch. 8) both increase quite early on in pregnancy by about 50%. Consequently the renal tubules are presented with increased amounts of solutes to be recovered. Sodium and water recovery are both enhanced by the actions of aldosterone and AVP/ADH (see below) to more than match the increased load delivered but the transport of glucose and amino acids is not. Indeed the tubular transport maximum for both glucose and amino acids may decrease. Once the load of glucose and amino acids delivered to the tubules exceeds the tubular transport maximum (see Ch. 8) glucose and amino acids appear in the urine (glycosuria and aminoaciduria of pregnancy).

In the later stages of pregnancy when the fetal skeleton is growing at its fastest (see Ch. 31), absorption of calcium by the renal tubules increases and more calcium is recovered from the filtrate. Tubular reabsorption of calcium is stimulated by parathyroid hormone which is secreted in increasing amounts by the parathyroid glands (see Ch. 14) as maternal blood calcium concentration falls.

Control mechanisms

The renin–angiotensin system (see Ch. 12) is stimulated with the result that aldosterone secretion by the adrenal cortex increases. The secretion of aldosterone is also enhanced by increased secretion of ACTH by the anterior pituitary. This gland enlarges by about 40% during pregnancy. As aldosterone promotes the renal tubular absorption of sodium, more sodium accumulates in the body.

Extra water is retained too as a result of the thirst-promoting effects of angiotensin II (and possibly prolactin) as well as by an increase in the sensitivity of the osmoreceptors in the hypothalamus to changes in osmotic pressure. This leads to a lowering of maternal plasma osmolality by about 10 mosmoles/kg H_2O after 3 months.

Nutrient balance

The fetus requires adequate supplies of all nutrients to support its growth, relying chiefly on glucose for energy. Maternal dietary requirements are increased also by the growth of her reproductive tissues and the increased energy costs of her daily activities. The adjustments made to meet these demands include changes in:

- food intake
- digestive function
- metabolism.

Food intake

Appetite is stimulated early on in pregnancy probably by the effects of hormones such as progesterone on the feeding centres in the hypothalamus as well as by the stimulus provided by the 10% decrease in fasting plasma glucose concentrations that occurs in the first 3 months of pregnancy. Sometimes women experience cravings for unusual foods and substances (a condition known as pica), and distaste for other foods that were previously enjoyed.

In early pregnancy, the intake of food exceeds immediate needs and consequently fat is laid down and provides an energy store for the mother in the later

Table 30.2 Increases recommended in daily dietary intake in pregnant women*

Nutrient	% Increase
Calcium	+ 140
Folate	+ 100
Zinc	+ 30
Iodine	+ 25
Protein	+ 11
Iron	+ 8

* Compiled from Truswell 1986.

stages of pregnancy when the demands of the growing fetus reach their peak.

There is an increased requirement for various nutrients during pregnancy (Table 30.2). If these requirements are not met the fetus draws on the mother's reserves at her expense.

Digestive function

The functioning of the digestive organs is affected by the change in hormonal balance during pregnancy. Chief among these is a reduction in tone and motility of the tract which is believed to contribute to:

- heartburn (see Ch. 9)
- feelings of nausea
- constipation.

Because of the reduction in motility it takes longer for food residues to pass through the gut. This does little to increase the absorption of nutrients such as glucose, amino acids and fats because these are already practically fully digested and absorbed in the non-pregnant state (see Ch. 9). However, it may enhance the absorption of water and salt in the colon, making the faeces harder.

The secretion of gastric acid decreases in the first half of pregnancy. This and the slower transit of food materials enhances the absorption of iron and calcium in the upper small intestine. Calcium absorption is also increased by calcitriol such that by 6 months calcium absorption is twice that of the non-pregnant state.

Metabolism

The mother's metabolism is readjusted so that energy stores in the form of fat are built up in the early stages of pregnancy and then drawn upon later. By using fatty acids in preference to glucose in the later stages of pregnancy, glucose is spared for the fetus. Extra glucose is also generated from amino acids by gluconeogenesis (see Ch. 10).

Some common problems of pregnancy

Many women sail through pregnancy in the best of health; others are plagued by a variety of minor ailments, such as constipation and heartburn. To the mother, these ailments can be very distressing, for example the young woman who finds that her breasts and abdomen are covered in stretch marks (striae gravidarum). These marks are caused by the stretching and tearing of layers of tissue in the dermis. They are red at first when the mother's size increases, and they persist as silvery lines after the pregnancy. The application of creams and moisturizers during pregnancy does not always prove effective in preventing the appearance of stretch marks. If a woman values the perfection of her body, this type of disfigurement may cause her to resent her baby.

Constipation during pregnancy has two probable causes:

- progesterone-induced relaxation of the bowel
- pressure on the bowel from the growing fetus.

Change in eating habits may also be involved. Prevention should be the aim – more fibre-containing foods, more water to drink and more exercise such as walking. Apart from causing discomfort, constipation may aggravate small haemorrhoids which are already present.

Heartburn (see Ch. 9) may also be troublesome. Progesterone relaxes the oesophageal sphincter of the stomach and allows reflux of the stomach contents into the oesophagus. Later in pregnancy, the condition is exacerbated by the increasing size of the uterus and the baby, which displaces abdominal organs such as the stomach, making it easier for gastric contents to be squeezed into the oesophagus. An old wives' tale states that heartburn means that the baby will be born with a lot of hair!

Other ailments attributed to the relaxing effects of hormones and the increasing size of the baby are backache and varicose veins.

Women who have Raynaud's disease may find that their condition is less troublesome when they are pregnant. Circulating vasodilator substances help to preserve blood flow to their hands and feet.

Waste disposal

The fetus produces many metabolic waste products including:

- CO_2
- urea, creatinine and uric acid
- unconjugated bilirubin.

All of these are eliminated via the placenta. In each case the substance diffuses across the barrier and is then eliminated via maternal excretory systems. Very little urea is formed by the fetus simply because the growing baby is in positive nitrogen balance (see Ch. 15). Bilirubin is formed from the turnover of red cells. Its production may increase if fetal red cells are destroyed by maternal antibodies.

Temperature regulation

A woman's body temperature rises by 0.5 to 1.0°C after ovulation (see p. 496) and remains elevated until mid-pregnancy if conception occurs. Thereafter it returns to its original level. Blood flow to the skin, particularly of the hands and feet, increases progressively during pregnancy and helps to dissipate heat. The increased blood flow may be caused by circulating vasodilator substances.

Posture and movement

Posture is affected in two ways:

- altered weight distribution
- softening of ligaments.

The increasing weight carried abdominally by the woman has to be supported by a change in posture, and the spine becomes increasingly curved. Several hormones including progesterone and relaxin cause softening of the ligaments at joints, and therefore loosens the skeleton. This is important in making pelvic structures more flexible at the time of birth but can cause problems and discomfort in the later stages of pregnancy.

Mood

Along with the considerable physical changes occurring within a woman's body as a result of the altered secretion of many hormones come changes in mood and in sense of well-being. Some women in the middle stages of pregnancy can have a sense of never

These metabolic effects are produced by the actions of several hormones including cortisol and the placental hormone human chorionic somatomammotrophin (HCS). HCS is secreted in increasing amounts during pregnancy (Fig. 30.18). It is similar in many ways to growth hormone and is therefore sometimes referred to as the 'maternal growth hormone of pregnancy'. Like growth hormone and cortisol, it has an anti-insulin effect which shifts metabolism towards the breakdown of fat stores (lipolysis) and the release of fatty acids into the bloodstream.

having felt so well before. There can be a heightened sense of awareness with many sensations appearing more vivid than hitherto. These passive changes in mood are intermingled with the normal anxieties and reactions associated with coming to terms with the new status of motherhood and the anticipation and fears associated with the imminent birth of a child.

PARTURITION

By convention, the length of gestation is timed from the first day of the last menstrual period prior to conception. Parturition occurs after an average of 40 weeks gestation. During this time the uterus develops to accommodate the growing fetus but then, at term, it provides the muscle power to expel the newborn baby from the mother's body through the dilated cervix. The signals initiating the process of parturition in humans are not yet fully understood.

Uterine contraction

Like most other smooth muscle, uterine muscle can contract spontaneously. However, during most of pregnancy its contractile activity is held in check by the inhibitory action of progesterone. As pregnancy proceeds, ripples of contraction begin to occur once more (Braxton Hicks' contractions), causing very small changes in intrauterine pressure. As the levels of oestrogen rise towards the end of pregnancy (Fig. 30.18) these contractions become more frequent and more powerful.

The increasing level of oestrogen affects the uterine smooth muscle in two ways. It increases the number of:

• gap junctions between cells
• receptors for oxytocin.

The gap junctions (see Ch. 4B) allow excitation to spread from cell to cell and therefore allow larger, concerted contractions to occur. Simultaneously, the increase in numbers of receptors to oxytocin allows the smooth muscle to become more sensitive to circulating levels of this hormone and more powerful contractions are produced that can raise intrauterine pressure to between 4 and 12 kPa (30–90 mmHg). These waves of contraction tend to begin at the top of the uterus, where some cells may act as a pacemaker, and sweep down towards the lower segment of the uterus (Fig. 30.21). These contractions, occurring during pregnancy before the cervix dilates, are usually painless but can be uncomfortable.

Cervical dilation

Towards the end of pregnancy the connective tissue of which the cervix is composed softens and the cervical

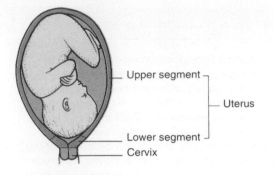
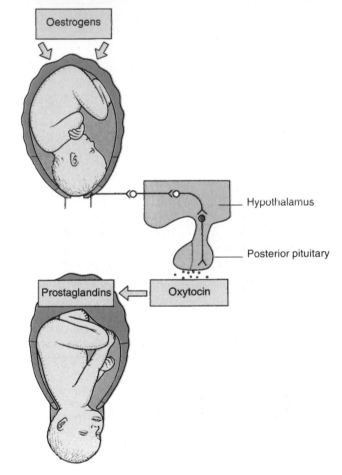

Figure 30.21 Parturition: hormonal control.

opening dilates. The connective tissue softens probably under the action of several hormones such as oestrogens and relaxin. Dilation occurs under the pressure exerted by the fetus as it is squeezed towards the opening by uterine contractions (Fig. 30.21). Softening and dilation proceed fairly slowly.

As the cervix dilates, sensory receptors within it are excited. Some reflexly stimulate the secretion of oxytocin from the posterior pituitary; others give rise to the sensation of pain. The oxytocin secreted by the pituitary promotes further waves of contraction, which distends the cervix even more, and consequently even more oxytocin is secreted (positive feedback). Oxytocin increases uterine contractions by stimulating the formation of prostaglandins as well as by acting directly on its own receptors.

Delivery

Eventually the baby is expelled from the uterus which contracts down and the muscle fibres permanently shorten. This causes the placenta to be stripped away from the wall. Bleeding from the torn vessels is checked by contraction of the uterine muscle fibres around them. Further contractions of the uterus squeeze the placenta out into the vagina. The whole process from the beginning of labour to delivery of the placenta can take anything from a couple of hours to a couple of days.

Placenta praevia

The placenta develops at the site of implantation of the trophoblast, which, ideally, takes place in the upper uterine segment (see Figs 30.7 and 30.21). Occasionally, the placenta develops either wholly or partially in the lower uterine segment (placenta praevia; see Figs 30.21 and 30.22). Depending on the area of the placenta attached to the lower segment, this is potentially a life-threatening condition. This is because, as the lower uterine segment grows and stretches after the 12th week of pregnancy, the placenta is likely to become separated from the uterine wall, causing bleeding from the maternal venous sinuses. Bleeding from the vagina after the 28th week of pregnancy is known as antepartum haemorrhage, and placenta praevia is one of the causes.

There are four types of placenta praevia:

- Type I is the least serious with only a small portion of the placenta attached in the lower segment. Normal delivery is possible and bleeding is usually minimal.
- Type II will allow normal delivery, but bleeding is likely to be moderate and the baby may suffer from hypoxia.
- Type III makes normal delivery impossible because the placenta is so placed that it would deliver first. Severe bleeding is likely to occur in late pregnancy.
- Type IV means that the placenta is attached centrally across the inner mouth of the cervix (internal os). Normal delivery is impossible and, when the placenta begins to separate, bleeding is torrential.

Placenta praevia can be diagnosed early for those women who attend antenatal clinics regularly and an elective caesarean section (see p. 508) can be planned. Those who do not have any antenatal care, for whatever reason, are at risk.

PUERPERIUM

The puerperium is defined as the time from the end of the last stage of labour until most of the systems that changed as a result of pregnancy have reverted to their prior state. This takes about 6 weeks, at which time the first menstrual period postpartum may occur in a woman who is not breast feeding her child. Resumption of ovulation and menstrual periods is delayed, however, by lactation, which continues well beyond the end of the puerperium, from 4 to 18 months, or even longer.

Reproductive organs

At term, the uterus weighs about 1 kg. This reduces to the 50 to 100 g of the non-pregnant state by degeneration and shrinkage of cells and tissue. The muscle continues to contract spontaneously in response to oxytocin. This occurs particularly during breast feeding when oxytocin secretion is increased (see p. 509).

The degenerating lining tissues of the uterus, particularly around the placental site, are shed and leak out through the vagina for a few days after parturition. After a week the vaginal discharge (lochia) consists simply of mucus, leucocytes, epithelial cells and exudate. This secretion has a protective effect and guards against ascending infection.

A new endometrial lining then develops and, once ovulation occurs, undergoes the characteristic menstrual cycling of proliferation, secretion and shedding again (Fig. 30.13).

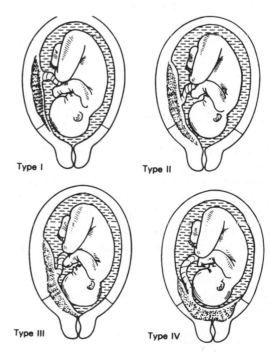

Figure 30.22 Types of placenta praevia. (From Chamberlain & Dewhurst 1986, with permission of Elsevier.)

Newly delivered mothers are taught, and encouraged to continue, postnatal exercises. These exercises improve circulation in the legs, strengthen the pelvic floor muscles (to avoid future stress incontinence), ease backache and help return the abdominal muscles to the pre-pregnant condition. The exercises are beneficial to almost any woman, whether a mother or not, especially for easing backache and keeping the pelvic floor muscles in good condition.

Caesarean section

Sometimes a baby cannot be delivered per vaginam. The alternative is to perform a caesarean section, an operation so named because Julius Caesar is said to have been delivered by that method. There are two types of caesarean section – classical and lower segment.

Caesarean section in the lower part of the uterus (lower uterine segment) is more commonly used because healing takes place more quickly and successfully. There is also less likelihood of rupture during future pregnancies because there is more fibrous tissue than muscle in this part of the uterus. The classical approach through the upper part of the uterus (upper uterine segment) is used before 32 weeks gestation because there is not a clear division between the two segments at that stage of the pregnancy.

Caesarean sections are elective (i.e. planned before labour begins) for the following reasons:

- disproportion between the baby's head and the mother's pelvis
- types III and IV placenta praevia (possibly type II also) (see Fig. 30.22)
- three or more fetuses.

Depending on the mother's health during pregnancy and the condition of the fetus, caesarean section may also be planned if there is breech presentation (buttocks and feet in position to deliver first), hypertension due to pregnancy (pre-eclampsia), diabetes mellitus, antepartum haemorrhage or retarded growth of the fetus.

Emergency caesarean section would be performed during labour for the following reasons:

- prolapse of the umbilical cord
- eclampsia (untreated pregnancy-induced hypertension or rapid onset of hypertension)
- rupture of the uterus
- disproportion discovered during labour
- fetal distress
- failure of the labour to progress.

Body systems

The fluid retained during pregnancy is lost within a few days, resulting in blood volume returning quickly to the non-pregnant state. Cardiac output reverts at the same time. With the sudden decrease in the concentration of vasodilator substances, such as progesterone, the tone of the muscle in the blood vessels increases. Veins that became varicose during pregnancy, because of this loss of tone, gradually recover. Similarly there is recovery of tone in the smooth muscle of the gut and of the bladder, though, for the first few days, a woman may have some problems with constipation and retention of urine, exacerbated by the effects of childbirth on pelvic organs and muscles. Renal function (GFR, blood flow and structural changes) also gradually reverts to the non-pregnant state.

Mood

The sudden drop in the concentration of steroid hormones has a rebound effect on mood in many women and can result in a short period of depression just after the baby is born. If there were pre-existing tendencies to psychological disturbance then the effects may be more marked and more long lasting (postnatal depression).

LACTATION

Milk is formed by the mammary glands. The mammary glands grow at puberty (see Ch. 31). Further development and enlargement of the glands occurs during pregnancy. After parturition the formation of milk is stimulated and milk is expelled from the ducts of the gland in response to suckling.

Development of glands

The breasts develop during pregnancy under the combined action of several hormones including:

- oestrogens
- progesterone
- HCS/HPL.

Some milk is formed during pregnancy but the amounts are small compared with the surge of production occurring after parturition. HCS/HPL (human placental lactogen) inhibits the production of prolactin (which promotes the formation of milk) and the fetoplacental steroids inhibit its milk-producing effects. Once the levels of these hormones have dropped dramatically postpartum, the action of prolactin is unrestrained.

Table 30.3 Composition of milk (per litre)*

	Human	Cows'
Energy (kcal)	700	670
Protein (g)	11	35
Fat (g)	40	37
Carbohydrate (g)	73	50
Sodium (mmol)	7	22
Calcium (mg)	350	1200
Vitamin C (mg)	38	15
Vitamin D (μg)	8	1.5

* Compiled from Truswell 1986.

Composition of milk

Human breast milk contains a mixture of nutrients and electrolytes. Its composition differs in a number of respects from cows' milk (Table 30.3). Notably it contains less sodium and calcium but is richer in vitamins C and D. Human breast milk also contains large quantities of IgG which are important in combating many microorganisms to which the baby will be exposed. After about a week, IgA predominates in the milk and this confers some protection against microorganisms entering the baby's digestive system.

Suckling

The secretion of prolactin, which stimulates milk formation, and of oxytocin, which promotes milk ejection, are both stimulated by suckling (Fig 30.23). During pregnancy, the skin receptors around the nipples of the breasts are not as sensitive as they are after the baby's birth. The stimulus of the baby's sucking reflexly excites the secretion of prolactin and oxytocin from the pituitary (Fig. 30.23). Prolactin secretion from the anterior pituitary is controlled by two hormones, prolactin releasing hormone (PRH) and prolactin inhibiting hormone (PIH) secreted by nerves of the hypothalamus into the portal hypophyseal blood vessels (see Ch. 11). Prolactin inhibits the action of LHRH on the secretion of FSH and LH by the pituitary as well as the actions of these hormones on the ovary. Consequently, ovulation and the return of menstrual cycles is inhibited. If suckling occurs frequently and regularly, ovulation does not reoccur in many women until breast feeding has ceased.

Breast feeding

It is the role of *every* healthcare practitioner to advocate breast feeding as the right way to feed infants. This premise is due to two issues:

- Breast milk contains many anti-infective components which are not replicated in artificial milks. As infants have an immature immune system for the first 18–24 months of life, breast feeding gives very positive advantages in reducing the risk of infection. In addition, breast milk contains nutrients in amount and quality tailored to meet a baby's needs. Breast feeding an infant reduces the risk of infant allergies, gastrointestinal problems and conditions such as eczema.

- The Baby Friendly Initiative (BFI) is part of a global campaign by the World Health Organization and the United Nations Children's Fund to ensure that mothers and infants benefit from the evidence-based physiological and psychosocial advantages of breast feeding. The initiative has an award incentive given to hospitals which have implemented the *Ten Steps to Breast Feeding* (policy and practices in place to promote breast feeding) and have achieved specific outcomes: the UK Standard is awarded where the breast feeding rate is 50–75% and all ten steps have been implemented. A Certificate of Commitment is given where a hospital is working towards the ten steps.

Ten Steps to Successful Breast Feeding

- Breastfeeding policy available which is communicated to all staff.
- All healthcare staff are trained to implement the policy.
- All pregnant mothers are informed of the benefits and management of breast feeding.
- Mothers are assisted to commence breast feeding within half an hour of delivery.
- Education of mothers in breast feeding and the maintenance of lactation is given, even if they are separated from their babies (i.e. the baby is in the Special Care Baby Unit).
- Neonates are to be given nothing other than breast milk unless medically necessary.
- 24 hour 'rooming-in' of mother and baby together in hospital.
- Breast feeding is managed on a 'demand from baby' basis.
- No teats or pacifiers are to be given to breastfeeding babies.
- Breastfeeding support groups are established to support women, particularly in the community.

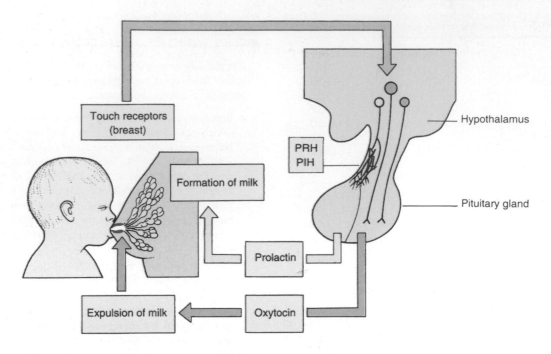

Figure 30.23 Hormonal control of milk secretion and ejection during breast feeding (PRH, prolactin releasing hormone; PIH, prolactin inhibiting hormone).

REFERENCES AND FURTHER READING

Anawalt B D, Amory J K 2001 Advances in male hormonal contraception. Annals of Medicine 33(9): 587–595

Andrade-Rocha F R 2001 Sperm parameters in men with suspected infertility: sperm characteristics, strict criteria sperm morphology analysis and the hypo-osmotic swelling test. Journal of Reproductive Medicine 46(6)(June issue): 577–582

Bancroft J 1989 Human sexuality and its problems, 2nd edn. Churchill Livingstone, Edinburgh

Bennett V R, Brown L K (eds) 1999 Myles' Textbook for midwives, 13th edn. Churchill Livingstone, Edinburgh

British Medical Journal 2001 Clinical evidence: A compendium of the best available evidence for effective health care. Issue 5, June 2001. BMJ Publishing Group

Carr B R, Blackwell R E 1993 Textbook of reproductive medicine. Appleton & Lange, Norwalk, CT

Chamberlain G, Dewhurst J 1986 A practice of obstetrics and gynaecology, 2nd edn. Churchill Livingstone, Edinburgh, p 39

Cox I, Melloni J, Sheld H H 2000 Melloni's Illustrated Dictionary of Obstetrics & Gynaecology. Parthenon Publishing, London

Hellerstedt B A, Pienta K J 2002 Testicular cancer. Current Opinion in Oncology 14(3)(May issue): 260–264

Hytten F, Chamberlain G 1991 Clinical physiology in obstetrics, 2nd edn. Blackwell, Oxford

Rogers A W 1992 Textbook of anatomy. Churchill Livingstone, Edinburgh, p 121

Truswell A S 1986 ABC of nutrition. British Medical Association, London

Williams P L, Warwick R, Dyson M, Bannister L H 1989 Gray's Anatomy, 37th edn. Churchill Livingstone, Edinburgh

Wright T C, Cox J T, Massad L S, Twiggs L B, Wilkinson E V 2002 2001 Consensus Guidelines for the management of women with cervical cytological abnormalities. Journal of the American Medical Association 287(16)Apr 24: 2120–2129

31 Development from conception to maturity

As you sit reading this book, you may marvel at the fact that all the information needed to direct your growth to the person you are now was once contained within a single cell (Fig. 31.1). Your personal development from conception to adulthood has been determined by the genetic blueprint contained within the nucleus of that cell. Expression of the genetic code led rapidly to differentiation of cell function in utero resulting in the baby that was born.

At birth, your environment changed abruptly. Within only a short space of time you adapted to totally new circumstances, leaving the wet, warm and sheltered environment of the uterus for a world in which you had to breathe air, adjust to hot and cold environments and begin to fend for yourself. After this momentous event you embarked upon roughly two decades of gradual, though no less important, change as you grew through infancy and childhood to maturity. The final burst of development taking you from childhood into adulthood was adoles-

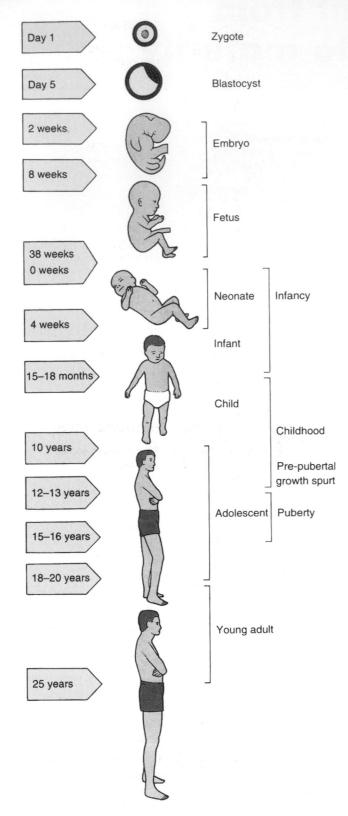

Figure 31.1 Stages of life from conception to adulthood.

cence. During this period your reproductive system matured, enabling you to pass on your genes to another generation.

FIRST STAGES OF LIFE

Your unique development plan was once tightly packed as 46 chromosomes (see Ch. 1) within a single cell. The expression of this genetic information played a major part in dictating the way you developed in utero from that cell to an embryo, a fetus and ultimately a newborn baby.

DEVELOPMENT AND FUSION OF THE GAMETES

Each new person is created by the fusion of one male and one female gamete (spermatozoon and ovum) (see Ch. 30). The primitive cells (spermatogonia and oogonia) that develop into mature spermatozoa and ova are produced in the fetal ovaries and testes. Each mature spermatozoon and ovum contains 23 chromosomes, only half the number present in other human cells. This halving of chromosomal number occurs as a result of meiosis during development of the gametes. When the gametes fuse, the resulting cell, the zygote, contains the full complement of 46 chromosomes. Spermatozoa and ova are both produced by meiosis but the staging of development differs between the two sexes.

If gametogenesis or fertilization is impaired, zygotes may form, containing a different number of chromosomes, resulting in altered development.

Meiosis

Each human cell including the primitive gametes (spermatogonia and oogonia) contains 46 chromosomes (23 pairs). Each pair of chromosomes consists of two structurally similar chromosomes (homologues), one of maternal origin, the other paternal (Fig. 31.2).

The first event in the process of meiosis (Fig. 31.3) is the replication of DNA in each homologue to form double-stranded DNA. The two chromosomes of each pair come together and some reshuffling of genetic material occurs between them. When the first meiotic division begins, the 23 pairs of chromosomes line up around the middle of a spindle of microtubules formed between the two poles of the cell (compare with mitosis; Ch. 1). The members of each pair of chromosomes separate, 23 being drawn to one pole of the cell and 23 towards the other. The cell divides, forming two daughter cells each containing only 23 chromosomes, half the usual number (haploid cell).

The daughter cells divide for a second time (second meiotic division). The chromosomes again line up at the middle of the spindle of microtubules but this time the two strands of DNA in each chromosome separate and

Autosomes

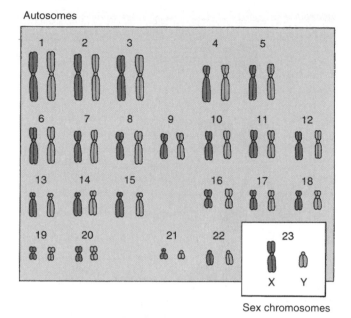

Figure 31.2 The 46 chromosomes of a human cell arranged in 23 pairs. (After Williams et al 1989, with permission of Elsevier.)

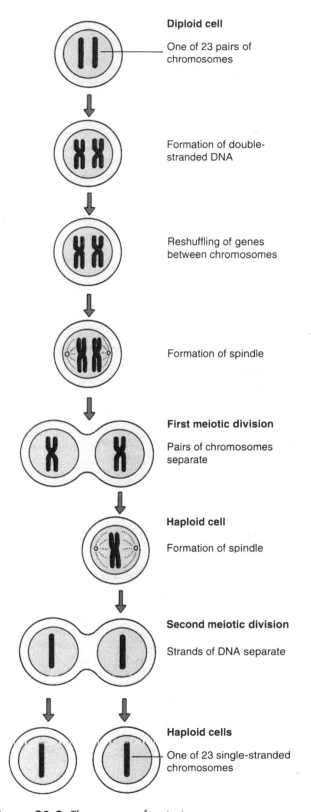

Figure 31.3 The process of meiosis.

each is drawn to opposite poles of the cell along the spindle and the cell divides forming two daughter cells. The second meiotic division is similar to mitosis (see Ch. 1) but differs from it in that only 23 chromosomes are involved from start to finish instead of 46. The resulting daughter cells are the mature gametes (spermatozoa and ova).

Male

In the male, meiotic division of the spermatogonia begins in the testes at puberty (see p. 536) when the reproductive organs reach maturity. From then on, sperm production continues prolifically throughout life.

Female

In the female, immature egg cells (oocytes) begin their first meiotic division whilst still in utero in the fetal ovaries. It is at this very early stage of life that reshuffling of genes inherited from parents occurs. Meiosis stops part way and the cells remain in this arrested state until they are stimulated by ovulation many years later to complete the process. Unlike the process in the male, when this first division occurs, the cell divides unequally yielding one large cell and a much smaller one, known as the first polar body (Fig. 31.4).

The second meiotic division takes place at fertilization when a sperm penetrates the ovum. Division again occurs unequally yielding one large cell (the mature ovum) and a much smaller one (second polar body) Simultaneously the first polar body also divides

creating a third polar body. Material from the first polar body can now be used in pre-implantation genetic diagnosis (PGD).

Spermatogenesis

Oogenesis

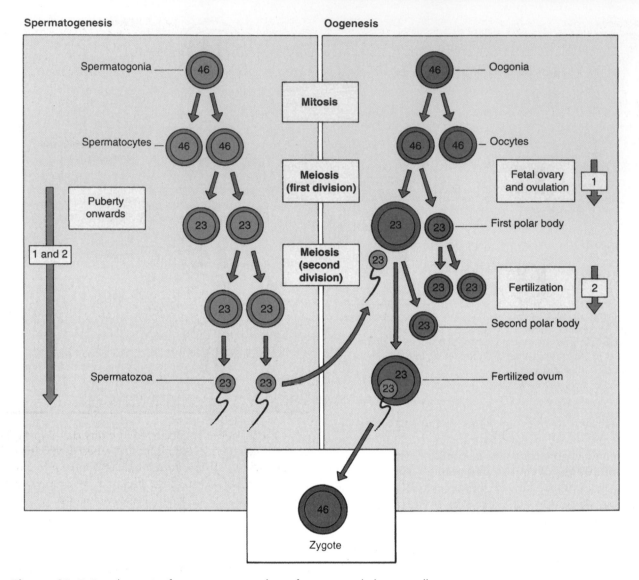

Figure 31.4 Development of spermatozoa and ova from primordial germ cells.

Altered development

The 46 chromosomes present in the fertilized ovum (zygote) consist of one pair of sex chromosomes, XX in the female and XY in the male, and 22 pairs of others (autosomes) (Fig. 31.2). Each pair of chromosomes and the genes within it determine different characteristics of the maturing adult. If meiosis or fertilization is disordered, zygotes that contain an abnormal number of chromosomes may form, resulting in altered development. Usually this precipitates spontaneous abortion at an early stage of pregnancy but sometimes the embryo may survive and a baby be born with congenital malformation. Abnormal numbers of chromosomes can result from:

• one or more chromosome pairs failing to separate during meiosis (nondisjunction)

• more than one sperm fertilizing the ovum (polyspermy).

Nondisjunction

If a pair of homologous chromosomes fails to separate, the two gametes formed will contain 24 and 22 chromosomes respectively. When these aberrant gametes fuse with a normal gamete the resulting zygote will possess either 47 or 45 chromosomes.

If nondisjunction occurs with the sex chromosomes a variety of aberrant chromosomal patterns may result. For example, the pattern could be XXX if there was one sex chromosome too many or X alone (XO) if there was one missing (Table 31.1).

Nondisjunction can also occur with the autosomes. The most common is nondisjunction of chromosome 21

Table 31.1 Examples of aberrant chromosomal patterns (karyotypes) resulting from nondisjunction of the sex chromosomes, and their consequences

Karyotype		Sex	Consequences	Name of syndrome	Incidence (per no. of live births of that sex)
Chromosome numbers	Sex chromosomes				
45	XO	Female	Impaired sexual development	Turner's	1:5000
47	XXX	Female	Minor		
47	XXY	Male	Impaired sexual development	Klinefelter's	1:500
47	XYY	Male	Minor		

An XO chromosomal pattern gives rise to Turner's syndrome, in which abnormalities are detectable at birth and there is abnormal maturation of the reproductive organs. An XXX pattern, however, tends not to give rise to observable abnormality until adolescence when the reproductive organs enter their final stage of maturation.

A hydatidiform mole is a conceptus consisting chiefly or entirely of placental tissue. A *complete hydatidiform mole* (all placental tissue and no embryo) results when the nucleus of the zygote consists entirely of paternal chromosomes, the maternal nucleus having disappeared before fertilization. Complete hydatidiform mole occurs in about 1 in 500 pregnancies. A *partial mole* (some embryonic development) results when the nucleus contains twice the normal number of paternal chromosomes plus the normal number from the mother.

giving rise usually to an ovum with three (trisomy) rather than two chromosome 21s. The result is the development of Down syndrome.

Less common congenital abnormalities resulting in the development of grossly abnormal fetuses arise from nondisjunction of chromosomes 18 and 13.

Polyspermy

In the unlikely event that two sperm simultaneously penetrate the same ovum, the resulting zygote possesses a total of 69 rather than 46 chromosomes. This causes severe developmental disturbances, for example partial hydatidiform mole. Most result in early spontaneous abortion.

Very soon after fertilization, an immunosuppressant protein (early pregnancy factor) appears in the mother's blood. The detection of this protein is used as an early indicator of pregnancy.

THE FIRST 2 WEEKS OF LIFE

Once fertilization has occurred, the tiny developing ball of cells has just a fortnight to embed itself into the endometrium of the uterus and turn on the hormonal mechanisms that stop menstruation from occurring (see Ch. 30). If it fails, it will be aborted in the menstrual fluid.

Day 1

In the upper reaches of a uterine tube, a single spermatozoon penetrates an ovum (fertilization) prompting the egg to undergo its second meiotic division (see p. 513 and Figs 31.3 and 31.4). The spermatozoon loses its tail, and its nuclear material is drawn towards the nucleus of the ovum. Twelve hours after penetration of the ovum by the spermatozoon, the maternal and paternal nuclei fuse and the genetic blueprint deciding the size, shape, sex and personality of the new individual is in place. Twelve hours later, at the end of the first day, the zygote divides, forming two daughter cells, and the process of development has begun.

Days 2 to 14

Cell division and differentiation

Cell division occurs every 12 to 15 hours with the result that 3 to 4 days after fertilization the conceptus consists of a cluster of about 16 to 32 cells (morula) (Fig. 31.5). The cells are still enclosed by the zona pellucida (see Ch. 30) and by some associated nutrient cells (corona

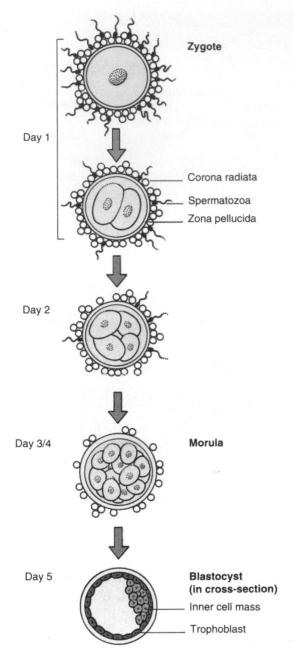

Figure 31.5 Stages of development in the first few days of life.

Twins

Twins may be identical or non-identical. Identical twins develop from the same fertilized ovum (monozygotic twins) whereas non-identical twins form as a result of the release and fertilization of two ova (dizygotic twins).

Most monozygotic twins develop as a result of division of the inner cell mass into two parts at about the end of the first week of life. If division is incomplete, Siamese twins develop. These twins are joined together to a greater or lesser extent, and sometimes can be successfully separated by surgery after birth.

Some monozygotic twins develop as a result of the division of the cluster of primitive cells into two morulae, or two blastocysts, in the first few days of development.

radiata). The zona pellucida helps to prevent polyspermy by barring the entry of other sperm once the ovum has been fertilized. It also stops the conceptus attaching itself prematurely to neighbouring tissue such as the wall of the uterine tube.

At about 4 days of life, a space appears within the ball of cells. Simultaneously, the first signs of cell differentiation appear. Within the ball of cells and to one side is a small mass of cells (inner cell mass) destined to become the embryo (Fig. 31.5). At this stage, the ball of cells is termed a blastocyst and the cells forming its wall

are referred to as the trophoblast. The blastocyst is swept into the uterine cavity by the action of cilia and the contraction of muscle of the uterine tubes.

Implantation

When the trophoblastic cells developing next to the inner cell mass make contact with the wall of the uterus (endometrium) they differentiate into two layers (Fig. 31.6):

- syncytiotrophoblast
- cytotrophoblast.

The cells of the syncytiotrophoblast burrow into the endometrium, implanting the blastocyst into the wall of the uterus. Implantation begins around day 6 or 7 and continues throughout the next few days so that the conceptus is completely embedded within the endometrium by the end of the first fortnight.

The syncytiotrophoblast digests its way through endometrial tissues, including blood vessels, secretory glands, and cells packed with stores of glycogen. Consequently at this very early stage the conceptus is surrounded by a highly nourishing environment.

Spaces (lacunae) appear within the syncytiotrophoblast, filled with maternal blood. These are the beginnings of the placental circulation.

Within the conceptus, differentiation and development is occurring. A space (amniotic cavity) develops between the inner cell mass and the cytotrophoblast. The original cavity of the blastocyst forms the yolk sac (Fig. 31.6).

The crucial events at this stage of development are those guaranteeing proper implantation of the conceptus. This depends on the endometrium and how it has developed under the action of hormones secreted by

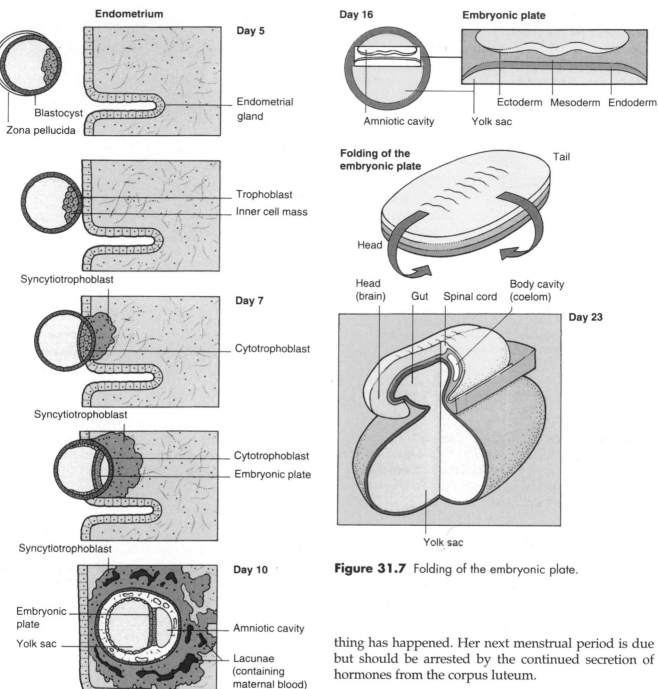

Figure 31.6 Implantation of the conceptus in the wall of the uterus.

Figure 31.7 Folding of the embryonic plate.

the corpus luteum (see Ch. 30). If development is deficient, implantation may not occur and the conceptus is aborted. At this very early stage of development the mother might only just be suspecting that some-

thing has happened. Her next menstrual period is due but should be arrested by the continued secretion of hormones from the corpus luteum.

EMBRYONIC LIFE

From the third week of life to the eighth, the conceptus is termed an embryo. Many crucial developments take place during this time.

Weeks 3 and 4

In weeks 3 and 4 there is an astonishingly rapid development of the cells of the embryonic plate. At the beginning of the third week the embryonic plate differentiates into three layers (Fig. 31.7):

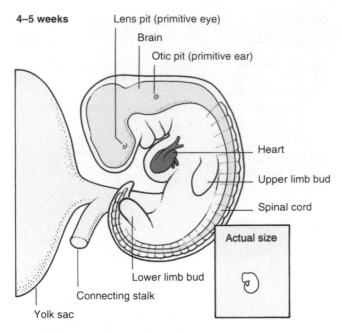

Figure 31.8 Structure of the human embryo – 4 to 5 weeks of age (inset: actual size).

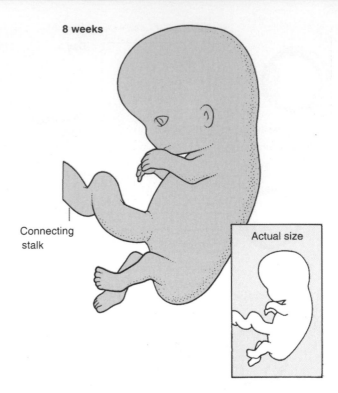

Figure 31.9 The human embryo – 8 weeks of age (inset: actual size).

- ectoderm
- mesoderm
- endoderm.

The growth of this 'sandwich' of tissues accelerates, some parts overtaking others in their speed of expansion. As a result tissues fold lengthwise and horizontally so that the embryonic tissue is converted from a flat plate of cells into a C-shaped cylindrical body (Fig. 31.7).

By 4 to 5 weeks the flat plate has been transformed into a tiny embryo (Fig. 31.8) possessing:

- a primitive heart and circulation
- the beginnings of a nervous system
- embryonic eyes and ears
- the first suggestion of developing limbs.

All this is occurring at a time when the mother-to-be has only just realized that she may be pregnant. This and the month following are critical periods of development. So much is happening so very quickly. Any disturbances of development, caused by drugs, radiation or viruses, will at these early stages have profound effects and can lead to serious congenital malformations.

Weeks 5 to 8

During the second month of life the basic structure of each of the systems of the body is formed and by 8 weeks of life the tiny embryo looks recognizably human (Fig. 31.9).

As a result of the folding of the embryonic plate, the amniotic cavity that was above the embryonic plate enfolds the embryo so that by 8 weeks the embryo is suspended in a fluid-filled cavity (Fig. 31.10A & B). A connecting stalk links the embryo with the developing placenta (see Ch. 30). The stalk becomes the umbilical cord containing:

- two umbilical arteries
- one umbilical vein.

Parts of the cavity of the yolk sac below the embryo (Fig. 31.7) develop into the digestive tract. Outpouchings from the yolk sac become the:

- lungs, trachea and larynx
- liver and digestive glands
- bladder and urethra of the urinary system.

The three distinct layers (ectoderm, mesoderm and endoderm) of the embryonic plate develop into different types of cells and tissues (Table 31.2). Organs usually consist of a mixture of these cell types. For example, the stomach is composed of neural, contractile, haemopoietic, epithelial and endocrine cells.

Each cell influences the growth and differentiation of its neighbours. As a result, development proceeds in an orderly and predetermined way. If the process is arrested, structures normally developing from that point may not form at all. For example the drug thalidomide, used in the 1960s as a sedative but now banned from use in pregnant women in some countries including the UK, critically arrests the development of the limbs and can affect the ear and the heart, structures that are forming simultaneously early in development (see Fig. 31.8).

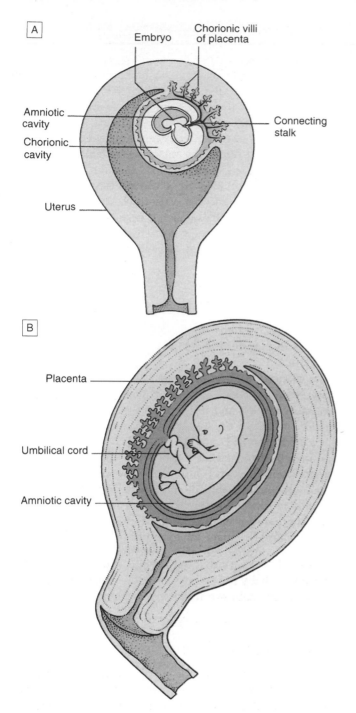

Figure 31.10 Uterus and conceptus. A, 4 to 5 weeks. B, 8 weeks.

FETAL LIFE

The fetal period is defined as that from the beginning of the ninth week of development to the time of birth (normally at 38 weeks). Considerable growth occurs

Table 31.2 Embryonic origins of cells and tissues

Cell type	Germinal layer		
	Ectoderm	**Mesoderm**	**Endoderm**
Neural	CNS ANS Sensory receptors	–	–
Contractile	–	Muscle – skeletal – cardiac – smooth	–
Support cells	–	Cartilage Bone Skin – dermis	–
Haemopoietic	–	Erythrocytes Immune system	–
Epithelial	Skin – epidermis – glands – nails/hair Eye – lens	Blood vessels Renal tubules	Gut Respiratory tract Pancreas Liver
Endocrine	Pituitary gland Adrenal medulla	Adrenal cortex Ovaries Testes	Thyroid Parathyroids

Key: CNS, central nervous system; ANS, autonomic nervous system.

during this period (see Fig. 31.16). The systems established in the first 2 months of life continue to mature, such that by about 6 months (26 weeks) the fetus is capable of independent existence, should it be born prematurely. In the last 3 months, further maturation occurs and stores of fat are built up in readiness for the transition from uterine to extrauterine life.

3 to 6 months

At about weeks 9 to 12, the fetal kidneys begin to produce urine. This is excreted into the amniotic cavity. The fluid in the cavity (amniotic fluid) is ingested by the fetus, absorbed by the developing digestive system and then re-excreted.

Bones grow and ossification begins (see p. 534). As the nervous system develops, the fetus becomes active, makes movements and becomes capable of reflex responses. As the fetus becomes larger the mother usually becomes very aware of fetal movements.

Genitalia develop. In the female, the developing ovaries begin to produce primordial follicles ready for the next generation to be conceived (see Fig. 31.4). By the fifth month of life the fetal ovaries have manufactured all the 5 million ovarian follicles the woman-to-be will ever possess.

Also in the fifth month, the fetus becomes covered with soft downy hair (lanugo) and brown fat begins to form.

In the sixth month, the fetal lungs begin to produce surfactant, a substance extremely important in breathing (see Ch. 7) that must be present in sufficient quantities for the baby to be able to breathe easily after birth. Without surfactant the lungs are extremely difficult to expand.

7 to 9 months

Maturation continues. Babies born from now on can survive, with assistance, but each remaining week in utero helps the fetus to build up its reserves (Table 31.3) and become more able to cope with the challenges it will meet at and immediately after birth. The nervous system is still developing. Each day that passes heralds the appearance of new responses, and better coordination of function and control.

The hair that had begun to grow all over the body in the fifth month is now well established and a head of hair is forming. As fat is laid down under the skin, the wrinkly 5-month-old fetus is transformed into the usually chubby looking full-term baby. By the time the baby is born, at about 38 weeks of age, body fat makes up 15 to 16% of its total body weight of 3.4 kg.

Table 31.3 Growth of fetal energy stores towards the end of gestation

Stores	Weeks of gestation					
	20	28	31	33	34	38
Body fat content (%)*	1	3.5	–	–	8	15
Body carbohydrate content (g)*	–	–	–	9	–	34
Liver glycogen (%)†	–	–	1	–	–	4

* From Widdowson (1981).
† From Shelley (1964).

Fetal movements are an important indication that the fetus is alive and not distressed. Patterns of movements vary; one fetus may be more active during the day and another may start exercising just as the mother is going to sleep! A change in pattern, reduced frequency or cessation of movements should be reported to the midwife immediately. Occasionally an active fetus will get the umbilical cord wound round its neck. Once the baby's head is born, the midwife always checks to make sure that the cord is not around the neck. If necessary, the cord is either loosened or clamped and cut before delivering the baby's body.

Normal, regular respirations are usually established within 60 seconds of delivery. Most midwives routinely clear the baby's mouth and nose of mucus, amniotic fluid etc., using a specially designed mucus extractor. This is usually sufficient intervention to encourage the baby to take his first breath; occasionally further steps have to be taken, for example to remove meconium from the airway. Holding the baby up by his ankles and slapping him is painful and dangerous – the spine is hyperextended, the intracranial pressure increased and the baby may be dropped.

ADAPTING TO LIFE OUTSIDE THE WOMB

At birth, momentous changes occur in the functioning of different parts of the body. During the first few days and weeks of life the newborn baby (neonate) has to adapt to its completely new surroundings. Within the uterus it was supplied with oxygen, nutrients, minerals and vitamins through the placental circulation and waste materials were eliminated through the same route. It was surrounded by a warm cushion of fluid, protecting it from external variations in temperature and limiting the stimuli to which it was exposed.

Once the baby has been born the functions of the placenta are taken over by three major systems:

• respiratory
• digestive
• urinary.

Each of these systems began to function in utero, but each has to mature and adapt for the baby to survive after birth.

The changes in these systems, particularly the respiratory system, necessitate major changes also in the circulatory system and in its control. Relative sizes and positions of major organs of the thorax, abdomen and pelvis are shown in Figure 31.11A & B.

Although detached at birth from its mother, the human cannot survive independently of its parents, unlike some other creatures. This is because the neural and musculoskeletal systems are very immature. Regulatory mechanisms maintaining internal stability in the face of external change, for example temperature regulatory mechanisms, are also immature. Consequently the neonate is more vulnerable to many external threats than the adult.

MAINTAINING OXYGEN SUPPLIES

In utero, oxygen and carbon dioxide were exchanged between maternal and fetal blood vessels of the placenta (see Ch. 30). Although breathing movements occur in the fetus no significant exchange of gases occurs across the developing alveoli because it is amniotic fluid, not air, that is being moved into and out of the fetal lungs. At birth, when the baby takes its first breath, the lungs expand, the flow of blood through the lungs increases and the way the blood is routed through the heart changes. Change also occurs in the production of red cells and in the synthesis of haemoglobin.

Fetal and neonatal circulation

The main features of the fetal circulation are shown in Figure 31.12A. There are three pathways which are open

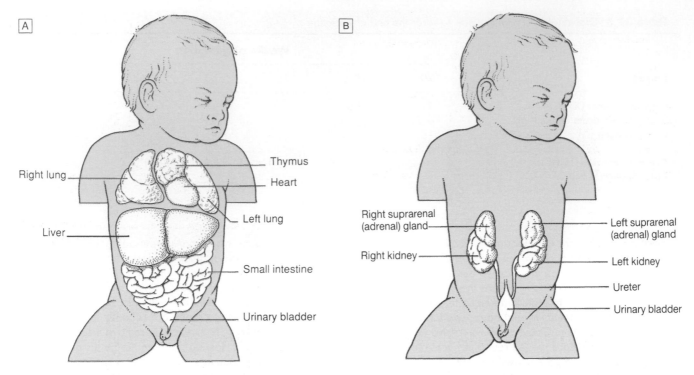

Figure 31.11 Major organs of the thorax and abdomen in the neonate. A, Thoracic and abdominal organs. B, The urinary system and adrenal glands. (From Rogers 1992, with permission of Elsevier.)

in the fetal circulation and which begin to close at birth and normally remain closed in the adult. These are:

• foramen ovale
• ductus arteriosus
• ductus venosus.

Foramen ovale

The foramen ovale is a hole in the wall between the two atria. It is covered in the left atrium by a loose flap of tissue. Because the foramen ovale is directly opposite the openings of the veins, blood returning to the heart from the superior and inferior vena cava mostly passes straight through this hole into the left atrium. From there it is pumped into the left ventricle and then via the aorta to the organs and tissues of the body.

Relatively little blood passes from the right atrium through the right ventricle into the pulmonary circulation because the resistance to blood flow in the pulmonary vessels is high. This is partly because the lungs are not expanded, and the pulmonary blood vessels as well as the alveoli are relatively small in size, and partly because of the effects of local factors, such as oxygen and carbon dioxide concentrations, on smooth muscle in the pulmonary vessels (see Ch. 12).

When the neonate takes its first breath, the pulmonary blood vessels expand because the pressure surrounding them (intrathoracic pressure; see Ch. 7) falls,

and because local chemical conditions change. The resistance to blood flow drops and more blood passes through the pulmonary veins into the left atrium (Fig. 31.12B). This increases the blood pressure in the left atrium and forces the flap covering the foramen ovale tightly against the wall, closing off the opening. Continued pressure maintains this contact and eventually in most people the hole is sealed off permanently by the growth of connective tissue.

Ductus arteriosus

The ductus arteriosus is a short vessel linking the pulmonary artery and the aorta (Fig. 31.12A). It is open in the fetus, diverting some of the blood pumped out of the right ventricle away from the lungs and into the systemic circulation.

The smooth muscle in the wall of the ductus arteriosus is very sensitive to the concentration of oxygen in the blood. When this rises (Fig. 31.13), after the baby has taken its first breath, the smooth muscle contracts and the vessel constricts. This reduces the flow of blood through the ductus arteriosus, encouraging more blood to flow through the pulmonary circulation. Consequently, the pressure of blood in the left atrium increases, pressing the flap covering the foramen ovale more tightly against the wall that separates the atria (septum).

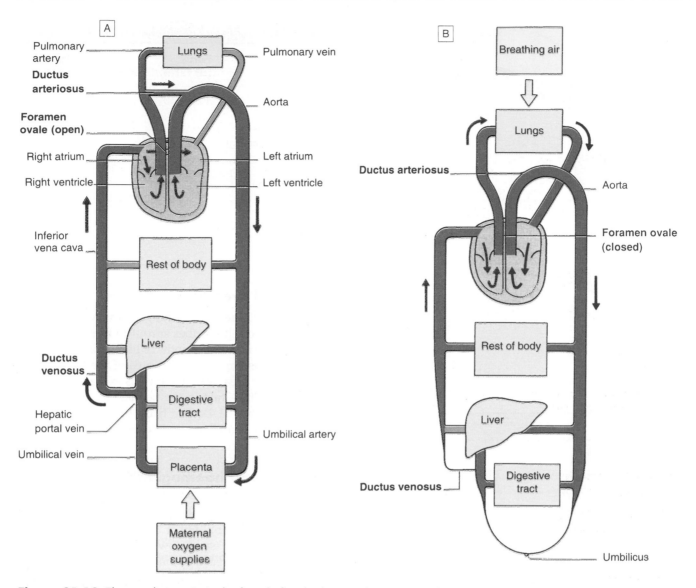

Figure 31.12 The circulation. A, In the fetus before birth. B, In the neonate after birth.

Neonatal hypoxia

If the baby should become hypoxic after birth, the muscle of the ductus arteriosus relaxes, the vessel dilates and blood is again diverted away from the pulmonary circulation. This is potentially serious because the fall in pressure in the left atrium may cause the foramen ovale to open up, allowing deoxygenated blood back into the left side of the heart. The lowered oxygen concentration makes the ductus arteriosus dilate even more and the situation becomes even worse with even less blood going to the lungs.

Ductus venosus

The ductus venosus is a vessel taking blood from the hepatic portal vein directly to the inferior vena cava (Fig. 31.12A). It diverts some of the blood coming from the placenta away from the liver.

When the flow of blood through the placenta is reduced by uterine contractions of labour (see Ch. 30), and later when the umbilical cord is cut, the quantity of blood flowing into the hepatic portal vein is reduced considerably and less blood passes through the ductus venosus (Fig. 31.12B). In due time the vessel shrinks, becoming just a small band of connective tissue (ligamentum venosum).

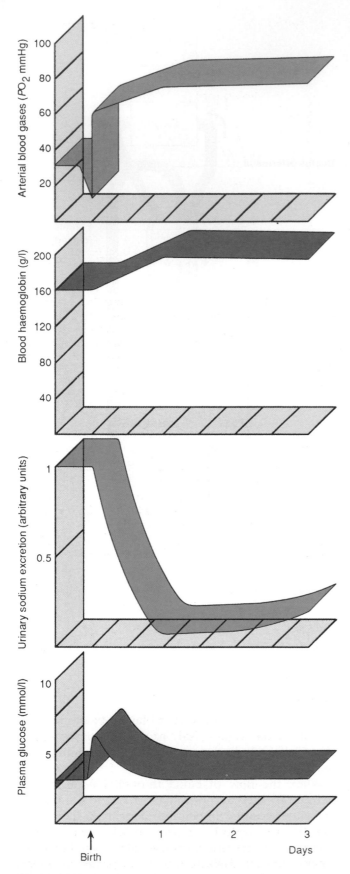

Table 31.4 Cardiorespiratory values compared

	Fetus (at term)	Neonate	Young adult
Heart rate (beats/min)	120–140	95–145	60–80
Blood pressure (systolic) (mmHg)	–	70–80	110–120
Respiratory frequency (breaths/min)	–	30–40* 40–80†	10–15

* Sleeping.
† Awake.

Lungs and breathing

After the first breath, the lungs grow very fast. The primitive conducting tubes sprout to form many more alveoli. In the first few months of life there is, as a result, a huge increase in the surface area of the lungs, vastly increasing the area available for gas exchange.

The respiratory rate in the neonate is higher than in the adult (Table 31.4). The baby breathes through its nose, cleverly managing to suckle and breathe at the same time.

Red cells and haemoglobin

At the time of birth, the haemoglobin concentration is normally higher than that in the adult (Fig. 31.13 and Ch. 3), and rises for a day or two because of the loss of extracellular fluids (see below).

The sudden increase in the concentration of oxygen in the blood (Fig. 31.13) suppresses the secretion of erythropoietin. Consequently the production of red blood cells (see Ch. 3) decreases and the blood haemoglobin concentration falls over the first few weeks after birth. Simultaneously the type of haemoglobin synthesized changes from the fetal form (HbF), which avidly binds oxygen at low partial pressures of oxygen (Fig. 31.14), to the adult form (HbA), requiring higher pressures to become fully saturated (see also Ch. 7).

FLUID AND ELECTROLYTE BALANCE

In utero, the fetus was enveloped in amniotic fluid and its need for water and electrolytes was met by the mother via the placenta. For a few days after birth, the baby loses more fluid via the skin and the kidneys than it is able to replace from its feeds. Consequently it loses weight. As the kidneys and regulatory mechanisms mature and as feeding becomes established, a more

Figure 31.13 Some of the changes occurring at and after birth. (After Case 1985.)

Apgar score

The Apgar score was devised by Virginia Apgar, an American anaesthetist. The scoring system is an assessment of the baby's physical condition, carried out by the midwife at 1 minute and 5 minutes after birth. There are five signs, each of which is awarded a score of 0, 1 or 2. A normal baby scores 7 to 10. The signs assessed (in order of importance) are:

- heart rate
- respiratory effort
- muscle tone
- reflex response to stimulus
- colour.

The screening for colour is not always used, reducing the range of the normal score to from 6 to 8; this is recorded as 'Apgar minus colour' to avoid confusion. Scores below 7 (or 6) indicate a varying degree of asphyxia requiring resuscitation. The criteria used to score each sign are as follows:

Sign	0	1	2
Heart rate	Absent	<100 beats/min	>100 beats/min
Respiratory effort	Absent	Slow, irregular	Good or crying
Muscle tone	Limp	Some flexion of limbs	Active
Reflex response to stimulus	None	Minimal grimace	Cough or sneeze
Colour	Blue/pale	Body pink, extremities blue	Completely pink

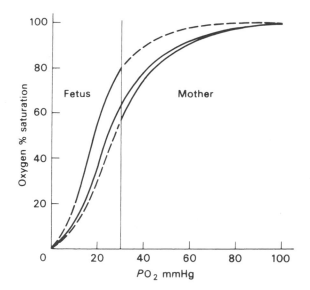

Figure 31.14 Oxygen–haemoglobin dissociation curves of fetal and maternal blood. The unbroken, continuous line in the centre is the curve for normal adult blood. (From Hytten F, Chamberlain G 1991 Clinical physiology in obstetrics, 2nd edn, Figure 18.1, by permission of Blackwell Scientific Publications Ltd.)

When the delivery of a baby is managed by a midwife, or doctor, the umbilical cord is clamped and cut sometime before the delivery of the placenta (third stage of labour). If the baby arrives quickly at home, or in a public place, without professional help, then it is safest not to tamper with the cord because the risk of infection and haemorrhage would be high. The baby (and the placenta if it has been expelled) should be wrapped warmly and professional help sought.

secure balance is achieved between input and output of water and electrolytes.

Before birth

The fetus consists largely of water (more than 80% of body weight) (compare adult values; Ch. 14). During fetal development most of this fluid is extracellular, but by 38 weeks the ratio of extracellular to intracellular fluid is about 50:50.

The fetal kidneys produce urine from 9 to 12 weeks of life. The urine formed is excreted into the amniotic cavity, contributing to the amniotic fluid enveloping the baby. The amniotic fluid also consists of fluid from the lungs and the skin. Amniotic fluid provides the baby with some freedom to exercise its growing limbs, which is important for proper development of the musculo-skeletal system.

Amniotic fluid is swallowed by the fetus, and its components are absorbed by the digestive tract and re-excreted.

At birth

At birth, the fluid present in the lungs is squeezed out as the fetus is pushed through the narrow birth canal. After the baby has been delivered, blood may drain from the placenta into the fetus (placento-fetal transfusion). As about 33% of fetal blood volume is contained within the vessels of the placenta this transfusion may be quite large. The size of the transfusion depends on how quickly the cord is clamped. The volume transfused affects the neonate's blood pressure (pressure depends partly on blood volume) and the total number of red cells in the fetal circulation.

After birth

After birth, the baby loses water through its skin, which is much thinner than in the adult, and water and electrolytes through the kidneys. As these losses are not immediately matched by an equivalent increase in fluid intake, the baby loses weight (up to 10% of its birth weight within the first few days). Most of this loss is from the extracellular fluid compartment (interstitial fluid and plasma).

As endocrine and renal systems (see Chs 11 and 8) adapt to new circumstances, the kidneys conserve more water and salt, and urinary losses decrease (Fig. 31.13). Simultaneously the intake of fluid increases as oral feeding begins and a new balance is established.

Over the first 2 to 3 years of life the power of the kidneys to conserve water and salts, and to excrete waste increases, with the result that the growing child is better able to tolerate disturbances in fluid and electrolyte balance. Until then, babies and young children are at greater risk of dehydration than an adult, especially during episodes of diarrhoea and vomiting.

NUTRIENT SUPPLIES

In the last few months of fetal life, stores are built up, providing the neonate with reserves to draw upon immediately after birth. After birth the digestive system (see Ch. 9) rapidly adapts to processing milk instead of amniotic fluid, and endocrine control systems gradually adapt to meet the challenges posed by intermittent feeding, increased activity and other stresses.

Before birth

In utero, all nutrients were supplied to the fetus through the placenta. Fetal glucose concentration is about half that in the mother and varies with her plasma glucose concentration. Towards the end of fetal development stores of fat and carbohydrate build up (Table 31.3).

At birth

The stress of birth increases activity in the sympathetic nervous system, and large amounts of adrenal medullary hormones (adrenaline and noradrenaline) are secreted. These hormones promote the breakdown of glycogen to glucose, and fats to fatty acids (see Chs 11 and 18). This increases plasma glucose concentration immediately after birth (Fig. 31.13), helping to maintain energy supplies when the supply of nutrients through the placenta ceases.

After birth

The neonatal digestive system rapidly adapts to processing a diet of milk. Digestive enzymes are synthe-sized and secreted to break down the constituents of milk. Of these, lactase is extremely important as it digests the main carbohydrate in milk, lactose. Movements of the gut propel the ingested milk through the digestive tract and push out accumulated waste materials. The first stool to be passed consists of epithelial cells, undigested mucus, and bile pigments (collectively referred to as meconium). The stool is black or dark green in colour due to the presence of bile pigments (see Ch. 10). In a few days the stools become greeny-brown. Eventually, as breast feeding is established and the digestive system develops, the soft stools become yellowish. Bowel motions occur very frequently, up to seven times a day in breast-fed babies, and evacuation occurs reflexly.

One of the major changes occurring after birth is increased secretion of many gastrointestinal hormones, including gastrin, CCK-PZ, motilin and GIP (see Ch. 9). These hormones:

- promote the growth of the digestive system
- stimulate digestive activity
- promote the secretion of insulin.

DEFENCE AND WASTE DISPOSAL

The newborn baby has to develop its ability to deal with bacteria, viruses, toxins and other environmental chemicals. As with the other systems, there are at first some short-term measures tiding the neonate over while its own systems of immunity and waste disposal develop.

Immunity

Before birth, some antibodies (IgG class; see Ch. 16) cross the placenta from mother to fetus, providing the neonate with some protection against bacterial infection. After birth, the neonate acquires more maternal antibodies (IgG, IgA and IgM) from breast milk.

Lymphoid tissue forms early in development (from the fifth week of life) and develops through fetal and neonatal life, infancy and childhood until puberty. Tonsils and adenoids reach their maximum size at about the age of 6 years, whereas the thymus, though already relatively large at birth (Fig. 31.11A), attains its maximum size around puberty.

Disposal of liposoluble waste

One of the problems faced by the newborn is the elimination of liposoluble waste materials, such as bilirubin. In utero, these substances passed across the placenta by passive diffusion and were processed by the mother's liver, before being excreted in her urine (see Chs 10 and 8). At birth, the capacity of the neonatal liver to process such substances is low. This contributes to the

Infant immunization schedules

Prior to the introduction of wide-scale immunization in the 1950s, the prevalence of childhood infectious diseases was responsible for the high infant mortality rate. In 1940 there were 46 281 cases of diphtheria with 2480 deaths; between 1979 and 1986 there were 26 cases and 1 death. The cases of paralytic polio were reduced from 4000 in 1955 to 35 between 1974 and 1978 – this included 25 cases in 1976–1977 when infection occurred in unvaccinated people. Since the introduction of immunization against measles in 1968, the number of notified cases has dropped from hundreds of thousands each year to an average of less than 100 000 – but up to 1992 there was still an average of 13 deaths a year. The most recent immunization to be introduced protects against Hib (*Haemophilus influenzae* type b) infection. This bacterium causes several illnesses, including one type of meningitis, severe croup, pneumonia, and joint, blood and bone infections. In 1992, Hib was the commonest cause of meningitis in children under 4 years old – about 65 died each year and about 150 were left with permanent brain damage (HEA 1992).

All children need help to fight against infectious diseases. The continuing death rate caused by measles is probably due to the reluctance of some parents to allow their children to be immunized. Unless there are contraindications specified by a doctor, all children should be immunized. The recognized schedule is as follows:

Vaccine	Age
Diphtheria/tetanus/pertussis, oral polio, Hib	1st dose: 2 months
	2nd dose: 3 months
	3rd dose: 4 months
Measles/mumps/rubella	12–18 months
Diphtheria/tetanus, oral polio	4–5 years

The presence of maternal antibodies in breast milk is just one of the reasons why it is the most suitable nourishment for the human baby. Modified cows' milk contains all the nutrients required by the baby but does not provide any protection against early infections.

jaundice occurring in some babies shortly after birth as a result of the breakdown of large numbers of red cells. After birth, enzyme systems, such as conjugases metabolizing liposoluble substances, increase in activity, with the result that waste products such as bilirubin are converted to water soluble products, and jaundice disappears, normally within a week.

It is important that the delivery room is comfortably warm, that the baby is dried, and is insulated from the cooler environment by clothing, or by nestling against its mother.

TEMPERATURE REGULATION

At birth, the baby is expelled from the relatively stable environment of the mother's uterus, into one which may be hot or cold and which may suddenly change from one to the other. The neonate's ability to thermoregulate is very limited.

Before birth

The fetus produces heat through metabolism, and in the later stages of pregnancy from the exercise it has kicking and moving inside the uterus. Fetal temperature (38°C) is above that of the amniotic fluid (37°C). Surplus heat is carried away in the blood flowing through the placenta. In utero the danger to the fetus is usually one of overheating. If the mother's body temperature rises in a fever, fetal temperature rises too.

At birth

At birth, there is usually very rapid heat loss. There can be a fall of 1°C every 5 minutes in some circumstances, for example in an exposed, very low birth weight (1 kg) baby, resulting rapidly in hypothermia. In a cold environment the baby loses heat by:

- conduction and convection to the cooler air
- evaporation of water from its skin
- radiation to colder objects such as windows and walls.

After birth

Temperature regulating mechanisms (see Ch. 17) gradually mature in the first few years of life but during this time the infant or young child is especially vulnerable to extremes of temperature, and depends on the caregiver for protection.

Heat production

The neonate generates heat in several ways:

- basal metabolism (high basal rate; see Ch. 17)
- assimilation and metabolism of food
- physical activity
- metabolism of brown adipose tissue (BAT).

Of these, the main source of extra heat in a cold environment is BAT. There is brown adipose tissue over the shoulders, around the kidneys and over the heart. BAT is a useful source of energy but it is only an emergency mechanism. Energy from the diet which is used to generate heat reduces that available to power growth.

Heat loss

Newborn babies lose heat relatively easily because of:

- large surface:volume ratio
- transepidermal water loss.

For its mass, a baby has a proportionately larger skin surface area than an adult and consequently loses relatively more heat by convection, conduction and radiation. Also the skin of the newborn is very thin, particularly in premature infants. A lot of water is lost through it and heat is used up in evaporating this water from the skin surface. However, adaptation of the skin occurs rapidly in the weeks after birth and water losses decrease.

Maintaining body temperature

The thermoneutral zone (see Ch. 17) for babies is about 32 to 36°C. Below this range of environmental temperatures, the naked baby maintains core temperature chiefly by increased metabolism of brown fat (non-shivering thermogenesis; see Ch. 17 and Fig. 31.15). Blood flow to the skin, and therefore heat loss, is reduced by vasoconstriction. However, the best insulation for a baby in a cold environment is suitable clothing and bedding.

Losing heat in a hot environment is also a problem for the newborn in that sweating mechanisms are not yet very effective. The number of active sweat glands increases steadily up to the age of about 2 years.

REFLEXES, AWARENESS AND ABILITIES

Although considerable development of the nervous system occurs before birth, maturation of the nervous system continues for many years afterwards. Maturation is visible to parents and friends in the almost daily changes occurring in the baby's and young child's awareness, behaviour and abilities. The newborn baby responds to the stimuli of light and sound and touch by simple reflexes. As maturation occurs during the first year of life, the infant develops the ability to make more complex movements and begins to make sense of the stimuli around it. Skills and understanding develop further in the second year of life when the infant begins to talk and to take charge of its own behaviour.

The first few months

The newborn baby responds reflexly to many different stimuli. In response to:

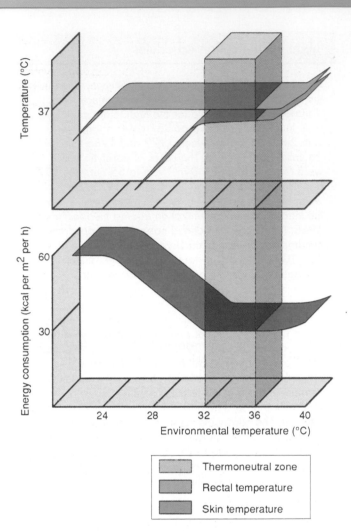

Figure 31.15 Maintenance of core body temperature in the naked neonate by cutaneous vasoconstriction and non-shivering thermogenesis. (After Rutter 1992 and Turner 1988, with permission of Elsevier.)

> If a baby's rectal temperature is normal but its skin feels cool, the baby is probably maintaining its body temperature by metabolizing brown fat and is therefore using up extra energy to stay warm.

- bright light – it blinks
- a sudden sound – it startles
- oral stimuli – it sucks
- an object pressed against its palm – it grasps
- backward movement of its head – it extends its arms (Moro reflex).

These are just a few of the many simple reflexes that can be elicited. The presence of the reflexes shows that the sense organs are functioning and that simple neural links have been established between sensory and motor systems.

As the baby grows older, and the nervous system matures, behaviour and capabilities change as reflex responses become more complicated. Whereas the newborn baby is simply startled in response to a sudden sound, the 3- to 4-month-old baby turns its head to face the source of the sound. Whereas a newborn baby simply gazes at a face, following every movement with its eyes, a 4- to 6-week-old baby responds to a familiar face (such as its mother's) by smiling.

Coordinated reflex activity of different muscle groups develops, enabling the baby to sit up, stay sitting and keep his head erect. What the baby lacks in his first few months of life and develops later is the careful control exercised by higher centres in the brain (cerebrum and cerebellum) over spinal and brain stem mechanisms (see Ch. 25). For example, when a baby of 3 to 4 months old reaches out for an object he usually misjudges where it is, rather like an adult with cerebellar dysfunction (see Ch. 25). A 6-month-old infant can voluntarily grasp an object in his hand but he has yet to develop the skill of picking things up with his fingers. He makes sounds but cannot yet form them into words. These skills of manipulation and speech rely on the maturation of function of the motor areas of the cerebral cortex and adjacent association areas, as well as the stimulation provided by the infant's environment.

The first year (infancy)

In the second 6 months of life the cerebellum and the cerebral cortex develop more control over posture and movement, and many neural links are forged within the association areas of the cerebral cortex (see Ch. 20).

Posture and movement

The infant progressively develops the ability to raise his head, sit, stand and then to walk, albeit in a tottering way. Control over head movements develops first, followed by control over arms and hands and then legs, the same sequence of maturation as in utero. As manipulative skills develop, the clumsy grasp is replaced by 1 year of age by a careful picking up of objects between finger and thumb. Coordination develops too so that the 9-month-old infant can, with some success, use a spoon to feed himself.

Understanding

At 7 months of age an infant usually responds to his name. Sufficient learning of the sound and the associated stimuli has occurred for him to respond appropriately. By 9 to 12 months of age he is able to imitate sounds and has understanding of the associations (meanings) of some of the complex sounds (words) he hears.

Occasionally, an infant becomes so adept at using gestures instead of sounds/words, and his parents equally adept at interpreting the gestures, that the development of speech is delayed. The infant knows the correct words and can say them, but pointing and grunting are often quicker and easier!

The second year (early childhood)

The developmental programme for the nervous system continues to unfold and to delight and surprise parents and friends with new behaviour and communication. Movements become more skilled, understanding develops, and the infant takes more control over what he does.

By about 13 months of age the infant can usually walk unaided but, rather like someone with Parkinson's disease (see Ch. 25), he has difficulty changing direction, for example when turning corners. He uses his hands a lot to build, pick up objects, and feed himself. He imitates his mother's actions. Sounds that he makes become strung together into language, at first unintelligible (to parents, that is) but then forming simple sentences. These new behaviours reflect the development of Wernicke's and Broca's areas (see Ch. 26).

By the age of 2 years, the child develops some understanding of the sensations associated with defecation and urination and begins to take deliberate action in response to them. This and other similar behaviours represent the beginnings of purposeful voluntary activity. More and more control is exercised over primitive reflex behaviours as the cerebrum increasingly dominates the activities of the brain stem and spinal cord.

GROWTH

Growth has been defined as 'the progressive development of a living being or part of an organism from its earliest stage to maturity, including the attendant increase in size' (Butterworths Medical Dictionary 1978). It includes therefore the changes occurring in the structure and properties of different cells as well as overall increases in the size of the body and its constituent parts. These changes follow a genetically determined pattern but are influenced by other factors including nutrition and hormones.

BODY SIZE

The most rapid period of growth occurs in utero (Fig. 31.16). Thereafter, there is steady growth in height

Developmental assessments

The health visitor carries out a series of developmental assessments until the child reaches school age. These assessments are usually carried out at home because a truer picture of the child's abilities is seen when he is in his own, familiar environment. Some assessments, such as hearing tests, may be performed at the health clinic because two experienced people are needed to test hearing accurately; all children have a hearing test when 8 to 9 months old. Health visitors receive special training in this skill.

Children can be assessed using the following broad headings:

- *Infant stimulation/motor (gross and fine)* – how a baby responds to his environment and progresses through sitting, crawling and walking, at the same time developing more precise skills, such as doing up buttons.
- *Cognitive* – general understanding, for example plays pat-a-cake, stacks blocks.
- *Development of language* – which is closely associated with hearing and vision.
- *Self-help* – how the child learns to feed, dress and wash himself.
- *Socialization* – how the child responds to others, parents, siblings, strangers.

These areas of development are all interrelated and must be used to form a whole picture of the child's development. For example, if a child has not developed the appropriate motor skills to stack blocks, it does not mean that he is lacking in understanding; similarly, a deaf or blind baby will not be able to respond in the normal way but is not necessarily lacking in intelligence.

Parents and those associated with childcare look for essential developmental milestones, for example the first smile at 4 to 6 weeks, and if these are not attained at the appropriate age further investigations may be necessary.

The following is a brief list of the main milestones:

4 to 6 weeks	Smiles – usually at mother
12 to 16 weeks	Turns head to sound
	Holds object placed in hand
12 to 20 weeks	Watches own hands – hand regard
20 weeks	Reaches for and grabs objects
26 weeks	Transfers objects from hand to hand
	Sits – supported by hands
	Chews and feeds self with a biscuit
	Lifts head when supine
9 to 10 months	Uses index finger to investigate objects
	Uses thumb and forefinger to pick up small objects
	Crawls/creeps
	Plays pat-a-cake, waves bye-bye
	Holds out arm for coat etc. when being dressed
13 months	Casting – throwing toys from cot, high chair
	Walks unaided
	Two to three single words
15 months	Stops casting
	Feeds self
	Stops putting objects in mouth (mouthing)
15 to 18 months	Mimics household tasks (e.g. dusting)
18 months	Becomes aware of toilet needs
21 to 24 months	Joining two to three words
2 years	Dry by day – occasional 'accident'
3 years	Dry by night
	Able to dress self except for difficult fastenings
	Able to stand, briefly, on one foot.

and weight until 'the adolescent' growth spurt preceding adulthood.

Height

Almost all of the height (97–98%) of the body is due to the bones of the skeleton and the intervening fibrocartilaginous discs. Growth in height therefore represents growth of bones and joints. Height depends also on posture and muscle strength.

Weight

The weight of the body depends largely on three tissues:
- bone
- muscle
- adipose tissue.

Body weight increases more or less in line with the increase in height, but whereas linear growth stops in adulthood because bones stop increasing in size, weight can continue to increase as a result of physical training, which develops muscle tissue, or of overeating, which increases fat stores (see Ch. 15).

Development of bones and teeth

Process

The connective tissue that is ultimately transformed into bone makes its appearance during the fifth week of life. It forms a model for the bone formation (ossification) beginning in the succeeding weeks.

The Portage home teaching scheme

Sadly, some children do not follow the normal pattern of mental development, and remain retarded throughout their lives. Early in the twentieth century these children were admitted to special hospitals for the mentally deficient where they received little, if any, stimulation. The Mental Health Act of 1960 abolished from legal usage the term 'mental deficiency' together with the classifications of idiot, imbecile and feeble minded. Since then, the terms 'mental subnormality' followed by 'mental handicap' have been used. More recently, the study of learning theories has increased the understanding of the problem, and affected children are referred to as having specific learning disabilities – in other words, they are no longer graded and labelled. Most people with learning disabilities are not physically ill and whenever possible they are cared for in the community, preferably at home. There are various schemes for helping the pre-school child who has a learning disability; one is known as the Portage Home Teaching Scheme.

Portage is the name of a town in Wisconsin, USA where the model was first developed by David and Martha Shearer and their colleagues. It is a home teaching service for pre-school children with specific learning disabilities. To qualify for home teaching, the child has to be at least 1 year behind the normal development expected for his age, except in the case of babies born with known handicapping disorders such as Down syndrome. For Down syndrome babies, the teaching is commenced as soon as the diagnosis is confirmed; for example the mother is shown how to provide extra stimulation of all the senses and to note the baby's responses. This helps to identify areas where the baby's learning may be particularly slow.

The home teaching team is usually led by a senior clinical psychologist and the teachers may be professional people, for example health visitors, social workers or others trained to use the system. After assessment of the child by the psychologist, the teacher visits on a weekly basis, setting precise tasks for the mother (or carer) to carry out with the child each day. The teacher assesses the child's ability to achieve the task and sets criteria for attainment; for example 'Ben will pull off socks', to be carried out four times a day, success criterion – three times out of four. Ben will have had previous tasks where he has pulled off his socks with help; now he is expected to manage unaided. These tasks cover all areas of development – socialization, language, self-help, cognitive and motor ability. The children's progress is discussed with the team at weekly meetings, ideas are exchanged and the psychologist gives advice.

Opinions vary regarding the efficacy of this type of teaching. It is not possible to have a control group because learning disabilities in children cannot be matched, for example no two children with Down syndrome are alike in their abilities. Undoubtedly there are remarkable improvements in some children, but the exact reason cannot be defined; is it the teaching, the intensive visiting, the support for the carers, or a bit of each? Some find the form of teaching unacceptable – it is based on operant conditioning which can be seen as learning tricks for rewards. Whatever the opinions of normal people, many children with specific learning disabilities have been helped to reach their full potential and to integrate well into the school environment.

The first centres of ossification to become established are termed primary centres. These are followed by secondary centres (epiphyses) (Fig. 31.17). In each developing bone the epiphyses are separated from the primary centres by a layer of cartilage termed the epiphyseal plate.

As growth proceeds the cartilage is gradually replaced by bone, including that between the primary and secondary centres. The latter event is termed fusion of the epiphyses. When it occurs in the long bones (of the legs and arms) at 16 to 21 years of age it marks the end of their longitudinal growth. The stage of development of the bones can be used to assess the developmental stage a child has reached (Figs 31.18 and 31.19).

Rates of growth

When bones grow, they do not grow at a uniform rate all over. In the limb bones, for example, more growth usually occurs at one end than the other. This can be important in deciding management of a fracture in a child. Also different bones mature at different rates. The development of the bones of the pelvis and lower limbs lags behind that of the upper limbs and shoulder girdle. Some of the last bones to complete development are those of the vertebral column and those of the base of the skull which continue to mature until about the age of 25 years.

Skull

In the infant, the bones of the skull are not fused together. There are gaps between them (the largest termed fontanelles) filled with fibrous connective tissue (Fig. 31.20). These gaps allow movement, which is important especially at the time of birth. The largest gap, the anterior fontanelle, is filled in by the end of the second year of life.

The shape of the skull changes greatly from infancy to adulthood, largely because of the growth still occurring

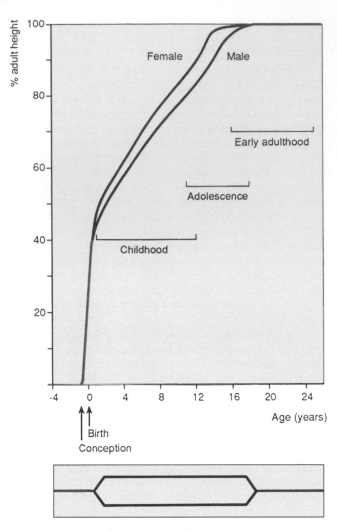

Figure 31.16 Growth in height from conception to maturity: boys and girls in the UK. (After Moore 1988 and Tanner 1989.)

Care of a child's teeth should begin as soon as the teeth erupt. A small, soft toothbrush moistened with water is usually sufficient until the child is able to cooperate with spitting out toothpaste – an activity enjoyed by most children. Initially the aim is for the child to get used to having the brush put in his mouth. If the gums are sore because more teeth are erupting, then it might be necessary to stop using the brush for a day or two. Conservation of primary teeth, apart from maintaining the normal function of biting and chewing, helps the growing jaw to retain a good shape and may avoid crooked eruption of the permanent teeth.

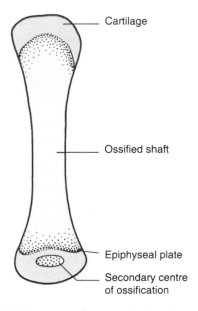

Figure 31.17 Structure of a growing long bone.

at the base of the skull and the development of the teeth. This is one of the reasons why facial features change so much during childhood, adolescence and early adulthood.

Teeth

The primary teeth begin to calcify at 4 to 6 months of fetal life. In the infant, the first teeth to erupt are usually the mandibular incisors. The secondary teeth develop inside the jaw bones and begin to push through and displace the primary teeth at about 6 years of age (Fig. 31.21). Whereas the second permanent molar erupts consistently at about 12 years of age (apparently used in the UK at one time to indicate when a child could be put to work!) the third molars (wisdom teeth) come through at any age from 18 years onwards or may not erupt at all.

CONTROL OF GROWTH

The main factors influencing growth are:

- genetic
- hormonal
- nutritional
- environmental.

Genetic factors

The developmental sequence and its expression is predetermined by the instructions coded in our DNA. There are separate genes coding for different aspects of body shape and form, and a huge variety of genes leading to differences in features between different individuals. For example, there are different genes responsible for determining the growth of the long bones as compared with other parts of the body.

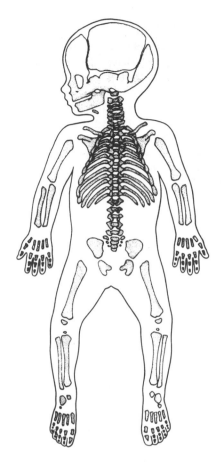

Figure 31.18 Ossification of the skeleton in a newborn baby. (From Sinclair D 1989 Human growth after birth, 5th edn, Figure 4.2, by permission of Oxford University Press.)

A defect in the gene controlling the length of the long bones gives rise to achondroplasia, a form of dwarfism in which only growth of the limbs is deficient. Other parts of the body grow normally.

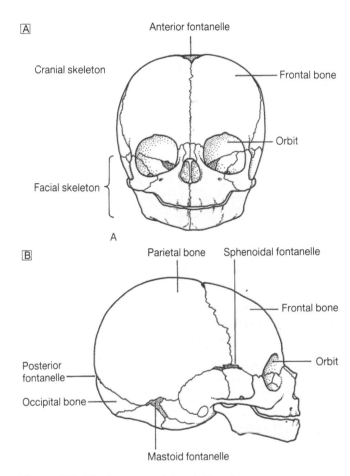

Figure 31.20 Structure of the skull in the neonate. A, From the front (anterior view). B, From the side (lateral view). (From Rogers 1992, with permission of Elsevier.)

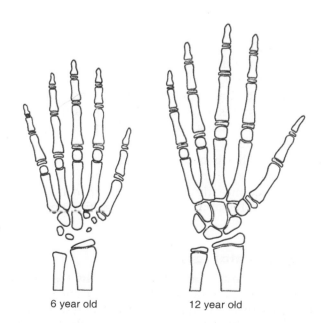

6 year old   12 year old

Figure 31.19 Development of the bones of the wrist and hand in a 6 year old (left) and a 12 year old (right). (After Rogers 1992, with permission of Elsevier.)

The unique combination of genes each person possesses (identical twins excepted) leads to individual differences between people. An obvious difference in the genetic blueprint is that between males and females. Differences in only 240 bases in a molecule of DNA (see Ch. 1) give rise to the different characteristics of male and female persons including the different timescale of development between the sexes (see p. 536) as well as ultimate differences in height, body composition and form.

Hormonal factors

Hormonal factors of importance include:

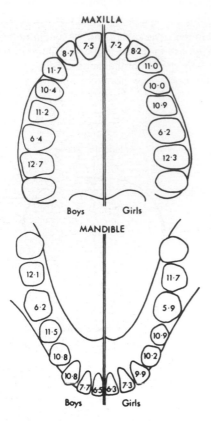

Figure 31.21 Average times of eruption (in years) of the secondary teeth. The times of eruption of the third molars (wisdom teeth) are not shown because they are so variable. (From Sinclair D 1989 Human growth after birth, 5th edn, Figure 5.2, by permission of Oxford University Press.)

- human chorionic somatomammotrophin (HCS)
- androgens (fetal, adrenal and gonadal)
- thyroxine
- somatotrophin.

The importance of each of these varies at different stages of life from that in utero, through childhood and into adolescence.

In utero

The factors controlling growth at this stage are not well understood. It is probable that at very early stages of life, growth and development are determined by substances secreted locally by all cells. As tissues differentiate, regulators of growth produced by specific endocrine glands and tissues become important, for example:

- HCS secreted by the placenta
- androgens secreted by the fetal adrenal glands
- thyroid hormones.

HCS (also known as placental lactogen; see Ch. 30) stimulates the production of somatomedins by all fetal tissues. These hormones promote growth.

Infancy and childhood

The fetal adrenal glands (Fig. 31.11B) regress after birth and the zone in the cortex that secretes androgens shrinks in size. However, other endocrine glands, including the pituitary and the thyroid, grow steadily. Thyroid hormones (see Ch. 11) are important for maturation of bones, teeth and the brain. Deficiency of thyroid hormones in childhood leads to cretinism.

Somatotrophin (human growth hormone) secreted by the anterior pituitary (see Ch. 11) has a major role in determining growth after birth. It:

- stimulates cell division
- stimulates the formation of DNA
- maintains protein synthesis
- stimulates somatomedin production by liver and kidney.

Somatomedins stimulate the proliferation of cartilage and therefore affect the linear growth of bones.

Adolescence

The beginning of adolescence is marked by increased secretion of the gonadotrophins, follicle stimulating hormone (FSH) and luteinizing hormone (LH). These hormones stimulate the ovaries and the testes to mature and increase their secretion of oestrogens and testosterone respectively (see p. 535). Simultaneously, the secretion of adrenal androgens is increased in both sexes. The secretion of androgens stimulates growth, and the secretion of gonadal hormones leads to the different characteristics expressed in male and female individuals, including differences in height and build.

Nutritional factors

Growth requires an adequate supply of raw materials. If there is malnutrition, growth is retarded. Malnutrition can occur in utero in the final stages of fetal development as a result of placental inadequacy, or, after birth, as a result of deprivation. All tissues are not affected to the same extent. The supplies to some tissues seem to be protected at the expense of supplies to others. In childhood, catch-up growth of height and weight usually occurs once adequate food is provided, but deprivation early in life may permanently affect development by limiting supplies at critical periods of growth.

Environmental factors

Before birth (antenatally) the baby's environment is dictated by the conditions in utero, and the mother's state of health and well-being. After birth (postnatally), environment in its widest sense can include any external stimuli affecting the baby whether these be opportunities to run and play, disturbances of family life affecting the infant's emotional development, or other physical factors such as time of year.

Antenatal

Babies that are 'small for dates' may have experienced retardation of growth because of impaired nutrition or because of the toxic effects of substances present in the mother's bloodstream. It is now well known that mothers who smoke or who drink alcohol regularly tend to give birth to babies that are smaller than expected.

Postnatal

Children who experience emotional upset may not grow as well as those who grow up in a secure environment. This is likely to be mediated via the hypothalamus and limbic system (see Ch. 20).

Interestingly, children grow at different rates at different times during the year. The rate of growth in height tends to be greatest in the springtime whereas the rate of growth in weight is greatest in the autumn. These annual changes in growth rate may be related to the changes in length of daylight during the year. Light and dark is known to affect various body systems.

ADOLESCENCE AND PUBERTY

Adolescence is the period of time during which the developing human undergoes his/her final stages of physical maturation. Puberty is that time during adolescence when secondary sexual characteristics appear and the reproductive system matures sufficiently for reproduction to be possible. These changes are triggered by increased secretion of the gonadotrophins by the anterior pituitary gland. The gonadotrophins excite the gonads to secrete steroid hormones, such as oestradiol and testosterone, that have widespread effects on many body cells and tissues including the reproductive organs.

The timing of development varies between individuals with the result that, during the teenage years, individuals of exactly the same age may have attained very different stages of development.

HORMONAL CHANGES AND EFFECTS

During childhood, the pituitary gland secretes small amounts of the gonadotrophins. The beginning of adolescence is marked by the start of pulsatile secretion of gonadotrophin releasing hormone (GnRH – also known as LHRH) from the hypothalamus (Fig. 31.22), which brings about pulsatile secretion of the gonado-

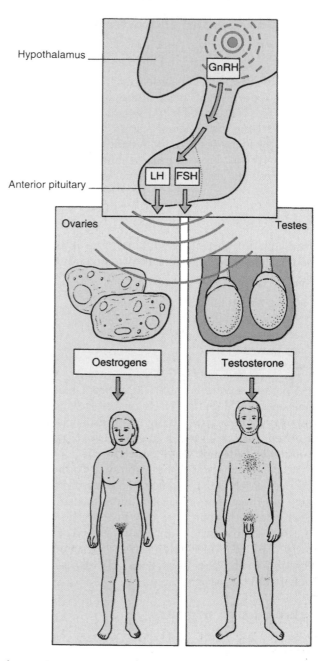

Figure 31.22 Hormonal control of puberty.

trophins, FSH and LH. These hormones in turn promote the development of the gonads, increasing their secretion of oestrogens in girls and testosterone in boys. Simultaneously the secretion of androgens by the adrenal gland increases, due possibly to another, as yet unidentified, pituitary hormone.

Together these hormones affect cellular function in many different tissues, resulting in:

- development of the secondary sexual characteristics
- maturation of the reproductive organs
- changes in psyche and behaviour.

Secondary sexual characteristics

Female

In girls, the first external evidence of the radical changes that are about to take place is the development of the breasts. This is followed by growth of pubic and axillary hair. Simultaneously there is a spurt in the growth rate, and height increases rapidly. As adolescence proceeds, the growth of bones, muscle and adipose tissue accelerates, and the characteristic female proportions develop.

Male

The changes occurring in boys are more extensive. The vastly increased secretion of testosterone from the testes affects:

- body growth
- external genitalia
- vocal cords
- hair growth
- sebaceous glands.

The broad-shouldered, muscular proportions of the male are caused by the effect of testosterone on bone and muscle tissue. Eventually this androgen also causes fusion of the epiphyses in the long bones, resulting in termination of longitudinal bone growth.

The penis grows and the scrotum becomes wrinkly and pigmented. As in women, the body becomes more hairy but there is more of it in more places, including the chest and the chin.

Growth of the larynx and enlargement of the vocal cords leads to deepening of the voice. Increased secretion from the sebaceous glands predisposes adolescent boys to acne.

Reproductive organs

Female

Internally, oestrogens facilitate growth of the ovarian follicles and promote the development of the muscle,

Acne is a distressing condition for the adolescent. It affects both boys and girls, being at its worst in girls between 16 and 17 years, and in boys between 17 and 19 years. It occurs at a time when self-confidence is often low and one's appearance is very important. Understanding of the misery it causes is needed, rather than a dismissive 'you'll grow out of it'. There are a variety of treatments available, including locally applied gels, antibiotic therapy, the drug isotretinoin which reduces sebum secretion, and hormonal treatment.

blood vessels and secretory lining of the uterus. The fact of this maturation becomes evident at the first menstrual bleed (menarche) when the lining, built up under the action of oestrogens, breaks down. Initially, menstrual cycles are not accompanied by ovulation (anovulatory cycles) but, after 12 to 18 months, ovulation becomes a regular feature, progesterone is secreted, and the adult pattern of hormonal change and events in the menstrual cycle is established (see Ch. 30). From this time on, the woman is fertile and reproduction is possible.

The time at which puberty begins may be linked to the attainment of a predetermined weight for height. As nutrition and health care has improved enormously in the Western world over the last 150 years, that weight has been attained at ever earlier ages. It is believed that this is the reason that the average age of puberty has declined over the last 150 years in the UK and USA from about 17 to 13 years. Menarche does not occur in girls until after the peak spurt of growth in height is over.

Male

At the start of adolescence, the testes begin to enlarge. Within them, the primitive germ cells, spermatogonia, are stimulated by FSH and testosterone to mature into fully fledged spermatozoa. Simultaneously the glands of the male reproductive system enlarge and secrete increased amounts of the fluids supporting the sperm. The seminal glands for example begin to secrete fructose, a sugar which sperm cells use for nourishment.

Psyche

At puberty the divergent physical development in young men and women is paralleled by divergence in behaviour. Young men tend to be more aggressive than women and this appears to be related to the level of secretion of testosterone. During adolescence the interaction between the sexes alters. Most young men begin to find a developing interest in young women and vice versa. These changes in behaviour are complex and depend on the social context as well as changing levels of hormones.

Some people do not develop heterosexual attractions and instead find people of the same sex to be sexually attractive (homosexuality). The reasons for this are still unclear. Genetic, psychological and social factors may all be involved, the particular blend of influential factors probably differing from one person to another.

Another significant change in adolescence is in socialization – the growth in understanding of interactions between people and the ability to communicate in more subtle ways. One disorder of mental development that may emerge in a small minority of people in their late teens is schizophrenia. It may be due to abnormality in the development of neural pathways involved in social interaction.

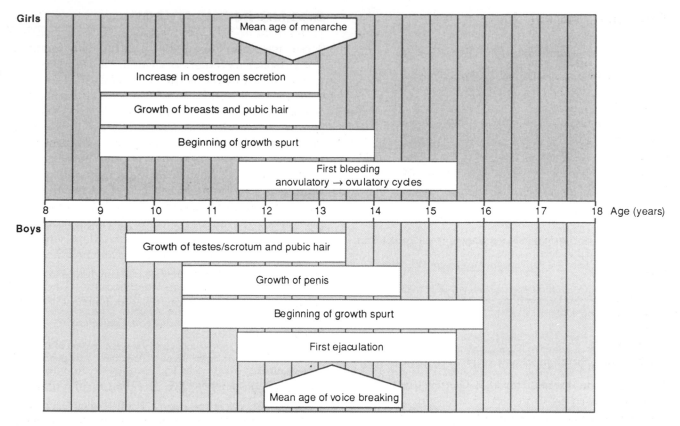

Figure 31.23 Timing of onset of various events during adolescence in girls and boys showing the wide range in age of onset. (After Bancroft 1989, with permission of Elsevier.)

EARLY AND LATE DEVELOPERS

The onset of puberty in boys and girls varies considerably between individuals (Fig. 31.23) with the result that teenagers of the same age may be at very different stages of sexual development. In a group of 14-year-olds there will be some who have barely begun pubertal change as well as those who have fully matured sexually. Those who are quick to mature physically tend also to score better on intelligence tests than those of the same age who have not reached the same stage of physical development.

These temporary biological differences can give rise to many psychological problems ranging from an unwarranted sense of inferiority in the late developer, to a feeling of frustration in the early developer, mature in body but constrained by society's definitions of 'age of maturity'.

PHYSIOLOGY OF THE CLIMACTERIC

A marked reduction occurs in the secretion of ovarian hormones in women in their late forties and early fifties, resulting in atrophy of reproductive organs and tissues in addition to affecting other systems and structures such as the cardiovascular system and the skeleton. The term menopause denotes the permanent cessation of menstruation in women. However, this is only one aspect of the climacteric – the years over which these major changes occur in the structure and function of the reproductive organs resulting in diminished reproductive capacity. During this time women experience endocrine, somatic and psychological changes due to physiological factors related to generic ageing and oestrogen depletion due to ageing specific to the ovaries.

The average age of the menopause, which has not changed since ancient times, is 51 years of age. However, approximately 4% of women undergo a *natural* menopause *prior* to 40 years of age. With a trend of increase in life expectancy in women in the Western world, a significant amount of a woman's lifetime will be following the climacteric. It is important, therefore, to increase understanding of the climacteric to ensure that women can continue to lead healthy and productive lives. The onset of the climacteric does not appear to be delayed by any factor such as

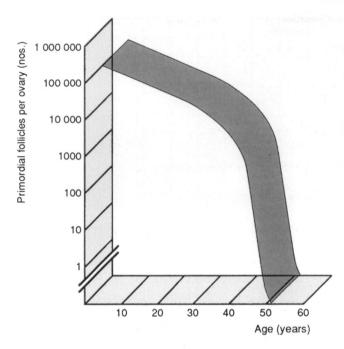

Figure 31.24 Decline in the number of primordial follicles with age. (After Richardson et al 1987, incorporating data of Block 1952.)

experiencing several pregnancies, hormonal contraceptive use or where there is hypothalamic amenorrhoea. Neither is the onset of the climacteric related to the onset of the menarche, race, height, weight or socio-economic conditions. It may be, however, that the menopause occurs earlier in women who smoke.

The ageing process of the ovary begins during fetal development. Although approximately seven million oogonia are present at 20 weeks' gestation, this number has decreased to 700 000 at birth. Following birth, the number again declines before the onset of puberty. During the adult reproductive years, successive cycles of ovulation and atresia deplete the ovaries of their follicles, so that by age 50, few if any are left (Fig. 31.24). This results in a decrease of oestrogen secretion and eventually cessation of menses. The appearance of the ovary in postmenopausal women demonstrates a reduction in size, a weight of less than 2.5 grams and a wrinkled, prune-like surface.

The decline in ovarian function during the climacteric impacts on two main components:

• troublesome conditions which have a perceived negative impact (i.e. hot flushes, psychological symptoms and urogenital atrophy)
• ill-health conditions which have a serious effect on female morbidity and mortality (i.e. osteoporosis and atherosclerosis).

AGEING IN THE OVARY

Successive cycles of ovulation and degeneration in the ovary deplete its content of ovarian follicles. This leads to the menopause, the final episode of bleeding in women. For several years prior to the menopause, oestradiol and progesterone production decline despite the occurrence of ovulatory cycles. This waning of ovarian oestrogen and inhibin secretion reduces the negative feedback inhibition on the hypothalamic–pituitary system, which in turn results in a gradual increase in FSH levels (Fig. 31.25). However, the residual ovarian follicles are increasingly less responsive to FSH, with the menopause occurring when these follicles do not respond to elevated levels of FSH. Postmenopausal women do have some circulating oestrogen despite this depleted ovarian follicle source – an adrenal androgen (androstenedione) undergoes change in peripheral tissues to oestrone.

Vasomotor flushes

One of the most common and negatively perceived symptoms for women at the climacteric are vasomotor flushes. Hot flushes are the result of cutaneous vasodilation that is caused by an acute lowering in the hypothalamic thermoregulatory set point. A sudden reduction in oestrogen levels serves to destabilize the thermoregulatory centre through multiple effects on neurotransmitters. More than 80% of women will experience hot flushes within 3 months of a natural or surgical menopause, with the majority having these for over 1 year. A woman may suddenly feel very hot, have a flushed skin, and begin to sweat (hot flushes). As this is followed by vasoconstriction, she may then feel chilled. Symptoms may continue for a while after the menopause as tissues are still adapting to fluctuating levels in hormones.

Genital atrophy

The tissues of the lower vagina, labia, urethra and trigone (of the bladder) are all oestrogen dependent; thus the loss of oestrogen at the menopause causes multiple effects. The protective elements of vascularity, elasticity and an acidic pH in the vagina are lost due to atrophic changes and loss of glycogen in the atrophied walls of the vagina. As a result, women may complain of dyspareunia and symptoms secondary to vaginal ulceration or infection. The urethra and urinary trigone experience similar atrophic changes which can result in dysuria, urgency, frequency and suprapubic discomfort.

Osteoporosis

This is progressive reduction in bone mass which in women is mainly caused by oestrogen deficiency. It

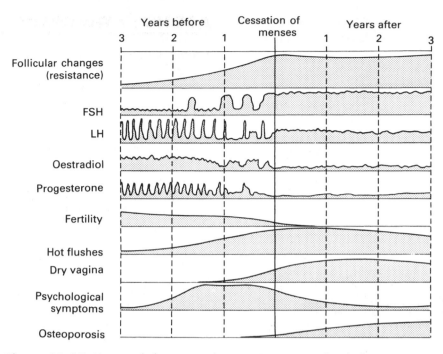

Figure 31.25 Hormonal changes and symptoms associated with the menopause. (From Bancroft 1989, with permission of Elsevier.)

develops when the rate of bone resorption exceeds the rate of bone formation. Oestrogen receptors are present in bone, thus oestrogen may act directly on bone to promote bone formation and reduce bone resorption. In addition, it is suggested that oestrogen decreases the sensitivity of bone to parathyroid hormone and increases calcitonin levels.

Peak bone mass is achieved at around age 30. After age 40, bone mass decreases but increasingly so at the time of the menopause (Fig. 31.26). Thus acute reduction in oestrogen levels during the menopause causes osteoporosis in susceptible women at a higher risk (white Caucasians, Orientals, thin women and those with a genetic or dietary predisposition to osteoporosis). Significantly, *once osteoporosis is established, it cannot be reversed*; thus an objective of health promotion agencies is to screen and initiate treatment in women showing early bone loss using hormone replacement therapy before fractures occur, commonly in the vertebral bodies, distal radius, femoral neck or hips.

Atherosclerosis

Research has suggested that oestrogens protect against the incidence of cardiovascular disease (CVD) because women experience a lower incidence of CVD than men across all age groupings. However, there is a rapid increase in female mortality from CVD after the menopause. Currently, various mechanisms are postulated as to why this premenopausal protective element is lost during the climacteric. These focus on the following:

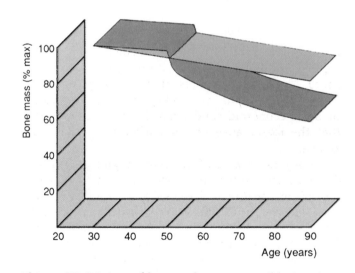

Figure 31.26 Loss of bone with age in men (blue) and women (purple). (Constructed from data in Rowe & Besdine 1988, and Hukins & Nelson 1987.)

- loss of oestrogens from the ovary exacerbates the oxidation of low-density lipoproteins, which increases atherogenecity
- lack of oestrogens alters prostaglandin metabolism, decreasing prostacyclin levels and increasing thromboxane levels, all of which promotes vasoconstriction
- lack of oestrogen acts on vessel walls to produce vasoconstriction.

Further research is required to establish the integrated effects of reduction in oestrogen levels in the climacteric period.

Psychological symptoms

Changes in steroidal levels are associated with alterations in mood. During the climacteric, when the secretion of steroid hormones declines, women may experience a variety of psychological symptoms:

- difficulty in concentration
- forgetfulness
- anxiety
- loss in confidence
- feelings of unworthiness.

These symptoms may persist for a time following the menopause when hormonal levels may be fluctuating. When symptoms have become problematic, medical treatment may be used with varying success.

Treatment of menopausal symptoms

Current debate in recent years has focused on the possible advantages, efficacy and adverse effects of various treatments for menopausal women:

- Randomized controlled trials have found that oestrogen replacement therapy relieves symptoms of urogenital atrophy and vasomotor symptoms and improves the quality in the short term.
- Pooled findings from various studies indicate that long-term use of oestrogen is associated with an increased risk of thromboembolic disorders, endometrial and breast cancers.
- In relation to drug therapy, progestogens relieve vasomotor symptoms when used in high doses; tibolone relieves vasomotor symptoms and improves sexual symptoms; clonidine reduces hot flushes.
- Other drug therapies using e.g. testosterone, antidepressants have not been shown to be effective in treating menopausal women.
- There is limited research evidence to suggest that soya flour, which contains phytooestrogens, is effective in relieving vasomotor menopausal symptoms.

MEN AND REPRODUCTIVE AGEING

In contrast to women, there is no age at which reproductive function naturally ceases. There are well-attested instances of men's ability to father children even into their nineties. However, changes do occur, albeit very gradually and to differing extents between individuals:

HORMONES

It is common, though not universal, for a decline in testicular function to occur as men grow older. This results in a decrease in testosterone secretion. Simultaneously, plasma concentrations of FSH and LH increase.

SEXUAL FUNCTION

Sperm continue to be produced throughout the life span. However, the speed and intensity of responses to sexual stimulation and frequency of sexual activity decreases with age.

REFERENCES AND FURTHER READING

Bancroft J 1989 Human sexuality and its problems, 2nd edn. Churchill Livingstone, Edinburgh
Very useful authoritative book on all aspects of human sexuality, including its biological basis and development

Behrman R E, Kleigman R 1990 Nelson's Essentials of paediatrics. W B Saunders, Philadelphia

Bennett V R, Brown L K (eds) 1993 Myles' Textbook for midwives, 12th edn. Churchill Livingstone, Edinburgh

Block E 1952 Quantitative morphological investigation of the follicular system in women. Acta Anatomica 14: 108

Campbell A G M, McIntosh N 1992 Forfar & Amell's Textbook of paediatrics, 4th edn. Churchill Livingstone, Edinburgh

Carr B 1993 The ovary. In: Carr B, Blackwell R. Textbook of reproductive medicine. Appleton & Lange, East Norwalk, CT

Case R M (ed) 1985 Variations in human physiology. Manchester University Press, Manchester
Contains a useful chapter giving more detailed information about physiological changes before and after birth

Critchley M (ed) 1978 Butterworths medical dictionary, 2nd edn. Butterworths, London

Davis J A, Dobbing J 1981 Scientific foundations of paediatrics, 2nd edn. Heinemann, London

Falkner F, Tanner J M 1986 Human growth. Plenum Publishing, New York
Authoritative three volume specialist review of human growth

HEA 1992 Protect your child with the new Hib immunisation. Health Education Authority Leaflet, Department of Health, London

Hukins D W L, Nelson M A 1987 The ageing spine. Manchester University Press, Manchester

Hytten F, Chamberlain G 1991 Clinical physiology in obstetrics, 2nd edn. Blackwell Scientific Publications, Oxford
Reference text. Further information on placental function

Illingworth R S 1987 The development of the infant and young child: normal and abnormal, 9th edn. Churchill Livingstone, Edinburgh
Authoritative specialist text, detailing the characteristics of the developing child and what the paediatrician looks for and why. Useful for reference

Illingworth R S 1991 The normal child, 10th edn. Churchill Livingstone, Edinburgh

Larsen W J 1993 Human embryology. Churchill Livingstone, Edinburgh
Well-illustrated detailed text, written for medical students. Useful source of further information

Leaflet MM/005/889/A200a A parent's guide to immunisation, 2nd edn. Merieux UK

Miller G A 1992 Psychology. The science of mental life. Pelican Books, London

Moore K L 1988 The developing human, 4th edn. W B Saunders, Philadelphia
Clinically oriented textbook of embryology written for medical students. Provides an overview of development, as well as detailed descriptions of the development of each system

Nillson L, Hamberger L 1990 A child is born. Doubleday, London
A beautiful book written for the general public with astonishing photographs of all stages of human development from conception to birth

Richardson S J, Senikas V, Nelson J F 1987 Follicular depletion during the menopausal transition: evidence for accelerated loss and ultimate exhaustion. Journal of Clinical Endocrinology and Metabolism 65: 1231–1237

Robertson N R C (ed) 1992 Textbook of neonatology. Churchill Livingstone, Edinburgh

Rogers A W 1992 Textbook of anatomy. Churchill Livingstone, Edinburgh, p 148, 150

Rowe J W, Besdine R W 1988 Geriatric medicine, 2nd edn. Little Brown, Boston, p 515

Rutter N 1992 Temperature control and its disorders. In: Robertson N R C (ed) Textbook of neonatology, 2nd edn. Churchill Livingstone, Edinburgh, p 217–231

Rymer J, Morris E 2001 Women's health section: Menopausal symptoms. In: the BMJ's Clinical evidence: A compendium of evidence-based care, Volume 5. BMJ Publications, London, p 1303–1310

Scharden J L 1993 Chemically induced birth defects, 2nd edn. Marcel Dekker, New York
Valuable reference work, cataloguing over 3300 drugs and chemicals with respect to their teratogenicity

Shelley H J 1964 Carbohydrate reserves in the newborn infant. British Medical Journal i: 273–275

Sinclair D 1989 Human growth after birth, 5th edn. Oxford University Press, Oxford
A lucidly written book providing a broad introduction to all aspects of growth for all students of health care

Singer S 1985 Human genetics, 2nd edn. W H Freeman, New York
Clearly presented fundamentals of human genetics

Tanner J M 1989 Foetus into man, 2nd edn. Castlemead Publications, Ware
Authoritative, yet concise and clearly written account of the results of research on human growth. Includes a very good bibliography

Turner T L, Douglas J, Cockburn F 1988 Craig's Care of the newly born infant, 8th edn. Churchill Livingstone, Edinburgh

Valman H B 1988 ABC of one to seven. British Medical Journal, London
Collection of short articles reprinted from the British Medical Journal

Valman H B 1989 The first years of life, 3rd edn. British Medical Journal, London
Collection of short articles reprinted from the British Medical Journal

Walsh B W, Schiff I 1993 Physiology of the climacteric. In: Carr B, Blackwell R. Textbook of reproductive medicine. Appleton & Lange, East Norwalk, CT

Widdowson E M 1981 Nutrition. In: Davis J A, Dobbins J (eds) Scientific foundations of paediatrics, 2nd edn. Heinemann, London, p 41–43

Williams P L, Warwick R, Dyson M, Bannister L H 1989 Gray's Anatomy, 37th edn. Churchill Livingstone, Edinburgh

32 Death and dying

Death may occur suddenly due to illness or accidents or be 'expected' due to the progression of illnesses such as circulatory diseases and cancers (malignant neoplasms). People die as the result of the failure of one or more body systems through injury, disease or ageing.

Personal experiences of dying depend upon its cause, its circumstances and the support provided. Healthcare professionals play an important role in ensuring patient and family needs are identified and met. Whilst the needs of patients and families may vary due to the circumstances surrounding death, there are likely to be physical problems which require to be dealt with, psychosocial and spiritual needs to meet and a need for open and honest communication.

DEATH

MAIN CAUSES OF DEATH

Patterns of health and disease differ in the United Kingdom and around the world. These patterns have changed over time and our understanding of the factors that influence patterns of health and illness has increased. It is important to explore the connections between length of life that people in different countries or social groups can expect and what they are likely to die of.

In the United Kingdom at the turn of the twentieth century, infectious diseases were the biggest killer but since then there has been a dramatic fall in deaths from infections due to improved water supplies, better hygiene, and the discovery and use of antibiotics. However, infectious diseases remain a major cause of death in some developing countries, especially amongst children, and considerable differences exist between infant mortality and life expectancy in different countries of the world (Table 32.1).

In the United Kingdom major causes of death include:

- developmental abnormalities in infants
- accidents and injury in young adults
- circulatory diseases and cancers in older persons.

Patterns of death change over time as can be seen from the earlier analysis in Figure 32.1.

Table 32.1 Infant deaths and life expectancy in different countries

Country	Under-1 mortality (per 100 000 live births)	Life expectancy (in years)
Argentina	2087.4	64
Croatia	802.8	64
France	476.8	71
Japan	376.8	74
Romania	2229.5	62
United Kingdom	609.0	70
United States of America	732.0	67

Source: WHO 1997.

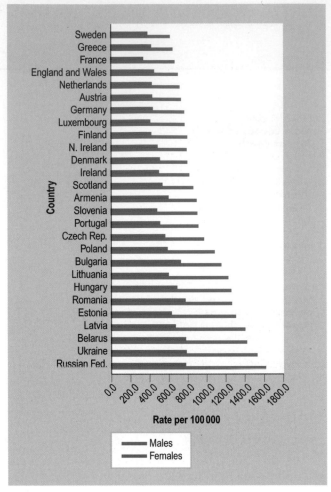

Figure 32.2 1996 age-standardized all-cause mortality rates per 100 000 population by sex. (WHO, 1996.)

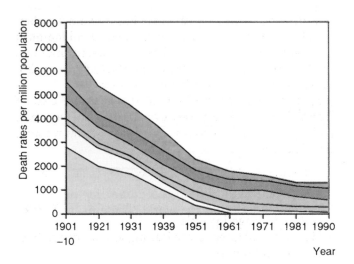

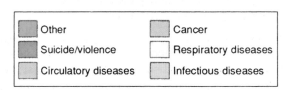

Other	Cancer
Suicide/violence	Respiratory diseases
Circulatory diseases	Infectious diseases

Figure 32.1 Mean annual death rates by major cause of death among males aged 25 to 44 years in England and Wales from 1901 to 1990. (Courtesy of S. Donnan, Department of Public Health and Epidemiology, University of Manchester. Source: OPCS.)

AGE AT DEATH

Several different measurements are used to describe the patterns of life and death within a population:

- mortality rates
- survival curves
- life expectancy.

Mortality rates

The mortality rate is the number of people, per given unit of population, dying in a given year (Fig. 32.2). Mortality is highest at the beginning and the end of our lives, times when we are most vulnerable either because of the immaturity of our body systems or because of their deterioration.

Survival curves

Survival curves show the percentages of people in a population who have survived to different ages. The differences in the shapes of the curves in countries such as England and Wales at the beginning and the end of the twentieth century, and between Western and developing countries reveal the effects of different social conditions including water supplies, housing and diet. In developing countries many deaths occur in childhood through malnutrition and infectious disease, whereas in other countries over 75% of the

Table 32.2 HALE (estimates for 2000) for a selection of the 191 member states of WHO

Rank	WHO member state	HALE in years		
		Overall	Male	Female
1	Japan	73.8	71.2	76.3
3	France	70.7	68.5	72.9
6	Italy	71.2	69.5	72.8
8	Switzerland	72.1	70.4	73.7
14	United Kingdom	69.9	68.3	71.4
24	United States of America	67.2	65.7	68.8
39	Argentina	63.9	61.8	65.9
68	Kuwait	64.7	64.6	64.8
89	Malaysia	61.6	59.7	63.4
140	Bangladesh	49.3	50.6	47.9
191	Sierra Leone	29.5	29.7	29.3

population can anticipate a long life of 70 years or more (Table 32.2).

However, better social conditions seem not to have had much effect on the maximum life span, which in all communities of the world is still about 100 to 110 years of age. Cerebrovascular disease and malignant neoplasms are significant causes of death in most European countries (Figs 32.3 and 32.4). These trends are predicted to continue to increase due to a range of factors such as sedentary lifestyle, tobacco smoking and a diet high in saturated fats.

Healthy life expectancy

The World Health Organization's (WHO) Healthy Life Expectancy (HALE) summarizes the expected number of years individuals can expect to live in the equivalent of 'full health'. Table 32.2 details the HALE (estimates for 2000) for a selection of the 191 member states of WHO and illustrates the considerable differences which exist in HALE for individuals. Previously, life expectancy was calculated in terms of years an individual could expect to live rather than years lived in good health.

Japan has the longest healthy life expectancy of 74.5 years amongst the 191 member states against a healthy life expectancy of less than 30 years in the lowest ranking country of Sierra Leone. The stark inequalities that exist between the nations of the world in healthy life expectancy are evident. The bottom 10 countries are all in sub-Saharan Africa where life expectancy has dropped over the last ten years due to the HIV-AIDS epidemic. AIDS has surpassed malaria, tuberculosis, pneumonia and diarrhoeal illness as the main cause of death in this region.

Japan is number 1 in the rankings due to the low rate of heart disease associated with a low fat diet. However,

lifestyle changes in Japan including a changing diet, which includes more red meat, and the long-term effects of the increased popularity of tobacco smoking, are likely to result in increased mortality from cardiovascular disease and malignant neoplasm.

A surprise is the position of the United States of America who rank relatively low amongst the wealthier nations. A number of reasons contribute to this ranking (WHO 2000):

- the ethnic mix and inner city poor, i.e. the divide between rich and poor
- the HIV epidemic and the resulting deaths of young and middle-aged people
- high levels of tobacco use leading to tobacco-related cancers and illness
- high levels of coronary heart disease
- fairly high levels of violence.

Understanding how lifestyle factors can influence life expectancy is important for healthcare workers who all have a role to play in health promotion. Changing trends in mortality, morbidity and life expectancy should inform healthcare planning at all levels. Understanding the health issues, which exist in a given area, is crucial if provision is to meet individuals' identified needs.

DEFINITIONS

Throughout our lives, cells die within our bodies either because they have come to the end of their natural life span or because they have been fatally injured. In that sense, death is a natural part of the process of living. Cells that die are usually replaced by others. Consequently the life of the body continues. As we age, the

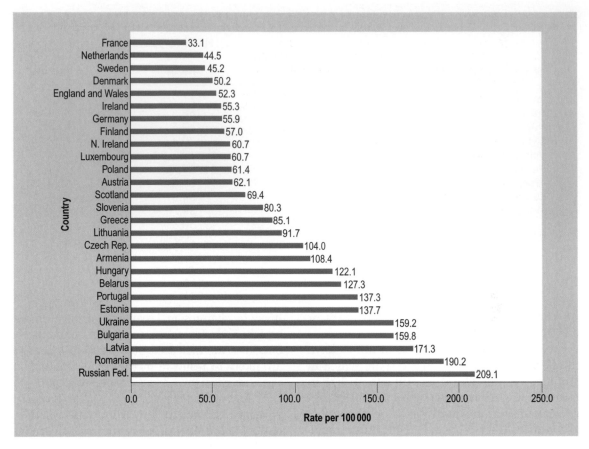

Figure 32.3 Age-standardized mortality rates for cerebrovascular disease per 100 000 population for selected European countries. (WHO, 1966.)

replacement of cells occurs more slowly and, as a result, different aspects of body function deteriorate.

The body continues to live as long as internal stability is maintained. Individual organs and tissues contribute to homeostasis and their failure upsets one or more key constituents of the interstitial fluid, altering the internal environment and impairing the function of other organs and tissues. Once this leads to failure of cardiac function and circulation of the blood stops, the life of the body as a healthy cooperative society of organs and tissues ceases. As the internal environment deteriorates even further all the cells of the body gradually cease to function too.

Death therefore is a process beginning with the failure of one part of the body which leads to failure of the life of the body as a whole.

Difficulties arise in deciding the stage in this process at which a person can be declared to be 'dead', particularly when there is loss of brain function. Loss of cerebral function results in loss of personality leading to the circumstances in which someone's body may continue to live, or to be maintained on a respirator, although awareness and purposeful activity no longer exist. Medically, distinctions are made between three states (Table 32.3):

- the vegetative state
- brain death
- certified death.

Vegetative state

Someone whose cerebral cortex is irreversibly damaged, but whose brain stem is intact, may live for many years in a state in which any awareness of the surrounding environment and purposeful activity is totally absent even though most of the body remains alive. Breathing occurs spontaneously, the heart beats, blood circulates and reflex movements occur but there is no understanding, communication or voluntary activity.

In this state, someone's personality has been irretrievably lost, with the result that it can be said that the 'person' has died even though the body remains alive. The fact that eyes open and many reflexes remain intact, especially those affecting hands, face and eyes can falsely give the impression that conscious awareness still exists.

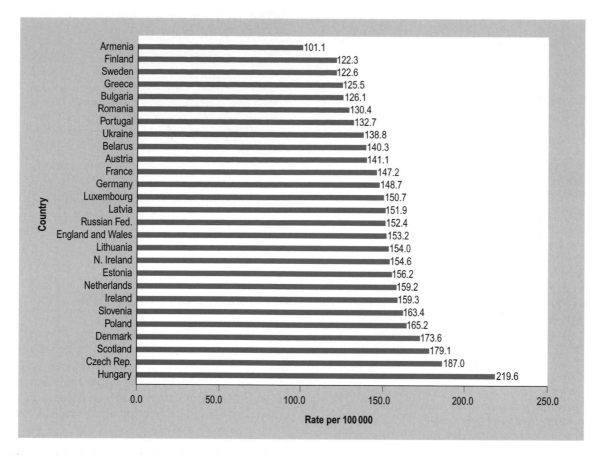

Figure 32.4 Age-standardized mortality rates for malignant neoplasms per 100 000 population for selected European countries. (WHO, 1996.)

Table 32.3 Role of different parts of the nervous system (CNS) in different behaviours and the consequences of loss of functions

Part of CNS	Role	Consequences of loss		
		State	**Features**	
Cerebral cortex	Awareness Understanding Purposeful behaviour	Vegetative state	Eyes open and move Breathes spontaneously May grimace, grasp and groan No voluntary movement	
Brain stem	Maintains consciousness Controls breathing, swallowing Reflex control of muscles (e.g. eyes, face, larynx, limbs) Autonomic control of circulation	Brain death	Coma Breathing stops Involuntary limb movement Incontinence	
Spinal cord	Reflex control of muscles (e.g. limbs) Autonomic reflexes	Death		

Brain death

Someone whose brain stem is irreversibly damaged will be in coma (see Ch. 21) and breathing stops (see Ch. 7). Life can be maintained by artificial ventilation as the heart continues to beat. Absence of detectable activity in the EEG (see Ch. 21) suggests brain death but is not proof of it.

The relatives and friends of a patient whose brain is permanently damaged may find it difficult to accept that recovery is impossible. This is particularly so when reflexes persist, especially the reflex grasping of a hand. When a grieving relative says, 'But he knows I'm here – he squeezed my hand', it takes knowledge and empathy to explain the situation.

Coping with death

Caring for dying patients and their families is challenging and places many stresses on professional carers. Repeated exposure to the death of people we have cared for, and formed relationships with, is difficult and can stretch personal coping resources. Similarly, practitioners may become disillusioned if they are unable to deliver 'excellent' care due to lack of knowledge, resources or conflict within the team.

When caring for dying patients there can be preoccupation with the physical aspects of care and symptom management. Of course controlling symptoms to help patients achieve optimum quality of life is crucial. However, evidence from patients and families repeatedly emphasizes the importance of good communication and interpersonal skills. Perhaps the most important role for healthcare professionals caring for dying patients and their families is being able to spend time with them and the ability to 'be with them' and not just 'doing' things for them.

There are a number of strategies which can help the professional carer to cope with repeated exposure to death. These include supportive team-working, adequate resources, realistic goals, and the willingness to accept support from other professionals.

Brain death is confirmed if it is impossible to elicit any brain stem reflexes and if all factors that could temporarily depress brain stem function, such as drugs and hypothermia, have been excluded. Reflexes tested include:

- pupillary and corneal reflexes (see Ch. 24)
- cough reflex and CO_2-induced respiratory movements (see Ch. 7).

When someone is brain dead it is still possible to elicit spinal reflexes (see Ch. 25) as the spinal cord is still functioning.

Certified death

Legally, a person is certified as dead once circulatory and respiratory function has ceased irreversibly. Loss of circulatory function is judged to be irreversible once the ECG (see Ch. 6) has shown no sign of activity for

Transplants

Organs should be removed as soon as possible after circulation and respiration have ceased, and death has been confirmed. Cells and tissues remain viable for a short time after death and therefore can be transplanted successfully into another body. Cooling arrests deterioration and helps to preserve normal function.

at least 5 minutes. If there is uncertainty over whether the heart has stopped beating, artificial ventilation is maintained for at least 2 hours after signs of life have ceased.

CHANGES POST-MORTEM

Once the circulation has ceased, the internal environment deteriorates rapidly, affecting cells and tissues and leading to alterations in a person's body and appearance. For example stiffening of the body (rigor mortis) occurs a few hours after death. Discoloration and softening occur later as decomposition begins to occur.

Rigor mortis

Stiffening of the body is caused by the binding of actin to myosin in muscles as a result of a gradual increase in intracellular calcium concentration and depletion of ATP (see Ch. 4B). As muscle cells die after death, ions such as sodium and calcium leak into the cytoplasm from the extracellular fluid and from intracellular organelles. These ions cannot be evicted and relaxation cannot occur because the ATP needed for these processes is depleted.

Rigor mortis begins 2 to 4 hours after death, the face stiffening before the hands and feet. Maximal stiffness develops between 12 and 48 hours depending on the environmental temperature, but then wears off over the next day or two as lysosomal enzymes (see Ch. 1) digest cellular proteins. These changes in the body are used by the pathologist and coroner as indicators of the probable time of death, should this not be known, for example if someone dies alone, or in unusual circumstances.

Decomposition

Blood drains from the surface structures of the body to accumulate in the dependent parts in the hour or two after death. As cells die, lysosomal enzymes begin the process of digestion that eventually disrupts red cells (haemolysis) and softens and finally liquefies the tissue. Bacterial contamination hastens the digestive process and produces iron sulphide which stains the tissues green and black. However, if the body is kept in a cold environment discoloration and decomposition are considerably delayed.

In preparing the body for burial or cremation undertakers replace the blood with an embalming fluid that destroys bacteria and preserves the tissues. As a result the corpse of a non-coloured person usually has a waxy white appearance unless make-up has been applied.

DYING AND PALLIATIVE CARE

An individual's personal experience of dying will depend on a number of factors including the:

- events of the death
- the nature of the support provided and how this fits with patient and family needs
- communication between those involved.

Death may occur suddenly and unexpectedly as the result of illness or an accident, or be gradual and expected as in life-threatening illnesses such as cancers and neurological disease.

SUDDEN, UNEXPECTED DEATH

Sudden death is due to lack of blood flow to the brain (cerebral ischaemia). This can be caused in several ways including cerebral haemorrhage (stroke) or cardiac arrest. In each case, the person rapidly loses consciousness because of the loss of blood supply to the brain. Someone having a heart attack may also experience a sharp crushing pain in the chest as a result of ischaemia of the cardiac tissues.

When a person dies suddenly family members and those closest to the deceased are likely to experience intense feelings including profound shock, numbness and disbelief. Outwardly they may appear to have accepted the death and seem to be coping 'well'. However, the reality of the death may not have fully penetrated their awareness and it is likely they will require time and, in some cases, professional support to work through the grieving process. Untimely, unexpected and disturbing deaths are more likely to cause severe and prolonged grief for the bereaved. Healthcare professionals need to be aware of sources of bereavement support to help people come to terms with their loss. Cruse Bereavement Care is one the leading charities in the United Kingdom, which exists to promote the well-being of bereaved people and help them to understand their grief and cope with their loss. (Contact details are given at the end of this chapter.)

GRADUAL DEATH

Death occurs gradually when there is failure of one or more of the organs and systems that maintain the composition of the internal environment. The quality of the internal environment gradually deteriorates, leading to malfunction of other cells and tissues. For example, in respiratory failure hypoxia and hypercarbia develop, leading to the failure of other organs such as the brain and heart. In renal failure, plasma potassium and hydrogen ion concentrations increase (see Ch. 14), disturbing cardiac function. In liver failure (see Ch. 10) toxic substances such as ammonia and bilirubin accumulate, poisoning other tissues including the brain.

EXPECTED DEATH AND PALLIATIVE CARE

Improving the quality of life of those dying presents a considerable challenge to healthcare professionals. Palliative care is recognized as a basic human right when curative treatment is no longer possible and combines holistic, patient and family focused care whilst remaining scientific or evidence based.

A useful, and widely accepted, definition of palliative care has been suggested by the World Health Organization (WHO):

Palliative care is the active total care of patients whose disease is not responsive to curative treatment. Control of pain, of other symptoms, and of psychological, social and spiritual problems is paramount. The goal of palliative care is best possible quality of life for patients and their families. (World Health Organization 1990).

Palliative care:

- affirms life and regards dying as a normal process
- neither hastens nor postpones death
- provides relief from pain and other distressing symptoms
- integrates the psychological and spiritual aspects of patient care
- offers a support system to help patients and relatives live as actively as possible until death
- offers a support system to help the family cope during the patient's illness and in their own bereavement.

Palliative care is a relatively new specialty, and in the United Kingdom evolved from the work of Dame Cicily Saunders and the recognition that many of the needs of patients suffering non-curative illness and their families were unmet. Patients with non-curative illness may be cared for in a range of clinical settings in acute hospitals or in the community. Only a very small percentage of patients die in specialist palliative care settings such as hospices although palliative care is often associated exclusively (wrongly) with cancer and hospice care. Patients suffering from neurological and cardiovascular disease are likely to need care based on the principles of palliative care. Palliative care is therefore 'everybody's business' and all healthcare professionals, regardless of the healthcare setting in which they work, require underpinning knowledge of palliative care.

The principles of palliative care are applicable earlier in the course of illness such as cancer in conjunction with potentially curative treatments including radiotherapy, chemotherapy and surgery. However, undoubtedly palliative care becomes of upmost importance as the illness progresses and the emphasis of care switches towards symptom relief and helping patients and families to achieve optimum quality of life.

Coping with the symptoms of advanced illness

Patients with life-threatening illnesses are likely to experience a range of symptoms as Table 32.4 illustrates.

The nature and severity of symptoms and problems experienced by individuals relates to the original illness, side effects from drugs and treatments such as chemotherapy and radiotherapy, and the physical and psychosocial impact of the illness. Symptoms are made worse by factors such as insomnia, exhaustion, anxiety and depression. Patients with life-threatening illnesses are likely to suffer a combination of symptoms and ongoing assessment of each symptom is crucial to the

Table 32.4 Common symptoms in advanced disease

Symptom	%
Weakness	95
Anorexia	80
Pain	80
Constipation	65
Dyspnoea	60
Insomnia	60
Sweats	60
Oedema	60
Dry/sore mouth	50
Nausea	50
Vomiting	40

Source: Kaye 1994.

management process. Assessment should incorporate three main questions:

1. What is the underlying pathological mechanism?
2. What has been tried and failed?
3. What is the impact of the symptom on the patient's life?

It is beyond the scope of this chapter to give detailed information about approaches to symptom management. There are numerous sources of information and further reading is suggested at the end of the chapter. Management of nausea and vomiting and pain are discussed here in greater detail as these symptoms impact severely on an individual's quality of life. However, it should be remembered that the patient is the most important judge of what is affecting *their* quality of life and healthcare professionals should ensure opportunities are given for patients to express their concerns.

Nausea and vomiting

Nausea and vomiting may be caused by gastric stasis, intestinal obstruction, raised intracranial pressure, drugs including opioids, biochemical changes, such as hypercalcaemia, or anxiety. Careful assessment of the patient is required to ascertain the causes of nausea and vomiting. There are three main pathways that trigger nausea and vomiting:

- chemoreceptor trigger zone – CTZ – chemical triggers
- vomiting centre – VC – cerebral trigger and/or visceral trigger
- gastrointestinal disturbances.

Reversible causes such as drugs, constipation, hypercalcaemia, cough, anxiety and gastric irritation should be identified and treated. The anti-emetic regimen should be prescribed regularly and as required and reviewed every 24 hours. If the patient is vomiting or oral absorption is in doubt, the subcutaneous route (syringe driver) or rectal route should be used.

Patients need support and reassurance and, for many patients, nausea and vomiting can be controlled by the use of four first line anti-emetics (Table 32.5).

Pain

Pain is a feared symptom of advanced disease. In cancer, it is estimated that pain is present in one-third of patients at the time of diagnosis, rising to more than two-thirds of patients in the terminal stages of illness. This means that one-third of cancer patients do not experience pain. Of the two-thirds who do experience pain, approximately 88% should have their pain adequately controlled by the application of basic pain management principles ('Principles of pain manage-

Table 32.5 Use of first line anti-emetics

Anti-emetic	Indications for use
Prokinetic anti-emetic: Metoclopramide, 10 mg PO stat and q.d.s. or 10 mg stat and 40–100 mg/24 hour SC infusion	Gastritis, gastric stasis, functional bowel obstruction
Anti-emetic acting in chemoreceptor trigger zone: Haloperidol, 1.5–3 mg by mouth immediately and at bedtime or 2.5–5 mg SC stat and 2.5–10 mg/24 hour SC infusion	Most chemical causes of vomiting including morphine, hypercalcaemia and renal failure
Antispasmodic and antisecretory anti-emetic: Hyoscine butylbromide, 20 mg stat and 80–160 mg/24 hour SC infusion	Cases of bowel colic and/or need to reduce gastrointestinal secretions
Anti-emetic acting principally in the vomiting centre: Cyclizine 50 mg PO stat and b.d.–t.d.s. or 50 mg SC stat and 100–150 mg/24 hour SC infusion	For organic bowel obstruction, raised intracranial pressure and motion sickness

Source: Twycross 1999.
Abbreviations used: PO: by mouth; stat: immediately; q.d.s.: four times a day; SC: subcutaneous; b.d.: twice daily; t.d.s.: three times daily.

Principles of pain management

More than 30 years ago Dame Cecily Saunders introduced the concept of 'total pain'. She recognized that pain is multifactorial, unique to the individual and comprises physical, psychological, social and spiritual elements.

Regular and comprehensive assessment of the physical, functional and spiritual impact of pain is essential. Use of a simple formal assessment tool is recommended.

Medication should be given by the:

Mouth: oral route is preferred for analgesics including strong opioids

Clock: regular analgesia should be prescribed as pain is difficult to control if frequent breakthrough is allowed to occur. 'As required' medication has no place in palliative care

Ladder: analgesics should be selected following assessment and dose titrated as a result of ongoing assessment. A patient's treatment should start at the step of the WHO ladder appropriate for the severity of the pain (Fig. 32.5).

WHO 1990, SIGN 2000, Twycross 1999, SPA 2000.

ment' box). There is convincing evidence that poor pain management remains a problem in some clinical areas in around one-third of patients. Furthermore, patients, family carers and health professionals share myths and misconceptions about the use of opiates such as morphine. These include fears of addiction and respiratory depression, the inevitability of cancer pain and the belief that strong opioids should be kept for 'really bad' pain.

Pain is an individual experience and, as with other symptoms in advanced disease, requires an individual assessment to establish how best to manage the problem. In order to ensure comprehensive assessment the following should be assessed:

- *physical* effects and manifestations of pain
- the *functional* effects – how the pain interferes with daily living
- *psychosocial* factors such as anxieties and fears, mood, cultural influences, effects on interpersonal relationships and consideration of factors affecting pain thresholds
- *spiritual* aspects of pain are difficult to define. Spiritual needs are often associated with religious aspects. However, spirituality is focused on the individual experience of illness which may result in spiritual disintegration, isolation and loss of meaning or purpose in life.

WHO suggest a three-step approach to analgesic choice which follows a gradual increase in strength of analgesic (Fig. 32.5). For mild pain, paracetamol is an example of a step 1 non-opioid analgesic. Patients who have moderate pain progress to step 2 and may be given a weak opioid such as codeine. Severe pain (step 3) is treated with strong opiates including morphine and diamorphine. A patient's treatment should commence at the appropriate step of the WHO ladder.

Medication to control pain should be given by the oral route providing the patient does not have difficulties swallowing or active vomiting. If the patient suffers from one or more of the following, the syringe driver,

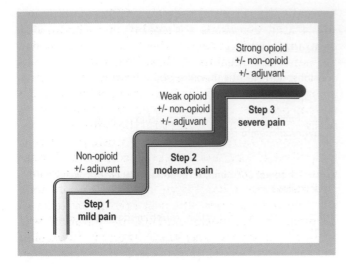

Figure 32.5 The WHO analgesic ladder. (Reproduced with kind permission of SIGN).

which can deliver high doses of analgesia via the subcutaneous route, should be considered.

Indications for using the subcutaneous route:

- persistent nausea and vomiting
- dysphagia
- gastrointestinal obstruction
- uncontrolled pain using other modes of administration
- decreased conscious level.

Diamorphine is the analgesic of choice for subcutaneous infusion due to its high solubility in water. Several drugs can be given in combination with diamorphine (at certain doses) such as anti-emetics and anticonvulsants. The compatibility of drugs must always be checked prior to administration. When transferring patients from the oral to the subcutaneous route of morphine administration, the oral dose should be divided by one-third to determine the starting dose.

Whenever regular opioid analgesia is used, laxatives *must* be prescribed as constipation may influence pain tolerance and cause disabling nausea and vomiting.

Caring in the last stages of life

Recognizing when a patient is nearing the end of life can be difficult but there are a number of signs which indicate the end is near. These are:

- *altered appearance* – translucency of skin, cool cyanosed extremities, gaunt facial features and glazed, distant and hollow eyes
- *decreased physical functioning* – profound weakness (bed-bound), drowsiness and longer periods of sleep, disinterest in food and fluid and difficulty in swallowing, day-to-day deterioration

Caring for the dying person and those closest to them

Holistic palliative care is multidimensional and multiprofessional in focus and embraces the needs of patients and those closest to them. A range of healthcare professionals will be involved in caring for the patient and family although nurses normally deal with the day-to-day tasks of helping patients and families cope with the physical, social and psychological impact of illness. The role of the nurse is therefore central to organization of care and, alongside other healthcare professionals, incorporates supportive and therapeutic roles. Therapeutic care is associated with treatment aimed at managing physical needs and difficult symptoms, and supportive care involves helping the person and family adapt to, and cope with, the resulting role and lifestyle changes.

The therapeutic and supportive roles of healthcare professionals are interwoven and the boundaries between them unclear. Similarly illness has physical, practical and psychosocial consequences for the patient and family which are also interwoven. For example, pain is a feared consequence of advanced illness and if a patient is extremely anxious due to family concerns, it may be more difficult to control their pain. Quality of life is an underpinning principle of palliative care. However, it is very difficult to help people achieve optimum quality of life if they are suffering from uncontrolled pain or nausea and vomiting.

The role of healthcare professionals in providing palliative care to meet the needs of patients and families is therefore challenging. Patients requiring palliative care are cared for in most healthcare settings so all professionals involved need knowledge of the palliative care approach which incorporates symptom management and the knowledge and communication skills to meet psychosocial care needs.

- *alterations in mental functioning* – poor concentration, disorientation, confusion, restlessness
- *altered vital signs* – changes in pulse rate and breathing rate, rhythm and volume.

At this stage the symptoms may be more difficult for the family to cope with than the patient as the patient may have lost consciousness and symptoms such as pain and oedema reduced in severity.

If renal failure occurs, the build-up of waste products such as urea and potassium in the blood may affect the brain and cause confusion, restlessness and sometimes hiccups. Secretions, which can no longer be coughed up, may accumulate in the airways making breathing irregular and very noisy (known as Cheyne–Stokes respiration and the 'rattle' respectively). The problem of noisy breathing is distressing for families and staff and to date, little is known about the effect on the patient of this under-researched symptom. Anticholinergic drugs such as hyoscine hydrobromide, which is also a sedative, may be given subcutaneously to reduce secretions.

Medication should be reviewed in the last stages of life and non-essential drugs stopped. Analgesics, anticonvulsants, tranquillizers and anti-emetics are essential drugs in this stage of the illness. The requirements for care of the mouth, eyes, bowel/bladder and pressure areas should be individually assessed. The needs of the family are paramount as the events surrounding death can influence how they cope with the bereavement in the longer term. Explanation of the possible causes of symptoms and intended treatment is crucial in order to support family members.

Caring for the family

Healthcare professionals have a responsibility to help family members whose problems might include: watching the patient suffer and deteriorate, adapting to changes in family dynamics and roles, getting adequate support and respite provision, dealing with social isolation and the financial implications of illness.

The needs of family members in relation to the following should be considered:

- information about the illness and treatments
- instruction and support in providing physical care
- support and encouragement
- assistance with practical and financial needs
- the opportunity to share their feelings and concerns.

ETHICAL CONCERNS

As in all areas of health care, ethical issues at the end of life are complex and require consideration. Ethical issues at the end of life can be separated into those that are the responsibility of the healthcare professional, and those governed by law, societal and cultural values. Decision-making in palliative care should be governed by the four ethical healthcare principles of:

- respect of autonomy: allowing people to make free, independent choices
- beneficence: doing good
- non-maleficence: avoiding harm
- justice: treating people with fairness.

Consent, confidentiality, honesty and resource allocation are issues common to all clinical decisions. At the end of life, artificial hydration, CPR, extraordinary versus futile treatments, withholding and withdrawing treatments and hastening death are issues which present ethical dilemmas to those involved.

For example, homeostasis is important in maintaining the normal cellular functioning of the body. If a patient becomes dehydrated with no opportunity to hydrate, then cellular metabolism becomes anaerobic. This leads to increasing toxicity of waste products in the patient's blood and to cerebral confusion, drowsiness and eventual death. In palliative care, the effects of hydration are inconclusive as dehydration may improve the analgesic effects of opioids by relief of oedema. In dyspnoeic patients, dehydration will reduce pulmonary secretions thereby increasing comfort and reducing the need for suctioning. Problems resulting from dehydration may include dry mouth and increased risk of pressure sore formation – arguably, both of these issues can be addressed by good care. Additionally there are psychological and emotional aspects of hydration which need to be considered alongside the physiological effects. In palliative care, starting intravenous fluids should be considered carefully, then regularly reviewed taking account of the patient's condition, prognosis and wishes.

Advances in medical science, increasing demands and finite health care resources for palliative care demands an ongoing debate as to the permissibility of actions or inaction when caring for people at the end of life.

CONCLUSIONS

In conclusion, caring for individuals who are dying and their families is a challenging, but rewarding, aspect of health care. The potential to manage symptoms associated with life-threatening illnesses is continually improving. However, effective communication is central to high quality palliative care and inadequate communication can cause distress and prevent adjustment to advanced, life-threatening illness. Cancer and other life-threatening illnesses may cause social isolation for patients and families and supportive communication may be all that is left when other therapeutic options are exhausted. Good communication can improve outcomes for patients and families in terms of psychological distress and an important role for the healthcare professional is that of 'being alongside' or 'being a companion' to those who are dying.

USEFUL ADDRESSES

Cruse Bereavement Care
Cruse House
126 Sheen Road
Richmond, Surrey TW9 1UR
Tel: 020 8940 4818 (Admin)
0870 167 1677 (Helpline)
Fax: 020 8940 7638

Hospice Information Service
St Christophers Hospice
51–59 Lawrie Park Road
Sydenham, London SE26 6DZ
Tel: 020 8778 9252
Fax: 020 8768 4662/3

Macmillan Cancer Relief
89 Albert Embankment
London SE1 7UQ
Tel: 020 7840 4600
Fax: 020 7840 7841

Marie Curie Cancer Care
89 Albert Embankment
London SE1 7TP
Tel: 020 7599 7777
Fax: 020 7599 7788

National Council for Hospice and Specialist Palliative Care Services
First Floor, 34–44 Britannia Street
London WC1X 9JG
Tel: 020 7520 8299
Fax: 020 7520 8298

Scottish Partnership for Palliative Care
1A Cambridge Street
Edinburgh EH1 2DY
Tel: 0131 229 0538
Fax: 0131 228 2967

REFERENCES AND FURTHER READING

Addington-Hall J, McCarthy M 1995 Dying from cancer: results of a national population-based investigation. Palliative Medicine 9: 295–305

Atkinson J, Virdee A 2001 Promoting comfort for patients with symptoms other than pain. Palliative nursing. Bringing comfort and hope. S Kinghorn and R Gamlin. Baillière Tindall, Edinburgh, 2 43–62

Beauchamp T, Childress J 1994 Principles of biomedical ethics. Oxford University Press, New York

Clark D, Hockley J, Ahmedzai S (eds) 1997 New themes in palliative care. Open University Press, Buckingham

Cleeland C, Gonin R, Hatfield A, et al 1994 Pain and pain treatment in outpatients with metastatic cancer: the Eastern Co-operative Oncology Group's Out-patient Pain Study. New England Journal of Medicine 330: 592–596

Doyle D, Hanks G, Macdonald G (eds) 1995 Oxford textbook of palliative medicine. Oxford University Press, Oxford

Doyle D, Hanks G, Macdonald G (eds) 1997 Oxford textbook of palliative medicine, 2nd edn. Oxford University Press, Oxford

Ferrell B, Johnston E, Grant M, et al 1993 Pain management at home. Cancer Nursing 16(3): 169–178

Field D, Clark D, Corner J, et al (eds) 2001 Researching palliative care. Open University Press, Buckingham

Gordon T 2001 A need for living. Wild Goose Publications, Glasgow

Jennett B 1987 Brain death and the vegetative state. In: Weatherall D J, Ledingham J G G, Warrell D A (eds) Oxford textbook of medicine, 2nd edn. Oxford University Press, Oxford, p 21.48–21.51
Clear description of distinctions made between different states

Kaye P 1994 A–Z Pocketbook of symptom control. EPL Publications, Northampton

Kennedy C, Lockhart-Wood K, Fielding H 1999 Use of the syringe driver in the community setting. International Journal of Community Nursing 4(5): 250–257

Lamb D 1985 Death, brain death and ethics. Croom Helm, Beckenham

Murray C 2000 Press Releases 2000: WHO issues new healthy life expectancy rankings, World Health Organization http://www.who.int/inf-pr-2000. 17 January 2002

National Council for Hospice and Specialist Palliative Care Services 1994 Guidelines for managing cancer pain in adults. National Council for Hospice and Specialist Palliative Care Services, England

National Council for Hospice and Specialist Palliative Care Services 1997 Changing gear – Guidelines for managing the last days of life in adults. National Council for Hospice and Specialist Palliative Care Services, Northamptonshire

National Council for Hospice and Specialist Palliative Care Services 1998 Guidelines for managing cancer pain in adults. National Council for Hospice and Specialist Palliative Care Services, Northamptonshire

Ogilvie C (ed) 1981 Brich's Emergencies in medical practice, 11th edn. Churchill Livingstone, Edinburgh

Pallis C 1983 ABC of brain stem death. British Medical Journal, London
Collection of short articles from the British Medical Journal

Redmond K 1998a Barriers to effective management of pain. International Journal of Palliative Care 4(6): 276–283

Redmond K 1998b Barriers to effective pain management in a community setting. Oncology Nurses Today 3(2): 10–13

Ritchie A C 1990 Boyd's Textbook of pathology, 9th edn. Lea & Febiger, Philadelphia

Robbins M 1997 Assessing needs and effectiveness: is palliative care a special case? New themes in palliative care. D Clark,

J Hockley and S Ahmedzai. Open University Press, Buckingham, p 13–33

Scottish Intercollegiate Guidelines Network 2000 Control of pain in patients with cancer. SIGN 44 Scottish Intercollegiate Guidelines Network, Edinburgh

Scottish Intercollegiate Guidelines Network online. Available: http://www.sign.ac.uk

Scottish Partnership Agency for Palliative and Cancer Care 1994 Palliative Cancer Care Guidelines Scottish Partnership Agency with the Clinical Resource and Audit Group, Edinburgh

Scottish Partnership Agency for Palliative and Cancer Care 2000 Relief of pain and related symptoms. Scottish Partnership Agency for Palliative and Cancer Care, Edinburgh

Twycross R 1999 Introducing palliative care. Radcliffe Medical Press, Oxon

Wilkinson S 1999 Schering Plough Clinical Lecture Communication: It makes a difference. Cancer Nursing 22(1): 17–20

World Health Organization 1990 Report of a WHO Expert Committee. Technical Report Series 804 Cancer pain relief and palliative care. World Health Organization, Geneva

World Health Organization 1997 Table 2: Infant deaths. http://www3.who.int/whosis/whsa

World Health Organization 2000 Press Releases 2000: WHO issues new healthy life expectancy rankings 4 June 2000. WHO, Geneva

World Health Organization 2002 Annex Table 4 Healthy Life Expectancy (HALE) in all member states, estimates for 2000. http://www.who.int/whosis/17 February 2002

Index

To make the index more useful for the reader, the following conventions have been used:
bold page numbers = main discussion of a subject
italic page numbers = boxed information
Where a reference refers to either a table or a figure, this has been noted (in parentheses) after the page number.

N

U

V